Metabolic Disorders and Critically Ill Patients

Carole Ichai • Hervé Quintard
Jean-Christophe Orban
Editors

Metabolic Disorders and Critically Ill Patients

From Pathophysiology to Treatment

Springer

Editors
Carole Ichai
Intensive Care Unit
Hôpital Pasteur 2
Centre Hospitalier Universitaire de Nice
Université Côte d'Azur
Nice
France

Hervé Quintard
Intensive Care Unit
Hôpital Pasteur 2
Centre Hospitalier Universitaire de Nice
Université Côte d'Azur
Nice
France

Jean-Christophe Orban
Intensive Care Unit
Hôpital Pasteur 2
Centre Hospitalier Universitaire de Nice
Université Côte d'Azur
Nice
France

Original French edition published by Springer-Verlag France, Paris, 2012,
ISBN 978-2-287-99026-7

ISBN 978-3-319-64008-2 ISBN 978-3-319-64010-5 (eBook)
https://doi.org/10.1007/978-3-319-64010-5

Library of Congress Control Number: 2017959327

Printed on acid-free paper

This Springer imprint is published by Springer Nature
The registered company is Springer International Publishing AG
The registered company address is: Gewerbestrasse 11, 6330 Cham, Switzerland

Contents

Part I

Fluid and Electrolytes Disorders

Water and Sodium Balance

1

Carole Ichai and Daniel G. Bichet

1.1 Introduction

Water is the major constituent of the body. It represents the unique solvant of various molecules (electrolytes) of our body. Although sodium is largely extracellular and potassium is intracellular, body fluids can be considered as being in a single "tub" containing sodium, potassium and water, because osmotic gradients are quickly abolished by water movements across cell membranes [1]. As such, the concentration of sodium in plasma water should equal the concentration of sodium plus potassium in total body water:

$$\left[\mathrm{Na}^{+}\right] \text{in plasma } \mathrm{H_2O} = 1.11 \times \left[\left(\mathrm{Na}^{+}\mathrm{e} + \mathrm{K}^{+}\mathrm{e}\right)\right] / \text{total boby } \mathrm{H_2O} - 25.6$$

This theoretical relationship was validated empirically by Edelman et al. [2] who used isotopes to measure exchangeable body cations and water. This equation has an intercept (−25.6); the regression line relating plasma sodium to the ratio of exchangeable ($Na^+ + K^+$) to total body water does not pass through zero because not all exchangeable sodium is free in solution. Exchangeable sodium is the major extracellular cation and sodium bound in polyanionic proteoglycans is also found in bone, cartilage and skin [1].

C. Ichai (✉)
Intensive Care Unit, Hôpital Pasteur 2, 30 Voie Romaine, 06001 Nice, Cédex 1, France

IRCAN (INSERM U1081, CNRS UMR 7284), University of Nice, Nice, France
e-mail: ichai@unice.fr

D.G. Bichet
Medicine and Molecular and Integrative Physiology, University of Montreal, Montréal, QC, Canada

Hôpital du Sacré-Cœur de Montréal, 5400 Boul Gouin O, Montréal, QC, Canada, H4J 1C5

C. Ichai et al. (eds.), *Metabolic Disorders and Critically Ill Patients*,
http://doi.org/10.1007/978-3-319-64010-5_1

Both water and sodium balances are physiologically strictly regulated by numerous hormonal, neuronal, and mechanical complex mechanisms in order to maintain intracellular and extracellular volumes constant.

1.2 Body Compartments and Water Shifts

1.2.1 Body Compartments and their Composition

Total body water (TBW) accounts for 50–70% of the total body weight in healthy adults. This proportion varies according to numerous parameters, such as age, sex and the lean mass/fat mass ratio (lean mass is very poor in water). TBW distributes for 2/3 in the intracellular volume (ICV), and the remaining 1/3 in the extracellular volume (ECV) [3–10].

The ICV is about 40% of total body weight. Potassium (K^+) is the most abundant intracellular cation (120 mmol/L), but large amount of proteins contribute also substantially to generate the oncotic pressure. The ECV is distributed into the plasma volume and the interstitial one. In normal physiological conditions, that is, in the absence of heart failure, cirrhosis and nephrotic syndrome, the plasma volume is equivalent to the "effective arterial blood volume" (EABV) which represents 1/4 to 1/3 of ECV, and 5% of the total body weight. In physiological situations, EABV is composed at 93% by water that contains various solutes. Some of them are ionized (anionic and cationic electrolytes) while others are not dissociated (blood urea nitrogen [BUN], glucose). Sodium (Na^+) is the most abundant plasma cation and, together with accompanying anions, are the major determinants of the osmotic force developed in the plasma. Non dissociated solutes (albumin, globulins and lipids) contribute for 7% of the plasma volume. The interstitial volume is 3/4 to 2/3 of the ECV, i.e. 15% of the total body weight. Contrary to the plasma volume which is anatomically limited by the capillary endothelium, the interstitial compartment is a less well defined space located around cells, lymph and conjunctive tissues. In terms of composition, the interstitial fluid is an ultrafiltrate of the plasma. Consequently, its composition is close compared to plasma, but due to its negligeable concentration in protein, sodium is quite lower and chloride higher in the interstitial compartment. For the same reasons, and because proteinates are impermeant solutes in the cells, the intracellular concentration in diffusible cations and in total ions is higher in cells: this is the Gibbs-Donnan equilibrium which creates an electrical difference in the membrane potential (Table 1.1).

1.2.2 Water and Electrolytes Shifts between the Body Compartments [3–10]

1.2.2.1 Movements across Intracellular and Extracellular Fluids

Water moves freely across the semi-permeable cell membranes according to the osmotic gradient leading to a shift from the low to the high osmotic volume until reaching a transmembrane osmotic equilibrium (Fig. 1.1) [4, 11–15]. Therefore,

Table 1.1 Main solutes and water composition of the body compartments

	Extracellular volume		Red blood cells	Intracellular volume
Solutes (mEq/L)	Blood plasma	Interstitial fluid		
Na^+	142	137	19	10
K^+	4	3	9.5	155
Mg^{++}	2	2	5	10
Ca^{++}	1	1	–	–
Cl^-	105	111	10	10
HCO_3^-	26	30	15	11
$HPO_4^{2-}/H_2PO_4^-$	2	2.3	110	105
SO_4^{2-}	1	1.2	–	2
Blood urea nitrogen	5	5	–	–
Glucose	5	5	Variable	Variable
Organic acids$^-$	5	5	–	–
Proteinates$^-$	17	0	320	74

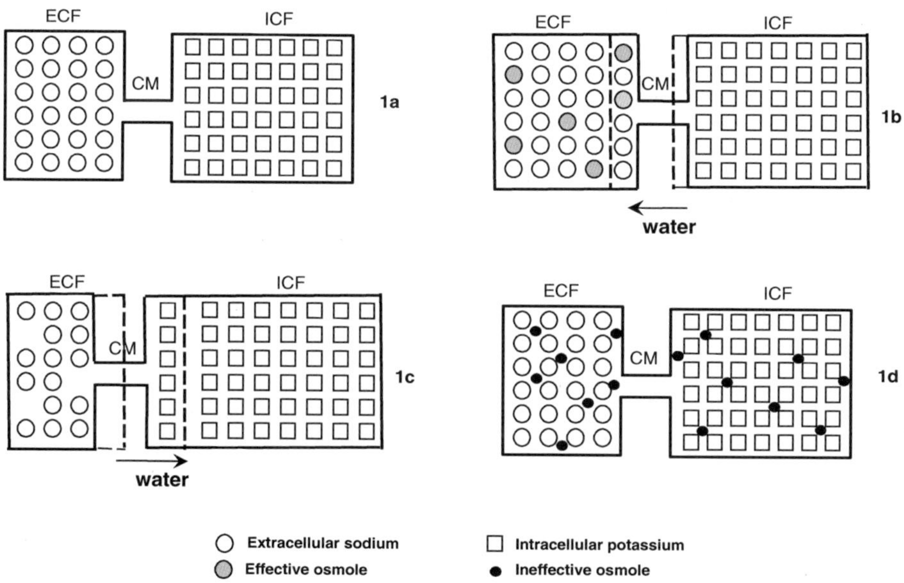

Fig. 1.1 Water movements between the extracellular (ECV) and intracellular volume (ICV) through the cell membrane (CM). (**a**) Normal volume and distribution of water in the ECV and ICV. The osmotic forces produced by the extracellular effective osmoles (mainly sodium) and the intracellular ones (mainly potassium) are equal, so that there is no osmotic gradient and consequently no water shift across the cell membrane. ECV and ICV are isoosmotic and isotonic. (**b**) Decrease (dehydration) of ICV. The accumulation of effective solutes (sodium or glucose) in the ECF creates an transmembrane osmotic gradient which induces water to cross cell membrane from the ICV to the ECV until reaching the osmotic equilibrium between both compartments. (**c**) Increase (hyperhydration) of ICV. The loss of effective solutes (sodium or glucose) in the ECV creates a transmembrane osmotic gradient which induces water to cross cell membrane from the ECV to the ICV until reaching the osmotic equilibrium between both compartments. (**d**) Normal volume and distribution of water in the ECV and ICV. Ineffective solutes such as urea distributes equally between the ECV and ICV. Thus, osmotic forces developped by the extracellular effective and ineffective osmoles and the intracellular ones are equal, so that there is no osmotic gradient and consequently no water shift across the cell membrane. ECV and ICV are isotonic but hyperosmotic

cell volume (hydration) depends on the solute movements and concentrations between the intracellular and extracellular fluids. Na^+-K^+-ATPase expressed in all plasma membranes restricts Na^+ to the extracellular volume compartment while K^+ is maintained intracellularly. This active, ATP-dependent phenomenon, activates a two Na^+ efflux for a three K^+ influx and creates a transmembrane potential. Because Na^+ is the dominating cation in plasma, sodium concentration is the major determinant of plasma osmolality (Posm) and consequently of ICV. Other Na^+ cotransporters, symport (with glucose), antiport (with Ca^{++} or H^+) are involved in various cell functions such as contractility, pH regulation, but not in the intracellular volume.

Not only Na^+, but many particles in the ICV and the ECV generate an osmotic force. However, their ability to induce an osmotic gradient and thus water shifts, depends on their capacity to distribute across the cell membrane [4, 11–15]. Diffusive or "ineffective" solutes such as urea and alcohols, which distribute equally in the ESV and the ICV are unable to promote any substantial osmotic gradient and do not modify cell volume. On contrary, non diffusive or "effective" extracellular solutes, i.e. Na^+ and its associated anions, are responsible for a transmembrane osmotic gradient leading to water efflux and cell shrinkage. The osmotic effect of glucose depends on the nature of tissues. Specific transporters (GLUT transporters), allow glucose to penetrate freely in non-insulin requiring tissues like blood cells, immune cells and brain cells. In this case, glucose behaves as an ineffective solute. By contrast glucose requires insulin to enter in the cells of insulin-dependent tissues (myocardium, skeletal muscle, adipose tissue) and is therefore here an effective osmoles that creating an osmotic gradient and ICV dehydration in case of hyperglycemia (insulin deficiency or resistance).

Total plasma osmolarity is defined as the concentration of all solutes (effective and ineffective) in a liter of plasma (mosm/L). Plasma osmolality is also the concentration of all solutes but in a kilogram of plasma water (mosm/kg). Both are very close in physiological situations and usually merged, because water plasma accounts for 93% of 1 l of plasma. Total plasma osmolality can be measured (mPosm [mosm/kg]) in the laboratory using the delta cryoscopic method (freezing point of the plasma) which provides a global value of all osmoles present in the plasma, regardless their normal or abnormal presence and their transmembrane diffusive properties. Posm can be easily calculated at bedside (cPosm [mosm/L]) considering the major electrolytes contained in plasma by the following formula: cPosm [mosm/L] = ([$Na^+ \times 2$] + glycemia + urea) (mmol/L) = 280–295 mosm/L. Because this calculation overrides abnormal (not usually measured) and minor plasma osmoles, mPosm is slightly higher than cPosm. The difference between these two parameters is known as the osmotic gap (OG = mPosm − cPosm), its value is around 10 mosm/L. Plasma tonicity (or effective osmolarity) refers to only major effective osmoles and is calculated using the following formula: P tonicity = [$Na^+ \times 2$) + glycemia] (mmol/L) = 270–285 mosm/L. P tonicity is therefore the best practical parameter for evaluating accurately the ICV [4, 10, 11].

For practical reasons, mPosm which is rarely obtained and cPOsm not calculated in most emergency situations since they are not accurate tools for determining ICV. Plasma tonicity, however, easily evaluates the intracellular hydration (Fig. 1.1). Plasma hypertonicity induces a water efflux from the cells to the ECV across the cell

Table 1.2 Permeability properties of main plasma osmoles and their impact on osmolarities and intracellular volume

Solutes	mPOsm (mOsm/kg)	cPOsm (mOsm/L)	P tonicity (mOsm/L)	Intracellular volume
"Effective" osmoles				
Glucose, glycine-glycerol, Histidine-tryptophan-ketoglutarate, hyperosmolar radiocontrast media	Hyperosmolality	Hyperosmolarity	Hypertonicity	Decreased (dehydration)
"Ineffective" osmoles				
Urea alcohol, ethylene glycol, Methanol[a]	Hyperosmolality Hyperosmolality	Hyperosmolarity Isoosmolarity	Isotonicity Isotonicity	Normal Normal

mPosm measured total plasma osmolality, *cPosm* calculated plasma osmolarity
[a]solutes associated with an increased mPosm and osmotic gap

membrane and always indicates a decrease in ICV (Fig. 1.1b). On the opposite, an increased in ICV with cell oedema is secondary to a water influx in cells due to plasma hypotonicity (Fig. 1.1c). The increased plasma concentration of diffusible osmoles induces a comparable hyperosmolarity in both extracellular and intracellular compartments without any osmotic gradient nor water shift as plasma is isotonic (Fig. 1.1d). In this latter situation, mPosm and OG will be useful and guide the diagnosis indicating the presence in plasma of high concentration of abnormal osmoles such as ethylene-glycol, methanol, mannitol, glycine or alcohols (Table 1.2). The precise identification of the additional solute is based on the clinical history and the specific biological measurement not always available in smaller centers.

1.2.2.2 Movements Across Interstitial and Plasma Fluids

Water shifts within the ECV between the interstitial and plasma compartment through the capillary endothelial cells. In physiological situations, this barrier is permeable to water and dissolved solutes, but totally impermeable to proteins which remain in the vascular bed. According to the Starling law, the direction of water movements between these two compartments is determined by the filtration pressure [4, 11–15]. This pressure depends on two opposite forces, the transmural hydrostatic and oncotic pressures: Filtration pressure = (Pc − Pi) - (πp − πi) (mmHg), Pc and Pi are respectively capillary and interstitial hydrostatic pressures, πp and πi are respectively plasma and interstitial oncotic pressures. Because protein remains in the plasma (πp = 10 mmHg), πi is negligeable. Hydrostatic pressures lead to extrude water, while oncotic ones to retain it. Thus, the direction of water flux is different among the localisation of capillary:

- on the arterial side, the high Pc is > Pi + πp and water shifts from the plasma to the interstitial space, allowing the distribution of oxygen, nutriments, hormones to the tissues

- on the venous side, the low Pc is < Pi + πp and the direction of water shift is inverted from the interstitial to the plasma volume allowing the elimination of various tissue wastes.

Interstitial oedema refers to an abnormal extracellular water distribution characterized by a sodium and water accumulation in the interstitial volume. These pathological situations can be the consequence of abnormal filtration pressure as frequently observed in severe hypoalbuminemia (cirrhosis, malnutrition) or abnormal increased vascular permeability related to endothelial cell dysfunction as observed in systemic inflammation or sepsis.

Plasma tonicity is the only accurate tool to assess the intracellular volume. Plasma hypertonicity always indicates an intracellular dehydration and hypernatremia is usually considered as the parameter allowing to assess intracellular volume. If natremia indicates always plasma hypertonicity, this is not the case for hyponatremia which can be associated with iso-, hypo- and hypertonicity (see chapter on dysnatremias). Total body sodium (quantity) which differs from natremia (plasma concentration) is the determinant of extracellular volume. A decreased in total body sodium indicates a low extracellular volume, with low effective arterial blood volume, i.e. hypovolemia.

1.3 Body Water Balance and Its Regulation

Preservation of cell volume is fundamental to maintain cell functions and avoid cell death. Variations in cell volume mainly result from changes in extracellular tonicity, but sometimes from modifications in intracellular osmoles concentration induced by metabolic derangements such as hypothermia or hypoxia/ischemia. Therefore, ECV tonicity must be maintained in a stable range thanks to a very narrow control of TBW volume. A close equilibrium between water intake and output allows such a strict regulation resulting in the control of body water homeostasis.

In a 70 kg-male adult, exogenous water is ingested orally and represents 1500–2500 mL/day, which is mostly reabsorbed (for about 90%) in the digestive tube. Daily water excretion is essentially performed by the kidney which produces a mean urine output of 1000–2000 mL/day (0.5–1 mL/kg/day). Water faecal losses are normally negligeable (50–100 ml/day) and insensible water losses (pulmonary and cutaneous) represent 500–1000 mL/day (Fig. 1.2) [4, 6, 11–13].

Body water homeostasis is controlled by three essential mechanisms: (1) the neurohormonal effect of vasopressin which regulates water urinary excretion and the renal sympathetic nerve activity [16], (2) the behavioral sensation of thirst which controls water intake and (3) the capacity of the kidneys to excrete diluted or concentrated urine. These three factors maintain plasma isotonicity despite wide daily variations in salt and water intake. Vasopressin and thirst are mainly triggered by osmotic and baro-volumic neurohormonal stimuli but many non osmotic- non baro/volumic stimuli have also been described [17].

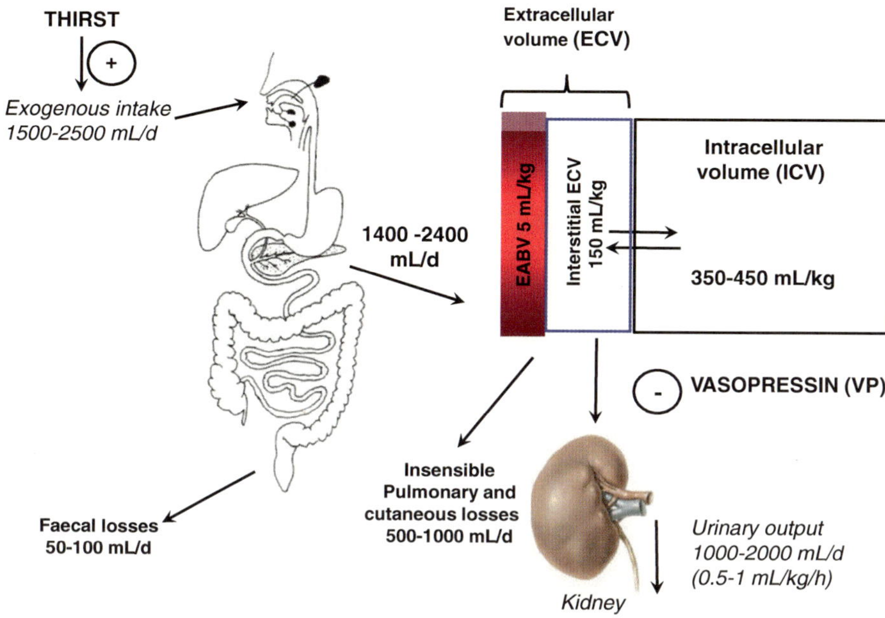

Fig. 1.2 Water balance and its major regulating mechanisms in a 70 kg adult. Water intake coming essentially from the exogenous drinks is equilibrate by water output. By regulating urine output, kidney plays an essential role in total body water balance. After its ingestion, water is massively reabsorbed by the gastrointestinal system and is further distributed in body compartments. Water homeostasis is mainly maintained thanks to vasopressin which controls urine output, and thirst which controls water oral intake

1.3.1 Regulation of Vasopressin Release and Thirst

1.3.1.1 Osmotic Regulation

Vasopressin, a nonapeptide hormone, is synthetized by magnocellular neurons located in the supraoptic (SOV) and paraventricular nuclei (PVN) of the anterior hypothalamus. Vasopressin is then transported along axons to be stored and released in the posterior pituitary. Vasopressin is also released from dendrites in the PVN and alters the function of pre-autonomic neurons in the PVN [18]. Specialized osmoreceptor structures are located at the BBB interface in the lamina terminalis in the anterior and dorsal wall of the third ventricle. Among these circumventricular organs (CVOs), the subfornical (SFO) and the organum vasculosum of the lamina terminalis (OVLT) are strategically placed to sense plasma osmotic signals. Tonicity is perceived specifically by these neuronals groups. All cells of an organism are responding to dehydration or to hyperhydration by changing their volume but cells of the subfornical organ (SFO), organum vasculosum of the lamina terminalis (OVLT), median preoptic nucleus (MnPO) are "perfect" osmoreceptors, that is, their changes in volume are maintained as long as the osmotic stimulus persists [19] (Fig. 1.3a). Cell shrinking during dehydration is mechanically coupled to the activation of Transient Receptor Potential Vanilloid (TRPV) channels through a denseley

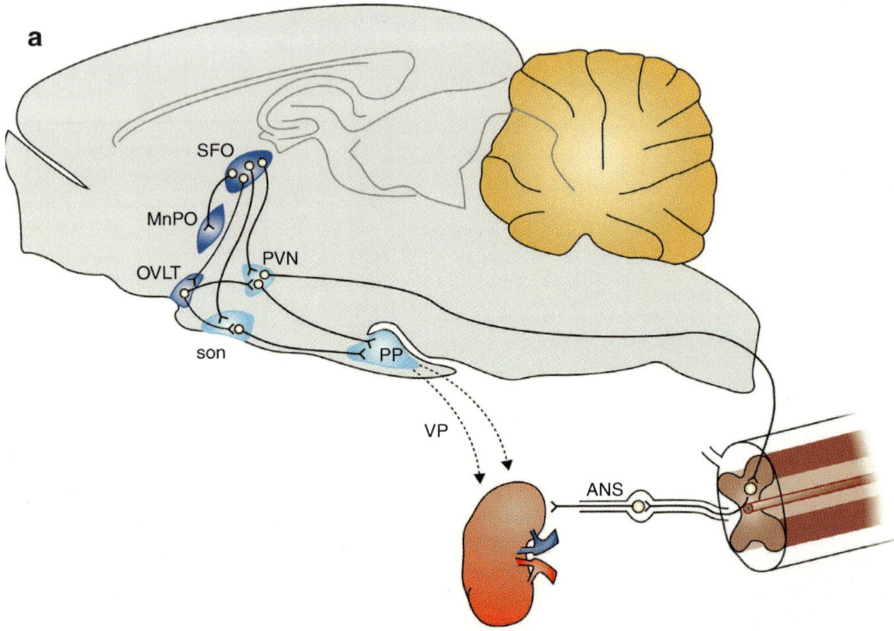

Fig. 1.3 Major osmoregulatory areas and pathways, of the central nervous system involved in mamalian. (**a**) Schematic representation of the osmoregulatory pathway of the hypothalamus (sagittal section of midline of ventral brain around the third ventricle in mice). Neurons (*lightly filled circles*) in the lamina terminalis (OVLT), median preoptic nucleus (MnPO) and subfornical organ (SFO) - that are responsive to plasma hypertonicity send efferent axonal projections (*black lines*) to magnocellular neurons of the paraventricular (PVN) and supraoptic nuclei (SON). The axons of these magnocellular neurons form the hypothalamo-neurohypophyseal pathway that courses in the median eminence to reach the posterior pituitary, where neurosecretion of vasopressin and oxytocin occurs. Dendritic vasopressin release during dehydration will stimulate sympathetic preautonomic cells in the PVN and directly increased renal nerve stimulation, a central integrated response to restore tonicity and volume. Modified from Wilson Y et al. [67] with permission. (**b**) Cell autonomous osmoreception in vasopressin neurons. Changes in osmolality cause inversely proportional changes in some volume. Shrinkage activates transient receptor vanilloid-type (TRPV1) channels and the ensuing depolarization increases action potential firing rate and vasopressin (VP) release from axon terminals in the neurohypophysis. Increased VP levels in blood enhance water reabsorption by the kidney (antidiuresis) to restore extracellular fluid osmolality toward the set point. Hypotonic stimuli inhibit TRPV1. The resulting hyperpolarization and inhibition of firing reduces VP release and promotes diuresis. Modified from Prager-Khoutorsky M et al. [19] with permission. (c) Osmoregulatory circuits in the mammalian brain and the periphery. Neurons and pathways are color-coded to distinguish osmosensory, integrative and effector areas. Afferent pathways from the OVLT to ACC are responsible for thirst perception. Central preautonomic neurons in the PVN are responsible for the increased renal sympathetic activity mediated by perception of dehydration by magnocellular cells in closed proximity (see Fig. 1.3a). *ACC* anterior cingulate cortex, *AP* area postrema, *DRG* dorsal root ganglion, *IML*, intermediolateral nucleus, *INS* insula, *MnPO* median preoptic nucleus, *NTS* nucleus tractus solitarius, *OVLT* organum vasculosum laminae terminalis, *PAG* periaqueductal grey, *PBN* parabrachial nucleus, *PP* posterior pituitary, *PVN* paraventricular nucleus, *SFO* subfornical organ, *SN* sympathetic nerve, *SON* supraoptic nucleus, *SpN* splanchnic nerve, *THAL* thalamus, *VLM* ventrolateral medulla. Reproduced from Bourque CW [17] with permission

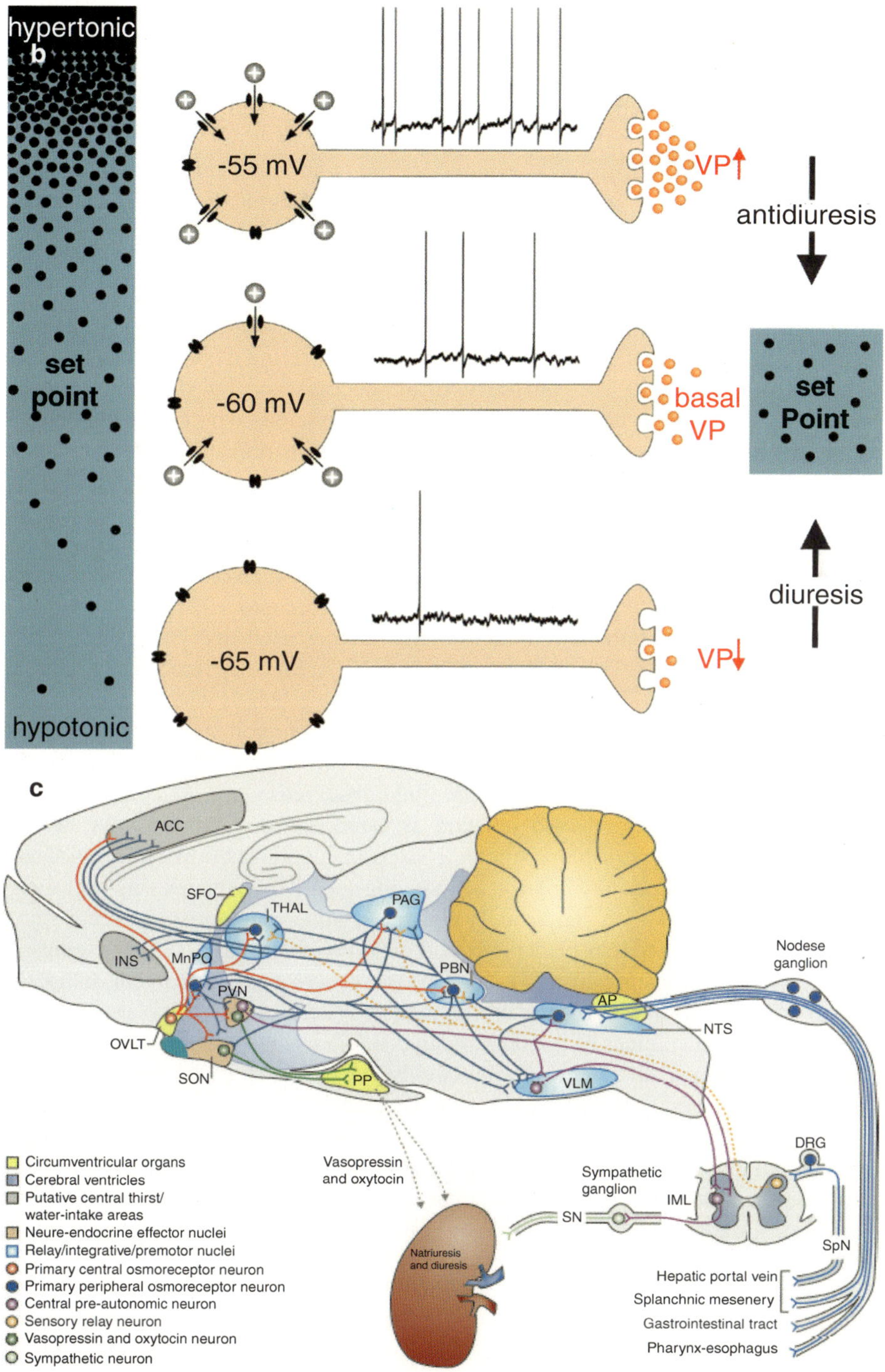

Fig. 1.3 (continued)

interweaved microtubule networks present only in osmosensitive cells [19] including excitatory thirst neurons from the SFO [20]. These excitatory SFO neurons project to the magnocellular cells of the SON and PVN producing vasopressin and, as a consequence, these neurosecretory cells will be depolarized and vasopressin will be released both from axonal and dendrites terminals. Dendritic vasopressin release during dehydration will stimulate sympathetic pre-autonomic cells in the PVN and directly increased renal nerve stimulation, a central integrated response to restore tonicity and volume [16]. Vasopressin producing cells in SON and PVN also bear TRPV1 channels, they depolarize during dehydration and hyperpolarize during overhydration. The net result of depolarization will be vasopressin release (Fig. 1.3b).

Thirst cells of the anterior wall of the third ventricle also project to two concious areas, the anterior cingulate cortex and the insula delivering a concious assessment of the dehydration state and, probably, of the necessary water volume to quench thirst. This is a unique situation where tonicity is consciously perceived, analogous to the hunger perception. Also thirst promoting neurons transmit negative valence teaching signals that are actively avoided in experimental animals [22] (Fig. 1.3c).

The OVLT, SFO, MnPO and the pituitary gland do not have a blood brain barrier, that is their capillary endothelium is fenestrated and allows a full exposure to plasma osmotic and hormonal variations including angiotensin II. Excitatory thirst neurons of the SFO specifically expressed AT1 angiotensin receptors [21] most probably explaining the osmoregulatory gain observed with increased circulating plasma levels of angiotensin [23]. This osmoregulatory gain is clinically important since, for the same osmotic stimulus, more vasopressin will be released when plasma angiotensin II is elevated, a common situation seen with hypotension and decreased effective blood volume of heart failure and decompensated cirrhosis, where hyponatremia with high vasopressin levels are often observed.

Hepatic sensory neurons also function as osmoreceptors: they express TRPV4 channels and signal hypo-osmotic stimuli from portal blood via the thoracic dorsal root ganglia with connections to vasopressin producing cells. This explains why liver transplant patient's osmolality is significantly higher as compared to normal subjects, since, in these liver denervated transplant patients, there is no inhibition of central vasopressin release by portal hyposmolality [24]. These portal osmoreceptors can signal changes in blood osmolality well before water intake impacts systemic blood osmolality.

Because of the confines of the skull, brain cell tolerance to volume changes is very narrow and only a small degree of brain swelling or shrinkage is compatible with life. As underlined recently by Sterns [1], although osmotic disturbances affect all cells, clinical manifestations of hyponatremia and hypernatremia are primarily neurologic, and rapid changes in plasma sodium concentrations in either direction can cause severe, permanent, and sometimes lethal brain injury. Tonicity changes as small as 1–2% alter vasopressin release with a threshold around 280 mOsm/kg in humans and a progressive increase with increasing osmolality. Under a value of 280 mosm/kg, plasma vasopressin concentration is below the detection limit of sensitive radio-immunoassays. The threshold of thirst sensation, using a visual analogue scale, has been reported for a long time to be 10 mOsm/kg higher than the vasopressin release one, i.e. 290–295 mOsm/kg [4, 11, 24, 25]. However, recent data strongly suggest that both are very close. As observed with vasopressin release, thirst sensation increases linearly with the increase

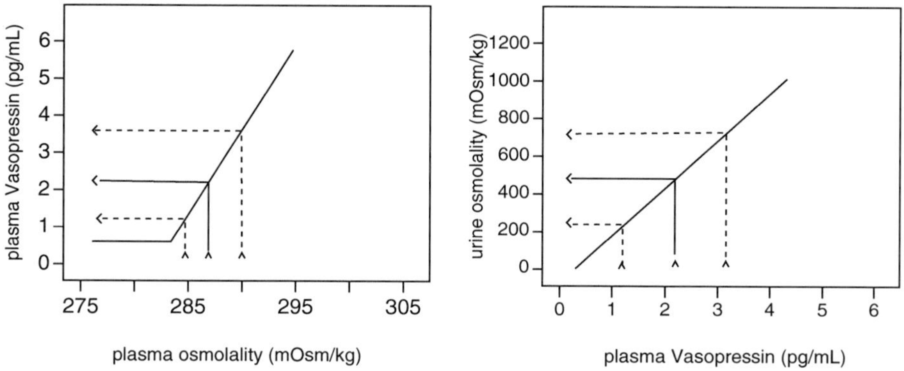

Fig. 1.4 Schematic representation of the effect of small alterations in the basal plasma osmolality on (*left*) plasma vasopressin and (*right*) urinary osmolality in healthy adults. Modified from Robertson GL et al. [68] with permission

in systemic tonicity [30]. The exquisite sensitivity and gain of the osmoreceptor–AVP–renal reflex is given by the following example (Fig. 1.4). A normally hydrated man may have a plasma osmolality of 287 mmol/kg, a plasma vasopressin concentration of 2 pg/mL and a urinary osmolality of 500 mmol/kg. With an increase of 1% in total body water, plasma osmolality will fall by 1% (2.8 mmol/kg), plasma AVP will decrease to 1 pg/mL and urinary osmolality will diminish to 250 mmol/kg. Similarly, it is only necessary to increase total body water by 2% to suppress the plasma AVP maximally (<0.25 pg/mL) and to maximally dilute the urine (<100 mmol/kg). In the opposite direction, a 2% decrease in total body water will increase plasma osmolality by 2% (5.6 mmol/kg), plasma AVP will rise from 2 to 4 pg/mL and urine will be maximally concentrated (>1000 mmol/kg). Thus, in the context of these sensitivity changes, a 1 mmol rise in plasma osmolality would be expected to increase plasma AVP by 0.38 pg/mL and urinary osmolality by 100 mmol/kg. Such a small change in plasma osmolality (measured by freezing point depression) or plasma AVP (by radioimmunoassay) may be undetectable yet of extreme physiological importance. For example, a patient with a 24-h urinary solute load of 600 mmol must excrete 6 l of urine with an osmolality of 100 mmol/kg to eliminate the solute; however, if the urine osmolality increases from 100 to 200 mmol/kg (due to an undetectable rise of 1 mmol in plasma osmolality and 0.38 pg/mL in plasma AVP), the obligatory 24-h urine volume to excrete the 600 mmol solute load decreases substantially from 6 to 3 l. The upper limit for water intake is dependent of the total osmoles to be excreted and of the minimal urine osmolality: 24 liters per day could be excreted if minimal urine osmolality is 60 with 1200 mOsm to be excreted. During dehydration, with the same osmotic load to be excreted and a maximal urine osmolality of 1200 mOsm, 1 l of urine will be excreted. As a consequence, the development of severe systemic hypertonicity is rare, except in case of primary abnormalities of thirst sensation (hypo- or adipsia) or in patients who have no access to water (coma, digestive aspiration).

There are differences in sensitivity of VP release depending on the sex. It is now well established that male presents a higher osmotic sensitivity than female, regardless their menstrual cycle. Despite an accepted role of gonadal steroids hormones, the precise mechanism of these differences remain complex. Testosterone has been reported to increase VP synthesis and release, while estrogen seems to confer opposite effects. This could be in relation with the presence of two types of estrogen receptors in the magnocellular neurons (ER α and β) and the level of exposure to both oestradiol and progesterone. However, estrogen lowers renal tubular sensitivity to VP in the same time. Vasopressin release and thirst are not equally sensible to all solutes. Indeed sodium and its cations confer a strongest osmotic powerful stimulation than non ionic osmoles (glucose for example).

1.3.1.2 Baroregulation

It is now well established that afferent neural impulses arising from stretch receptors in the left atrium, carotid sinus and aortic arch inhibit the secretion of vasopressin. Conversely, when the discharge rate of these receptors is reduced, vasopressin secretion is enhanced (for review, see Norsk [26]). Moreover, the relative potency of the cardiac and sino-aortic reflexes in the release of vasopressin appears to vary among species. For example, the increase in plasma vasopressin that occurs during moderate hemorrhage in the dog is attributable primarily to reflex effects from cardiac receptors; sino-aortic receptors appear to exert only minor influences on vasopressin release in this situation. In contrast, sino-aortic receptors appear to play the dominant role in eliciting vasopressin secretion during blood loss in nonhuman primates and humans [26]. In humans, blood pressure reductions of as little as 5%, induced by the ganglion blocking agent trimetaphan, significantly altered plasma arginine vasopressin concentration [27]. Furthermore, an exponential relationship between plasma vasopressin and the percentage decline in mean arterial blood pressure has been observed with large decreases in blood pressure (Fig. 1.5). Since an interdependence exists between osmoregulated and baroregulated arginine

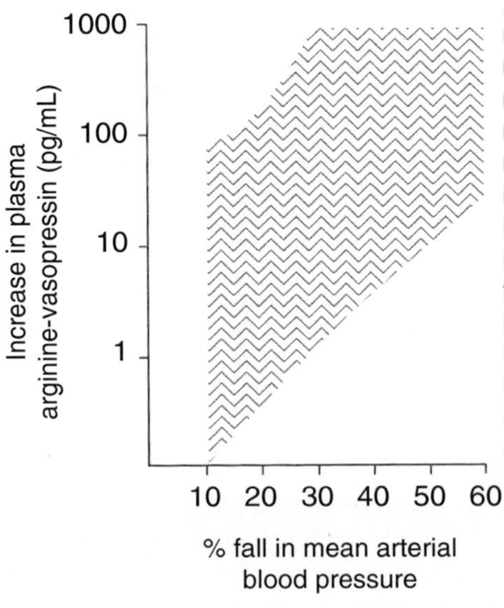

Fig. 1.5 Increase in plasma arginine vasopressin AVP during hypotension. Note that a large diminution in blood pressure in normal humans induces large increments in AVP. Reproduced from Zerbe GL et al. [69] with permission

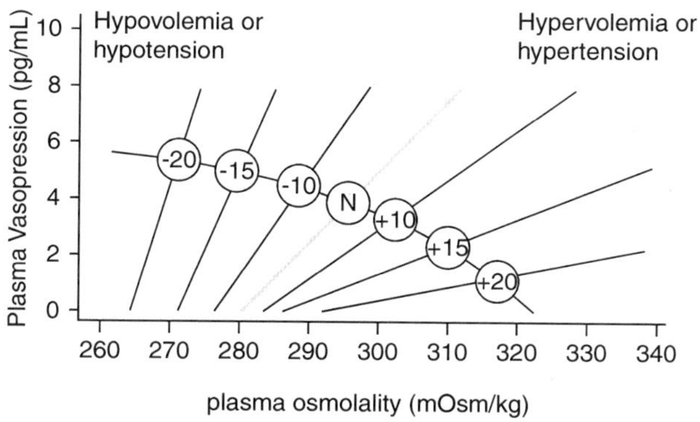

Fig. 1.6 Schematic representation of the relationship between plasma vasopressin and plasma osmolality in the presence of differing states of blood volume and/or pressure. The line labeled N represents normovolemic normotensive conditions. Minus numbers to the left indicate percent fall, and positive numbers to the right, percent rise in blood volume or pressure. Reproduced from Vokes TP et al. [70] with permission

vasopressin secretion [28] (Fig. 1.6), under conditions of moderate hypovolemia, renal water excretion can be maintained around a lower set-point of plasma osmolality, thus preserving osmoregulation. As hypovolemia becomes more severe, plasma arginine vasopressin concentrations attain extremely high values and baroregulation overrides the osmoregulatory system. An enhanced osmoreceptor sensitivity, but blunted baroregulation, has been described in elderly subjects [29].

1.3.1.3 Hormonal Influences on the Secretion of Vasopressin

Studies on the direct effects of various peptides and other biological substances on the release of vasopressin may be confounded by the hemodynamic effects of these substances, which indirectly modulate vasopressin release via the cardiovascular reflexes. For example, the infusion of pressor doses of norepinephrine increases both arterial blood pressure and left atrial pressure. Each of these changes is capable of eliciting a reflex inhibition of vasopressin release which should reduce plasma vasopressin. However, the inhibitory effects of the sino-aortic and cardiac reflexes on vasopressin release seem to be offset by the direct stimulatory effect of circulating norepinephrine. A similar situation may exist with the possible stimulation of vasopressin release by angiotensin. The direct stimulatory effect of angiotensin may be offset by inhibitory influences elicited from the cardiovascular reflexes. Angiotensin is a well-known dipsogen and has been shown to cause drinking in all the species tested [30]. Morton et al. [31] submitted six normal subjects to a 3-day diet containing 10 mmol of sodium and 60 mmol of potassium per day. The mean cumulative sodium loss (±SD) for the six subjects was 208 ± 94 mmol. Sodium restriction had no effect on serum sodium concentrations. Sodium depletion increased the circulating concentrations of angiotensin II more than fivefold ($p < 0.001$), but had no effect on plasma arginine vasopressin concentrations. In short, physiologic concentrations of angiotensin II do not cause an increase in plasma vasopressin concentration in normal subjects.

The presence of endogenous opioid peptides and opioid receptors in the neural lobe has led to the suggestion that opioid peptides play a role in the release of neurohypophyseal hormones [32]. It is now recognized that opioid drugs exert their pharmacologic effects through an interaction with specific receptors. These receptors are classified into several types: μ, δ, σ and κ. μ Agonists such as morphine and methadone are responsible for the classical opiate effects of analgesia, respiratory depression, and physical dependence. They typically cause an antidiuresis in hydrated animals and humans [33]. In contrast, κ agonists have analgesic properties, but do not cause respiratory depression nor physical dependence at the dose required for analgesia. They have been shown to cause a water diuresis in experimental animals and in humans, probably by the inhibition of vasopressin secretion [34]. *K* opioid agonists could have potential therapeutic benefits in the treatment of hyponatremia secondary to increased arginine vasopressin secretion.

Neuropeptides such as neurotensin or cholecystokinine activates the stretch-inactivated cation channels mainly by a G-protein cellular transductive message and cause vasopressin release and thirst. A very rapid and robust release of arginine vasopressin is seen in humans after cholecystokinin (CCK) injection [35]. Nitric oxide is an inhibitory modulator of the hypothalamo–neurohypophysial system in response to osmotic stimuli [36]. Vasopressin secretion is under the influence of a glucocorticoid-negative feedback system and the vasopressin responses to a variety of stimuli (haemorrhage, hypoxia, hypertonic saline) in normal humans and animals appear to be attenuated or eliminated by pretreatment with glucocorticoids [37]. Finally, nausea and emesis are potent stimuli of arginine vasopressin release in humans and seem to involve dopaminergic neurotransmission [38]. The osmotic stimulation of arginine vasopressin release by dehydration or hypertonic saline infusion, or both, is regularly used to test the arginine vasopressin secretory capacity of the posterior pituitary (Fig. 1.7a). This secretory capacity can be assessed directly by comparing the plasma arginine vasopressin concentration measured sequentially during a dehydration procedure with the normal values and then correlating the plasma arginine vasopressin with the urinary osmolality measurements obtained simultaneously [39]. Copeptin, the C-terminal part of the arginine vasopressin precursor peptide, has been found to be a stable surrogate marker of arginine vasopressin release [40] and a useful measurement in the differential diagnosis of polyuric states [41]. The AVP release can also be assessed indirectly by measuring plasma and urine osmolalities at regular intervals during the dehydration test [42] (Fig. 1.7b). The maximum urinary osmolality obtained during dehydration is compared with the maximum urinary osmolality obtained after the administration of 1-desamino[8-D-arginine]vasopressin [desmopressin (dDAVP]) (1–4 μg sc or intravenously during 5–10 min). The nonosmotic stimulation of AVP release can be used to assess the vasopressin secretory capacity of the posterior pituitary in a rare group of patients with the essential hypernatremia and hypodipsia syndrome [43]. Although some of these patients may have partial central diabetes insipidus, they respond normally to nonosmolar AVP release signals such as hypotension, emesis, and hypoglycemia. In all other cases of suspected central diabetes insipidus, these nonosmotic stimulation tests will not give additional clinical information.

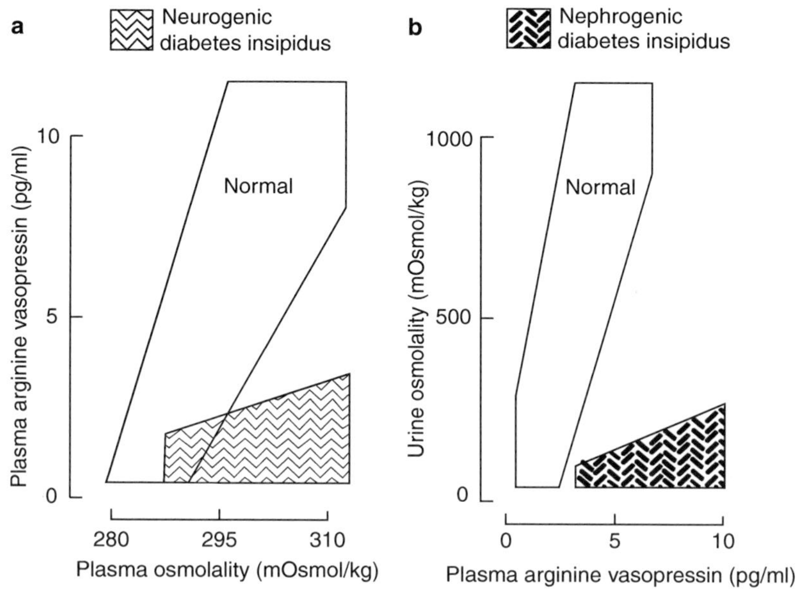

Fig. 1.7 Direct, measurements of vasopressin, and indirect, measurements of urine osmolality, evaluations of vasopressin secretion during dehydration (**a**) or hypertonic saline infusions testing (**b**)

In summary, vasopressin secretion and thirst perception and quenching, and the ability of the kidney to respond to vasopressin are key regulators of water balance. In the thirst centers, cell shrinking during dehydration is mechanically coupled to the activation of Transient Receptor Potential Vanilloid (TRPV) channels and lead to the depolarization of vasopressin neurosecretory neurons and to the central and systemic release of vasopressin. These tonicity and vasopressin producing cells are outside the blood brain barrier and angiotensin II is augmenting the gain of osmoreceptors cells, that is, augmenting vasopressin release for the same osmotic stimulus. Low blood pressure and its perception by other stretch receptors is also a potent baro-regulator of vasopressin release during hypotension or low effective arterial blood volume. Thus, over and above the multifactorial processes of excretion water balance is dependent of a complex multiple control system orchestrated by the brain.

1.3.2 Regulation of Renal Water Excretion by Vasopressin

After its release in the systemic circulation, VP is delivered to the kidneys to control water excretion via urine output. Water reabsorption in the proximal convoluted tubule is passive, but the cell membrane becomes impermeable in the distal tubule while sodium reabsorption persists. Vasopressin activates an active free-water reabsorption by renal cells of the limb of Henle and distal tubule thanks to a binding with three types of receptor [44]. Vasopressin acts mainly through renal V2 receptors (V2R), which are located on the basal cell membrane of the collecting duct. Vasopressin binding to these receptors is coupled with a G-protein activation. This promotes a cascade of reactions resulting in an increased intracellular cyclic AMP (cAMP) production and the expression of water channels; i.e. aquaporins. Aquaporins were first identified in the 1990s [45]. This large ubiquitous family of transmembrane proteins is mainly involved in water and neutral solute trafficking. Based on their functional properties and their primary aminoacid sequences, AQPs are divided into three subgroups: (1) AQP 0, 1, 2, 4, 5, 6, 8 are water channels; (2) AQP7 is an aquaglyceroporin permeable to small neutral molecules; (3) AQP3, 7, 9, 10 are implicated in urea, glycerol, and water movements; (4) AQP11, 12 are superaquaporins [46, 47] (Fig. 1.8). All of the AQPs are characterized by a common tetrameric structure which includes six transmembrane domains, an alpha helix connected by five loops, intracellular amino- and carboxyl-terminal domains associated with twofolded loops. This represents the intrasubunit of each subunit. Water passes essentially through the central pore in the middle of the tetramer subunit, while ions may cross the channel through individual subunit pore pathways [8, 46, 48].

Vasopressin-regulated channels responsible for water permeability of collecting duct are AQP2. They are highly selective and specific water channels (Fig. 1.9).

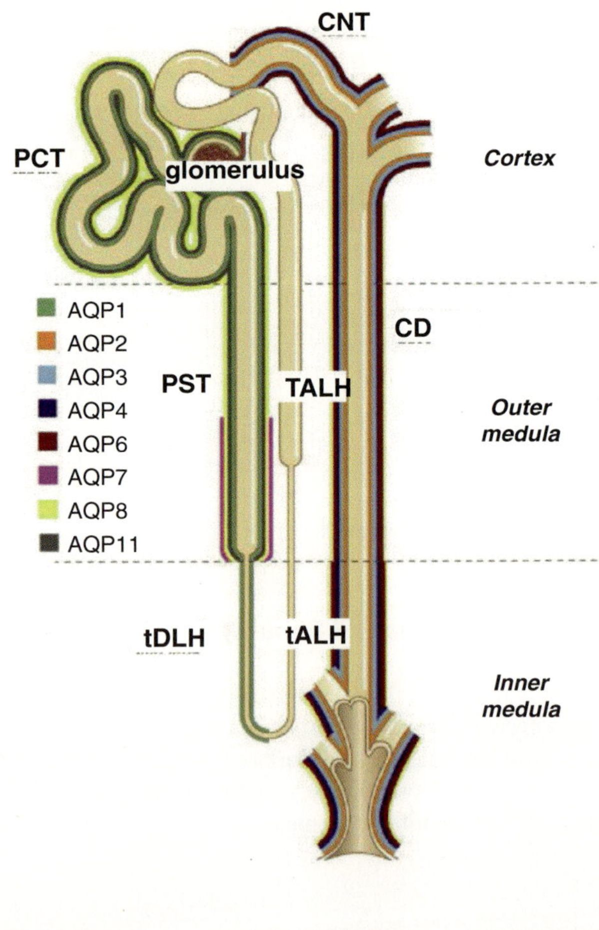

Fig. 1.8 Expression of renal aquaporins along the nephron. *CD* collecting duct, *CNT* connecting tubule, *PCT* proximal convoluted tubule, *PST* proxima straight tubule, *tALH* thin ascending loop of henle, *tDLH* thin decending loop of Henle, *TALH* thick ascending loop of Henle. Modified from Kortenoeven ML et al. [50] with permission

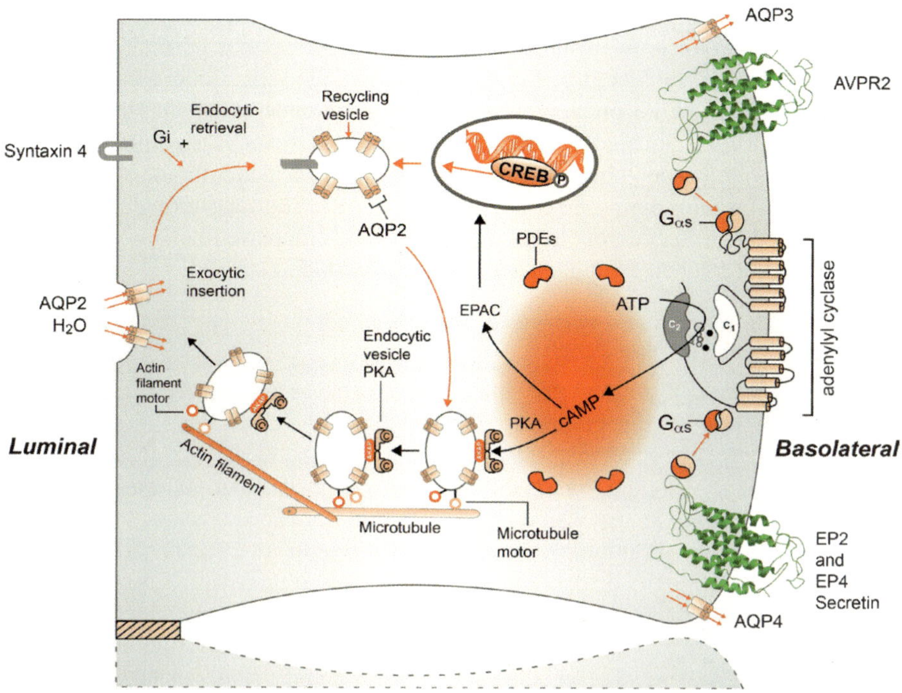

Fig. 1.9 Schematic representation of the effect of arginine vasopressin (AVP) to increase water permeability in the principal cells of the collecting duct. AVP is bound to the V_2 receptor (a G-protein-linked receptor) on the basolateral membrane. The basic process of G-protein-coupled receptor signaling consists of three steps: a hepta-helical receptor that detects a ligand (in this case, AVP) in the extracellular milieu, a G-protein that dissociates into alpha subunit bound to GTP and beta and gamma subunits after interaction with the ligand-bound receptor, and an effector (in this case, adenylyl cyclase) that interacts with dissociated G-protein subunits to generate small-molecule second messengers. AVP activates adenylyl cyclase increasing the intracellular concentration of cyclic adenosine monophosphate (cAMP). The topology of adenylyl cyclase is characterized by two tandem repeats of six hydrophobic transmembrane domains separated by a large cytoplasmic loop and terminates in a large intracellular tail. Generation of cAMP follows receptor-linked activation of the heteromeric G-protein (G_s) and inter-action of the free G_{as}-chain with the adenylyl cyclase catalyst. Protein kinase A (PKA) and possibly the Exchange factor directly activated by cAMP (EPAC) are the target of the generated cAMP. On the long term, vasopressin also increases AQP2 expression via phosphorylation of the cAMP responsive element binding protein (CREB), which stimulates transcription from the AQP2 promoter. Cytoplasmic vesicles carrying the water channel proteins (represented as homotetrameric complexes) are fused to the luminal membrane in response to AVP, thereby increasing the water permeability of this membrane. Microtubules and actin filaments are necessary for vesicle movement toward the membrane. The mechanisms underlying docking and fusion of aquaporin-2 (AQP2)-bearing vesicles are not known. The detection of the small GTP binding protein Rab3a, synaptobrevin 2, and syntaxin 4 in principal cells suggests that these proteins are involved in AQP2 trafficking [71]. When AVP is not available, water channels are retrieved by an endocytic process, and water permeability returns to its original low rate. Internalized AQP2 can either be targeted to recycling pathways or to degradation via lysosomes. AQP3 and AQP4 water channels are expressed on the basolateral membrane)

VP exerts its regulation in two ways. The short-term regulation is the result of AQP2 trafficking and relocation in the renal cell membrane. Under normal conditions, AQP2 channels are restricted within the cytoplasm. VP-V2R binding first activates the expression of AQP3 on the basal membrane of renal cells. This triggers the transport of AQP2 located in intracellular vesicles (exocytosis) [44, 49, 50]. Therefore, the activated phosphorylated AQP2 on the apical membrane allows water reabsorption through the pore [8, 44, 46, 48, 51, 52]. The long-term regulation of AQP2 related to vasopressin occurs as a result of an increased half-life and abundance of AQP2 by increasing its transcription [44, 51–53].

In summary, renal AQP2 activation following vasopressin secretion represents the central key for controlling urine dilution/concentration and consequently water balance. Thus, the collecting duct permeability to water varies according to plasma vasopressin concentration: in case of a low concentration of vasopressin, urines are highly diluted (minimal urinary osmolality is about 100 mosm/L); if vasopressin release increases, urinary concentration in a linear fashion with vasopressin due to a large amount of water reabsorption. However, despite a continuous increase in vasopressin concentration, urine concentration reaches a maximum value of 1000–1200 mosm/L. Usually, the kidney is able to equilibrate a 1000–2000 mL per day of water ingestion through urine concentration/dilution. Urea, sulfates, phosphates and other substrates issued from the cellular metabolism are responsible for a 600 mosm per day which requires an obligatory and minimal water excretion of 500 mL per day by the kidney. AQP2 dysregulation is recognised to be responsible for various water disorders: mutations of V2R or AQP2 cause polyuric pathologies, especially nephrogenic diabetes insipidus; increased AQP2 expression leads to abnormal water retention as observed in the syndrome of inappropriate antidiuretic hormone secretion (SIADH) [10, 53–56].

Vasopressin enables also to control water balance through the activation of various solutes co-transporters [44, 57]. The bumetamide-sensitive sodium-chloride cotransporter is located in the thick ascending limb of Henle. vasopressin stimulates its activity leading to increase the active reabsorption of sodium-chloride. The resulting medullary interstitial accumulation of solutes promotes water reabsorption from renal ducts. Vasopressin also promotes water reabsorption by triggering the epithelial sodium channel (ENaC) activity in the collecting duct, in an aldosterone-independent way [58] (see infra). The subsequent increase in sodium reabsorption facilitates water reabsorption [44, 58–60].

1.4 Body Sodium Balance and Its Regulation

1.4.1 Sodium Balance

Sodium is a monovalent cation and a strong base. Its molecular weight is 23, chloride molecular weight is 35.4 and 1 g of NaCl contains 17 mmol of Na. Total body sodium is 60 moles per kg. Forty percent is located in the bones [61]. Plasma sodium concentration is 140 ± 2 mmol/L and 144 ± 2 mmol/L in the interstitial compartment and freely crosses the capillary membrane. Intracellular sodium concentration varies but remains very low (<20 mmol/L) due to Na^+-K^+-ATPase enzyme activity which continuously extrudes sodium from cells. Due to its high extracellular content, sodium is the prime determinant of the volume of this compartment. In other words, body sodium content regulates the ECV and arterial pressure, while natremia, which is the plasma sodium concentration, determines plasma tonicity and consequently the ICV. In pathological situations, the presence of oedema indicates an increased ECV (interstitial), due to the accumulation of Na (and water). It is important to underline that interstitial and EABV ("volemia") vary in an opposite way in most clinical situations. For example, patients with congestive cardiac or renal insufficiency or ascitic cirrhosis present oedema and low EABV. In these situations, ECV volume is abnormally high due to the increased sodium content in the interstitial volume, while EABV is low. The treatment of these water and electrolyte abnormalities is difficult because sodium vascular loading is essential to maintain effective circulation, but worsens oedema.

In physiological situations, the exogenous oral intake of Na is higher than the needed one. The difference depends on food habits. The obligatory losses by the skin and the intestinal tractus correspond to the minimal intake required (10 mmoles per day). Despite variations in Na intake, total Na balance is usually constant due to an equilibrium between sodium intake and renal excretion. The kidney represents the key organe of this tight regulation [62]. Total sodium renal elimination is >95% of that excreted. Quantitatively, this represents 500 g of sodium extracted from plasma per day. This regulatory mechanism is the major energetic and expenditure challenge of the tubular epithelium (Fig. 1.10).

As reviewed recently, the kidney filters vast quantities of Na at the glomerulus but excretes a very small fraction of this Na in the final urine [62]. Although almost every nephron segment participates in the reabsorption of Na in the normal kidney, the proximal segments (from the glomerulus to the macula densa) and the distal segments (past the macula densa) play different roles. The proximal tubule and the thick ascending limb of the loop of Henle interact with the filtration apparatus to deliver Na to the distal nephron at a rather constant rate. This involves regulation of both filtration and reabsorption through the processes of glomerulotubular balance and tubuloglomerular feedback. The more distal segments, including the distal convoluted tubule (DCT), connecting tubule, and collecting duct, regulate Na reabsorption to match the excretion with dietary intake.

Sodium filtration is passive, while its reabsorption is an energy-consuming process. The total sodium entering the glomerus is filtered, i.e. 25 moles per day. Sixty to seventy percent is reabsorbed along the proximal convoluted tubule (PCT). This isotonic process is performed by Na^+/H^+ exchangers (NHE3) [60]. The thick ascending limbs of the loop of Henle (TALH) are responsible for 25–35% of sodium reabsorption. This active process is mediated by Na-K-2Cl (NKCC) cotransporters. Only 8–10% of sodium filtered enters the distal convoluted tubule (DCT) and 6–10% is finally reabsorbed. The pathways of sodium transport differ according to the part of DCT: in the proximal part, reabsorption is performed by Na-Cl (NCC)

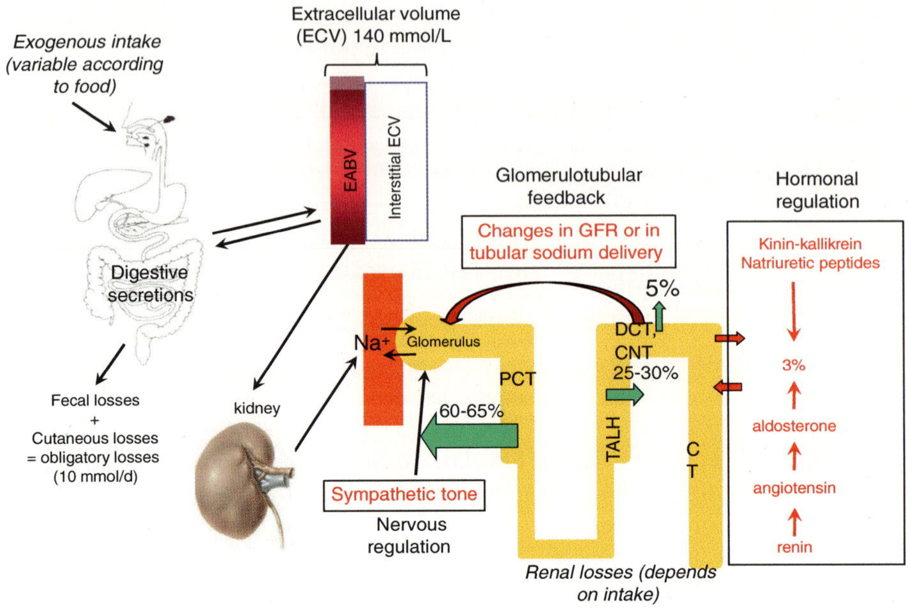

Fig. 1.10 Sodium balance and its major regulating mechanisms in a 70 kg adult. Sodium intake coming essentially from the exogenous food is equilibrate by urinary sodium output. By regulating sodium excretion, kidney plays an essential role in total sodium balance. After its ingestion, sodium is massively reabsorbed by the gastrointestinal system and is further distributed in body compartments. Sodium homeostasis is mainly maintained thanks to the hormonal renin angiotensin aldosterone system axis which globally triggers renal sodium reabsorption in the collecting tubule. Natriuretic peptides and the kinin-kallikrein systems behaves as natriuretic effectors. Besides the hormonal system, sodium balance regulation is controlled by the glomerulotubular feedback which is mediated by sodium tubular delivery and glomerular filtration rate (GFR), and a sympathetic nervous pathway. *CNT* connecting tubule, *CT* collecting tubule, *DCT* distal convoluted tubule, *EABV* effective arterial blood volume, *ECV* extracellular volume, *PCT* proximal convoluted tubule

cotransporters; in the distal tubule sodium is reabsorbed through the Epithelial sodium channel (ENaC). In the final, a very low content of filtered sodium reaches the collecting duct (CD). However, due to large variations in sodium excretion, the CD plays a major role to maintain sodium balance. The intestinal tract participates strongly in sodium exchanges: sodium excretion through biliary, pancreatic and intestinal secretion are important. But, in physiological situations, almost all excreted sodium is reabsorbed. This phenomenon explains why patients presenting severe intestinal losses (gastric suctioning or intestinal fistula) are hypovolemic.

1.4.2 Regulation of Sodium Balance

The mechanisms involved in sodium balance regulation consist in loops (Table 1.3): a peripheral or central signal activates receptors which trigger an afferent

Table 1.3 Major factors and mechanisms of sodium balance regulation

	Afferent mechanisms	stimuli	Efferent mechanisms	Effects
Hormonal factors				
– angiotensin	– decrease in renal perfusion pressure	– renin	– increase in the sympathetic nerve tone	– renal Na PCT reabsorption
		– hyperkalemia	– increase in GFR	– renal Na DCT and CD reabsorption
			– aldosterone release	
– aldosterone	– renin	– angiotensin	– activation of the epithelial channel ENaC	– renal Na DCT and CD reabsorption
			– activation of the Na-K-ATPase pump	– renal K DCT and CD excretion
			– activation of the epithelial channel ROMK	= Antinatriuretic and kaliuretic effect
– natriuretic peptides	– hypertension	– sympathetic nervous tone	– systemic and renal vasoconstriction	= hypotensive effect
	– hypervolemia		– increase in GFR	= natriuretic effect
			– decrease in PCT and CD Na reabsorption	
– bradykinin	– kallicrein		– systemic and renal vasodilation	
– prostaglandins	– sympathetic nervous tone	– PGE2, PGI2	– modulation of GFR and RBF	= modulation of natriuresis and urine output
Mechanical factors				
– GFR	– decrease in renal perfusion pressure		– stimulation of renin and aldosterone	= antinatriuretic effect
			– inhibition of angiotensin	
			– decrease in the SRAA activation	
– tubuloglomerular feedback		– decrease in tubular Na delivery		= natriuretic effect

CT collecting tubule, *ENaC* epithelial sodium channel, *GFR* glomerular filtration rate, *K* potassium, *Na* sodium, *DCT* distal convoluted tubule, *PCT* proximal convoluted tubule.

transmission to a central or peripheral command; an efferent transduction of the signal through efferent pathways reaches effectors (organs). Kidneys and vessels are the most important.

1.4.2.1 Afferent Pathways

Two pathways are activated [6]:

- the activation/inhibition of mechanoreceptors which depends on volemia and arterial pressure. In case of hypervolemia or arterial hypertension, these stretch receptors are activated, leading to an inhibition of the central signal and consequently to decrease the neurendocrine and sympathetic response. Baroreceptors are located in the high pressure arterial system (aortic arch, carotid sinus) and sensored modifications in pressure. Various organs contain low pressure receptor: pulmonary artery circulation, atrial and ventricular walls and portal vessels (voloreceptors). Regardless their situation, these receptors are activated or inhibited by changes in parietal stretch. The signal issued from the systemic arterial circulation is conducted along the vagus (X) and the glossopharyngial (IX) nerves to the central nervous system (Fig. 1.11).

mechanical mechanisms such as a decrease in GFR or in sodium delivery in the tubule. An increased amount of sodium delivered in the juxtaglomerular apparatus

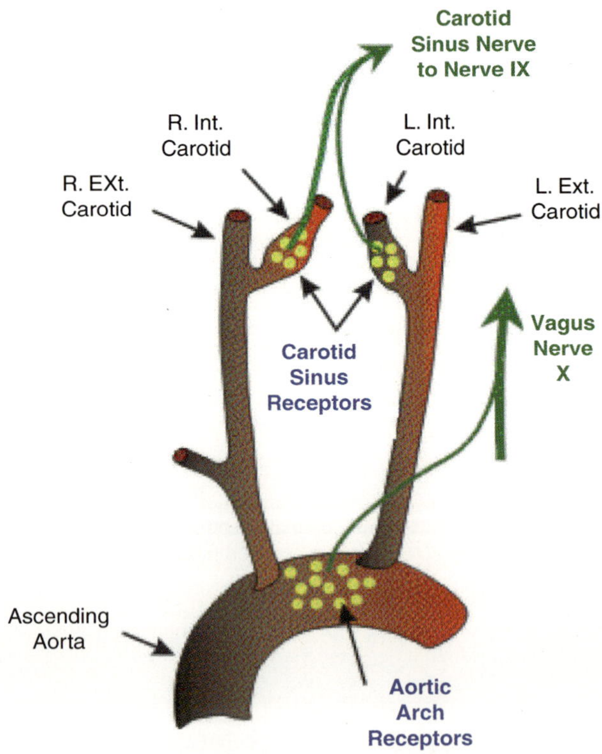

Fig. 1.11 Major peripheral mechanoreceptors and pathways implicated in the renin-angiotensin-aldosterone and vasopressine release. *Ext* external, *I* internal, *L* left, *R* right

induces a decrease in GFR, leading in return to a decrease in sodium delivery. This is the famous "tubuloglomerular feedback" which is mediated by a vasoconstriction of glomerular afferent arterioles.

1.4.2.2 Efferent Pathways

The transmission (transduction) of the signal is conducted through three pathways: the hormonal, neuronal pathways and the sodium and potassium dietary.

- *The hormonal system* plays a key role in the regulation of sodium balance. Sodium excretion is precisely controlled thanks to several hormone systems responsible in sodium renal reabsorption or excretion.
  - Renin-Angiotensin-Aldosterone system (RAAS) axis: this is the most important system of sodium balance regulation. Renin is synthetized by the epithelial cells of the afferent arteriole of the juxtaglomerular apparatus located in the DCT. Renin release is mainly activated by a decrease in renal perfusion pressure which triggers the receptors located on the juxtaglomerular afferent arterioles. Hyperkalemia, hyponatremia and an increase in sympathetic nerve activity also stimulate renin synthesis. Non active angiotensinogen is synthetized by the liver, then converted into the inactive angiotensin I in the kidney thanks to renin. The converting enzyme allows the conversion of angiotensin I into the active angiotensin II. This latter molecule binds to specific transmembrane receptors and triggers consequently several peripheral and central effects: release of aldosterone, thirst, vasoconstriction (Fig. 1.12). The final results is always to control sodium

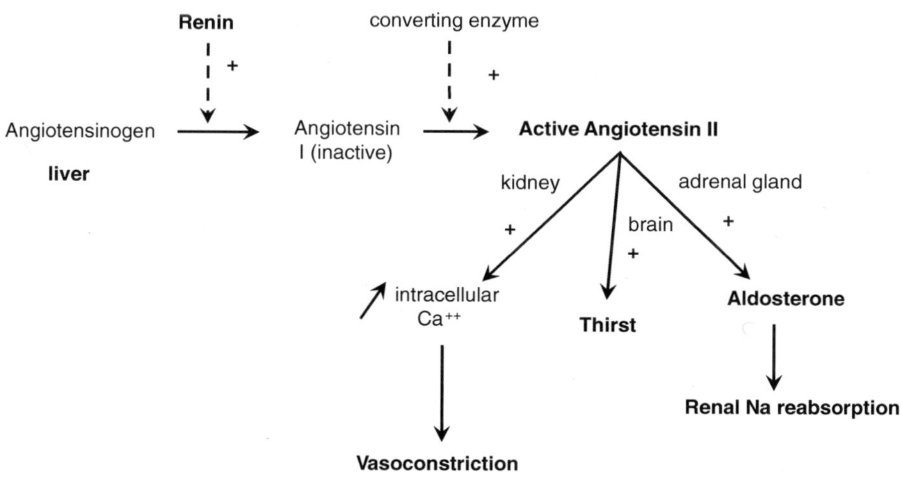

Fig. 1.12 The renin-angiotensin-aldosterone system axis. Renin is synthetized by renal cells of the juxtaglomerular apparatus, angiotensinogen is synthetized by the liver and aldosterone by the adrenal gland. The activation of renin synthesis and release by hypovolemia/arterial hypotension converts angiotensinogen (inactivate molecule) in angiotensin 1 (inactivate molecule). The converting enzyme conducts to the release of the active angiotensin II. This latter triggers several effects on different organs: vasoconstriction, renal sodium reabsorption and thirst

balance (renal excretion or reabsorption). Aldosterone, the final molecule of the RAAS axis, is synthetized and released by cells of the juxtaglomerular apparatus. Late DCT, connecting tubule (CNT) and cortical collecting duct (CCD) represents the aldosterone-sensitive distal nephron. Aldosterone binds intracellular to mineralocorticoid receptors, migrates to the nucleus and upregulates sodium (and water) reabsorption and potassium excretion. Sodium reabsorption caused by aldosterone is mediated by ENaC which is located essentially in the apical membrane of the CD. This effect is controlled by a negative feedback of the RAAS axis [58]. In the same time, aldosterone stimulates sodium basal reabsorption thanks to an increased Na^+-K^+-ATPase pump activity and increases ATP production by mitochondria. Aldosterone is also involved in potassium balance. It has a kaliuretic effect due to the activation of the permeability renal out-medullary potassium channel (ROMK). This channel which is located on the apical membrane promotes potassium excretion. All of these effects are rapidly effective in 30–60 min. Aldosterone enables to activate directly sodium reabsorption by an upregulation of the thiazidique sensitive-Na-Cl transporter in the DCT [44].

Angiotensin II enables to increase arterial pressure by different mechanisms independently from the aldosterone action [63]. This effect is due to several actions: i) a direct sodium reabsorption secondary to a direct ENaC activation; ii) a systemic vasoconstriction due to an increased in the sympathetic nerve activity; iii) an increased thirst sensation and water renal reabsorption induced or not by VP secretion. Recent data have shown that angiotensin can deliver a signal from a central nervous activation. The first step of this signal is a binding of angiotensin on central transmembrane AT1 receptors. According to their isoform, the transduction pathway and signal differs [64, 65]. Briefly, AT1a which are present in the SFO and OVLT and SFO structures, activates phospholipase C which induces the production of inositol triphosphate (IP3) and diacylglycerol (DAG). This traditional pathway induces the release of intracellular stores of calcium, and triggers water intake. AT1b activation stimulates a mitogen-activated protein kinase (MAPK) leading to increase NaCl intake. AT1b are located in the cerebral cortex and the hippocampus. Thus, it seems that central stimulation of NaCl reabsorption and water intake may be triggered directly by angiotensin, but follows separate signal transduction and gates.

– Natriuretic peptides (NP): NP synthesis is activated by stretching disseminated mecanoreceptors located on cardiac walls (atrial NP [ANP]) and central nervous system (CNP). Half-life varies between 4 and 20 min according to the type of peptide. NP provides vascular effects and renal sodium exchanges. The systemic vascular impact consists in vasodilation which contributes to decrease arterial pressure. On kidneys, NP induces vasodilation of the afferent glomerular arteriole coupled with a vasoconstriction of the

efferent glomerular arteriole, leading to an increased GFR without any modification of RBF. As a consequence, NP promotes sodium renal filtration and its excretion. NP produces its natriuretic effect by other mechanisms: sodium renal reabsorption induced by RAAS activation is counteracts by NP in the PCT and the CD and by transmembrane sodium channels inhibition. NP enables also to trigger renal sodium excretion via a direct stimulation of stretch receptors and a signal transduction from CNS. The final global action is a natriuretic one [6]. Thus variations in volemia exerts a feedback on NP release: hypovolemia reduces NP release and consequently renal sodium excretion, and conversely.
  - Kinin-kallicrein system: kallicrein is a serine protease produced by collecting tubule cells. It converts kininogen into bradykinin. This system controls several ion channels in the CNT and CCD. His effect is globally an inhibition of sodium reabsorption which results from an inhibition of ENaC activity [60]. In the same time, bradykinin induces vasodilation and an increase in capillary permeability. Finally, this system more modulates than regulates sodium balance and arterial pressure.
  - Prostaglandins (PG): they are synthetized by kidneys and exerts a modulating effect on sodium balance. According to their nature and their localisation, some of them provide vasodilation or vasoconstriction with a final goal of preserving GFR and RBF. They can inhibit renin release promoting a natriuretic effect.
  - Vasopressin: vasopressin contributes by itself to sodium balance regulation. This hormone upregulates a thiazidique sensitive-sodium-chloride cotransporter which is located in the DCT and causes urine dilution. VP also binds on V1 receptors which are expressed in the renal medullar vasculature. This activation mediates renal blood flow and consequently renal Na reabsorption aiming to control volemia and arterial pressure.
- *Sodium and potassium dietary* participates also to sodium balance regulation. Low dietary sodium increases aldosterone release and consequently sodium reabsorption. A high potassium dietary associated with a constant sodium intake reduces directly renal sodium reabsorption in the PCT, TALH and DCT thanks to an activation of angiotensin II. Potassium triggers also sodium reabsorption as a consequence of aldosterone release independently of the angiotensin II one.
- *Long-term sodium balance* has been recently evoked. Some new experimental data have shown that when maintaining sodium intake constant for several weeks, sodium excretion is directly related to cortisol which might modify tissue sodium storage [66]. Sodium is bound to proteoglycans which are constitutive of skin, bones and conjonctive tissues. This stored sodium represents an important reservoir which can modifiy independently of sodium plasma concentration. Adverse effects of chronic hyponatremia might be related to changes in this sodium reservoir: loss of calcium from bones, increase in the osteoclasts activity which might be responsible for osteoporosis and fractures

In summary, total sodium pool is the determinant of extracellular volume, especially the effective arterial blood volume, i.e. volemia. Sodium balance is physiologically maintained constant to preserve arterial pressure and volemia. The RAAS axis plays the major role of this regulation thanks to vascular (and central) stretch receptors. By sensing modifications in parietal vascular stretch, both angiotensin and aldosterone modify renal sodium reabsorption. Indeed, hypotension or hypovolemia stimulates angiotensin-aldosterone release which causes sodium reabsorption. This effect is completed by VP release, and intrarenal modifications in sympathetic nerve tone. Besides these sodium reabsorption effect, other hormonal systems including natriuretic peptides, kinin-bradykinin and prostaglandin systems exerts natriruretic effects.

Conclusion

Water and sodium are inseparable. Natremia which determines usually plasma tonicity, is the major determinant of intracellular volume. Body sodium content mainly determines the extracellular volume according to variations in effective arterial blood volume (volemia) and arterial pressure. Water and sodium balances are strictly regulated to maintain cell volume and volemia constant. Water balance is classically maintained thanks to vasopressin hormone and thirst which cause respectively renal water reabsorption and oral intake. Sodium balance is regulated by the renin-angiotensin-aldosterone system axis which is considered as the classical hormonal system responsible of renal sodium reabsorption and several natriuretic systems including natriuretic peptides, kinin-kallicrein and prostagladins systems. In all cases, the kidney is the principal trigger and effector of these effects.

However, recent data showed that water and sodium homeostasis are determined by very complex additional mechanisms mediated by hormonal, neuronal, intrinsic neurogenic pathways. These different pathways often cause potentialized effects aiming to maintain water and sodium balances. Nowadays, considering its major role in centralizing peripheral informations and in determining integrative neuronal informations, the central nervous system must be considered as a very effective complex neural network

References

1. Sterns RH (2015) Disorders of plasma sodium--causes, consequences, and correction. N Engl J 372:55–65
2. Edelman IS, Leibman J, O'Meara MP, Birkenfeld LW (1958) Interrelations between serum sodium concentration, serum osmolarity and total exchangeable sodium, total exchangeable potassium and total body water. J Clin Invest 37:1236–1256
3. Mount DB (2010) Hyponatremia. Semin Nephrol 29:1–317
4. Orban JC, Ichai C (2012) Hyponatrémies en réanimation. Encycl Med Chir (Anesthésie-Réanimation) 36-860-A-05:16

5. Danziger J, Zeidel ML (2014) Osmotic homeostasis. Clin J Am Soc Nephrol 10:852–862
6. Patel S (2009) Sodium balance - an integrated physiological model and novel approach. Saudi J Kidney Dis Transplant 20:560–569
7. Antunes-Rodrigues J, Ruginsk SG, Mecawi AS et al (2014) Neuroendocrinology of Hydromineral homeostasis. In: De Luca LA Jr, Menani JV, Johnson AK (eds) Neurobiology of body fluid homeostasis: transduction and integration. CRC Press, Boca Raton (FL). Chapter 3
8. Noda Y (2014) Dynamic regulation and dysregulation of the water channel aquaporin-2: a common cause of and promising therapeutic target for water balance disorders. Clin Exp Nephrol 18:558–570
9. Ferguson AV (2014) Circumventricular organs: integrators of circulating signals controlling hydration, energy balance, and immune function. In: De Luca LA Jr, Menani JV, Johnson AK (eds) Neurobiology of body fluid homeostasis: transduction and integration. CRC Press, Boca Raton (FL). Chapter 2
10. Spasovski G, Vanholder R, Allolio R et al (2014) Hyponatraemia guideline development group. Clinical practice guideline on diagnosis and treatment of hyponatraemia. Intensive Care Med 40:320–331
11. Orban JC, Ichai C, Quintard H (2014) Troubles hydroélectrolytiques et acidobasiques. In: Fourcade O, Geeraerts T, Minville V, Samii K (eds) Traité d'Anesthésie et de Réanimation. Lavoisier, Paris, pp 847–892
12. Harring TR, Deal NS, Kuo DC (2014) Disorders of sodium and water balance. Emerg Med Clin North Am 32:379–401
13. Adrogue HJ, Madias NE (2014) Diagnosis and treatment of hyponatremia. Am J Kidney Dis 64:681–684
14. Verbalis JG (2006) Whole-body volume regulation and escape from antidiuresis. Am J Med 119:S21–S29
15. Petitclerc T (2013) Disorders in sodium-water balance. Nephrol Ther 9:38–49
16. Son SJ, Filosa JA, Potapenko ES et al (2013) Dendritic peptide release mediates interpopulation crosstalk between neurosecretory and preautonomic networks. Neuron 78:1036–1049
17. Bourque CW (2008) Central mechanisms of osmosensation and systemic osmoregulation. Neuroscience 9:519–531
18. Bichet DG (2014) Central vasopressin: dendritic and axonal secretion and renal actions. Clin Kidney J 7:242–247
19. Prager-Khoutorsky M, Bourque CW (2015) Mechanical basis of osmosensory transduction in magnocellular neurosecretory neurones of the rat supraoptic nucleus. J Neuroendocrinol 27:507–515
20. Oka Y, Ye M, Zuker CS (2015) Thirst driving and suppressing signals encoded by distinct neural populations in the brain. Nature 52:349–352
21. Betley JN, Xu S, Cao ZF et al (2015) Neurons for hunger and thirst transmit a negative-valence teaching signal. Nature 521:180–185
22. Zhang Z, Bourque CW (2008) Amplification of transducer gain by angiotensin II-mediated enhancement of cortical actin density in osmosensory neurons. J Neurosci 28:9536–9544
23. Lechner SG, Markworth S, Poole K et al (2011) The molecular and cellular identity of peripheral osmoreceptors. Neuron 69:332–344
24. Zerbe RL, Robertson GL (1987) Osmotic and nonosmotic regulation of thirst and vasopressin secretion. In: Narins RG (ed) Maxell & Kleeman's clinical disorders of fluid and electrolyte metabolism. Mc Graw Hill Inc, New York, pp 61–78
25. Verbalis JG (2003) Disorders of body water homeostasis. Best Practice & Research Clin Endocrinol Metab 17:471–503
26. Norsk P (1989) Influence of low- and high-pressure baroreflexes on vasopressin release in humans. Acta Endocrinol 121(Suppl 1):3–27
27. Baylis PH (1983) Posterior pituitary function in health and disease. Clin Endocrinol Metab 12:747–770
28. Robertson GL (1983) Thirst and vasopressin function in normal and disordered states. J Lab Clin Med 101:351–371

29. Rowe JW, Minaker KL, Sparrow D, Robertson GL (1982) Age-related failure of volume-pressure-mediated vasopressin release. J Clin Endocrinol Metab 54:661–664
30. Rolls B, Rolls E (1982) Thirst (problems in the behavioural sciences). Cambridge University Press, Cambridge, UK
31. Morton J, Connell J, Hughes M, Inglis G, Wallace E (1985) The role of plasma osmolality, angiotensin II and dopamine in vasopressin release in man. Clin Endocrinol 23:129–138
32. Martin R, Voigt KH (1981) Enkephalins co-exist with oxytocin and vasopressin in nerve terminals of rat neurohypophysis. Nature 289:502–543
33. Giarman NJ, Mattie LR, Stephenson (1953) Studies on the diuretic action of morphine 117:225–226
34. Yamada K, Nakano M, Yoshida S (1990) Inhibition of elevated arginine vasopressin secretion in response to osmotic stimulation and acute haemorrhage by U-62066E, a kappa-opioid receptor agonist. Br J Pharmacol 99:384–388
35. Abelson JL, Le Melledo J, Bichet DG (2001) Dose response of arginine vasopressin to the CCK-B agonist pentagastrin. Neuropsychopharmacology 24:161–169
36. Wang H, Morris JF (1996) Constitutive nitric oxide synthase in hypothalami of normal and hereditary diabetes insipidus rats and mice: role of nitric oxide in osmotic regulation and its mechanism. Endocrinology 137:1745–1751
37. Raff H (1987) Glucocorticoid inhibition of neurohypophysial vasopressin secretion. Am J Phys 252:R635–R644
38. Rowe JW, Shelton RL, Helderman JH, Vestal RE, Robertson GL (1979) Influence of the emetic reflex on vasopressin release in man. Kidney Int 16:729–735
39. Zerbe RL, Robertson GL (1981) A comparison of plasma vasopressin measurements with a standard indirect test in the differential diagnosis of polyuria. N Engl J Med 305:1539–1546
40. Balanescu S, Kopp P, Gaskill MB, Morgenthaler NG, Schindler C, Rutishauser J (2011) Correlation of plasma copeptin and vasopressin concentrations in hypo-, iso-, and hyperosmolar states. J Clin Endocrinol Metab 96:1046–1052
41. Fenske W, Quinkler M, Lorenz D et al (2011) Copeptin in the differential diagnosis of the polydipsia-polyuria syndrome--revisiting the direct and indirect water deprivation tests. J Clin Endocrinol Metab 96:1506–1515
42. Miller M, Dalakos T, Moses AM, Fellerman H, Streeten DH (1970) Recognition of partial defects in antidiuretic hormone secretion. Ann Intern Med 73:721–729
43. McKenna K, Thompson C (1998) Osmoregulation in clinical disorders of thirst appreciation. Clin Endocrinol 49:139–152
44. Knepper MA, Tae-Hwan K, Nielsen S (2015) Molecular physiology of water balance. N Engl J Med 372:1349–1358
45. Preston GM, Carroll TP, Guggino WB, Agre P (1992) Appearance of water channels in Xenopus oocytes expressing red cell CHIP28 protein. Science 256:385–387
46. Huber VJ, Tsujita M, Nakada T (2012) Aquaporins in drug discovery and pharmacotherapy. Mol Asp Med 33:691–703
47. Benga G (2012) On the definition, nomenclature and classification of water channel proteins (aquaporins) and relatives. Mol Asp Med 32:514–517
48. Yool AJ, Campbell EM (2012) Structure, function and translational relevance of aquaporin dual water and ion channels. Mol Asp Med 33:553–561
49. Brown D, Bouley R, Paunescu TG, Breton S, Lu HAJ (2012) New insights into the dynamic regulation of water and acid-base balance by renal epithelial cells. Am J Cell Physiol 302:C1421–C1433
50. Kortenoeven ML, Frenton RA (2014) Renal aquaporins and water balance disorders. Biochim Biophys Acta 1840:1533–1549
51. Wilson JL, Miranda CA, Knepper NA (2013) Vasopressin and the regulation of aquaporin-2. Clin Exp Nephrol 17:751–764
52. Sasaki S (2012) Aquaporin 2: from its discovery to molecular structure and medical implications. Mol Asp Med 33:535–546

53. Verbalis JG, Goldsmith SR, Greenberg A et al (2013) Diagnosis, evaluation, and treatment of hyponatremia: expert panel recommendations. Am J Med 126(suppl 1):S1–42
54. Adler SM, Verbalis JG (2006) Disorders of body water homeostasis in critical illness. Endocr Metab Clin North Am 35:873–894
55. Juul KV, Bichet DG, Nielsen S, Nørgaard JP (2014) The physiological and pathophysiological functions of renal and extrarenal vasopressin V2 receptors. Am J Physiol Renal Physiol 306:F931–F940
56. Holmes RP (2012) The role of renal water channels in health and disease. Mol Asp Med 33:547–552
57. Kortenoeven ML, Pedersen NB, Rosenbaek LL, Fenton RA (2015) Vasopressin regulation of sodium transport in the distal nephron and collecting duct. Am J Physiol Renal Physiol 309:F280–F299
58. Mironova E, Bugaj V, Roos KP, Kohan DE, Stockand JD (2012) Aldosterone-independent regulation of the epithelial Na^+-channel (ENaC) by vasopressin in adrenalectomized mice. Proc Natl Acad Sci 109:10095–10100
59. Stockand JD (2010) Vasopressin regulation of renal sodium excretion. Kidney Int 78:849–856
60. Staruschenko A (2012) Regulation of transport in the collecting tubule and cortical collecting duct. Compr Physiol 2:1541–1584
61. Hannon MJ, Verbalis JG (2014) Sodium homeostasis and bone. Curr Opin Nephrol Hypertens 23:370–376
62. Palmer LG, Schermann J (2014) Integrated control of Na transport along the nephron. Clin J Am Soc Nephrol 10:676–687
63. Weber MA (2002) Introduction: the hemodynamic and vascular effects of angiotensin II: managing the consequences. Am J Hypertens 15:1S–2S
64. Daniels D (2014) Diverse role of angiotensin receptor intracellular pathways in the control of water and salt intake. In: De Luca LA Jr, Menani JV, Johnson AK (eds) Neurobiology of body fluid homeostasis: transduction and integration. CRC Press, Boca Raton (FL). Chapter 5
65. Menani JV, Vieira AA, Colombari DSA et al (2014) Preoptic-periventricular integrative mechanisms involved in behavioral, fluid-electrolyte balance, and pressor responses. In: De Luca LA Jr, Menani JV, Johnson AK (eds) Neurobiology of body fluid homeostasis: transduction and integration. CRC Press, Boca Raton (FL). Chapter 4
66. Titze J (2015) A different view on sodium balance. Curr Opin Nephrol Hypertens 1:14–20
67. Wilson Y, Nag N, Davern P et al (2002) Visualization of functionally activated circuitry in the brain. Proc Natl Acad Sci U S A 99:3252–3257
68. Robertson GL, Shelton RL, Athar S (1976) The osmoregulation of vasopressin. Kidney Int 10:25–37
69. Zerbe RL, Henry DP, Robertson GL (1983) Vasopressin response to orthostatic hypotension. Etiologic and clinical implications. Am J Med 74:265–271
70. Vokes TP, Robertson GL (1985) Physiology of secretion of vasopressin. In: AGRP C (ed) Frontiers in hormone research: diabetes insipidus in man, vol 13. S. Karger, Basel, pp 127–155
71. Valenti G, Procino G, Liebenhoff U et al (1998) A heterotrimeric G protein of the G_i family is required for cAMP-triggered trafficking of aquaporin 2 in kidney epithelial cells. J Biol Chem 273:22627–22634

Sodium Disorders

2

Carole Ichai and Jean-Christophe Orban

2.1 Introduction

Dysnatremias are the most common electrolyte disorders, especially in critically ill and surgical patients. Brief notions of pathophysiology focused on the mechanisms and regulation of intracellular volume are needed to analyze dysnatremias. Such disorders may induce severe organ dysfunctions, especially cerebral dysfunction, and cause death. The practical diagnostic and therapeutic approach of hyponatremias and hypernatremias must follow safety rules of management to prevent iatrogenic complications. Because this book is dedicated to critically ill situations, we will focus essentially on acute and severe dysnatremias, especially for the treatment.

2.2 Pathophysiology Definitions

This paragraph is voluntary summarized because it is largely detailed in another chapter (see "Water and Sodium Balance" chapter).

2.2.1 Body Compartments

Total body water (TBW) is the most compound of total body weight in an adult (50–70%). TBW distributes for two-thirds in the intracellular volume (ICV), and the remaining one-third in the extracellular volume (ECV) [1–6]. ICV and ECV

C. Ichai (✉) • J-C. Orban
Intensive Care Unit, Pasteur 2 Hospital, 30 Voie Romaine, 06001 Nice, Cédex 1, France

IRCAN (INSERM U1081, CNRS UMR 7284), University Hospital of Nice, Nice, France
e-mail: ichai@unice.fr

C. Ichai et al. (eds.), *Metabolic Disorders and Critically Ill Patients*,
http://doi.org/10.1007/978-3-319-64010-5_2

are separated by cell membranes. ECV is divided into the plasma or the effective arterial blood volume (EABV) (25–30%) and the interstitial volume (70–75%). EABV is normally composed of 93% water that contains dissociated and non-dissociated solutes. Seven percent of the plasma volume is occupied by non-dissociated molecules (lipids and proteins) without water. As cell membranes are semipermeable, water crosses freely between the ICV and the ECV according to the osmotic transmembrane gradient [2, 7, 8]: water moves from the low to the high osmotic compartment until reaching the osmotic equilibrium. Therefore, ICV depends on the solute concentrations between both compartments. Only effective or impermeant solutes are able to create such an osmotic gradient across cell membranes, leading to water movements and changes in cell volume. Among them, sodium (Na^+) is the major impermeant solute of the ECV and potassium (K^+) of the ICV: thanks to the Na^+-K^+-ATPase pump located on cell membranes, Na^+ is restricted to the ECV, whereas K^+ is essentially located in the ICV. Therefore, total body sodium content (pool) is the major determinant of arterial pressure, while serum sodium concentration and its associated cations play a major role in determining plasma osmolality. Diffusive or ineffective solutes, i.e., urea and alcohols (ethanol, methanol, ethylene glycol), cross freely to the cell membrane and is distributed equally in the ICV and the ECV. Therefore, they are unable to create any change in cell volume. The osmotic effect of glucose depends on the nature of tissues: for non-insulin-mediated ones, glucose behaves as an ineffective solute; for insulin-mediated tissues in the presence of insulin, glucose remains a noneffective solute, but in case of insulinopenia or insulin resistance, glucose becomes an effective impermeant solute. At last, mannitol and glycerol, non-physiological solutes, are also extracellular effective solutes. Based on its osmotic properties, mannitol is one of the most popular treatments of cerebral edema (osmotherapy).

2.2.2 Osmolarities and Plasma Tonicity

Total plasma osmolarity is defined as the concentration of all osmotic solutes in a liter of plasma (mosm/L). Plasma osmolality is also the concentration of all solutes but in a kilogram of plasma water (mosm/kg). In normal conditions, both are very close as water contributes to 93% of 1 liter of plasma, but in case of severe hyperlipidemia or hyperprotidemia, the amount of plasma water decreases leading to an artificial decreased serum sodium concentration (see chapter "Plasma Tonicity and Hyponatremia"). Plasma osmolarity can be approached in different ways [1–3, 7–9]. The measured total plasma osmolality (mPosm [mosm/kg]), which is performed in the laboratory using the delta cryoscopic method, provides a global value of all osmoles present in the plasma, regardless of their normal or abnormal presence and their transmembrane diffusive properties. Posm can be easily calculated at bedside (cPosm [mosm/L]) considering the major electrolytes contained in plasma by the following formula: cPosm [mosm/L] = ([Na^+ × 2] + glycemia + urea) (mmol/L) = 280–295 mosm/L. Because this calculation overrides abnormal (not usually measured) and minor plasma osmoles, mPosm is slightly higher than cPosm. The difference between these two parameters is known as the osmolar gap (OG = mPosm - cPosm), and its value is around 10 mosm/L. Plasma tonicity (or effective osmolarity) refers to only major effective osmoles and is calculated using the following formula: P tonicity = [Na^+ × 2) + glycemia] (mmol/L) = 270–285 mosm/L. P tonicity is therefore the best practical parameter for evaluating accurately the ICV [2, 4, 7, 8]: a hypotonic stress always indicates an increased ICV (cell edema), whereas a hypertonic stress is always associated with a decreased ICV (cell shrinkage).

2.2.3 Body Water Balance and Its Regulation

Briefly, in physiological conditions, water intake and output are closely equilibrated, aiming to control TBW and consequently extracellular tonicity. This phenomenon allows to maintain a stable ICV and to avoid any changes in cell volume. Preservation of cell volume is fundamental to maintain cell functions and avoid cell death. Due to its essential contribution in plasma tonicity, serum sodium concentration, i.e., natremia, is the major parameter participating in TBW and cell volume. On the other hand, because body sodium is mainly extracellular, total body sodium amount determines ECV regulation.

TBW is controlled by three neurohormonal mechanisms: vasopressin (VP) or antidiuretic hormone (ADH), thirst, and the capacity of the kidney to concentrate or dilute urines. In physiological situations, thanks to these mechanisms, plasma tonicity remains stable despite wide daily variations in water intake or excretion [2–4, 8, 10]. VP and thirst are mainly triggered via an osmotic stimulus [1, 10, 11]. VP is synthetized by nuclei of the anterior hypothalamus, stored and released by the posterior pituitary. Tonicity is closely perceived by special neurons mainly located in the subfornical (SFO) and the organum vasculosum of the lamina terminalis (OVLT) of the circumventricular organs [3, 4, 6]. Such neurons are perfect osmoreceptors able to detect very low changes in plasma tonicity and cell volume. Modification in cell volume triggers the activation (cell shrinkage) or inhibition (cell edema) of some cationic protein channels, the transient receptor potential vanilloid (TRVP) of these osmoreceptors, leading finally to activate or inhibit VP release and thirst sensation [12–14]. Because any modification in cell volume is poorly tolerated (especially for the brain), VP release is modified for tonicity changes as small as 1–2%. In humans, above a threshold around 280 mosm/kg, VP secretion increases linearly with an increasing osmolality (from 280 to 330 mosm/kg); under this threshold, VP concentration remains undetectable in plasma [2, 15]. The threshold of thirst seems to be very close from that of VP, and its upper limit is very high depending on the total osmoles to be excreted (up to 25 l of urine output is possible with normal kidneys). VP release and thirst are also triggered by changes in arterial pressure and volemia via an activation of peripheral baro-/voloreceptors which are mainly located on the sino-aortic vascular walls [16, 17]. When both changes in osmolality and arterial pressure/volemia stimulate VP and thirst, there is an amplification of the phenomenon (e.g., hypotension and hyperosmolality). However, in case of opposite stimulus, the resulting effect depends on the severity of modification in volemia: only severe hypovolemia (of at least 5–10%) overrides the osmoregulation allowing extremely high VP concentrations [16, 17]. Other non-osmotic, non-volumic stimuli enable to activate VP release and thirst such as pain, morphinics, nausea, vomitings, and hypoxia.

Renal water excretion is mainly controlled by VP which promotes water renal reabsorption in the collecting tube. VP binds to its V2 receptors (V2R) which are located on the basal cell membrane [18]. The complex VP-V2R triggers a cascade of reactions, resulting finally in the expression and activation of water channels, i.e., aquaporins [5, 11, 19–21]. Aquaporin-2 activation allows high volume of water reabsorption by kidneys. In the absence of VP, urine is diluted with a maximum decrease in urine osmolarity of 50–100 mosm/L. The linear increase in VP concentration induces a linear increase in urine concentration with a maximal urine osmolarity of 1200 mosm/L. Above this value and despite a persistent increase in VP concentration, urine cannot concentrate more.

In summary: usually, thanks to VP and thirst mainly, TBW is maintained constant allowing to control plasma tonicity and consequently cell volume. The kidney is the central organ which regulates urine concentration or dilution according to plasma VP concentration and water intake. Thirst is the second major mechanism which allows to prevent the development of severe hypertonicity. Therefore, inappropriate secretion of ADH (SIADH) may be responsible for inappropriate water reabsorption by the kidney, leading to hypotonic hyponatremia. On the other hand, because thirst has no real upper limit, hypertonicity is theoretically impossible, except in case of abnormal thirst behavior (elderly patients) or difficulties to drink (prolonged gastric suctioning, coma, etc.) [18, 22].

2.2.4 Cell Volume Regulation-Osmoregulation

Cell volume modifications are poorly tolerated and a constant cell volume is essential to prevent cell damages and dysfunction. Cell edema secondary to a hypotonic stress can cause cell rupture; hypertonicity induces cell shrinkage which can promotes damages of the cytoskeleton, breaks in DNA, and apoptosis [13]. Because the brain is maintained in a non-extensible skull, brain swelling or shrinkage exposes to lethal brain injury, especially when changes in volume are rapid. Hypotonic-induced cerebral edema can be complicated by refractory intracranial hypertension and ultimately by brain death; hypertonic-induced brain shrinkage can cause intracerebral hemorrhage with poor neurological outcome or death too. This explains why clinical manifestations of hyponatremia and hypernatremia are primarily neurologic and life-threatening but nonspecific.

Fortunately, all but almost cerebral cells are not really perfect osmometers (except those responsible for VP stimulation located in the circumventricular organs). Indeed, brain cells enable to limit their volume changes related to an osmotic stress. Such protective effects, i.e., cerebral osmoregulation, result from an adjustment of the intracellular solute content to the extracellular one [1–3, 10, 13, 23]. This phenomenon aims to limit the development of a transmembrane osmotic gradient and consequently cell volume modifications. Cell volume regulation consists in a regulatory volume decrease (RVD) in response to hypotonic-induced cell swelling and of a regulatory volume increase (RVI) in response to hypertonic-induced cell shrinkage [24–30]. Two types of effective solutes, i.e., osmoprotective molecules, are implicated in this regulation: the inorganic are electrolytes (mainly Na, K, Cl), and the organic are idiogenic osmoles (or osmolytes) and consist in amino acids, polyols, and triethylamines. Chloride via its voltage-dependent channels (ClC) and its sodium (NCC), potassium (KCC), sodium/potassium (NKCC) cotransporters is also essential for regulating brain volume [31, 32]. NCC and NKCC favor sodium, potassium, and chloride entry in the cell and are inhibited by an increased intracellular chloride concentration. Plasma hypotonicity activates KCC3 leading to extrude potassium and chloride from the cell and to attenuate cerebral edema (RVD). On contrary, plasma hypertonicity activates NKCC1 which induces the entry of sodium, potassium, and chloride in the cell and finally decreases cell shrinkage (RVI). An acute hypotonicity triggers quickly in some minutes to 2–4 h an extrusion of inorganic osmoles. This phenomenon protects rapidly but moderately and incompletely the brain cell from volume changes. Only prolonged (chronic on 24–48 h) hypotonicity enables to strongly blunt the osmotic gradient and avoid relevant cell volume changes, thanks to the excretion of osmolytes. This mechanism takes a longer time required to obtain synthesis or metabolism of these organic solutes by cells. In this situation, cerebral osmoregulation is delayed but is strongly efficient and complete and restores the brain volume (Fig. 2.1). Cerebral osmoregulation induced by a hypertonic stress consists in opposite shifts of electrolytes and organic osmoles, leading also to control cerebral volume.

Aquaporin-4 channels (AQP4) are also largely involved in cerebral cell volume changes [25, 33, 34]. They are strongly present in the brain, located on glial cells which are close from arterial vessels and subarachnoid spaces, and in the supraoptic nucleus. Indeed, during hyponatremia, knockout animals for AQP4 show an intense reduction in cerebral edema and in mortality as compared with the control [35]. Hypertonic saline seems to induce its antiedematous effect, thanks to these perivascular AQP4 [34]. However, AQP4 are also responsible for a reabsorption of water in vasogenic edema related to brain tumor [36].

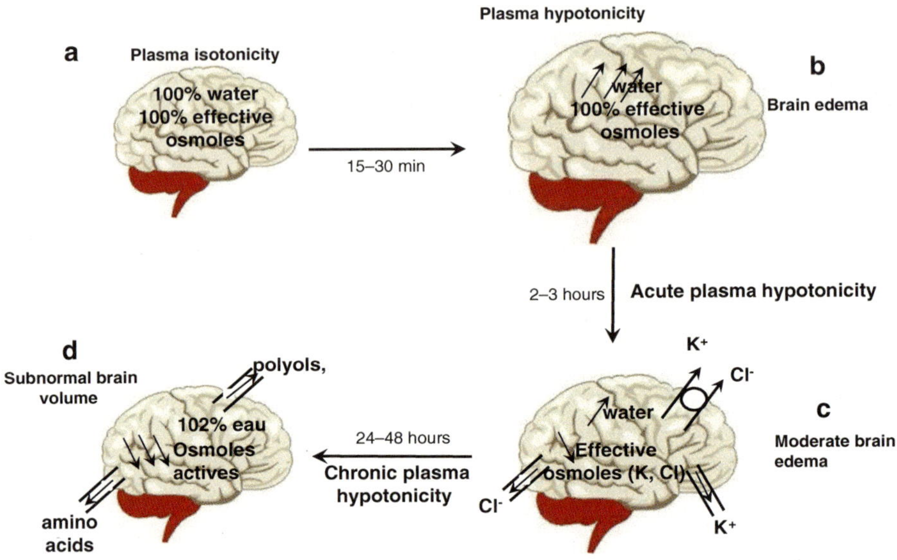

Fig. 2.1 Mechanisms of brain volume regulation during plasma hypotonic stress (osmoregulation). (**a**): *Normal brain volume*: water and effective osmole contents are 100% (**b**): *Immediate plasma hypotonicity*: plasma hypotonicity induces water extrusion from brain cells because the amount of intracellular effective osmoles cannot change immediately. The resulting high transmembrane osmotic gradient provokes brain edema. (**c**): *Acute plasma hypotonicity*: after 2–3 h of plasma hypotonicity, brain cells enable to reduce their amount of effective osmolytes by extruding electrolytes (inorganic osmoles including potassium and chloride essentially) and attenuate the transmembrane osmotic gradient. As a result moderate and incomplete brain edema develops. (**d**): *Chronic plasma hypotonicity*: after 24 h or more prolonged plasma hypotonicity, a substantial extrusion of organic effective osmoles (osmolytes such as polyols and amino acids) from brain cells blunts the transmembrane osmotic gradient. As a result, cerebral osmoregulation appears quasi-complete and the brain recovers a subnormal volume

Non-osmotic stress as ischemia-reperfusion, hypothermia, or acidosis enables to trigger cell volume changes [29]. Chloride, potassium channels, and sodium-potassium-chloride (NKCC) cotransporters seem to be involved in this phenomenon which is controlled by the intracrine renin-angiotensin system.

> In summary, the efficiency of cerebral osmoregulation depends strongly on the time of development and the duration of the osmotic disorder. Because of an incomplete cerebral osmoregulation, rapid dysnatremias are more often symptomatic and life-threatening and require an emergent aggressive treatment. Classically, longer development of hyponatremias, which is commonly associated with a quasi-complete cerebral volume regulation, is more usually asymptomatic or poorly symptomatic and thus does not require an emergent treatment. Moreover, due to a downregulation of transporters, the recovery of modifications in brain osmoles takes a longer time

when cerebral osmoregulation is complete. Therefore, a rapid treatment becomes an osmolar stress which exposes to a risk of overcorrection with an inverse osmotic gradient. Such a risk is particularly well known in patients presenting chronic hyponatremia which expose to the risk of osmotic demyelination syndrome if natremia normalizes too rapidly. Efficiency of osmoregulation is also affected by hypoxia and sex, female being less protected than male [37, 38].

2.3 Epidemiology: Prognosis

Dysnatremias are the most common electrolyte disorders [39–43]. Most studies reported a frequency between 25 and 50%, depending on the patient's conditions, the threshold of abnormal values, and on the delay of appearance of dysnatremia. Hoorn et al. [39] showed that 15–30% of hospitalized patients experienced moderate (130–135 mmol/L) and 3% severe (<125 mmol/L) hyponatremia. Among the severe one, 36% were symptomatic and only 20% of them survived. Most frequent causes of hyponatremia are the syndrome of inappropriate secretion of antidiuretic hormone (SIADH), surgical patients (especially neurosurgical patients), and drug-induced hyponatremia, while hypernatremia is frequently iatrogenic. Numerous studies found that dysnatremias, even moderate, are independently associated with an increased risk of in-hospital mortality [39, 41, 44]. A recent meta-analysis including 81 studies found that 17.4% of patients (n = 147,948) experienced a moderate hyponatremia (125–135 mmol/L), which was significantly associated with an increased risk of overall mortality (RR = 2.6) and morbidity [41]. Moreover, mortality was inversely correlated with the depth of hyponatremia.

Several recent studies are focused on dysnatremias in critically ill patients [45–49]. Most of them considered only dysnatremias at admission in intensive care unit (ICU) and showed that hyponatremia was more frequent than hypernatremia (11–26% vs. 2.5–9%, respectively). In a retrospective study performed in 77 ICUs over a period of 10 years, Funk et al. [47] showed that 24% of patients presented dysnatremias at admission, 17.3% were hyponatremic and 6.9% were hypernatremic. According to the level of serum sodium concentration, patients were distributed as follows: slight, moderate, and severe hyponatremia in 13.8%, 2.7%, and 1.2%, respectively, and slight, moderate, and severe hypernatremia in 5.1%, 1.2% and 0.6%, respectively. Hypo- and hypernatremia were independent risk factors of mortality and poor outcome. The risk is raised with the importance of serum concentration abnormality (OR from 1.32 to 1.81 for hyponatremia and from 1.48 to 3.64 for hypernatremia). The global incidence of ICU-acquired dysnatremias varies from 30 to 40% of patients, and hypernatremia seems to have twice the incidence of hyponatremia [46, 48]. Globally, hyponatremia developed and persisted within 1–3 days and hypernatremia within 1–5 days. The impact of ICU-acquired dysnatremias on morbi-mortality in critically ill patients remains controversial [45, 46, 48]. In a recent large cohort prospective observational study, hyponatremia at admission in ICU was found in 34.3% of patients, and 36.2% of them were caused by a SIADH [50]. Patients were diagnosed as euvolemic in 58.9%, hypervolemic in 26.3%, and hypovolemic in 14.8% of cases. The authors confirmed that hyponatremia was an independent risk factor for an increased mortality (HR = 1.61) and morbidity (longer length of stay and mechanical ventilation).

Finally, none of these studies proves the causality between dysnatremias and the increased morbi-mortality. Indeed, in a retrospective observational study, Chawla et al. [43] reported that more patients presenting a moderate hyponatremia (<120 mmol/L) died than those with severe hyponatremia (<110 mmol/L), with a peak of mortality between 120 to 124 mmol/L. The authors hypothesized that severe hyponatremias were essentially due to a drug-associated effect, while moderate ones were observed in patients with numerous comorbidities and severe illnesses. Therefore at this time, it is not possible to conclude if dysnatremia is a simple marker or the direct cause of death.

2.4 Hyponatremias

2.4.1 Hyponatremia and Plasma Tonicity

Hyponatremia not always reflects plasma hypotonicity with its related risk of brain edema. Therefore, the first step in the management of hyponatremia is to eliminate non-hypotonic hyponatremias [2, 9, 13, 23, 51, 52]:

- *Pseudohyponatremias* occur in case of a marked increase in lipid or protein plasma concentration. Hyponatremia is the result of a laboratory artifact due to the high volume occupied by excessive lipids or proteins in plasma and to the sample dilution before measurements [53]. In this situation, the total number of solute particle in the water phase of plasma is unchanged. Therefore, the direct measurement of serum osmolality (mosm/kg), which is performed on undiluted sample, confirms that hyponatremia is isotonic (Fig. 2.2). As a practical consequence, no shift of water occurs and there is no risk of brain edema.
- *False hyponatremias* are caused by the abnormal accumulation of effective solutes other than sodium in the ECV. The resulting plasma hyperosmolality causes an osmotic shift of water from the ICV to the ECV that induces in turn a dilutional hyponatremia. This hyperosmolar hyponatremia can be isotonic or hypertonic, depending on the severity of excessive effective osmoles and on the osmotic-induced polyuria. When associated with hypertonicity, hyponatremia conducts to cell shrinkage which requires rehydration, whereas isotonic hyponatremia has no impact on cell volume. The most common cause of hypertonic hyponatremia is hyperglycemia [1, 2, 9, 23, 30, 54, 55]. In this situation, calculation of plasma tonicity remains the easier and most accurate tool to estimate possible changes in ICV, regardless the actual serum sodium concentration. Alternatively, natremia can be corrected considering the glucose elevation. Corrected natremia [cNa^+], which estimates what would be natremia with nor-

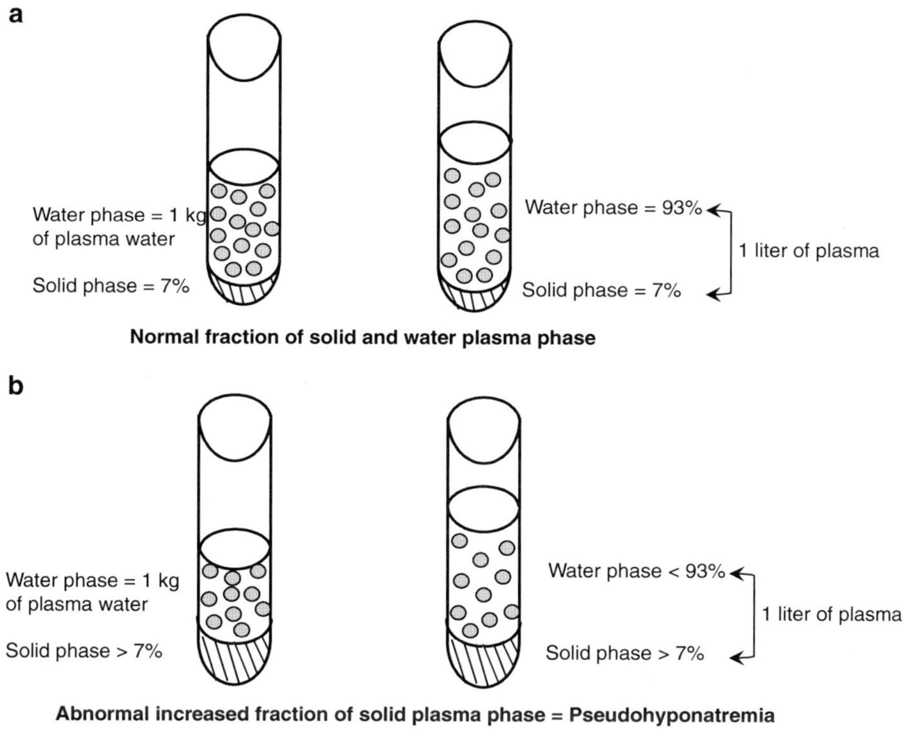

Fig. 2.2 Plasma sodium concentration in normal and increased fraction of solid plasma particles. (**a**): *Normal repartition of solid and water plasma phases*: 1 l of plasma distributes normally into 7% of solid phase (lipids and proteins) and 93% of water phase (containing electrolytes, especially sodium). Therefore, 1 kg of plasma water is very close from 1 l of plasma and normal plasma sodium concentration per kg, or per liter of plasma is also very close (140 ± 2 mmol/L). (**b**): *Increased solid plasma phase* (hyperlipidemia or hyperprotidemia): the increase in solid phase decreases in proportion of plasma water phase, and 1 kg of water plasma differs from 1 l of plasma. Therefore, if ion measurements assumed a constant distribution between the water and solid phase, sodium concentration per liter of plasma will be underestimated (related to a dilution effect), while sodium concentration per kilogram of plasma water remains normal: this is the isotonic pseudohyponatremia. Gray circles represent sodium particles

moglycemia, can be calculated using the following formula: [cNa^+] = (measured [Na^+] + [glycemia × 0.45 [mmol/L) (for every 5.5 mmol/L increase in glycemia, add 2.4 mmol/L to measured natremia) [54]. Other effective osmoles may accumulate in plasma and cause hypertonic hyponatremia: mannitol, glycerol/glycine surgical irrigant solutions, hyperosmolar radiocontrast media, histidine-tryptophan-ketoglutarate, and maltose. Due to the context, such situations are usually easily recognized. If necessary, an elevated osmolar gap, which is calculated by the difference between the measured and the calculated plasma osmolarity, will confirm the presence of excessive abnormal plasma effective osmoles.

– *Hypotonic hyponatremias* are those at risk of cerebral edema and require a specific treatment.

The following paragraphs will be focused on the sole hypotonic hyponatremias. The confirmation of hypotonicity is a prerequisite and the first step of the diagnosis of hyponatremia [2, 9, 13, 23, 30]. Therefore, the European clinical practice guidelines (ECPG) [9] and the American guidelines [23] recommend firstly to exclude hyperglycemic hyponatremias by measuring serum glucose concentration. Hyponatremia associated with a low measured osmolality always reflects hypotonicity. However, because it is not available everywhere and every time, such a measurement cannot be recommended. On the other hand, plasma tonicity which can be performed easily at bedside is accurate enough to diagnose hyponatremias at risk of brain edema and must be calculated in all situations associated with hyponatremia.

2.4.2 Definitions

Hyponatremia is consensually defined as a serum sodium concentration <135 mmol/L. The management of hyponatremic patients depends on its severity. Consequently, it is essential to define "severe" hyponatremia. Unfortunately, many definitions are reported in the literature [9, 13, 23, 30, 56, 57]. Hyponatremia below 120–125 mmol/L is usually considered as severe [13, 23, 55, 56]. The speed of development of hyponatremia is also a classical parameter of severity. Acute hyponatremia is defined by a rate of development <48 hours and is considered as severe due to the risk of brain edema, by opposition with chronic hyponatremia developed in more than 48 h. This classification is consistent with the pathophysiology of brain regulation and consequently with therapeutic strategies: acute hyponatremia requires an aggressive immediate treatment to limit brain edema, while chronic hyponatremia needs a slow correction aiming to avoid osmotic demyelination. Unfortunately, the speed of development of hyponatremia is not often known, especially in critical situations. However, some conditions and drugs are particularly associated with an acute decrease in natremia [9, 13] (Table 2.1). Among them psychotic polydipsia, exercise-induced hyponatremia, postoperative period, and intracranial injuries are frequent. After eliminating these situations, hyponatremia should be presumed as chronic despite no precise speed of its development.

The depth of hyponatremia as well as its delay of development is not only responsible for the efficiency of cerebral osmoregulation. Indeed, sex, age, hypoxia, and individual variations contribute also to this regulation [57]. For this reason, the ECPG [9] decided to provide three definitions of hyponatremia based on the (1) biochemical severity, (2) time of development, (3) and symptoms and their severity which is the first parameter to consider for the treatment (Table 2.2). These definitions were elaborated to avoid usual confusion by physicians and to recommend hierarchical therapeutic guidelines with successive steps.

Table 2.1 Major drugs and conditions associated with acute hyponatremia (non-exhaustive list)

Drugs	Conditions
– *Diuretics* • Thiazides • Amiloride, indapamide • Loop diuretics – *Anticancer* • Vincristine, vinstatine • Platinum agents • Cyclophosphamide – *Antidepressants* • Tricyclic antidepressants • Selective serotonin reuptake inhibitors • Monoamine oxidase inhibitors – *Antihypertensive agents* • Angiotensin converting enzyme inhibitors • Calcium antagonist agents – *Antiepileptic agents* • Carbamazepine, sodium valproate – *Antipsychotic agents* • Phenothiazine, butyrophenone – *Proton pump inhibitors*	– Postoperative period – Polydipsia (psychotic potomania) – Exercise-associated hyponatremia – Post-resection of the prostate, post-resection of endoscopic uterine surgery, or arthroscopy – Colonoscopy preparation

Table 2.2 Classification of major symptoms caused by hyponatremia according to their severity (non-exhaustive list)

Symptoms	Severity
– Severe (highly life-threatening) – Moderately severe – Mild (not life-threatening)	• Vomiting • Cardiorespiratory distress • Abnormal and deep somnolence • Seizures • Coma (Glasgow coma scale ≤ 8) • Confusion, delirium • Headache • Nausea without vomiting • Falls, gait instability • Falls-related fractures • Impaired attention, cognitive disturbances, cramps, fatigue

2.4.3 Pathophysiology and Classification

Hyponatremia is primarily a disorder of water balance indicating a relative excess of body water to body solute (sodium): water intake (or infusion) exceeds kidney free water excretion. In most clinical situations, both mechanisms, i.e., excessive water intake and impaired and inappropriate urine dilution, are associated. Nevertheless, based on the major mechanism of development, hyponatremias are classified into three categories that are associated with three ECV status [2, 23, 30, 56, 58–60]:

- *Euvolemic hyponatremias* are due to an absolute body water excess without change in total body amount. This is classically observed in case of inappropriate kidney water reabsorption (SIADH) or in case of excessive water intake (psychotic polydipsia).
- *Hypovolemic hyponatremias* are due to excessive sodium losses which cause volume depletion and in turn increase VP secretion creating ultimately water retention with hyponatremia despite plasma hypotonicity [58]. Such conditions may be provoked by gastrointestinal kidneys or skin disorders.
- *Hypervolemic hyponatremias* are due to excessive renal sodium and water reabsorption. In these situations, the effective arterial blood volume (EABV) is usually low, while the interstitial one is increased (as expressed clinically by peripheral edema). Effective hypovolemia triggers both VP and renin-angiotensin secretions, leading to renal water and sodium reabsorption, respectively. In such patients, both body water and sodium amount are elevated as observed in various congestive conditions (heart and liver failures, nephrotic syndrome, kidney diseases).

Such a classification is conceptually useful to understand major mechanisms according to the underlying cause of hyponatremia and in turn to select most appropriate therapies according to the ECV presentation. But in clinical practice, ECV assessment at bedside remains very difficult (except the increased ECV expressed by edema). Moreover, such clinical differentiations are not so clear-cut and depend on kidney function, drugs, and patient's conditions. For example, a patient with SIADH can be treated concomitantly with diuretics that cause effective hypovolemia. Nevertheless, causes of hyponatremia remain commonly classified considering the theoretical volume of the extracellular compartment (see paragraph "etiologic diagnosis").

2.5 Diagnosis

2.5.1 Clinical Symptoms

Because hypotonicity can induce cerebral edema, most clinical signs of hyponatremia are neurologic, but not specific [2, 10, 13, 23, 30, 56, 59]. The severity of hyponatremic encephalopathy depends on the importance of brain edema and its consequence, intracranial hypertension. Therefore, the severity of symptoms varies according to the efficiency of cerebral osmoregulation. Most symptoms are summarized in Table 2.2. In acute hyponatremia, various parameters are associated with an increased risk of cerebral edema expressed by clinical signs of encephalopathy: female (risk multiplied by 28), children, old female treated with thiazides, psychiatric polydipsia, and hypoxia [25, 26]. In all cases, the history and the context must be rigorously identified in order to confirm the causal relationship between clinical signs and hyponatremia. Complementary exams can be needed to eliminate other causes of encephalopathy (CT scan, EEG). Some studies reported that neurological signs associated with hyponatremia might be related not only to brain edema but also to alterations in brain excitability induced by a hypotonic-related neurotransmitter exocytosis (glutamate) [26].

For a long time, chronic hyponatremia has been thought to be asymptomatic and without any deleterious consequences. Since a decade, growing data show that mild chronic hyponatremia is an independent risk factor of various side effects including falls, gait instability, falls-related fractures, impaired attention, and death. These symptoms are independent from age and sex [61–65]. Kinsella et al. [63] found that the incidence of hyponatremia was higher in women presenting fractures than in those without fractures (8.7 vs. 3.2% or 2.25). Hoorn et al. [64] confirmed in elderly patients that chronic hyponatremia was an independent risk of fractures. Cognitive impairment may favor falls and fractures. Chronic hyponatremia is also responsible for a direct alteration in bone density. Indeed, bone, cartilage, and connective tissues serve as a sodium reservoir. Chronic hyponatremia stimulates directly the osteoclast activity, leading to a decreased bone mineral activity [63, 65, 66]. Moreover, decreased bone density correlates closely with the depth of hyponatremia.

In summary: chronic hyponatremia is highly more frequent than the acute one, but the latter is usually associated with moderate or severe neurological symptoms which need an emergent aggressive treatment aiming to prevent or reduce brain edema by increasing rapidly natremia. Many data suggest nowadays that mild chronic hyponatremia is not totally asymptomatic and is associated with cognitive impairment, falls, and fracture. This probably justifies to increase serum sodium levels to subnormal values, but always carefully at a slow rate to avoid osmotic demyelination syndrome (ODS).

2.5.2 Etiologic Diagnosis

The determination of the underlying cause of hypotonic hyponatremia is crucial, but may be impossible at admission and should not delay the emergent treatment of acute hyponatremias. In practice, such a diagnosis can be performed concomitantly with the treatment. In chronic asymptomatic/mild symptomatic hyponatremia, the determination of the underlying cause is needed and precedes the specific treatment. Therefore, the first step in the management of symptomatic acute hypotonic hyponatremia consists in increasing urgently serum sodium concentration, while the determination of the underlying cause is needed before beginning any treatment of chronic hypotonic hyponatremia [9]. For practical reasons, we decided to detail the etiologic approach in a paragraph before treatment, even not the order advised in practical algorithms.

Questions focused on treatments and history of the patient are crucial to approach the underlying cause of hyponatremia. The most common etiologic categorization is still based on the pathogenetic modifications in the ECV. But, despite a thorough

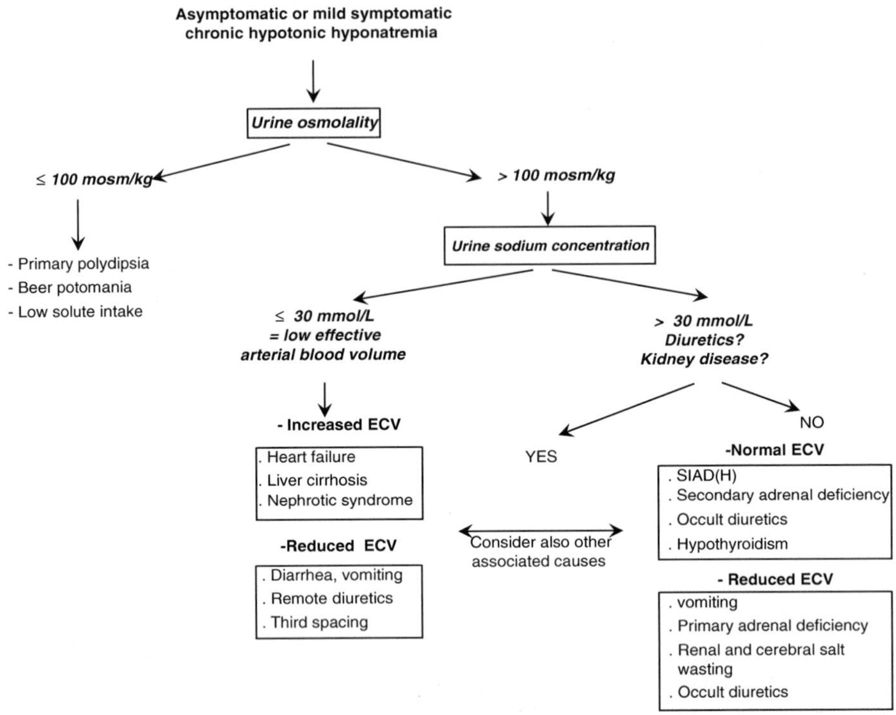

Fig. 2.3 Algorithm for determining the cause of hypotonic hyponatremia

clinical examination, this strategy is not realistic in clinical practice. The assessment of ECV is critical and not accurate (low sensitivity and specificity) leading to misclassifications [67]. Regardless of the parameters used, the diagnosis performance is always better with an algorithm than without [44, 68]. Both urine osmolality (Uosm) and sodium concentration (UNa) are needed, but the place of these parameters in the etiologic algorithm varies according to recommendations (Fig. 2.3) [9, 23].

A Uosm ≤100 mosm/L clearly indicates an excessive water intake. UNa with a threshold of 30 mmol/L has a good sensitivity and specificity to distinguish hypovolemia from euvolemia and hypervolemia. However, diuretics are responsible for an elevated UNa regardless of the ECV status [44, 68–71]. For an accurate interpretation, urine measurements must be performed as soon as possible (before any treatment if possible) on a spot urine sample taken simultaneously with a blood sample. Despite such recommendations, Uosm and UNa are measured in only 10% and 27%, respectively, leading to an absence of determination of the underlying cause of hyponatremia [44]. Other laboratory tests do not have to be performed systematically, but may be useful: serum copeptin, urea and acid uric concentrations, and fractional sodium and uric acid excretion [69, 72, 73]. Among them, fractional uric acid excretion <12% seems to be the most accurate to differentiate low effective arterial blood volume (EABV) from euvolemic hyponatremias. Fractional uric acid excretion might be used for ambiguous conditions such as diuretic treatments or differential diagnosis between SIADH and cerebral salt wasting syndrome. Diuretic treatment does not exclude the contribution of other causes of hyponatremia, especially if hyponatremia persists despite stopping diuretics. For all these reasons, the ECPG [9] who wanted a very pragmatic approach, decided to propose an etiologic algorithm based on the determination of Uosm, followed by UNa on priority before the ECV assessment (Fig. 2.3).

2.5.2.1 Urine Osmolality ≤100 mosm/kg

These situations are due to excessive water intake and low solute intake. The ECV is normal and VP secretion absent as expressed by the low Uosm which is the marker of the appropriate response of kidney: maximal dilution of urines in response to excessive water intake. Hyponatremia develops only when the kidney reaches its maximal possibility for diluting urines. Thus, such conditions require very high volume and rapid water intake (20–30 l per day), usually associated with an impairment in solutes and free water renal loss [9, 10, 49]. Most causes are psychotic polydipsia or self-water intoxication, beer potomania, and low solute intake. Polydipsia-related hyponatremia occurs in 60% of psychiatric patients.

2.5.2.2 Urine Osmolality >100 mosm/kg

Major causes of hyponatremias with a high urine osmolality are SIADH (30–40%) and diuretic treatments, especially thiazides (20%) [23, 44, 72, 74–77]. The determination of the underlying cause requires a further UNa determination which allows to distinguish situations with low UNa (≤30 mmolL) from those with high UNa (>30 mmol/L).

UNa ≤30 mmol/L

A low UNa strongly suggests a low EABV, even in patients on diuretics. Hypovolemic hyponatremia refers to patients with reduced global ECV. Clinical signs such as orthostatic hypotension, tachycardia, arterial hypotension, and dry mucus membrane suggest hypovolemia. Biological parameters of functional acute kidney injury can be helpful, but are neither sensitive nor specific, and can be altered by other factors. Correction of low volemia with 0.9% NaCl will correct concomitantly hyponatremia by stopping VP non-osmotic vasopressin secretion:

- *Hyponatremia with low ECV (hypovolemic)* can be caused by sodium losses issued from the gastrointestinal tract. In case of substantial vomitings, hyponatremia is classically accompanied by metabolic alkalosis (concomitant losses of chloride). By contrast, profuse diarrhea induces hyponatremia associated with metabolic acidosis. Large cutaneous sodium losses represent another cause of hypovolemic hyponatremia as observed in extensive burned patients. At least, hypovolemic hyponatremia can be caused by prolonged administration of diuretics and an excessive water intake/infusion that is frequently associated and which contributes to worsen hyponatremia.
- *Hyponatremia with high ECV (hypervolemic) but low EABV* is present in 25% of hyponatremic critically ill patients and is independently associated with an increased risk of morbi-mortality [78]. Modifications of ECV are complex, characterized by a

high global ECV related to the increased interstitial compartment while the EABV is reduced. Congestive heart failure and cirrhosis are classical causes of hypervolemic hyponatremia [49, 56, 60, 79–81]. In these conditions, the decrease in EABV is due to the reduction in cardiac output and vasoplegia. These modifications activate the sympathetic nervous system, the renin-angiotensin-aldosterone axis, and VP release, leading to sodium and water renal reabsorption and finally hyponatremia. Therefore, patients present signs of volume overload: pulmonary edema, ascites, and peripheral edema. The diagnosis is usually easy to make on the context. The reduced EABV is responsible for a secondary hyperaldosteronism with the low UNa, except for the frequent situation of patients receiving diuretics [49, 56, 60, 79]. In nephrotic syndrome, the reduction in EABV is usually attributed to hypoalbuminemia and the resulting low oncotic pressure and vasoplegia, leading to non-osmotic VP release. Hypervolemic hyponatremia is commonly worsened by diuretics and fluid absorption and infusion.

UNa >30 mmol/L

When UNa is elevated, a very pragmatic approach is to confirm or eliminate a possible treatment by diuretics or kidney disease, both conditions that frequently affect natriuresis independently of ECV and may conduct to erroneous diagnosis [76, 82]. Moreover, both situations do not eliminate possible other causes of hyponatremia. On the other hand, UNa can also be reduced despite diuretics (especially with long-term treatment) and kidney disease (Fig. 2.3). Therefore, regardless of diuretics or kidney disease, hyponatremia associated with a UNa >30 mmol/L can be classified according to the ECV which can be reduced or normal:

- *Hypovolemic hyponatremia* can be caused by gastrointestinal or renal losses. Vomitings are usual causes. Renal losses can be due to various causes. Cerebral salt wasting syndrome (CSW) is well documented in patients with intracranial injury such as subarachnoid hemorrhage, traumatic brain injury, brain tumors or infections, and neurosurgical postoperative period [49, 83–85]. Abnormal salt wasting may be related to kidney dysfunction (renal wasting syndrome, RWS) [82]. For some authors, regardless of the primary organ dysfunction, i.e., the brain or kidney, this is a unique syndrome, and the distinction between CSW and RSW is a simple semantic differentiation of a similar disorder which occurs in two different contexts [85, 86]. Primary adrenal mineralocorticoid deficiency (Addison disease) can cause hypovolemic hyponatremia associated with hyperkalemia due to renal sodium losses and potassium reabsorption.
- *Euvolemic hyponatremia*. The SIADH is the most frequent cause of euvolemic hyponatremia. The inappropriate antidiuresis may result from an inappropriate secretion of ADH from the pituitary gland or an ectopic site. It may also result from vasopressin receptors or aquaporin abnormalities (genetic or acquired mutations). Therefore, SIADH is one clinical setting of the large conditions of the syndrome of the inappropriate antidiuresis (SIAD) [23, 49, 72, 74, 87, 88]. ECV is usually normal because after an initial phase of increased total body water, renal sodium excretion is stimulated in response to natriuretic factors. Consequently, despite a persisting high plasma concentration in ADH, patients present hypotonic urines

Table 2.3 Diagnostic criteria for the syndrome of inappropriate antidiuresis (SIAD) or secretion of antidiuretic hormone (SIADH)

Absolute criteria	Relative criteria
– Plasma hypotonicity (<275 mosm/kg) – Antidiuresis: urine osmolality > 100 mosm/kg at some level of decreased plasma tonicity – Clinical euvolemia – Urine sodium concentration >30 mmol/L with normal salt and water intake – Absence of adrenal, thyroid, pituitary, or renal insufficiency – No recent treatment with diuretics	– Serum urea < 3.6 mmol/L – Serum uric acid < 0.24 mmol/L – Failure to correct hyponatremia after 0.9% saline infusion – Correction of hyponatremia with fluid restriction – Fractional sodium excretion > 0.5% – Fractional urea excretion > 55% – Fractional uric acid excretion > 12%

related to a decreased number of V2R and of AQP2 expression on the collecting tube: this is the "vasopressin escape phenomenon." Additional abnormalities of thirst sensation can contribute to worsen hyponatremia. The diagnosis of SIAD(H) is based on classical absolute (or essential) criteria that includes (1) hypotonic hyponatremia (plasma tonicity <275 mosm/kg), (2) urine osmolality >100 mosm/kg despite a decreased plasma tonicity (abnormal antidiuresis), (3) clinical euvolemia, (4) urine sodium concentration > 30 mmol/L with normal sodium and water intake and no diuretics, and (5) absence of adrenal, thyroid, pituitary, and renal insufficiency (Table 2.3). Relative (or supplemental) criteria include (1) (partial) correction of hyponatremia with fluid restriction, (2) failure to correct hyponatremia with 0.9% saline infusion, (3) serum uric acid <0.24 mmol/L, (4) serum urea <3.6 mmol/l, (5) fractional sodium excretion (FeNa) > 0.5%, (6) fractional urea excretion (Fe urea) >55%, and (7) fractional uric acid excretion(FeUA) > 12%. Calculation of fractional excretion is based on the following formula: Fe X (%) = (UX/PX) × (Pcreat/U creat) × 100, x being the substance and UX, PX, P creat, and Ucreat being the urine and plasma concentrations of X and creatinine, respectively. Plasma VP measurement does not frequently contribute to the diagnosis. Indeed, four situations have been observed in patients with SIADH receiving 0.9% NaCl: (1) type A or "random" SIADH, present in 30 to 40% of patients, is characterized by a constant ectopic raised VP plasma concentration, regardless of plasma tonicity; (2) type B or "leak" SIADH found in 30% of patients is characterized by a raised basal VP concentration which increases normally with plasma hypertonicity; (3) type C or "reset osmostat," also present in 30% of patients, is characterized by a decreased threshold of VP secretion leading to high VP plasma concentration despite low plasma tonicity; and (4) type D in 10% of patients is characterized by a normal VP secretion: this is the antidiuresis nephrotic syndrome which is observed in children and is due to abnormal activation of V2R (gene mutations) [17]. In clinical practice, because of difficulties to assess ECV and because SIADH and CSW appear in similar contexts, it is recommended to consider additional biological parameters such as FeNa and FeUA to distinguish them (Table 2.4). In all cases, SIAD(H) remains a diagnosis of exclusion. There are numerous causes of SIAD(H) (Table 2.5), including essentially cancers (digestive and pulmonary), central nervous system disorders, and pulmonary diseases [9, 70,

Table 2.4 Criteria to differentiate the syndrome of inappropriate secretion of antidiuretic hormone (SIADH) and cerebral salt wasting syndrome (CSW)

	SIADH	CSW
Clinical signs		
– Blood pressure – Cardiac frequency – Central venous pressure – Urine volume	– Normal – Normal – Normal – Normal	– Low/normal (orthostatic hypotension) – Normal/high – Low – High
Biological parameters		
– Serum urea – Serum uric acid – Fractional sodium excretion > 0.5% – Fractional urea excretion > 55% – Fractional uric acid excretion > 12%	– Normal/low – Normal/low	– Normal/high – Low

Table 2.5 Major causes of syndrome of inappropriate secretion of antidiuretic hormone (SIADH)

Disorders of the nervous central system
– Infections (bacterial, viral, mycotic, tuberculosis): encephalitis, meningitis, abscess
– Traumatic brain injury: Epidural and subdural hematoma, subarachnoid hemorrhage, brain edema
– Primary and secondary brain tumors
– Cavernous sinus thrombosis
– Cerebral atrophy, hydrocephalus
– Stroke, intracerebral hemorrhage, postanoxic encephalopathy
– Peripheral neuropathy, Guillain-Barré syndrome
– Acute intermittent porphyria, multiple sclerosis
– Delirium tremens, acquired immunodeficiency syndrome (AIDS)
Pulmonary disorders
– Small cell anaplastic cancer, mesotheliome
– Infection (bacterial, viral, mycotic, tuberculosis)
– Acute respiratory distress syndrome (ARDS)
– Chronic obstructive pneumopathy, artificial ventilation with expiratory positive pressure
– Asthma, cystic fibrosis
Malignant diseases
Carcinoma: lung, oropharynx, larynx, gastrointestinal tract, pancreas, stomach, genitourinary tract, bladder, prostate, thymoma, sarcoma
Other causes
– Drugs: vasopressin analogues, antidepressants, antidiabetic drugs, anticonvulsivants, anticancer drugs, antimitotics, antipsychotics, ecstasy
– Postoperative period, pain, nausea, vomitings, AIDS, idiopathic
– Exercise-associated hyponatremia

87, 88]. The perioperative period is considered to be at high risk of SIAD because VP secretion is triggered by several non-osmotic stimuli (nausea, vomitings, pain, hypoxia, morphinics, hypovolemia) (see paragraph "perioperative hyponatremia"). A lot of drugs enable to induce SIADH such as selective serotonin reuptake inhibitors, antidiabetics, and thiazides which are responsible of SIADH in 10–30% of treated patients [75, 77, 89–91]. Table 2.5 summarizes most drugs at risk for developing hypotonic hyponatremia with SIADH. Finally, the cause of SIAD(H) remains frequently unidentified [70].

- Endocrinological diseases: secondary adrenal insufficiency/glucocorticoid deficiency [49, 72, 87] because of low concentration of cortisol fails to suppress corticotrophin release factor leading to an increased release in ACTH and VP. Renal water excretion is also altered independently of VP [92]. Only severe hypothyroidism (myxedema) could cause hyponatremia because of a reduced cardiac output and glomerular filtration rate.

2.5.2.3 Special Conditions Associated with Hyponatremia

- *Exercise-associated hyponatremia* (EAH) [93–96]: EAH occurs in 5–28% of intense and prolonged physical activity (marathon). Risk factors involved in such disorder are combined: excessive water intake (hypotonic solutions) associated with a non-osmotic inappropriate secretion of ADH, long race duration (>4–6 h), and extreme temperatures. The production of IL6 (related to muscle glycogen depletion), stress, and nausea with hypovolemia triggers ADH secretion. Hyponatremia can be hyper-, hypo-, and euvolemic. Clinical presentation has no specific aspect and appears as an acute moderately or severely symptomatic life-threatening condition:

– *Postoperative hyponatremia*: it is the third cause of acute in-hospital acquired hyponatremia. It develops preferentially in children and women [39, 49, 84, 97]. Hyponatremia results from a non-osmotic stimulation of ADH and is precipitated by hypotonic fluid infusions and perioperative impairment in renal urine dilution [97–99]. Postoperative hyponatremia may reach 30% of patients in surgeries at risk such as neurosurgery and orthopedic and gynecologic surgeries. However, only 1–2% of them are severe. The incidence of hyponatremia in neurosurgical patients is elevated, depending on the underlying cause: 10–20% in patients undergoing surgery for brain hematoma, hypophysectomy, intracranial tumors, and traumatic brain injury; it reaches 50% in subarachnoid hemorrhage [49, 83, 100, 101]. Hyponatremia develops acutely within the 2–4 days following surgery and is frequently symptomatic. Clinical presentation may be amplified by a preexistent brain edema or injury. The mechanism of hyponatremia is complex, and the distinction between SIADH and CSW remains difficult [102, 103]. ACTH deficiency is an additional confusing factor. In this setting, the North American guidelines recommend to treat hyponatremia as soon as its concentration is below 131 mmol/L [83].

- *Transurethral resection of prostate (TURP) syndrome*: the irrigating solution for endoscopic surgery can be responsible of acute hyponatremia [104–106]. Large volume of hypotonic glycocolle solutions may be absorbed directly intravascularly or through the interstitial tissue. At the initial phase, hyponatremia is "translocational," i.e., hypertonic (due to glycocolle), and is associated with a transitory hypervolemia which may cause arterial hypertension and cardiac failure. Hypotonic hyponatremia occurs later when glycocolle is metabolized leading to an excessive volume of free water in the vessels. Neurologic symptoms are related to brain edema but also to a direct cerebral toxicity of glycocolle metabolites (ammoniac, glutamate, serine) [106, 107]. This syndrome was firstly described after prostatic surgery but can develop after endoscopic gynecologic or arthroscopic surgeries. The preventive strategy consists in accurate assessment of fluid volumes irrigated during the procedure, a close monitoring of sodium concentration within the intra- and postoperative period, and the use of 0.9% NaCl irrigating solutions with a bipolar electrode device [108].
- *Diuretic-induced hyponatremia*: all diuretics may cause hypotonic hyponatremia, but thiazides remain the most frequently implicated [75–77, 90, 91]. Leung et al. [91] have shown that 30% of the exposed patients to thiazide diuretics develop hyponatremia and that thiazides multiply the risk of hyponatremia by five. Female, black, age >70 years increase this risk. Hyponatremia develops rapidly within the 10–14 days following the first prescription, but the risk persists within the ten following years. Hyponatremia is usually accompanied by a severe and reversible hypokalemia within 2–5 days after stopping thiazides.

2.6 Treatment

The optimal specific treatment of hypotonic hyponatremia is still debated because of the risk of life-threatening cerebral edema in case of undercorrection of hyponatremia balanced by the risk of osmotic demyelination syndrome (ODS) provoked by a too excessive and rapid treatment (overcorrection) (Table 2.6) [9, 13, 23, 51, 58, 60, 109]. Four expert guidelines published within the last 3 years are available in the literature: North America [23], Spain [110], Europe [9], and the United Kingdom [88].

Table 2.6 Complications and risk factors associated with an inappropriate treatment of hyponatremia

Complications	Context	Exacerbating factors
Brain edema caused by a delayed or insufficient correction of hyponatremia	Severe or moderate symptomatic and acute hyponatremia	• Female, children • Postoperative period • Thiazide treatment • Psychotic polydipsia • Hypoxia
Osmotic demyelination syndrome caused by a too rapid or overcorrection of hyponatremia	Mild symptomatic or asymptomatic chronic hyponatremia	• Chronic alcoholism • Hypokalemia • Burn • Malnutrition

2.6.1 General Strategies

Major principles and strategies of treatment of hypotonic hyponatremia are consensual. However, some conflicting recommendations exist among countries due to various reasons: methodology (interpretation of the evidence), nature of the expert group, few strong evidence, recent data on chronic hyponatremia, and development of vaptans (different approvals among countries).

The first principle of treatment is to distinguish situations requiring an immediate and aggressive treatment aiming a rapid raised in natremia from that needing a slow increased natremia and favoring the etiologic treatment. This strategy is strongly supported by the risk of fatal brain swelling caused by "severe" hyponatremia, which overtakes on the induction of ODS. Acute hyponatremia which is defined by a speed of development in less than 48 h is usually accepted as being severe [23, 87, 110], by opposition to chronic hyponatremia developed in more than 48 h. However, from a practical point of view, the essential point is to identify patients with severe or moderate symptoms indicating brain edema, regardless whether hyponatremia is acute or chronic which is frequently difficult to determine [9, 23]. Moreover, it is helpful to know conditions that contribute to exacerbate cerebral edema [9, 10] (Table 2.6).

The second principle of treatment consists to identify patients at risk of ODS. Usually asymptomatic patients or those with mild symptoms may develop ODS, especially in case of chronic hyponatremia. Contrary to the previous conditions, an overcorrection or too rapid correction of these hyponatremia must be avoided, and the treatment consists firstly to stop and treat the underlying cause of hyponatremia as soon as possible, and consider alternative treatments if not sufficient.

The third principle consists in determining the most efficient and safety rate of correction depending on the symptoms and the rate of development of hyponatremia. In all cases, guidelines must define targets which are the expected goals and limits which do not have to be exceeded (Fig. 2.4) [9, 13, 51, 88].

Finally, the strategy can be elaborated considering (1) first the presence of symptoms and their severity and (2) second the acute or chronic development of hyponatremia. This leads to three situations: (1) hyponatremia with severe or moderate symptoms regardless of the speed of development of hyponatremia, (2) acute hyponatremia without severe or moderate symptoms, and (3) chronic hyponatremia.

2.6.2 Hyponatremia with Severe or Moderate Symptoms

The management of such patients requires an intensive care unit (ICU) or at least an environment where close biochemical and clinical monitoring can be provided. Regardless of whether hyponatremia is acute or chronic, the aim of the treatment is to raise rapidly serum sodium concentration by 4–6 mmol/L which is sufficient to reverse or avoid most serious complications (brain herniation). This can be achieved

	Severe/moderate symptomatic hyponatremia (regardless acute or chronic)	**Mild symptomatic/asymptomatic chronic hyponatremia**
Principles	. Immediate 3% hypertonic saline	. No hypertonic saline
	. If possible stop the underlying cause, threat the underlying cause	
Goals	. Avoid and prevent brain edema -Increase natremia by 4-6 mmol/L and improve symptoms within 1-2 hrs	. Avoid and prevent osmotic demyelination - Increase natremia by 4-6 mmol/L within 24 hrs in profound hyponatremia (<125 mmol/L)
Limits	. Do not exceed an increase of 6-10 mmol/l in the first 24 hrs and 8 mmol/L every 24 hrs thereafter . Always stop hypertonic saline when natremia reaches 130 mmol/L	. Do not exceed an increase of 8-10 mmol/L in the first 24 hrs and 8 mmol/L every 24 hrs thereafter . Consider relowering natremia if correction is too rapid (DDAVP or hypotonic fluids) with an expert
Practical management	. 150 mL 3% hypertonic saline i.v. over 15-20 min completed by 1 or 2 maximum additional boluses if goals are not reached . Management in ICU or structure allowing close clinical and biological monitoring . Establish the underlying cause	. Stop all factors that provoke or contribute to hyponatremia, especially diuretics if possible . Give the cause-specific treatment . Hypovolemic hyponatremia : give fluid infusion . Hyper-and euvolemic hyponatremia : give fluid restriction±loop diuretics or urea or vaptans

Fig. 2.4 Major principles of the strategy for treating hypotonic hyponatremia

with a 100–150 mL (2 ml/kg) intravenous (i.v.) bolus infusion of 3% hypertonic saline (or equivalent 3–4.5 g) over 15–20 min [9, 10, 13, 23, 111–113]. The next step of the treatment is guided by the evolution of the patient. If severe symptoms improve or natremia increases of 4–6 mmol/L within the following hours, it is recommended to infuse 0.9% saline (smallest volume) until the underlying cause treatment is started. An additional 3% saline i.v. can be repeated two or three times if there is not enough or no improvement. In all cases, serum sodium concentration must be closely checked 15–20 min after each bolus and every 4–6 h daily after stopping hypertonic saline bolus and until natremia stabilized. The safe limit that does not have to be surpassed is a total increase in natremia of 6–10 mmol/L during the first 24 h and 8 mmol/L during every 24 h thereafter. As soon as serum sodium concentration reaches 130 mmol/L, stop hypertonic saline infusion.

While treating the patient, it is recommended to perform additional explorations to establish the underlying cause and administer its specific treatment. Guidelines do not recommend the use of any predictive formulas which overestimate the speed of correction [9, 13, 113]. Indeed, formulas are static and do not integrate the fact that kidney capacity of dilution and the possible avoidance of a specific cause may vary during time, leading to unpredictable modifications in natremia. The clinical judgment, the history of the patient, the context, and the follow-up remain essential parameters needed to guide the strategy after the initiation of the emergent administration of hypertonic saline. In this way, additional hypertonic saline boluses must be very carefully indicated in rapidly reversible acute hyponatremia when the cause is stopped, such as in self-induced water intoxication or in the postoperative period after stopping hypotonic fluid infusion, EAH [23].

2.6.3 Acute Hyponatremia Without Severe or Moderate Symptoms

The first step is to eliminate an error in serum sodium concentration measurement. After confirming hypotonic hyponatremia, the absence of severe or moderate symptoms allows to recommend firstly a cause-specific treatment and to stop all factors that contribute or provoke hyponatremia (hypotonic fluids, drugs). A bolus of 3% hypertonic saline can be suggested in case of profound acute decrease in natremia exceeding 10 mmol/L always associated with a close monitoring of natremia [9].

2.6.4 Chronic Hyponatremia Without Severe or Moderate Symptoms

2.6.4.1 Principles and Risks

Loss of organic osmolytes during chronic hyponatremia protects the brain from edema but exposes to osmotic demyelination lesions when the increase in serum sodium concentration is too rapid. Indeed, the recovery of osmolyte content is not immediate and takes several days. This explains why rapid correction of hyponatremia behaves as a hypertonic stress leading to various injuries (apoptosis, blood-brain barrier disruption, and demyelination). There is a consensus to recommend against the administration of hypertonic saline in these patients. The strategy consists firstly to stop all factors (fluids, water intake, drugs) that contribute or provoke hyponatremia and to give a cause-specific treatment [9, 10, 13, 51, 87]. Aiming a raise in natremia is only recommended for profound (<125 mmol/L) or moderate (125–129 mmol/L) chronic hyponatremia [9]. The recommended goal is an increase of 4–6 mmol/24 h and an upper limit increase of <10 mmol/L during the first day and <8 mmol/L during the following day. Lower limits around 8 mmol/L can be advised in patients at risk of ODS (Table 2.6). ODS has been reported when speed correction of chronic hyponatremia exceeded 10–12 mmol/L per 24 h. At last, raising serum sodium concentration should not be aimed in mild chronic hyponatremia (<130 mmol/L).

Despite these recommendations, overcorrection commonly occurs and current guidelines recommend to relower serum sodium concentration if the limit is exceeded [114–117]. This goal can be reached using desmopressin (DDAVP) or electrolyte-free water. Such a strategy may be performed as a curative or rescue therapy of excessive serum sodium correction by the administration of DDAVP alone or in association with glucose solutions or as preventive administration of DDAVP combined with hypertonic saline. The lack of strong evidence does not allow to recommend a unique preferred strategy. DDAVP is administered initially with a dose of 1–4 μg (intravenously or parenterally), followed by repeated boluses according to the response on neurological function, urine output, and serum sodium concentration change. The interval between two doses should not be less than 6–8 h. The administration of hypotonic fluids is an alternative strategy which consists in a 3–10 mL/kg infusion [9, 23]. The preventive attitude is less consensual than the curative one, because DDAVP seems to be unlogical and inefficient in patients presenting SIADH [58]. Moreover, a recent meta-analysis has shown that there is only limited data and low evidence concerning such a strategy [114]. At last, the optimal timing, dose, and duration of DDAVP administration remain to be determined. Therefore, considering the risk and the clinical experience to relower natremia, the ECPG group [9] recommends to refer or consult an expert for this patient management.

ODS, also named central pontine myelinolysis (CPM), is characterized by a demyelination located on central pontine and extrapontine structures. For a long time, this syndrome has been attributed exclusively to a too rapid correction or overcorrection of chronic hyponatremia. However, other conditions have been reported to provoke or favor CPM: chronic alcoholism, malnutrition, hypokalemia, and burn patients [118–120]. Regardless of the cause, blood-brain barrier is altered and becomes permeable allowing an abnormal cerebral entry of cytokines and lymphocytes and finally demyelination. Clinically, the patient presents a classical biphasic evolution: the initial neurological improvement obtained with the correction of hyponatremia, is followed by a worsening neurological status within the following 1–8 days. Manifestations consist in nonspecific signs of encephalopathy including behavioral abnormalities, seizures, pseudobulbar palsy, quadriparesis, locked-in syndrome, permanent disability, or death. Brain resonance magnetic imaging enables to confirm the diagnosis, thanks to the identification of demyelination injury after a delay of 1 or 2 weeks. Prevention of ODS is commonly based on the respect of speed correction of hyponatremia. Uremia has been reported to prevent demyelination by accelerating the recovery of cerebral amount of organic osmolytes [121]. Myoinositol and minocycline enabled to improve rat survival following rapid correction of chronic hyponatremia [122, 123].

2.6.4.2 Additional Specific Treatments According to the Underlying Cause

Additional non-emergent treatment depends on the underlying cause and on the ECV status.

Besides the specific cause therapy, the first-line treatment of chronic hypovolemic hyponatremia consists in restoring ECV with an i.v. infusion of crystalloids (0.9% saline or balanced solutions) at a rate of 0.5 to 1 mL/kg.

Despite limited data, fluid restriction (800–1200 mL) is suggested in moderate or profound hyper- and euvolemic chronic hyponatremia as a first-line therapy. This can be complemented by the administration of a loop diuretic (furosemide), especially when urines are concentrated [9, 74, 87, 124]. Both demeclocycline and lithium may increase serum sodium concentration by inducing a nephrogenic insipidus diabetes [9, 74, 87, 124]. However, their beneficial effect is inconstant, unpredictable, and associated with important adverse effects (neurotoxicity, nephrotoxicity). Consequently, most experts do not recommend these drugs in SIADH.

Major conflicting recommendations refer to urea and vaptan therapies. Urea has been successfully administered in moderate and profound chronic hyponatremia without real side effects [107, 125, 126]. The ECPG suggests to administer a daily dose of 0.25–0.50 g/day urea as a second-line treatment (after fluid restriction) [9].

But urea is not commercialized and requires a pharmaceutical preparation with sucrose and sparkling water to avoid the bitter taste. Vaptans are non-peptidic antagonists of vasopressin receptors [23, 109, 127]. While VP binds at a superficial site, vaptans penetrate deeply into the membrane. Their main effect consists in an increase in solute-free water excretion by kidneys. Regardless of their affinity on vasopressin receptors, they increase urine output. V2R antagonists exert only renal effects and are called "aquaretics." V1a-V2R antagonists combine two properties, i.e., renal and vascular vasodilating effects. Currently, two molecules are commercialized and available in most countries: tolvaptan (Samsca®) is a selective V2R antagonist and conivaptan (Vaprisol®) is a mixed V1a-V2R antagonist. Pharmacokinetic characteristics are similar for both: high level of protein bound, half-life of 6–10 h, and metabolization by the hepatic cytochrome P450. Conivaptan may be administered intravenously at a dose of 40 mg daily for a maximum of 4 days because of its potential hepatotoxicity. Tolvaptan can only be prescribed orally at a dose of 15–60 mg daily. Indications of vaptans as a treatment of asymptomatic or mild symptomatic chronic hyponatremia remain a source of debate. Such a conflicting strategy can be explained by the difference in vaptan approval by agencies among countries, paucity of data with high level of proof, divergent interpretation of evidence-based medicine (efficiency vs. adverse events), expert's disclosure, and industry sponsorship (editorial dependence) [128, 129]. The FDA and the Canadian agencies state that vaptans may be indicated as a first-line therapy for hyper- and euvolemic chronic hyponatremia. This strategy is based on several arguments. There is no doubt that vaptans enable to increase natremia of 4–6 mmol/L in these patients [130–134]. These results have been confirmed in two recent meta-analyses [133, 134]. Rozen-Zvi et al. [133] included 15 randomized controlled studies comparing vaptans vs. placebo or no treatment (± associated with fluid restriction). They found that vaptans increased serum sodium concentration by 5.27 mmol/L early (after 1–7 days) and up to 1 month. Similar results from 11 randomized controlled studies were reported in a second meta-analysis with an increased natremia of 5.7 mmol/L at day 5 of treatment [134]. More than 3000 hyper- and euvolemic asymptomatic/mild symptomatic hyponatremic patients were collected in an international registry [135]. The authors confirmed that tolvaptan successfully increased natremia by a median of 4 mmol/L for up to 4 years. The last meta-analysis has been performed by the ECPG group including additional trials published between 2010 and 2013. The update data with 20 randomized controlled studies (2009 patients) also confirmed that vaptans enable to increase serum sodium concentration by 4.3 mmol/L within 3–7 days as compared with placebo [9]. No real difference in adverse or serious adverse events (CPM) related to a rapid increase in natremia has been reported [9, 133–135]. Moreover, fluid restriction which is still considered as the first-line alternative treatment can be ineffective and difficult to maintain in numerous patients [129]. Failure of fluid restriction to increase natremia commonly occurs in patients with high urine osmolality (>500 mosm/kg), low urine output (<1500 ml/day), and low increase in sodium after 2 days of treatment (<2 mmol/L). Because tolvaptan was recently reported to be associated with liver toxicity, the FDA recommends limiting its use to 30 days and not to use it in patients with liver disease (hypervolemic hyponatremia) [136]. Tolvaptan is not indicated in hypovolemic chronic hyponatremia because of a high risk of worsening vasodilating-related hypotension. Current recommendations in North America indicate that vaptans can be considered as an optional treatment in asymptomatic or mild symptomatic chronic non-hypovolemic hyponatremia, except for patients with liver disease [109]. Short-term indication is safe and simple in patients presenting hyponatremia <125 mmol/L, and as soon as natremia raises of 6–8 mmolL, water intake must be matched with urine output to prevent an excessive elevation in natremia. Vaptans may be indicated as a long-term optional strategy in patients with irreversible mild symptomatic euvolemic hyponatremia (<130 mmol/L) who fail or resist to fluid restriction. Tolvaptan must be initiated with low daily dose (15 mg) and progressively increased (to 60 mg daily) until reaching serum sodium concentration ≥135 mmol/L within 1 week. Natremia must be checked at least once a week at the beginning and monthly thereafter. Tolvaptan requires regular liver enzyme monitoring and must be stopped in case of elevated values (except for patients waiting for liver transplantation). European experts do not recommend the use of vaptans considering that the quality of the evidence is reduced due to the absence of comparative studies with alternative treatment and the absence of evaluation of major endpoints such as mortality or severe adverse events [9, 87]. Indeed, meta-analysis does not report any beneficial effects of vaptans on long-term survival or quality of life [9]. Moreover, the risk for a rapid sodium concentration increase is present (RR = 1.61) and has been pointed by drug agencies [9, 137–139], especially when vaptans are combined with hypertonic saline administration. Despite no published report of ODS, neurological injury has been indicated in patients receiving tolvaptan due to an excessive correction of hyponatremia [137]. Vaptans also enable to induce adverse events such as polyuria, thirst, mouth dryness, constipation, and hepatotoxicity [109, 140]. At last, patients presenting concentrated urines have a resistance to vaptans (as observed with fluid restriction): patients with high level of VP (some SIADH), with hypervolemic heart failure or cirrhosis because of the low EABV, excessive water intake related to "reset osmostat" SIADH, or nephrogenic syndrome of inappropriate antidiuresis. Therefore, the ECPG group considered that there is no proven beneficial effect of vaptans apart the increase in natremia while safety remains questioned [9]. This group recommended against vasopressin receptor antagonists in treating hyper- and euvolemic chronic hyponatremic patients and recommends fluid restriction as a first-line strategy for these patients [9].

In summary: only severely and moderately symptomatic hyponatremic patients require an immediate and aggressive treatment with i.v. hypertonic saline, aiming to prevent or avoid urgently life-threatening cerebral edema. The first therapy recommended for treating mild symptomatic chronic hyponatremia is to stop drugs and reversible situations that provoke hyponatremia (thiazides, excessive water intake), before considering vaptans which require a long delay of action. For these latter patients, the cause-specific treatment is the most appropriate and increasing natremia should not be the sole goal. Hypovolemic hyponatremia requires volume expansion. Alternative treatments of hyper- and euvolemic chronic hyponatremia remain controversial: fluid restriction firstly and no vaptans in Europe and vaptans firstly in North America. In case vaptans are indicated, an expert management is preferable with a regular monitoring of serum sodium concentration and liver enzyme levels because of both risks of overcorrection of natremia and hepatotoxicity. Vaptans and hypertonic saline should never be associated.

2.7 Hypernatremia

2.7.1 Definition: Pathophysiology

Hypernatremia is defined by a serum sodium concentration >145 mmol/L. Hypernatremia is always associated with plasma hypertonicity and consequently responsible for cell shrinkage (dehydration). Hypernatremias may be induced by three mechanisms which conduct to classify them according to the resulting changes in ECV (Fig. 2.5) [13, 141]:

- *Euvolemic hypernatremias* are due to "pure water" losses. Total body sodium content remains unchanged and maintains a normal ECV.
- *Hypovolemic hypernatremias* are due to hypotonic losses leading to a combination of cell shrinkage and a reduced ECV.
- *Hypervolemic hypernatremias* are due to an absolute sodium retention in the ECV which conducts to combine cell shrinkage and hypervolemia.

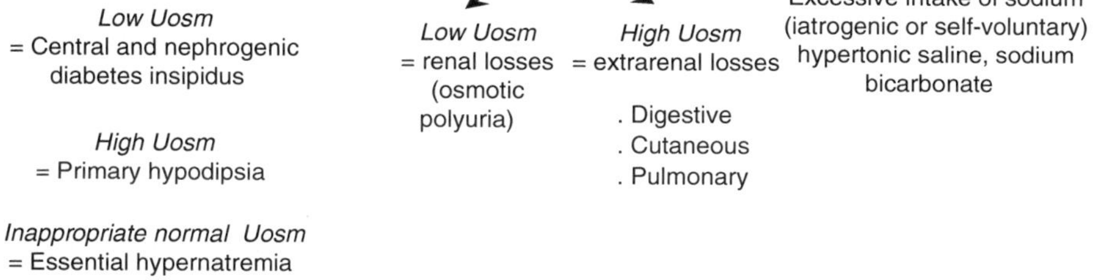

Fig. 2.5 Algorithm for determining the cause of hypernatremia

2.7.2 Diagnosis

2.7.2.1 Clinical Symptoms

Similarly with hyponatremia, severity of hypernatremia is essentially related to its impact on brain volume. Therefore, clinical manifestations are primarily neurologic but not specific, and their severity depends on the speed of development of the trouble. Acute hypertonic stress resulting from acute hypernatremia (<48 h) induces cerebral vascular injury and sudden brain shrinkage which induces intracranial hemorrhage, while symptoms are mild or absent in case of chronic hypernatremia. Severity of hypernatremia depends on the severity of neurological signs and on the presence of hypovolemia. The interpretation of symptoms must be integrated in the history, treatments of the patient, and the context which can be useful to distinguish acute symptomatic from chronic asymptomatic hypernatremia. Clinical signs are related to cell dehydration [13, 141]:

- *Neurological signs* are those of nonspecific encephalopathy including consciousness impairment, ataxia, nystagmus, hypertonia, stupor, seizures, profound coma, or those related to intracranial hemorrhage (hemiplegia) or thrombosis of dural sinus. Acute hypernatremia may lead finally to death.
- *Thirst* may be absent in case of hypodipsia and consciousness alteration.
- *Reduced body weight* allows to assess body water deficit, but it may remain stable or elevates when plasma hypertonicity is associated with an increased ECV.
- *Other signs* are fever, dyspnea, and rhabdomyolysis. However, it is commonly difficult to prove the causal relationship between those signs and hypernatremia.

In summary, there is no specific clinical sign, and treatment is delayed, explaining the high rate of morbi- mortality during hypernatremia which is also frequently associated with severe underlying causes [141].

2.7.2.2 Etiologic Diagnosis (Fig. 2.5)

Euvolemic hypernatremia: They include three major causes:

- *Diabetes insipidus* [142]: this syndrome is characterized by a common polyuria and polydipsia. Urines are abnormally diluted. Central diabetes insipidus is caused by a lack of ADH secretion which is due to central nervous system alterations. However, in most cases, this is also combined with an impairment in thirst sensation which results from alterations in receptors of thirst. Therefore, hypernatremia can develop only if both abnormalities are associated or in case of impossible water intake. Central and nephrogenic diabetes insipidus can be distinguished, thanks to an administration of desmopressin that will increase urine osmolality of 50% only in central diabetes insipidus. Numerous nervous central system lesions may induce central diabetes insipidus (trauma, stroke, hemorrhage, tumors, neurosurgery, etc.). Nephrogenic diabetes insipidus may be due to gene mutations of V2R VP-receptors or of aquaporin-2. It may be caused by acquired troubles such as hypokalemia, hypercalcemia, or some drugs (lithium, antifungic molecules, antibiotics, antiviral drugs, or antimitotics).

- *Primary hypodipsia* refers to an impairment in thirst behavioral while its stimulation is normal. Urine osmolality and density are elevated showing an appropriate response of kidneys to plasma hypertonicity.
- *Essential hypernatremia* is due to an abnormally elevated threshold of ADH and thirst secretion. Urine osmolality in relation with plasma hypertonicity is too low:
  - *Hypovolemic hypernatremia*: the diagnosis of the underlying cause is orientated by the context, electrolyte blood measurements, and above all Uosm. A low Uosm indicates losses from the kidney which are caused by osmotic polyuria due to the presence of glucose or urea in urines or to diuretic administration. A high Uosm is present when losses are caused by gastrointestinal or cutaneous alterations.
  - *Hypervolemic hypernatremia*: they are usually due to therapeutic errors or voluntary self-poisoning. Most frequent causes are infusions of hypertonic saline or concentrated sodium bicarbonate infusions. The clinical presentation consists in severe signs of cell dehydration due the acute speed of development of hypernatremia. The frequent pulmonary edema or congestive heart failure manifestations are related to the rapid extracellular fluid overload.
  - *Perioperative hypernatremia*: age, infection, and diuretics have a major role in the development of hypernatremia whatever the context and independently of the type of surgery. Indeed, the risk of perioperative hypernatremia strongly increased in elderly patients which present an impairment in thirst sensation and urine concentration capacity, frequently associated with severe comorbidities or dementia. Hypernatremia occurs in 22% of cases following neurosurgery and abdominal surgeries. In half of cases, it appears within the 5 days following surgery. Digestive surgery is at risk of excessive hypotonic losses from the gastrointestinal tract: preoperative digestive losses (vomitings, diarrhea), intraoperative water losses, and postoperative digestive losses (gastric aspiration, digestive fistulas) which are commonly insufficiently supplemented. About 18% of central diabetes insipidus are observed after neurosurgery or in traumatic brain injury and appear early within the 12 or 24 postoperative hours and disappear after 5–7 days.

2.7.3 Treatment

Both preventive and curative including the underlying cause treatments are needed. As recommended for hyponatremia, the appropriate strategy for reducing hypernatremia depends on the severity of symptoms, the ECV alteration, the speed of development of hypernatremia, and the reversibility of the cause. Therefore, the therapy aims to:

1. Maintain or restore the ECV especially in case of hypovolemia to avoid shock or tissue hypoperfusion (crystalloids). This is the first priority that must be reached before any correction of natremia [13, 141].
2. Correct plasma hypertonicity/hypernatremia with hypotonic solutions (5% dextrose or water when possible). In case of acute symptomatic hypernatremia, a rapid decrease in serum sodium concentration is needed to prevent or treat brain shrinkage and its consequences. This can be achieved with a rapid i.v. 5% dextrose infusion or renal removal therapy especially when patient presents kidney insufficiency. Oral water intake is insufficient and frequently impossible due to central nervous alteration. Despite the real proof of side effects of an excessive correction of hypernatremia, it is commonly advised to not exceed a reduction in plasma tonicity of 5 mosm/L/h or in natremia 2–2.5 mmol/L. Therefore, serum sodium levels must be closely and frequently (every 4–6 h) checked, and a clinical monitoring is also required. Such a treatment is maintained until severe neurological signs disappear and natremia is 145 mmol/L [13]. Asymptomatic chronic hypernatremia requires the replacement of water losses, the cause-specific treatment, and if necessary, a reduction of natremia that will not exceed 10 mmol/L per day. Oral water intake may be useful because it allows a safe regular and progressive decrease in serum sodium concentration, allowing to prevent overcorrection and the risk of brain edema. The speed of correction of hypernatremia must be lower in patients at risk such as elderly patients, children, and patients at risk of brain edema or intracranial hypertension.

Conclusion

Cell volume depends on the transmembrane osmotic gradient, i.e., on plasma tonicity which is determined by the sole effective plasma osmoles. Plasma hypertonicity always induces cell shrinkage and conversely plasma hypotonicity always induces cell edema. ADH and thirst are both major mechanisms that regulate closely plasma tonicity and consequently cell volume. Because of its location in the inextensible skull, modifications in brain volume caused by dysnatremias are responsible for the common neurological signs. Therefore, dysnatremias must be considered when severe as life-threatening conditions.

Hyponatremia can be associated with plasma hypertonicity (in case of hyperglycemia) and isotonicity (pseudohyponatremia in case of hyperprotidemia or hyperlipidemia), but only hypotonic hyponatremia can induce brain edema. Due to cerebral osmoregulation, the risk of hypotonic hyponatremia depends on the efficiency of this regulation. Therefore, the most pragmatic strategy to treat hypotonic hyponatremia is to consider the severity of neurological signs. Patients presenting severe neurological signs require an immediate and aggressive treatment aiming to increase rapidly natremia of 4–6 mmol/L using an i.v. infusion of 3% hypertonic saline and to prevent or reverse brain edema. Increasing serum sodium in asymptomatic or mild symptomatic chronic hyponatremic patients is not a real goal, and the treatment is essentially based on the cause-specific treatment. Besides such treatment, the raise of chronic hyponatremia can be reached using fluid restriction and the use of vaptans remains controversial. Overcorrection of chronic hyponatremia exposes to the risk of osmotic demyelination.

Hypernatremia is always associated with plasma hypertonicity and consequently with cell shrinkage. Therefore, hypernatremic patients commonly present central nervous system impairments. Treatment of hypernatremia depends also on the severity of symptoms. Besides, the underlying cause treatment and severe symptomatic hypernatremic patients require a rapid decrease in serum sodium concentrations using i.v. hypotonic solutions, whereas asymptomatic patients can be treated using oral water intake aiming a slow and progressive reduction in natremia.

References

1. Mount DB (2010) Hyponatremia. Semin Nephrol 29:1–317
2. Orban JC, Ichai C (2012) Hyponatrémies en réanimation. Encycl Med Chir (Anesthésie-Réanimation) 36-860-A-05:16
3. Danziger J, Zeidel ML (2014) Osmotic homeostasis. Clin J Am Soc Nephrol 10:852–862
4. Antunes-Rodrigues J, Ruginsk SG, Mecawi AS et al (2014) Neuroendocrinology of Hydromineral homeostasis. In: De Luca LA Jr, Menani JV, Johnson AK (eds) Neurobiology of body fluid homeostasis: transduction and integration. CRC, Boca Raton, FL. Chapter 3
5. Noda Y (2014) Dynamic regulation and dysregulation of the water channel aquaporin-2: a common cause of and promising therapeutic target for water balance disorders. Clin Exp Nephrol 18:558–570
6. Ferguson AV (2014) Circumventricular organs: integrators of circulating signals controlling hydration, energy balance, and immune function. In: De Luca LA Jr, Menani JV, Johnson AK (eds) Neurobiology of body fluid homeostasis: transduction and integration. CRC, Boca Raton, FL. Chapter 2
7. Harring TR, Deal NS, Kuo DC (2014) Disorders of sodium and water balance. Emerg Med Clin North Am 32:379–401
8. Petitclerc T (2013) Disorders in sodium-water balance. Nephrol Ther 9:38–49
9. Spasovski G, Vanholder R, Allolio R et al (2014) Hyponatraemia guideline development group. Clinical practice guideline on diagnosis and treatment of hyponatraemia. Intensive Care Med 40:320–331
10. Adrogue HJ, Madias NE (2014) Diagnosis and treatment of hyponatremia. Am J Kidney Dis 64:681–684
11. Knepper MA, Tae-Hwan K, Nielsen S (2015) Molecular physiology of water balance. N Engl J Med 372:1349–1358
12. Prager-Khoutorsky M, Bourque CW (2015) Mechanical basis of osmosensory transduction in magnocellular neurosecretory neurons of the rat supraoptic nucleus. J Neuroendocrinol 27:507–515
13. Sterns RH (2015) Disorders of plasma sodium: causes, consequences and correction. N Engl J Med 372:55–65
14. Ciura S, Liedtke W, Bourque CW (2011) Hypertonicity sensing in organum vasculosum lamina terminalis neurons: a mechanical process involving TRPV1 but not TRPV4. J Neurosci 31:14669–14676
15. Bourque CW (2008) Central mechanisms of osmosensation and systemic osmoregulation. Neuroscience 9:519–531

16. Daniels D (2014) Diverse role of angiotensin receptor intracellular pathways in the control of water and salt intake. In: De Luca LA Jr, Menani JV, Johnson AK (eds) Neurobiology of body fluid homeostasis: transduction and integration. CRC, Boca Raton, FL. Chapter 5
17. Robertson GL, Athat S (1976) The interaction of blood osmolality and blood volume in regulating plasma vasopressin in man. J Clin Endocrinol Metab 42:613–620
18. Juul KV, Bichet DG, Nielsen S, NØrgaard JP (2014) The physiological and pathophysiological functions of renal and extrarenal vasopressin V2 receptors. Am J Physiol Renal Physiol 306:F931–F941
19. Huber VJ, Tsujita M, Nakada T (2012) Aquaporins in drug discovery and pharmacotherapy. Mol Asp Med 33:691–703
20. Kortenoeven ML, Frenton RA (2014) Renal aquaporins and water balance disorders. Biochim Biophys Acta 1840:1533–1549
21. Wilson JL, Miranda CA, Knepper NA (2013) Vasopressin and the regulation of aquaporin-2. Clin Exp Nephrol 17:751–764
22. Holmes RP (2012) The role of renal water channels in health and disease. Mol Asp Med 33:547–552
23. Verbalis JG, Goldsmith SR, Greenberg A et al (2013) Diagnosis, evaluation, and treatment of hyponatremia: expert panel recommendations. Am J Med 126:S1–42
24. Bhardwaj A (2006) Neurological impact of vasopressin dysregulation and hyponatremia. Ann Neurol 59:229–236
25. Ayus JC, Achinger SG, Arieff A (2008) Brain cell volume regulation: role of sex, age, vasopressin and hypoxia. Am J Physiol Renal Physiol 295:F619–F624
26. Pasantes-Morales H, Lezama RA, Ramos-Mandujano G et al (2006) Mechanisms of cell volume regulation in hypo-osmolality. Am J Med 119:S4–11
27. Sterns R, Silver SM (2006) Brain volume regulation in response to hypo-osmolality and its correction. Am J Med 119(Suppl 7A):S12–S16
28. Sardini A, Amey JS, Weyland KH et al (2003) Cell volume regulation and swelling-activated channels. Biochem Biophys Acta 1618:153–162
29. De Mello W (2014) Regulation of cell volume and water transport – an old fundamental role of the renin-angiotensin aldosterone system components ate the cellular level. Peptides 58:74–77
30. Sterns RH, Hix JK, Silver SM (2013) Management of hyponatremia in the ICU. Chest 144:672–679
31. Verkman AS, Galietta LJV (2009) Chloride channels as drugs targets. Nature 8:153–171
32. Kahle KT, Staley KJ, Naheb BV et al (2008) Roles of the cation-chloride cotransporters in neurological disease. Nature Clin Parct 4:490–503
33. Badaut J, Fukuda AM, Jullienne A, Petry KG (2014) Aquaporin and brain diseases. Biochim Biophys Acta 1840:1554–1565
34. Zeynalov E, Chen CH, Froehener SC et al (2008) The perivascular pool of aquaporin-4 mediates the effect of osmotherapy in postischemic cerebral edema. Crit Care Med 36:2634–2640
35. Manley GT, Fukimura M, Ma T et al (2000) Aquaporin-4 depletion in mice reduces brain edema after acute water intoxication and ischemic stroke. Nat Med 6:159–163
36. Papadopoulos MC, Manley GT, Krishna S, Verkman AS (2004) Aquaporin-4 facilitates reabsoprtion of excess fluid in vasogenic brain edema. FASEB 18:1291–1293
37. Wenner MM, Stachenfeld NS (2012) Blood pressure and water regulation: understanding sex hormone effects within and between men and women. J Physiol 590:5949–5961
38. Sladek CD, Somponpun SJ (2008) Estrogen receptors: their roles in regulation of vasopressin release for maintenance of fluid and electrolyte homeostasis. Front Neuroendocrinol 29:114–127
39. Hoorn EJ, Lindemans J, Zietse R (2006) Development of severe hyponatraemia in hospitalized patients: treatment-related risk factors and inadequate management. Nephrol Dial Transplant 21:70–76
40. Thompson CJ (2010) Hyponatraemia: new associations and new treatments. Eur J Endocrinol 162:S1–S3

41. Corona G, Giuliani C, Parenti G et al (2013) Moderate hyponatremia is associated with increased risk of mortality: evidence from a meta-analysis. PLoS One 8:e80451
42. Sherlock M, Sullivan EO, Agha A et al (2009) Incidence and pathophysiology of severe hyponatraemia in neurosurgical patients. Postgrad Med J 85:171–175
43. Chawla A, Sterns RH, Nigwekar SU, Cappuccio JD (2011) Mortality and serum sodium: do patients die from or with hyponatremia? Clin J Am Soc Nephrol 6:960–965
44. Huda MS, Boyd A, Skagen K et al (2009) Investigation and management of severe hyponatraemia in a hospital setting. Postgrad Med J 82:216–219
45. Darmon M, Pichon M, Schwebel C et al (2014) Influence of early Dysnatraemia correction on survival of critically ill patients. Shock 41:394–399
46. Stelfox HT, Ahmed SB, Khandwala F et al (2008) The epidemiology of intensive care unit-acquired hyponatremia and hypernatremia in medical-surgical intensive care units. Crit Care 12:R162
47. Funk GC, Lindner G, Druml W et al (2010) Incidence and prognosis of dysnatraemias present on ICU admission. Intensive Care Med 36:304–311
48. Sakr Y, Rother S, Mendoca Pires Ferreira A et al (2013) Fluctuations in serum sodium level are associated with an increased risk of death in surgical ICU patients. Crit Care Med 41:133–142
49. Palmer BF (2009) Hyponatremia in the intensive care unit. Semin Nephrol 29:257–270
50. Padhi R, Panda BN, Jagati S, Patra SC (2014) Hyponatremia in critically ill patients. Ind J Crit Care Med 18:83–87
51. Sterns RH, Silver SM (2016) Complications and management of hyponatremia. Curr Opin Nephrol Hypertens 25:114–119
52. Thompson C, Berl T, Tejedor A, Johannsson G (2012) Differential diagnosis of hyponatraemia. Best Pract Res Clin Endocr Metab 26(suppl1):S1–S6
53. Turchin A, Seifter JL, Seely EW (2003) Clinical problem-solving. Mind the gap. N Engl J Med 349:1465–1469
54. Hillier TA, Abbott RD, Barrett EJ (1999) Hyponatremia: evaluating the correction factor for hyperglycemia. Am J Med 106:399–403
55. Sterns RH, Hix JK, Silver S (2010) Treating profound hyponatremia: a strategy for controlled correction. Am J Kidney Dis 56:774–779
56. Schrier RW, Bansal S (2008) Diagnosis and management of hyponatremia in acute illness. Curr Opin Crit Care 14:627–634
57. Arieff AI (2006) Influence of hypoxia and sex on hyponatremic encephalopathy. Am J Med 119(Suppl 7A):S59–S64
58. Adrogué HJ, Madias NE (2012) The challenge of hyponatremia. J Am Soc Nephrol 23:1140–1148
59. Thompson C, Hoorn EL (2012) Hyponatraemia: an overview of frequency, clinical presentation and complications. Best Pract Res Clin Endocr Metab 26(suppl1):S7–15
60. Lee JJ, Kilonzo K, Nistico A, Yeates K (2014) Management of hyponatremia. CMAJ 186:E281–E286
61. Ayus JC, Negri AL, Kalantar-Zadeh K, Moritz ML (2012) Is chronic hyponatremia a novel risk factor for hip fracture in the elderly? Nephrol Dial Transplant 27:3725–3731
62. Zaino CJ, Maheshwari AV, Goldfarb DS (2013) Impact of mild hyponatremia on falls, fractures, osteoporosis, and death. Am J Orthop 42:522–527
63. Kinsella S, Moran S, Sullivan MO et al (2010) Hyponatremia independent of osteoporosis is associated with fracture occurrence. Clin J Am Soc Nephrol 5:275–280
64. Hoorn EJ, Rivadeneira F, van Meurs JB et al (2011) Mild hyponatremia as a risk factor for fractures: the Rotterdam study. J Bone Miner Res 26:1822–1828
65. Verbalis JG, Barsony J, Sugimura Y et al (2010) Hyponatremia-induced osteoporosis. J Bone Miner Res 25:554–563
66. Hannon MJ, Verbalis JG (2014) Sodium homeostasis and bone. Curr Opin Nephrol Hypertens 23:370–376

67. Chung HM, Kluge R, Schrier RW, Anderson RJ (1987) Clinical assessment of extracellular fluid volume in hyponatremia. Am J Med 83:905–908
68. Fenske W, Maier SK, Blechschmidt A et al (2010) Utility and limitations of the traditional diagnostic approach to hyponatremia: a diagnostic study. Am J Med 123:652–657
69. Fenkse W, Störk S, Koschker AC et al (2008) Value of fractional uric acid excretion in differential diagnosis of hyponatremic patients on diuretics. J Clin Endocrinol Metab 93:2991–2997
70. Hsu CY, Chen CL, Huang WC et al (2014) Retrospective evaluation of standard diagnostic procedures in identification of the causes of new-onset syndrome of inappropriate antidiuresis. Int J Med Sci 11:192–198
71. Musch W, Decaux G (2001) Utility and limitations of biochemical parameters in the evaluation of hyponatremia in elderly. Int Urology Nephrol 32:475–493
72. Decaux G (2009) The syndrome of inappropriate secretion of antidiuretic hormone (SIADH). Semin Nephrol 29:239–256
73. Fenkse W, Störk S, Bleschschmidt A, Maier SG, Morgenthaler NG, Allolio B (2009) Copeptin in the differential diagnosis of hyponatremia. J Clin Endocrinol Metab 94:123–129
74. Peri A, Giuliani C (2014) Management of euvolemic hyponatremia attributed to SIADH in the hospital setting. Minerva Endocrinol 39:33–41
75. Ramos-Levi AM, Duran Rodriguez-Hervada A, Mendez-Bailon M, Marco-Martinez J (2014) Drug-induced hyponatremia: an update review. Minerva Endocrinol 39:1–12
76. Hix JK, Silver S, Sterns RH (2011) Diuretic-associated hyponatremia. Semin Nephrol 31:553–566
77. Rodenburg EM, Hoorn EJ, Ruiter R et al (2013) Thiazide-associated hyponatremia: a population-based study. Am J Kidney Dis 62:67–72
78. Bennani SL, Abouqal R, Zeggwagh AA et al (2003) Incidence, étiologies et facteurs pronostiques de l'hyponatrémie en réanimation. Rev Med Interne 24:224–229
79. Ichai C, Lena D (2008) Hyponatremia in the setting of acute heart failure syndrome. In: Mebazaa A, Gheorghiade M, Zannad FM, Parrillo JE (eds) Acute heart failure. Springer, London, pp 786–796
80. Angeli P, Wong F, Watson H, Ginès, Investigators CAPPS (2006) Hyponatremia in cirrhosis: results of a patient population survey. Hepatology 44:1535–1542
81. Gianotti RJ, Cardenas A (2014) Hyponatremia and cirrhosis. Gastroenterol Rep (Oxf) 2:21–26
82. Combs S, Berl T (2014) Dysnatremias in patients with kidney disease. Am J Kidney Dis 63:294–303
83. Rahman M, Friedman WA (2009) Hyponatremia in neurosurgical patients: clinical guidelines development. Neurosurgery 65:925–935
84. Kirkman MA (2014) Managing hyponatremia in neurosurgical patients. Minerva Endocrinol 39:13–26
85. Verbalis JG (2014) Hyponatremia with intracranial disease: not often cerebral salt wasting. J Clin Endocrinol Metab 99:59–62
86. Maesaka JK, Imbriano LJ, Ali NM, Ilamathi E (2009) Is it cerebral or renal salt wasting? Kidney Int 76:934–938
87. Hannon MJ, Thompson J (2010) The syndrome of inappropriate antidiuretic hormone: prevalence, causes and consequences. J Endocrinol Metab 162:S5–12
88. Grant P, Ayuk J, Bouloux PM et al (2015) The diagnosis and management of inpatient hyponatremia and SIADH. Eur J Clin Investig 45:888–894
89. Liamis G, Milionis H, Elisaf A (2008) A review of drug-induced hyponatremia. Am J Kideny Dis 52:144–153
90. van Blijderveen JC, Straus SM, Rodenburg EM et al (2014) Risk of hyponatremia with diuretics: chlortalidone versus hydrochlorothiazide. Am J Med 127:763–771
91. Leung AA, Wright A, Pazo V et al (2011) Risk of thiazide-induced hyponatremia in patients with hypertension. Am J Med 124:1064–1072
92. Schrier R (2008) Vasopressin and aquaporin 2 in clinical disorders of water homeostasis. Semin Nephrol 28:289–296

93. Armed Forces Health Surveillance Center (AFHSC) (2014) Update: Exertional hyponatremia, active component, U. S. armed forces, 1999-2014. MSMR 21:18–21
94. Hew-Butler T, Rosner MH, Fowkes-Godek S et al (2015) Statement of the 3rd international exercise-associated Hyponatremia consensus development conference, Carlsbad, California. Br J Sports Med 49:1432–1446
95. Urso C, Brucculeri S, Caimi G (2014) Physiopathological, epidemiological, clinical and therapeutic aspects of exercise-associated Hyponatremia. J Clin Med 3:1258–1275
96. Severac M, Orban JC, Leplatois T, Ichai C (2013) A near -fatal case of exercise-associated hyponatremia. Am J Emerg Med 813:e1–e2
97. Chung HM, Kluge R, Schrier RW, Anderson RJ (1986) Postoperative hyponatremia. A prospective study. Arch Intern Med 146:333–336
98. Gardner LB, Preston RA (2000) University of Miami Division of clinical pharmacology therapeutic rounds: the water-intolerant patient and perioperative hyponatremia. Am J Ther 7:23–30
99. Harris B, Schopflin C, Khaghani C et al (2015) Perioperative intravenous fluid prescribing: a multi-centre audit. Crit Care 4:15
100. Hannon MJ, Finucane FM, Sherlock M et al (2012) Clinical review: disorders of water homeostasis in neurosurgical patients. J Clin Endocrinol Metab 97:1423–1433
101. Hannon MJ, Thompson CJ (2014) Neurosurgical hyponatremia. J Clin Med 14:1084–1104
102. Kleindienst A, Hannon MJ, Buchfelder M, Verbalis JG (2015) Hyponatremia in neurotrauma: the role of vasopressin. J Neurotrauma 33(7):615–624
103. Gritti P, Lanterna LA, Rotasperti L et al (2014) Clinical evaluation of hyponatremia and hypovolemia in critically ill adult neurologic patients: contribution of the use of cumulative balance of sodium. J Anesth 28:687–695
104. Hahn RG (2006) Fluid absorption in endoscopic surgery. Br J Anaesth 96:8–20
105. Cooper JM, Brady RM (2000) Intraoperative and early postoperative complications of operative hysteroscopy. Obstet Gynecol Clin N Am 27:347–366
106. Ichai C, Ciais JF, Roussel LJ et al (1996) Intravascular absorption of glycine irrigating solution during shoulder arthroscopy: a case report and follow-up study. Anesthesiology 85:1481–1485
107. Decaux G, Andres C, Gankam KF, Kengne F, Soupart A (2010) Treatment of euvolemic hyponatremia in the intensive care unit by urea. Crit Care 14:R184
108. Tamman AE, Ahmed HH, Abdella AH, Taha SA (2015) Comparative study between monopolar electrodes and bipolar electrodes in hysteroscopic surgery. J Clin Diagn Res 9:QC11–QC13
109. Berl T (2015) Vasopressin antagonists. N Engl J Med 372:2207–2216
110. Runkle I, Navarro A, Pose A et al (2013) El tratamiento de la hiponatremia secundaria al sındrome de secrecion inadecuada de la hormona antidiuretica. Med Clin (Barc) 141:507.e1–507e10
111. Moritz ML, Ayus JC (2010) 100 cc 3% sodium chloride bolus: a novel treatment for hyponatremic encephalopathy. Metab Brain Dis 25:91–96
112. Rosner MH (2015) Preventing deaths due to exercise-associated hyponatremia. Clin J Sport Med 25:301–302
113. Mohmand HK, Issa D, Ahmad Z, Cappuccio JD, Kouides RW, Sterns RH (2007) Hypertonic saline for hyponatremia: risk of inadvertent overcorrection. J Am Soc Nephrol 2:1110–1117
114. MacMillan TE, Tang T, Cavalcanti RB (2015) Desmopressin to prevent rapid sodium correction in severe hyponatremia: a systematic review. Am J Med 12:1362.e15–1362.e24
115. Gharaibeh KA, Cgraig MJ, Koch CA et al (2013) Desmopressin is an effective adjunct treatment for reversing excessive hyponatremia overcorrection. World J Clin Cases 16:155–158
116. Rafat C, Schortgen F, Gaudry S et al (2014) Use of desmopressin acetate in severe hyponatremia in the intensive care unit. Clin J Am Soc Nephrol 9:229–237
117. Sood L, Sterns RH, Hix JK, Silver SM, Chen L (2013) Hypertonic saline and desmopressin: a simple strategy for safe correction of severe hyponatremia. Am J Kidney Dis 61:571–578

118. Singh TD, Fugate JE, Rabinstein AA (2014) Central pontine and extrapontine myelinolysis: a systematic review. Eur J Neurol 21:1443–1450
119. Norenberg MD (2010) Central pontine myelinolysis: historical and mechanistic considerations. Metab Brain Dis 25:97–106
120. Murase T, Sugimura Y, Takefuji S, Oiso Y, Murata Y (2006) Mechanisms and therapy of osmotic demyelination. Am J Med 119(suppl7A):S69–S73
121. Gankam-Kengne F, Couturier BS, Soupart A, Decaux G (2015) Urea minimizes brain complications following rapid correction of chronic hyponatremia compared with vasopressin antagonists or hypertonic saline. Kidney Int 87:323–331
122. Takagi H, Sugimura Y, Suzuki H et al (2014) Minocycline prevents osmotic demyelination associated with aquaresis. Kidney Int 86:954–964
123. Silver SM, Schroeder BM, Sterns RH, Rojiani AM (2006) Myoinositol administration improves survival and reduces myelinolysis after rapid correction of chronic hyponatremia in rats. Exp Neurol 65:37–44
124. Moritz ML, Ayus JC (2014) Management of hyponatremia in various clinical situations. Curr Treat Options Neurol 16:310
125. Soupart A, Coffernils M, Couturier B et al (2012) Efficacy and tolerance of urea compared with vaptans for long-term treatment of patients with SIADH. Clin J Am Soc Nephrol 7:742–747
126. Coussement J, Danguy C, Zouaoui-Boudjeltia K et al (2012) Treatment of the syndrome of inappropriate secretion of antidiuretic hormone with urea in critically ill patients. Am J Nephrol 35:265–270
127. Palmer BF (2013) The role of V2 receptor antagonists in the treatment of hyponatremia. Electrolyte Blood Press 11:1–8
128. Nagler EV, Vanmassenhove J, van der Veer SN et al (2014) Diagnosis and treatment of hyponatremia: a systematic review of clinical practice guidelines and consensus statements. BMC Med 12:231
129. Verbalis JG, Grossman A, Höybye C, Runkle I (2014) Review and analysis of differing regulatory indications and expert panel guidelines for the treatment of hyponatremia. Curr Med Res Opin 30:1201–1207
130. Verbalis JG, Adler S, Schrier RW, Berl T, Zhao Q, Czerwiec FS, For the SALT Investigators (2011) Efficacy and safety of oral tolvaptan therapy in patients with the syndrome of inappropriate antidiuretic hormone secretion. Eur J Endocrinol 164:725–732
131. Udelson JE, Bilsker M, Hauptman PJ et al (2011) A multicenter, randomized, double-blind, placebo-controlled study of tolvaptan monotherapy compared to furosemide and the combination of tolvaptan and furosemide in patients with heart failure and systolic dysfunction. J Card Fail 17:973–981
132. Hauptman PJ, Burnett JC Jr, Gheorghiade M et al (2013) Clinical course of patients with hyponatremia and decompensated systolic heart failure and the effect of vasopressin receptor antagonism with tolvaptan. J Card Fail 19:390–397
133. Rozen-Zvi B, Yahav D, Gheorghiade M, Korzets A, Leibovici L, Gafter U (2010) Vasopressin receptor antagonists for the treatment of hyponatremia: systematic review and meta-analysis. Am J Kidney Dis 56:325–337
134. Jaber BL, Almarzouqi L, Borgi L, Seabra VF, Balk EM, Madias NE (2010) Short-term efficacy and safety of vasopressin receptor antagonists for treatment of hyponatremia. Am J Med 124:977.e1–977.e9
135. Greenberg A, Verbalis J, Amin A et al (2015) Hyponatremia: current treatment practice and outcomes report of the hyponatremia registry: an observational multicenter international study. Kidney Int 88:167–177
136. Food and Drug Administration. FDA Safety Communications (2013) FDA limits duration and usage of Samsca (tolvaptan) due to possible liver injury leading to organ transplant or death. http://www.fda.gov/Drugs/DrugSafety/ucm350062.htm
137. Di Benedetto G, See M (2012) Direct Health-care Professional Communication on the risk of increases in serum sodium with tolvaptan (Samsca) which are too rapid. http://www.mhra.

gov.uk/home/groups/comms-ic/documents/websiteresources/con146921.pdf. Accessed 26 March 2011
138. Malhotra I, Gopinath S, Janca KC et al (2014) Unpredictable nature of tolvaptan in treatment of hypervolemic hyponatremia: case review on role of vaptans. Case Rep Endocrinol 2014:807054
139. Lehrich RW, Ortiz-Melo DI, Patel MB, Greenberg A (2013) Role of vaptans in the management of hyponatremia. Am J Kidney Dis 62:364–372
140. Gross P (2014) Panel recommendations on hyponatremia. Am J Med 127:e29
141. Adrogue HJ, Madias NE (2000) Hypernatremia. N Engl J Med 342:1493–1499
142. Garofeanu CG, Weir M, Rosas-Arellano MP et al (2005) Causes of reversible nephrogenic diabetes insipidus: a systematic review. Am J Kidney Dis 45:626–637

3 Potassium Disorders

Carole Ichai

3.1 Introduction

Potassium is the most abundant intracellular cation. It plays a major role in neuromuscular excitability, especially by maintaining electric resting and action potential of the membrane. In physiological conditions, the regulation of external and internal balances allows to control and maintain serum plasma concentration stable. The management of potassium disorders is based on a diagnosis and a therapeutic strategy. This chapter will focus particularly on critically ill patients presenting severe and symptomatic dyskalemias.

3.2 Potassium Metabolism

3.2.1 Body Potassium Distribution

Potassium (K^+) is the second most abundant cation which accounts for a total body amount of 50 mmol/kg, i.e., 4000–5000 mmoles for an adult of 70 kg. Ninety-eight percent of whole-body potassium is present in the cells, among which 80–90% is located in the muscle. Intracellular potassium concentration is between 100 and 140 meq/L (mmol/L). The remaining 2% are located in the extracellular compartment, and normal plasma K^+ level is 3.5–5 mmol/L (Fig. 3.1) [1–10]. Approximately 90% of total body potassium is exchangeable within 24 h.

C. Ichai
Intensive Care Unit, Hôpital Pasteur 2, 30 Voie Romaine, 06001 Nice, Cedex 1, France

IRCAN (INSERM U1081, CNRS UMR 7284), University Hospital of Nice, Nice, France
e-mail: ichai@unice.fr

C. Ichai et al. (eds.), *Metabolic Disorders and Critically Ill Patients*,
http://doi.org/10.1007/978-3-319-64010-5_3

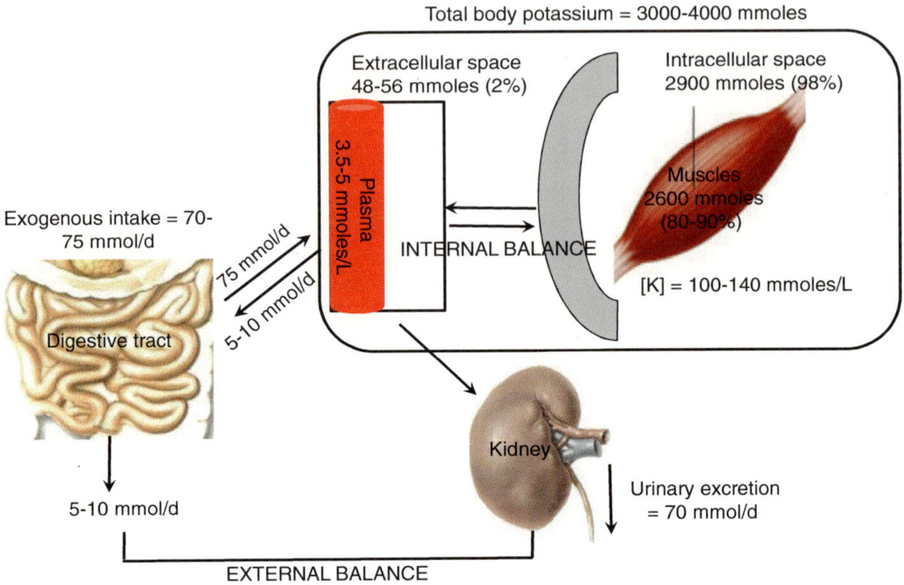

Fig. 3.1 Physiological distribution of potassium in the body and potassium balance (in an adult of 70 kg). Total body amount of potassium represents 3000–4000 mmoles, which are distributed for 98% in the intracellular volume. Intracellular potassium concentration is between 100 and 140 mmol/L, while normal plasma potassium level is around 3.5–5 mmol/L. The internal potassium balance consists in an asymmetric repartition of potassium between the intra- and the extracellular space, aiming to maintain a transmembrane potential and a normal value of kalemia. The external potassium balance aims to equilibrate potassium intakes and losses. Intakes come essentially from exogenous meal (around 75 mmoles). They are essentially equilibrated by an equivalent amount of losses by kidneys (very low losses produced by skin and colic tube)

3.2.2 Potassium Balance and Its Regulation

Extracellular/intracellular potassium ratio, [Ke]/[Ki], explains why mild absolute variations in kalemia may greatly impact on neuromuscular excitability. Therefore, it is not surprising to find a precise control for strictly regulating kalemia. To maintain kalemia and potassium homeostasis, two complementary systems are involved: the regulation of the internal and of the external balances.

3.2.2.1 Internal Potassium Balance

Internal potassium balance is the first line of immediate kalemia regulation. However, this is a transitory short-term regulation which consists in the maintenance of an asymmetric distribution of potassium between the intra- and the extracellular fluid [1, 4, 6, 11–13]. The physiological transmembrane gradient between extracellular potassium [Ke] and intracellular potassium concentrations [Ki] is maintained thanks to the transmembrane Na-K-ATPase, an enzyme that induces the entry of two K^+ into the cell while extruding three Na^+ out of the cell. This active phenomenon consumes one molecule of ATP. In the same time, some leakage currents compensate these active fluxes (Fig. 3.2a). Thanks to this Na-K-ATPase pump, [Ki] remains elevated between 100 and 140 mmol/L, while extracellular sodium concentration [Nae] is high around 140 mmol/L, and the resting potential of the membrane is around −60 to −80 mV (gradient of 20:1) (see infra).

The redistribution between the intra- and the extracellular potassium is modulated by several parameters. Among them, insulin and ß-adrenergic catecholamines are the most important controlling mechanisms. After binding on their own specific membrane receptors (R insulin, R-ß2-adrenergic), the Na-K-ATPase pump is activated and consequently K^+ entries from the extracellular fluid into the cell (Fig. 3.2b). The rapid and sudden increased kalemia stimulates insulin and endogenous catecholamine secretion. Adrenalin shows a biphasic effect: the initial hyperkalemia related to the alpha-adrenergic stimulation is followed by hypokalemia which results from the stimulation of ß2-adrenergic receptors. Stress-induced exogenous adrenergic secretion conducts to comparable hypokalemic effects. Such phenomenons may decrease kalemia by 0.5–1 meq/L. Other parameters enable to modulate

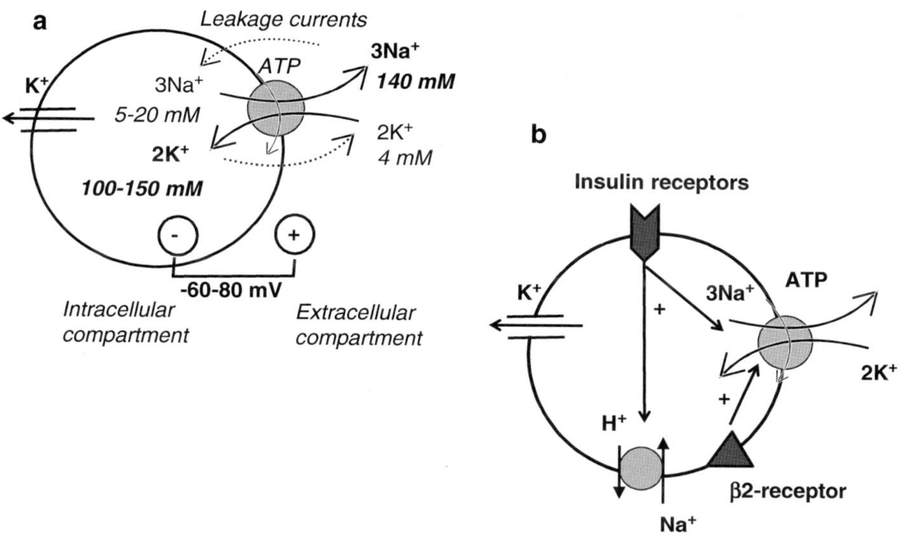

Fig. 3.2 Na-K-ATPase pump and its role in the intracellular potassium concentration. (**a**) The transmembrane Na-K-ATPase requires ATP energy to actively work. The resulting effect is the entry of three sodiums into the cell which are exchanged with the extrusion of two potassiums from the cell. Besides these major active exchanges, passive transmembrane leakage currents slightly attenuate these gradients of concentration. The final result is the presence of an electric membrane gradient, which is characterized by a negative charge inside the cell and a positive charge outside the cell: this represents the resting potential of the membrane of the cell which is around −60 to −80 mV. (**b**) When binding to its receptor, insulin activates the transmembrane Na-K-ATPase pump and simultaneously the sodium/proton pump, leading in turn to a greater entry of potassium in the cell and finally to hypokalemia (secondary to the transfer). ß2-Adrenergic agonists induce hypokalemia by a similar mechanism after binding to their own specific receptors

the internal potassium homeostasis. Aldosterone, which also activates the Na-K-ATPase pump, allows to redistribute potassium into the intracellular fluid. This phenomenon modifies kalemia only in case of a chronic secretion. Glucagon has a less known effect: after an initial hyperkalemia which is related to the efflux of potassium from hepatocytes, hypokalemia may develop due to an insulin stimulation. Consequently, the intestinal K^+ absorption during a meal should not induce hyperkalemia thanks to the potassium sequestration by the liver and muscles. During a fasted condition, kalemia remains constant thanks to the continuous K^+ extrusion from cells performed by the Na-K-ATPase pump.

Acid-base status enables also to modify potassium transmembrane transfers [14]. The classical relationship between acidosis and hyperkalemia is not constant and depends on the cause of acidosis. In case of hyperchloremic metabolic acidosis, the inorganic anion chloride (Cl^-) accumulates in the extracellular fluid. This change requires an electric neutralization which consists in an efflux of an intracellular cation, i.e., potassium with hyperkalemia. During organic metabolic acidosis, the organic anion (lactate$^-$, ketone bodies$^-$) enters into the cell and is metabolized, so that no efflux of potassium is required to maintain plasma electroneutrality. Respiratory acidosis does not induce hyperkalemia [15–17].

Skeletal muscle accounts for the higher content of whole-body potassium. For this reason, this organ plays also a major role in the short-term regulation of potassium transmembrane movements. Indeed, even moderate, the release of potassium by the muscle may conduct to significant variations of kalemia [2, 18]. Due to a high number of transmembrane potassium channels and Na-K-ATPase pumps, body muscles enable to intake 134 moles of potassium per minute, leading theoretically to exhaust the extracellular potassium content in 25 s with a full work. Therefore, hormonal- or drug-induced hyperkalemia and hypokalemia may be observed when the principal target is skeletal muscle (e.g., hyperkalemia induced by succinylcholine).

3.2.2.2 External Potassium Balance

Potassium intake comes essentially from the ingestion of meal which represents 70–75 mmol/day. Usually, the daily ingested amount exceeds the required one. The gut intake is exclusively and totally located in the small bowel [4, 19]. In physiological conditions, potassium excretion is balanced by potassium intake. The kidney is the major organ responsible for maintaining potassium balance by excreting most of potassium, while colic and cutaneous losses participate only for 10–15% of the total amount of potassium excretion (5–10 mmol/day) (Fig. 3.1) [11, 20, 21]. With a glomerular filtration rate (GFR) of 125 ml/min and a kalemia of 4.5 mmol/L, the total load of potassium which is filtered in the glomerulus reaches 810 mmoles, a value which is largely above the exogenous feeding intake. Indeed, more than 90% potassium that is filtered at the glomerulus is passively reabsorbed in the proximal tubule (around 66%) and in the ascending limb of the loop of Henle (around 29%). At the entry of the collecting duct, only 2% of the filtered potassium persists and will be regulated by hormonal and nonhormonal mechanisms. Potassium reabsorption in the proximal tubule is performed through paracellular spaces and is inversely proportional to the extracellular volume. In the ascending limb of the loop of Henle and along the aldosterone-sensitive distal nephron, sodium, potassium, and chloride transfers are closely linked and performed by various channels, cotransporters (sodium-potassium-chloride cotransporters, NKCC), or exchangers. Loop diuretic effects are mediated by NKCC2 which are located on the apical membrane. Therefore, renal potassium regulation is mainly performed through active excretion or reabsorption in the distal convoluted tubule (DCT), the connecting tubule, and the cortical collecting duct (Fig. 3.3). Apical principal cells of first part of DCT (DCT1) primarily reabsorb NaCl through a thiazide-sensitive NaCl cotransporter (NCC) [21]. Sodium apical entry activates basal sodium extrusion and potassium influx by the Na-K-ATPase pump. Simultaneously, the apical depolarization caused by sodium entry promotes (1) the apical potassium secretion through various channels and a potassium chloride cotransporter (KCC) and (2) the active basolateral cell sodium extrusion and potassium influx by the Na-K-ATPase pump. DCT2 (connecting tubule and collecting duct) cells sense potassium via an apical membrane voltage channel amiloride-sensitive epithelial sodium (ENaC). Apical sodium entry

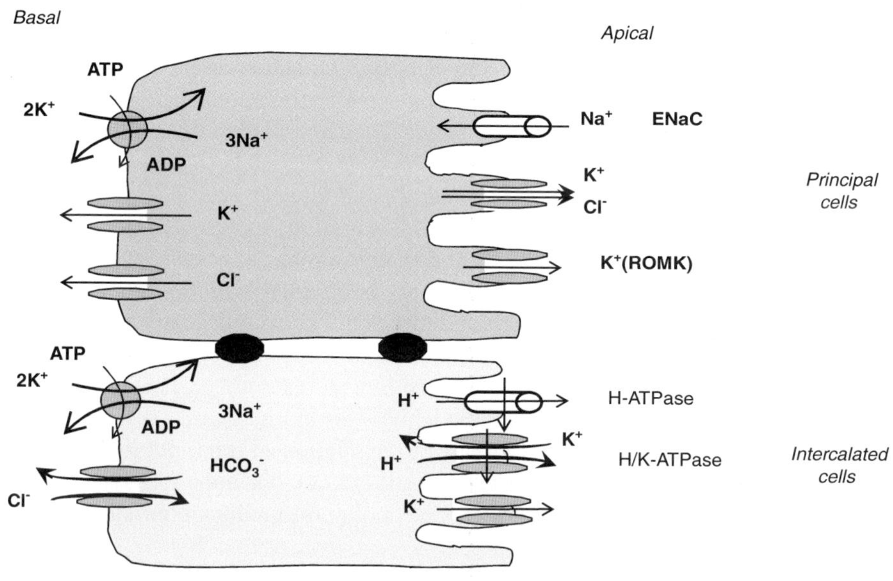

Fig. 3.3 Major mechanisms of potassium transport in the distal convoluted tubule and the collecting duct of the kidney. In principal cells, potassium is actively reabsorbed from the peritubular fluid by the Na-K-ATPase pump and is secreted at the apical membrane by potassium/chloride cotransporters (KCC). Epithelial channels participate to these exchanges on the apical side: sodium is reabsorbed by the epithelial sodium channel (ENaC), while potassium can be secreted by the renal outer medullary potassium channel (ROMK). Extrusion of potassium and chloride from the cell at the basal side is also performed by specific channels. At last, the net effect is an absolute loss of potassium in urines. In intercalated cells, potassium is also actively reabsorbed from the peritubular fluid by the Na-K-ATPase pump which is secreted at the apical membrane by potassium channels. Active secretion/reabsorption of potassium through proton/potassium ATPase exchangers is also possible to equilibrate the external potassium balance. *ADP* adenosine diphosphate, *ATP* adenosine triphosphate, *Cl* chloride, *H* proton, *K* potassium, *Na* sodium

induces several phenomenons: (1) activation of the basal Na-K-ATPase pump which leads to sodium extrusion and potassium uptake and (2) apical membrane depolarization which stimulates apical potassium extrusion via potassium channels. Potassium is also actively reabsorbed by the apical membrane of intercalated cells by a proton-potassium pump. Recent studies have shown that adrenal cells which produce aldosterone works in concert with connecting tubule and collecting duct which are aldosterone-sensitive segment of the nephron and with DCT cells which contain K^+ sensors leading to preserve K homeostasis [22]. Therefore, a low plasma K level sends the same signal to both cells: apical membrane hyperpolarization of adrenal cells which closes voltage-activated calcium channels and inhibits aldosterone release, while apical membrane hyperpolarization of DCT cells conducts to increase intracellular chloride content which inhibits NCC. The global resulting effect is a decrease renal potassium loss [22, 23].

Factors Controlling Kaliuresis and Potassium Balance: The Homeostatic Regulation

Aldosterone is the major hormonal system that regulates renal tubular secretion of potassium and therefore kalemia. In this way, its secretion is stimulated independently from the renin-angiotensin system. When kalemia increases, adrenal cortical cells that are responsible for aldosterone secretion are stimulated leading to increase kaliuresis and conversely. Aldosterone target is located essentially on the external cortical and medullar collecting renal cells. Aldosterone enters in the cell and binds to its basolateral cytosolic receptor. Aldosterone has three effects [2, 4, 6, 7, 20]: (1) on the apical side, activation of sodium reabsorption and potassium excretion through selective channels; (2) on the basolateral side, activation of the Na-K-ATPase pump and the resulting global effect is an increased potassium urinary excretion and sodium reuptake which underlines the close link between potassium and sodium (Fig. 3.4); and (3) in the principal cells of the collecting duct, activation of kaliuresis. Therefore, due to NaCl reabsorption, aldosterone plays a major role in maintaining arterial pressure and volemia while it is simultaneously responsible for the long-term regulation of kalemia thanks to regulation of renal potassium excretion/reabsorption. Both glucocorticoids and antidiuretic hormone (ADH) stimulate directly kaliuresis in the collecting duct. Catecholamines reduce potassium urinary excretion in the DCT.

Kalemia and potassium intake: an elevation in kalemia induces an increased kaliuresis which becomes linear above 4 mmol/L. Both aldosterone and a decreased potassium intake reduce potassium urinary excretion thanks to a direct inhibition of potassium channels which are located in the principal cells of the collecting duct.

Factors Controlling Kaliuresis Without Regulation of Potassium Balance: The Nonhomeostatic Regulation

Both sodium and chloride flux and contents in the DCT enable to modify urinary potassium secretion [14, 21]: any increase in tubular flux of these electrolytes rises kaliuresis and conversely. For a constant kalemia, an elevation in intraluminal sodium load or a reduction in intraluminal potassium load increases urinary

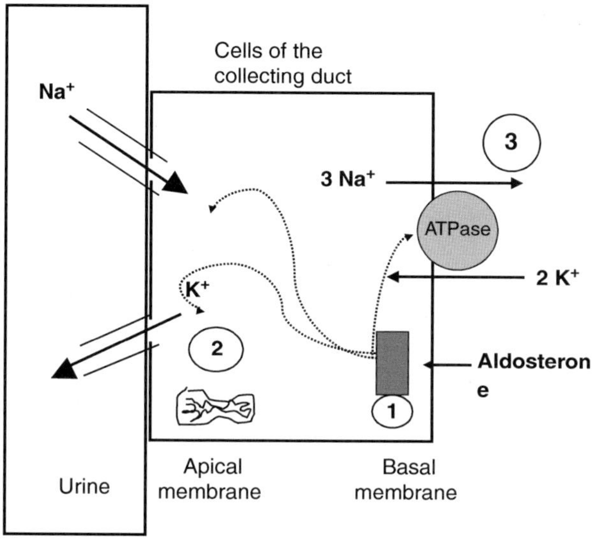

Fig. 3.4 Renal effects of aldosterone. The major site of action of aldosterone is located on the distal nephron, especially on the external cortical and medullary collecting tube. Aldosterone enters into the cell through the membrane and binds to its cytosolic receptor. This binding triggers several phenomenons: (1) stimulation of sodium (and chloride) reabsorption and potassium excretion through specific channels at the apical membrane, (2) stimulation of the Na-K-ATPase pump at the basal membrane, and (3) facilitation of the work of the Na-K-ATPase pump thanks to the increased production of ATP by the mitochondria. All of these effects contribute to promote hypokalemia and kaliuresis secondary to aldosterone release

potassium excretion. Acidosis, mineralocorticoid antagonists, and loop kaliuretic diuretics (furosemide) stimulate also kaliuresis.

3.2.2.3 Integrated Potassium Homeostasis

External potassium balance is performed by three control systems [21]. Two negative feedback control mechanisms react to kalemia changes and to the amount of potassium intake to maintain plasma potassium level and regulate potassium balance thanks to appropriate changes in urinary potassium excretion. The third system which has been described more recently consists in a predictive adaptation based on our circadian rhythm of meal and sleep-wake cycle.

External Balance and "Reactive" Negative Feedback Control

The best known system is the one which is activated by changes in kalemia: potassium excretion increases in response to hyperkalemia in order to normalize kalemia and conversely. The second reactive negative feedback system responds to changes in potassium oral intake (during meal), independent of kalemia: the stimulation of splanchnic receptors (located on the intestinal tube and the liver) during potassium intake would trigger potassium urinary excretion from a double signal, one coming from the intestinal tube and the other one coming from the central nervous system [24].

"Predictive" Adaptation According to a Circadian Rhythm
This adaptation is based on our physiological rhythm of food intake and consists in a modulation of the reactive systems to drive a most appropriate response of our circadian rhythm (for meal and for sleeping periods). This phenomenon is triggered by a central clock in the suprachiasmatic nucleus of the brain which controls numerous circadian rhythms. The night-light cycle activates this central oscillator which activates in turn renal intracellular oscillators leading finally to cyclic basal variations in potassium urinary excretion. Exercise and oral potassium intake amplify these oscillations aiming to minimize variations in kalemia. Precise mechanisms of such a regulation are still not really known as well as interactions with mineralo- and glucocorticoids [21].

In summary, hypo- and hyperkalemia may result from changes in potassium intake, alteration in potassium urinary excretion, or in transcellular shifts. Aldosterone is the major system implicated in the control of the external potassium balance.

3.2.3 Physiological Functions of Body Potassium

Potassium participates to numerous physiological functions. Among them, the gradient of intracellular [Ki] and extracellular [Ke] potassium concentration is essential for maintaining the resting potential of the membrane because cell membrane is not permeant to sodium but highly permeant to potassium. This membrane potential consists in a difference in the electric potential which results from the gradient of concentration between [Ki] and [Ke]. At the resting state, maintaining this gradient requires energy (ATP) to drive the membrane Na-K-ATPase pump. Therefore, the potential of the membrane depends on Ki/Ke ratio which is determined by variations in extracellular potassium concentration [2, 4, 6, 7, 9, 12]. The reflecting Ke by kalemia is the major determinant of this potential and can be calculated according to the Nernst formula: $Ek = -61 \log [Ki]/[Ke] = -80$ mV. Any elevation of kalemia reduces the potential of the membrane and conversely. Finally, kalemia, or more precisely the [Ki]/[Ke] ratio, determines the resting membrane potential and, in turn, the threshold for triggering the electric potential of action. This latter is characterized by a membrane depolarization induced by a profound elevation in the membrane permeability which allows a massive sodium entry in the cell. This phenomenon produces the conduction in nerves and the coupled muscular excitability-contractility (peripheral skeletal muscle and myocardium). In myocardium, pacemaker cells of the sinoatrial node are characterized by a higher resting membrane potential (around −60 mV) and a spontaneous diastolic depolarization which allows to initiate the depolarization and, in turn, the contraction of all other myocardial cells (Fig. 3.5a). Potassium is also highly involved in glycogen and protein synthesis and cellular metabolism.

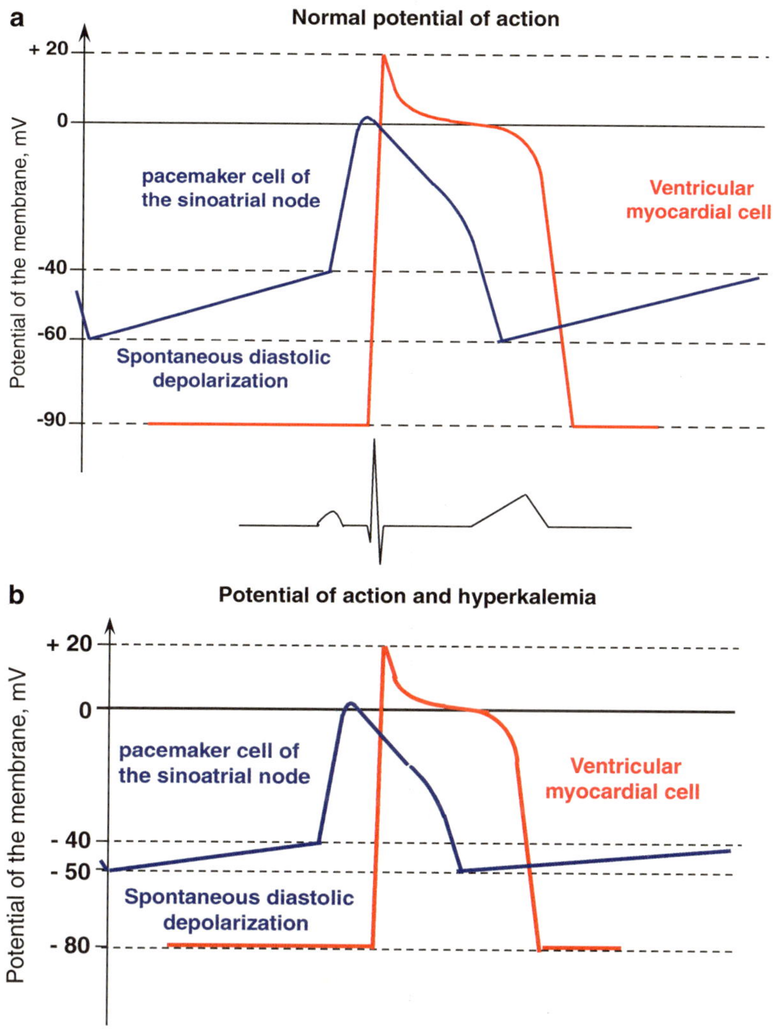

Fig. 3.5 Potential of action on cardiomyocytes and automatic pacemaker cells of the sinoatrial node. (**a**) Normal potential of action. The membrane depolarization consists in a massive entry of sodium into the cell (which corresponds to the QRS complex on the ECG); it is followed by a spontaneous repolarization (which corresponds to the T-wave on the ECG). Automatic pacemaker cells slightly differ as a spontaneous depolarization occurs that allows to trigger the potential of action. (**b**) Potential of action and hyperkalemia. Hyperkalemia increases myocyte excitability by decreasing the resting potential, by prolonging myocardial conduction and repolarization, and by reducing the potential of action. (**c**) Potential of action and calcium. Calcium infusion increases the number of sodium channels which in turn reduces the threshold of the potential of action and accelerates conduction. (**d**) Potential of action and hypokalemia. Hypokalemia elevates the resting potential which in turn decreases the membrane excitability and prolonged the potential of action

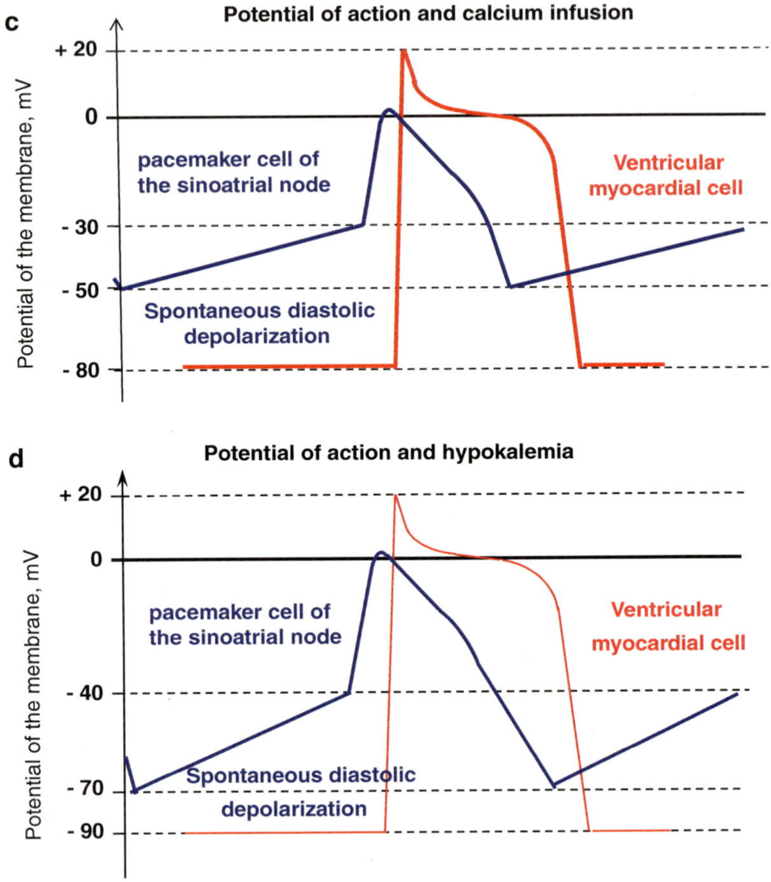

Fig. 3.5 (continued)

3.3 Epidemiology of Potassium Disorders

Potassium disorders are among the most common electrolyte abnormalities which can be responsible for life-threatening consequences such as cardiac arrest and severe cardiac arrhythmias [5, 6, 25–29]. Hyperkalemia is present in 1.1–10% of hospitalized patients [26–31], a higher frequency being observed in patients at risk as chronic kidney disease [32]. On the other hand, even frequent in intensive care units (ICU), its prevalence remains poorly evaluated [33]. A retrospective large observational study has shown that hyperkalemia is associated with an increased risk of mortality and that the odds ratio increased with the elevation of kalemia [34]. Severe hyperkalemia ($\geq$ 6.5 mmol/L) on admission or during hospitalization has been reported to require an emergent hospitalization in 68.8% of hyperkalemia. The most common cause was chronic kidney disease. Only 37.7% of them had typical abnormal ECG signs, and 20.3% present severe hyperkalemia at the time of cardiac arrest. Multiple organ failure was present in 24.5% patients when hyperkalemia was diagnosed [35]. Mortality rate of these patients was 30% and hyperkalemia was independently associated with mortality. Hyperkalemia is frequently induced or favored by drugs (heparin, potassium-sparing diuretics, angiotensin-converting enzyme inhibitors) or by some comorbidities such as chronic renal insufficiency or hypoaldosteronism [3, 25, 27, 28, 36–38]. Hypokalemia is observed in 20% of hospitalized patients [3]. This incidence exceeds 50% in polytrauma patients in the acute initial period. Around 40% of patients develop hypokalemia within 2–3 days following surgery.

3.4 Hyperkalemias

Hyperkalemia is defined as a serum potassium level exceeding 5 mmol/L. It is usually classified as mild between 5 and 5.0 mmol/L, moderate between 6 and 6.4 mmol/L, and severe (potentially fatal) if ≥6.5 mmol/L [5, 7].

3.4.1 Clinical Symptoms

Usually mild and moderate hyperkalemias are asymptomatic. However, clinical manifestations are not always related to the absolute value of kalemia but rather to its rate of development associated with the underlying condition. Most of the clinical manifestations are associated with alterations in excitability of neuromuscular and cardiac tissues [4–6, 7, 39–43].

- *Neuromuscular manifestations*: this can be associated with muscular weakness, asthenia, cramping, paresthesia, or hypotonic paralysis (abolition of reflexes) which may lead in turn to respiratory failure. Neither diaphragmatic or bilateral cranial nerve motor impairment nor sensitive manifestations are usually present [6, 8, 9, 14].
- *Cardiovascular and ECG signs*: hyperkalemia decreases the membrane potential which in turn induces a membrane hyperexcitability (Fig. 3.5b). Nevertheless, in case of prolonged hyperkalemia, membrane excitability will decrease due to an inactivation of membrane sodium channels which is related to depolarization. These effects are associated with a slowdown of conduction and a shortened potential of action. Cardiac alterations in response to hyperkalemia are not similar in all parts of the heart, and in a decreasing order are atria, ventricular cells, His bundle, and sinoatrial node, which explain the progressive abnormal ECG signs. It is classical to consider that ECG abnormalities are related with hyperkalemia severity (depth) (Fig. 3.6). The earlier sign consists in peaked T-waves, T-waves being narrow and sharp because of the faster repolarization. This abnormality is followed by prolonged PR intervals, flattened or absent P-waves, widened QRS, and shortened QT intervals, which are the witnesses of the reduced excitability. Most severe arrhythmias consist of a sinusoidal QRS aspect with a

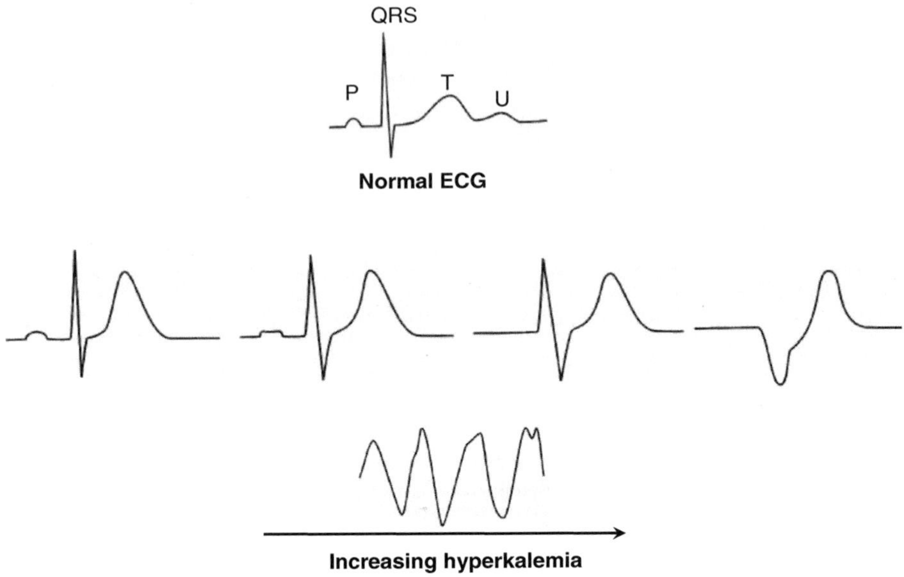

Fig. 3.6 ECG signs of hyperkalemia

merging of S- and T-waves to finally evolve toward cardiac arrest related to bradycardia, ventricular tachycardia/fibrillation, or asystole [44, 45]. This progression is not always observed because for a same level of hyperkalemia, high variability in ECG signs has been reported in humans [29]. In 127 patients presenting hyperkalemia between 6 and 9.3 meq/L, no severe arrhythmia was observed, and only 46% of the patients showed the classical hyperkalemic ECG abnormalities [28]. Another retrospective study underlines the low sensitivity of ECG to diagnose hyperkalemia [29]. Indeed, a normal ECG may be observed in patients presenting severe hyperkalemias while developing suddenly and immediately ventricular fibrillation (VF). The speed of hyperkalemia development can probably explain these variations in ECG signs. Moreover, hyperkalemic-related ECG abnormalities may be exacerbated by metabolic disorders such as hypocalcemia, acidosis, and hyponatremia [29]. Despite the weaknesses of ECG changes, ECG monitoring remains essential to manage hyperkalemia.

– *Metabolic manifestations*: hyperkalemia may induce hyperchloremic acidosis by increasing ammoniagenesis.

3.4.2 Etiologies

The first step for diagnosing the cause of hyperkalemia consists of eliminating pseudohyperkalemia which is defined as a relevant difference between plasma and serum potassium concentration (>0.4 mmol/L). Pseudohyperkalemia may occur in case of hemolysis, membrane abnormalities of red blood cell in children, elevated

Table 3.1 Major causes of hyperkalemias

Hyperkalemias caused by an excessive exogenous intake if associated with: – Chronic renal insufficiency – Cardiac insufficiency or failure – Diabetes – Dehydration, hypovolemia
Hyperkalemias caused by cell transfer: – Intensive physical exercise – Rhabdomyolysis, muscular trauma, burn, status epilepticus – Insulinopenia (± hyperglycemia) – Hyperchloremic metabolic acidosis – Drugs: ß-blockers, succinylcholine – Hyperkalemic familial periodic paralysis
Hyperkalemias caused by inappropriate urinary potassium reabsorption: *Reduction of the total amount of sodium delivered to the distal nephron* – Renal insufficiency (especially when associated with excessive intake) – Hypovolemia (dehydration, congestive cardiac insufficiency) *Hypoaldosteronism* – Primary: adrenal insufficiency (Addison's disease), tubular acidosis type 4 – Secondary: • Syndrome of hyporeninism-hypoaldosteronism • Drugs: potassium-sparing diuretics (spironolactone, triamterene, amiloride), trimethoprim, angiotensin-converting enzyme inhibitors, angiotensin receptor antagonists, heparins, nonsteroidal anti-inflammatory agents

leukocytes, or thrombocythemia [5, 46]. In these situations, potassium is released by lysed cells. The diagnosis can be suspected in the absence of ECG abnormalities despite severe hyperkalemia. Pseudohyperkalemia does not require any specific treatment. Except in case of acute and massive potassium load, hyperkalemia can result from only two mechanisms: transmembrane cellular shift characterized by a reduction in cell entry or an elevation in cell extrusion or a decrease in urinary excretion [1, 9, 39, 42, 43]. Regardless of the mechanism, iatrogenic drug-induced hyperkalemias are very frequent [3, 9]. Major causes of hyperkalemias are summarized in Table 3.1.

3.4.2.1 Tools Required for the Diagnostic Approach

The determination of the cause of hyperkalemia is based firstly on the clinical history, physical examination, and current treatments. Several biological exams are useful. Plasma electrolyte measurements as well as arterial blood gas, blood urea nitrogen, and creatininemia are essential. Urine electrolytes (including kaliuresis, natriuresis, and chloruresis), osmolarity, creatinine, and creatinine clearance are usually sufficient for establishing the cause of hyperkalemia. Some additional parameters may be useful.

- *Urinary potassium excretion*: 24-h kaliuresis allows to distinguish renal from extrarenal causes of hyperkalemia—a value >200 mmoles indicates an extrarenal origin of hyperkalemia.

- *Other parameters*: potassium transtubular gradient (KTTG) is calculated according to the following formula: (urinary K x plasma osmolality)/(plasma K/urinary osmolality). A value under 8 refers to a renal origin of hyperkalemia [27, 47]. Fractional potassium excretion (FeK) is calculated according to the following formula: [(urinary K/plasma K)/(urinary creatinine/plasma creatinine)] × 100%. A value <10% may suggest a renal origin.

3.4.2.2 Hyperkalemias Due to Excessive Exogenous Intake (Elevated Total Body Potassium)

A sole excessive exogenous intake cannot induce hyperkalemia, except when high amounts are administered rapidly or in patients with favoring underlying conditions [2, 3, 48]. Potassium supplementation might be implicated in the development of hyperkalemia in 15–40% of hospitalized patients [29, 41, 49]. Patient's conditions and drugs often favor this trouble. Drugs are identified as contributing factors in 4–20% of hospitalized patients [50, 51]. The most frequently concerned are potassium-sparing diuretics, nonselective ß-blockers, angiotensin-converting enzyme (ACE) inhibitors, heparin, succinylcholine, and nonsteroidal anti-inflammatory drugs (NSAIDs) [3, 5, 52]. Most frequently pathologies encountered are chronic renal insufficiency, cardiac insufficiency, diabetes, and dehydration.

3.4.2.3 Hyperkalemias Due to Cell Transfer (Normal Total Body Potassium)

- *Physical exercise*: potassium extrusion from cell during physical exercise is induced by two phenomenons. Muscle contraction refers to a membrane depolarization which is triggered by a sodium entry in the cell, while potassium is extruded in the interstitial space leading to its vascular entry. The efflux of intracellular potassium is facilitated by the reduction in intracellular ATP concentration which favors potassium channel opening. This phenomenon is usually short and transitory, followed by a returning intracellular entry of potassium when contraction stops [2, 46]. Potassium extrusion from cells is also favored by catecholamine and glucagon releases which induce an inhibition of insulin secretion. The degree of plasma potassium rise depends on the intensity, the duration, and the training of the patient. Hyperkalemia is strongly attenuated in trained individuals because of the increased number of muscular Na-K-ATPase pumps [2]. Kalemia increases around 0.3–0.4 meq/L for a mild exercise (slow walk), 0.7–1.2 meq/L for a moderate exercise, and up to 2 meq/L for an intensive exercise (marathon). This hyperkalemia is essentially localized to the muscle and seems to be beneficial as it induces arteriolar vasodilation which allows to increase the regional blood flow of the exercised muscle. On a pathophysiological point of view, hyperkalemias associated with muscular trauma, rhabdomyolysis, burn, and status epilepticus are very close from that of muscular exercise [53].
- *Depolarizing muscle relaxant* (*succinylcholine*) [53–55]: the first case was reported in 1967 in a burned patient. In the normal innervated muscle, succinylcholine depolarizes only the neuromuscular junctional receptors (AchRs) which are mostly located in this area. The resulting efflux of intracellular potassium is

limited to this area and conducts to a modest increase in kalemia of 0.5–1 mmol/L. All situations that conduct to a loss of contraction lead to increase markedly the density of these membrane receptors (upregulation) in the extra-junctional area. Moreover, all of these receptors present an abnormal structure (immature receptors) causing a massive efflux of intracellular potassium. This phenomenon persists because the molecule cannot be metabolized by acetylcholinesterase which is only present in the perijunctional area. Therefore, in this situation, hyperkalemia is profound and persistent. Most situations at risk of succinylcholine-induced hyperkalemia are (1) functional or anatomical denervation such as in motor neuron deficits, prolonged chemical denervation (muscle relaxants, magnesium, clostridium toxins), and neuromyopathies, (2) simple immobilization within 3–5 days, and (3) muscle injury due to a direct trauma, tumor, inflammation burn, and severe infection. Therefore, succinylcholine administration must be avoided from 48 to 72 h following a denervation state.

- *Insulinopenia* (*± hyperglycemia*): this represents one of the most frequent causes of hyperkalemia. As observed in nontreated or nonequilibrated diabetes, insulin deficit slows down the membrane Na-K-ATPase driven, which reduces the entry of intracellular potassium (Fig. 3.2b). Hyperglycemia exacerbates this phenomenon: due to hyperglycemic-associated plasma hypertonicity, the resulting intracellular shrinkage elevates [Ki] and creates a transmembrane potassium gradient which is favorable to a passive intracellular potassium efflux through selective channels.
- *Inorganic metabolic acidosis*: as described previously, exceeding plasma chloride cannot enter easily into the cell. Therefore, intracellular potassium is excreted and goes in the extracellular space to maintain plasma electroneutrality. It is classical to consider that a 0.1 reduction in pH induces a 0.7 meq/L elevation in kalemia (Burnell equation) [15, 16, 56]. However, organic metabolic and respiratory acidosis is usually not solely responsible for hyperkalemia. In this case, other causes of hyperkalemia such as insulinopenia, ß-blocker administration, or chronic renal insufficiency with a high potassium intake must be recognized.
- *Drug-induced hyperkalemias* [3, 36]: drugs frequently promote hyperkalemia as a primary cause or contributing factor in 35 to 75% of hospitalized patients [49]. Nonselective ß-blockers are associated with hyperkalemia in 4–17% of hospitalized patients [34]. The blocking effects on the selective receptors of the membrane Na-K-ATPase favor the extrusion of intracellular potassium (Fig. 3.2b). Nevertheless, hyperkalemia remains moderate (increase of 0.3–0.5 mmol/L) and transitory because exceeding plasma potassium will be rapidly eliminated in urines. Digoxin, by its binding on its membrane receptor, also blocks the transmembrane Na-K-ATPase pump. The resulting transmembrane potassium transfers are dose-dependent, so that hyperkalemia appears only in case of overdose or intoxications. Succinylcholine can provoke hyperkalemia which is induced by membrane depolarization and an efflux of intracellular potassium [39–41]. In this situation, the elevation of kalemia can reach 1 meq/L in 2–5 min. Even transitory, this hyperkalemia can have severe consequences and induce cardiac

arrest, especially in favoring conditions such as motor denervation (see previous chapter).

- *Hyperkalemic familial periodic paralysis*: this hereditary disease is rare and is due to an abnormal inactivation of voltage-dependent sodium channels—the prolonged opening of sodium channels induces an extrusion of muscular intracellular potassium [2].

3.4.2.4 Renal Hyperkalemia (Elevated Total Body Potassium)

The decrease in urinary potassium excretion may result from a reduction in sodium or water content which is delivered in the distal nephron as observed in case of renal insufficiency or hypovolemia. The second mechanism of renal hyperkalemia is hypoaldosteronism.

- *Renal insufficiency*: hyperkalemia results from several mechanisms. The loss of functional nephrons is responsible for an inherent decrease ability in potassium excretion. At the beginning of the disease, urinary potassium excretion compensates exogenous potassium intake. But when chronic renal insufficiency worsens, even in the absence of oligoanuria, hyperkalemia develops due to modifications in dietary (low sodium intake, substitution of salt by potassium salts, metabolic acidosis, anemia).
- *Circulating hypovolemia*: in this condition, the total amount of potassium which is delivered to the nephron decreases leading to reduce urinary potassium excretion. This is commonly observed in patients with congestive cardiac insufficiency.
- *Hypoaldosteronism*: this can be observed in pathologies that are characterized by a decrease in aldosterone production and defines primary hypoaldosteronism: Addison's disease or isolated hypoaldosteronism such as in hereditary, acquired, infection, or renal chronic disease (tubular acidosis type 4). Primary hypoaldosteronism is also frequently induced by drugs. ACE inhibitors or angiotensin receptor antagonists as sartans (ARA II) are implicated in the development of hyperkalemia in 9–38% of hospitalized patients [29]. They induce hypoaldosteronism thanks to an inhibition of the synthesis or of the action of angiotensin II. Heparin decreases the number and the affinity of angiotensin II and in turn a hypoaldosteronism which is observed in 7% of patients treated with this drug [57]. The increase in kalemia can reach 1.7 meq/L within 3 days following the beginning of treatment [57, 58]. NSAI drugs can also induce a primary hypoaldosteronism by reducing renin synthesis which results from a renal prostaglandin inhibition. Nevertheless, all of these treatments cannot induce real severe hyperkalemias if they are not associated with chronic renal insufficiency. Secondary hypoaldosteronism is characterized by a reduction in the effects of aldosterone. Among them, hereditary pseudohypoaldosteronism types I and II are rare. Acquired secondary pseudohypoaldosteronism can be observed in hypoaldosteronism-hyporeninism associated with chronic renal insufficiency. But, the most frequent causes are drug-induced hypoaldosteronism due to potassium-sparing diuretics (spironolactone, triamterene, amiloride) which acts by a competitive inhibition on

aldosterone [3]. These treatments can cause a fatal hyperkalemia in 10–20% of patients receiving these treatments. Trimethoprim has the same effect and can increase kalemia of 0.6–1 mmol/L.

3.4.3 Treatment

The specific treatment of the cause of hyperkalemia is the first needed one, but will not be developed in this chapter. Three lines of treatments are available according to the impact of hyperkalemia and the resulting emergent treatment that is needed.

3.4.3.1 Treatments

- *Emergency treatment = calcium (calcium chloride or gluconate)*: calcium directly antagonizes membrane excitability leading to a decrease in the threshold of the action potential [5, 60]. This effect conducts to stabilize myocardial excitability and in turn to reverse cardiac effects without lowering kalemia and without reducing kalemia (Fig. 3.5c). The efficiency of chloride and gluconate salts is similar for equivalent amount of calcium. Therefore, the choice between both presentations depends on practice: calcium gluconate is well tolerated when infused in a peripheral venous as compared with calcium chloride which may lead to severe vascular necrosis and extravasation. The onset of calcium action is very rapid, within 1–3 min after the infusion, and the duration of action is 30–60 min, allowing to act quickly while adding in the same time longer acting treatments that reduce kalemia. The efficiency of calcium requires a continuous ECG monitoring. The recommended dose is 1 g (10 ml of 10%) intravenously in 10 min. In the absence of ECG improvement, a new dose may be repeated in 5 min.
- *Intermediate-term efficient treatments = agents aiming to shift potassium into the cells* [2, 4, 5, 59]: these drugs decrease kalemia by inducing a rapid redistribution of K into the intracellular space.
  - Insulin provides a dose-dependent hypokalemic effect which is due to the activation of Na-K-ATPase pump (Fig. 3.2b). Except in case of hyperglycemia, insulin must be administered simultaneously with glucose to prevent hypoglycemia. Various strategies of administration are reported in the literature concerning the dose and the route. A recent systematic review has failed to perform a meta-analysis due to large methodological heterogeneities of studies. Briefly, no real difference was observed between the route of administration, i.e., intravenous bolus (15–30 min) or longer infusion (over 60 min). Different doses of insulin (10UI, 12UI in bolus, 20UI over 60 min) associated with various amounts of glucose from 25 to 60 g allowed to reach comparable mean reduction of 0.8 mmol/L with a peak decrease at 15 min [62, 63]. However, 18% of hypoglycemic episodes were observed, mostly when only 25 g of glucose was administered. Therefore, 20 UI of insulin with 60 g of glucose administered within 60 min should be a good alternative to the administration of 10 UI of insulin with 25 g of glucose [63]. Such a strategy is also efficient in patients with chronic renal insufficiency.

- ß-Adrenergic agonists [61, 62, 64]: salbutamol, a specific ß2-adrenergic agonist, decreases kalemia of 0.5–1 mmol/L within 30–60 min. Regardless of the route of administration, intravenously or by inhalation (10–20 mg), its effect is dose-dependent. The association with insulin-glucose conducts to additive hypokalemic effects which allow to reach a reduction of kalemia of 1.3 mmol/L, even in patients with renal insufficiency. However, regardless of patients who received ß-blockers, 40% of patients failed to respond to this therapy. Moreover, side effects such as tachycardia, tremor, and anxiety may be observed. For these reasons, a monotherapy using ß-adrenergic agonists should be prohibited.
- Sodium bicarbonate: even accepted as a very classical treatment, the efficiency of sodium bicarbonate to treat hyperkalemia is not really demonstrated and remains questioned, except in case of metabolic acidosis. Data clearly reported that short-term sodium bicarbonate infusion does not reduce kalemia. Only prolonged infusions (4 h) enabled to induce a mild decrease in kalemia (reduction of 0.3 mmol/L) [4].

Long-term treatments = agents aiming to remove potassium from the body [9, 10, 23, 60, 65]:

- Cation exchange resins: sodium polystyrene sulfonate (SPS) (Kayexalate®) is a nonselective sodium cation exchange resin which works on the colonic intestinal lumen, the preferential site of gastrointestinal potassium excretion. The onset of action of SPS is of 1–2 h with a peak of action of 4 h. The administration can be performed orally (suspension) or rectally (enema), but the oral one is the most efficient [66]. Its efficiency is finally moderate and above all not predictable. Globally, SPS enables to reduce kalemia of 0.4–1 mmol/L. This limited exchange capacity is explained by its simultaneous competitive effect on other cations (calcium, magnesium, and sodium). The posology is classically ranged between 15 and 60 g/day orally or 30–60 g/day rectally every 6 h. However, Mistry et al. [66] have recently demonstrated that the capacity of SPS to decrease kalemia is dose-dependent, the most efficient dose being 60 g/day orally which allowed to reduce kalemia of 0.9–1 mmol/L. It is important to underline that despite its large use since 60 years, SPS efficiency has never been evaluated in a randomized controlled study. Moreover, SPS treatment is associated with numerous adverse events related to its intestinal action. Most frequent side effects include constipation, diarrhea, nausea, and electrolyte disturbances (hypomagnesemia, hypocalcemia, excessive sodium load, metabolic alkalosis). The most serious adverse event is colonic necrosis which is observed in 2% of patients receiving this treatment. Two recent potassium-binding agents are now available: sodium zirconium cyclosilicate (waiting for the approval by medical agencies) and patiromer (Veltassa®). Patiromer is orally administered and provides exchanges between calcium and potassium in the distal colon, allowing its large capacity of potassium exchange. Reduction in kalemia appears in 7 h and maintained up to 48 h. The treatment can start with an initial dose of 8.4 g once daily and progressively increased up to a maximum of 25 g once daily to reach the maximum efficiency. Patiromer shows similar gastrointestinal side effects than SPS, but at this time, no serious adverse effect or electrolyte disturbances have been reported. In summary, due to their selective action, both new potassium-binding agents seem to offer more efficiency to reduce hyperkalemia and less adverse effects.

- Kaliuretic loop diuretics: their efficiency to treat hyperkalemia has never been really evaluated [23, 60]. We can consider them as an additional treatment useful in case of fluid and sodium overload, but they are contraindicated in patients with hypovolemia (which is frequent in critically ill patients). In this latter situation, diuretics will worsen hypovolemia and in turn renal potassium reabsorption, leading to an inverse effect on kalemia.
- Renal removal therapy: hemodialysis is the treatment of choice of severe hyperkalemia in chronic renal insufficiency [67–69]. This is the most efficient therapy allowing to reduce kalemia of 1 mmol/L from the first hour and further of 1 mmol/L more within the two following hours. Potassium removal can be increased by using dialysate solutions which contain no or low potassium, a high blood flow, or solutions buffered with sodium bicarbonate.

3.4.3.2 Strategies and Algorithm of Treatments of Hyperkalemia

Due to their various delays of action, several agents require usually to be associated [5, 70, 71]. There is no real data allowing to precise the threshold of hyperkalemia which requires a symptomatic therapy. Moreover, the low specificity of ECG signs does not permit to consider only this exam to decide the treatment too. Therefore, the first priority is to evaluate the need for an emergent treatment using a combination of history, clinical exam, ECG, and a repeated biological monitoring of kalemia [2, 4, 5, 9, 10, 43, 46, 59, 60]. The choice of treatments is therefore governed by the analysis of these parameters. Urgent treatment is indicated when symptoms are present (or severe hyperkalemia), abrupt changes in kalemia and ECG modifications especially when comorbidities are associated. Several strategies have been reported recently in a review [61]. But there is no real consensual guideline, and the strategy must always take into account hyperkalemia severity and other interfering metabolic disorders (calcemia, natremia, pH) or underlying worsening conditions (renal insufficiency, respiratory-cardiac arrest). No specific treatment is required for asymptomatic to mild hyperkalemia. It seems finally reasonable to administer an emergent treatment when hyperkalemia is >6–6.5 mmol/L and in patients with ECG signs. In these cases, the first approach consists of reversing the impact of hyperkalemia on the membrane excitability to avoid VT/VF and asystole. This is achieved by calcium salts which promote shift potassium into the cell, without waiting the measurement of kalemia. However, this temporary measure must be followed by an intermediate-term treatment which enhances the redistribution of potassium into the cells (insulin, ß-adrenergic agonists). A second approach allows to manage moderate asymptomatic or mild hyperkalemia. This long-term treatment consists to increase the elimination of potassium. This may be accomplished by loop diuretics, exchange resins, and renal removal therapies (hemodialysis). The choice between these therapies

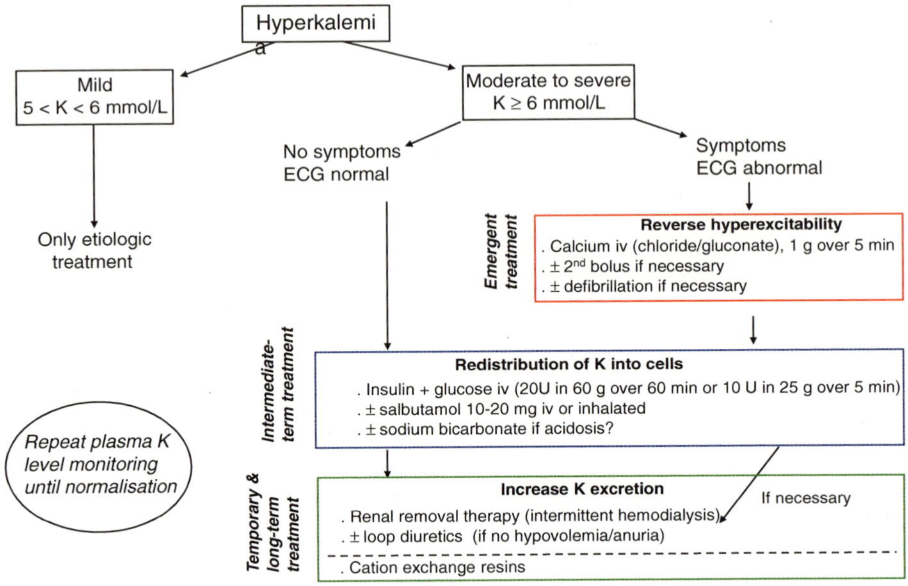

Fig. 3.7 Algorithm of treatment of hyperkalemias

depends on the cause of hyperkalemia and the condition of the patient [72, 73]. Hyperkalemia usually develops slowly in chronic renal insufficiency and is therefore associated with a good clinical tolerance. Nevertheless, in this situation, hyperkalemia >6.5 mmol/L needs to be treated, and the best choice is hemodialysis, except in case of real emergency [74, 75]. In patients with a persistent diuresis and no hypovolemia, loop diuretics may be tested, but are usually inefficient or not sufficient and are prescribed by waiting long-term treatments such as hemodialysis or exchange resins. Kalemia must be monitored to appreciate the efficiency of the treatment and to detect a potential rebound. In all cases, potassium exogenous load must be stopped as well as drugs which induce hyperkalemia. An algorithm of treatment is proposed in Fig. 3.7.

3.5 Hypokalemias

Hypokalemia is defined as a serum potassium level ≤3.5 mmol/L [4, 5, 7, 76]. It is usually classified as mild between 3 and 3.5 mmol/L, moderate between 2.5 and 3 mmol/L, and severe if >2.5 mmol/L.

3.5.1 Clinical Symptoms

Similar with hyperkalemias, hypokalemias remain asymptomatic in mild and moderate abnormalities. Clinical signs appear only in severe hypokalemias, especially if its development was rapid, or in particular favoring conditions such as cardiac insufficiency or myocardial ischemia [1, 2, 6, 8, 9, 12, 39–41, 51, 76].

- *Neuromuscular manifestations*: they are characterized by a muscular weakness, cramps, myalgias, paralysis, or tetraparesia without sensitive deficit.
- *Cardiovascular and ECG manifestations* are characterized by the appearance of a U-wave (positive deflection after the T-wave), a decrease in the T-wave amplitude, a ST segment depression, T-wave inversion, and sometimes a prolonged PR interval (Fig. 3.8). These signs are related to the increase in the potential of the membrane which reduces myocardial excitability and extends the potential of action. Ventricular extrasystoles (VES), atrioventricular blocks (AVB), and severe arrhythmias (VT, VF, asystole) occur when favoring factors such as myocardial ischemia or digitalic treatments are associated. A prolonged QT interval and "torsades de pointes" are the consequences of electrolyte disorders which induce a prolongation of ventricular repolarization (Fig. 3.5d). Therefore, such syndromes are present in case of hypokalemias and also of hypomagnesemias.

3.5.2 Etiologies

Hypokalemia can be caused by three mechanisms: a transmembrane shift of potassium into the cells, an insufficient exogenous intake of potassium, and excessive potassium losses.

3.5.2.1 Tools Required for the Diagnostic Approach

The diagnosis of hypokalemia requires initially to precise the clinical history and chronic treatments taken by the patient [1, 2, 6, 8, 9, 39–41, 51, 76]. Urinary

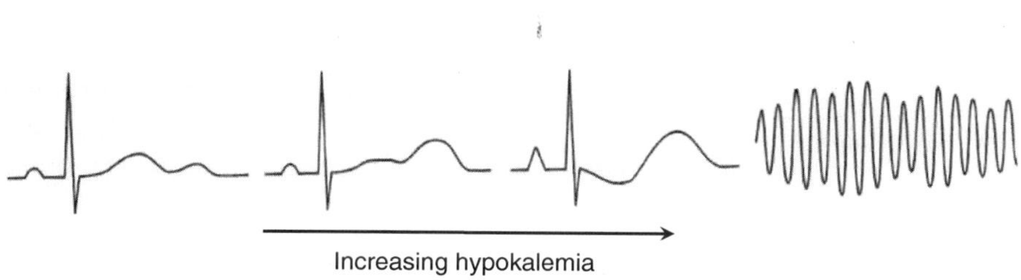

Fig. 3.8 ECG signs of hypokalemia

potassium losses allow to distinguish renal from nonrenal potassium losses. Additional biological exams such as plasma renin, aldosterone, or cortisol levels may be needed depending on the context.

3.5.2.2 Hypokalemias Due to Cell Transfer (Normal Total Body Potassium)

They result from similar mechanisms than hyperkalemia, but in the inverse direction. Potassium entry of K in the cell is usually transitory and responsible for moderate hypokalemias.

- *Hypokalemia secondary to a muscular exercise*: during a physical exercise, the release of endogenous catecholamines stimulates Na-K-ATPase pumps causing in turn the entry of potassium into the cells [2].
- *Drug-induced hypokalemia*: regardless of their mode of administration (inhalation or intravenous infusion), ß-adrenergic agonists may cause acute hypokalemia in a dose-dependent fashion (Fig. 3.2b). A sole dose of ß-adrenergic agonists can reduce kalemia of 0.36 mmol/L. Potassium entry into the cell which is stimulated by the activation of Na-K-ATPase pump is essentially located in the skeletal muscles. These abnormalities occur more frequently in pathologies associated with high concentrations in catecholamines such as in myocardial infarction, congestive cardiac insufficiency, or trauma patients [2]. These effects can also be present in patients with chronic renal insufficiency receiving inhaled ß-agonists leading to a possible decrease of kalemia which may reach 0.6 mmol/L [62]. ß1-Agonists such as dobutamine can also reduce kalemia of 0.5 mmol/L [3]. Theophylline and caffeine can be responsible of hypokalemia secondary to the stimulation of endogenous catecholamines. Insulin (± glucose) administration leads to similar effects. It is therefore essential to monitor closely kalemia when treating diabetic ketoacidosis or hyperglycemic hyperosmolar syndromes. In these situations, simultaneous potassium substitution is frequently needed rapidly to avoid the development of acute severe hypokalemia. Chloroquine and thiopental may cause hypokalemia by blocking the muscular potassium channels which in turn inhibit the efflux of potassium from muscular cells [2]. Hypokalemia can be observed in refeeding syndromes due to the reduction in Na-K-ATPase-driven pump. In this situation, hypokalemia is associated with moderate to severe hypophosphatemia.
- *Hypochloremic alkalosis*: the decrease in plasma chloride level favors the entry of potassium into the cell in order to maintain plasma electroneutrality [9, 15, 16, 56, 76].
- *Familial hypokalemic periodic paralysis or Westphal disease*: this is a familial dominant gene disease which is characterized by an abnormal membrane permeability. Such disorder conducts to acute hypokalemia. Clinical manifestations consist in flaccid paralysis crisis during several hours expressed by paraplegia or quadriplegia which are frequently triggered by a physical exercise or by a high-carbohydrate meal.

3.5.2.3 Hypokalemias Due to Low Exogenous Intake (Reduced Total Body Potassium)

The decrease in exogenous intake of potassium must be important (< 1 g/h) and cannot be responsible solely for a severe hypokalemia because renal excretion of potassium can decrease simultaneously to reach less than 15–25 meq/L. An insufficient potassium intake represents only a worsening factor associated with another cause of hypokalemia as in patients at risk (cardiac failure, hypertension, diabetes).

3.5.2.4 Hypokalemias Caused by Excessive Losses (Reduced Total Body Potassium)

Depending on urinary potassium excretion, it is possible to distinguish renal from extrarenal causes. The presence of arterial hypertension (AHT) and urinary chloride excretion is a useful data to determine the etiology (Fig. 3.9).

- *Hypokalemias related to extrarenal losses*: they are characterized by a low kaliuresis (< 20 meq/L), low chloruresis (< 10 meq/L), and no AHT. These hypokalemias can be due to high gastrointestinal losses as observed during profuse diarrhea, vomitings, intestinal fistula, villous adenoma, or digestive suctioning. In these situations, the mechanism of hypokalemia is frequently multiple due to the association of digestive and renal losses related to the secondary hyperaldosteronism. Laxative abuse or excessive administration of cation exchange resins enables to induce hypokalemia by increasing colonic potassium excretion [3]. When administered orally, the effect begins within the first 2 h to reach its maximum in 6 h. However, the hypokalemic effect is clinically relevant only in case of profuse diarrhea [4, 70].

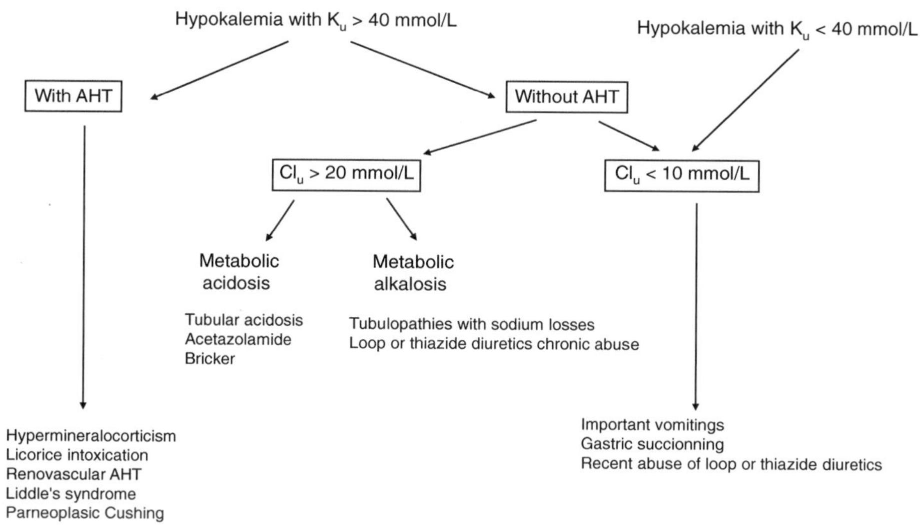

Fig. 3.9 Algorithm to determine the cause of hypokalemia. *AHT* arterial hypertension, *Clu* chloruresis, *Ku* kaliuresis

– *Hypokalemias related to renal losses*: they are characterized by a high kaliuresis >40 meq/L. The etiologic diagnosis is based on the presence or not of AHT and chloruresis.
  - Renal hypokalemias associated with AHT: the association of AHT, hypokalemia, and elevated urinary potassium expressed usually as endocrine abnormality is a primary hypermineralocorticism caused by an adrenal adenoma, a Conn's syndrome, or a Cushing's disease. The secondary hyperaldosteronism caused by a renal artery stenosis results from renovascular mechanisms of compensation: to maintain GFR despite the renal artery stenosis, the reduction of pressure of the afferent arteriole is associated with an increase of pressure of the efferent arteriole. Secondary hyperaldosteronism can also be iatrogenic caused by gluco- or mineralocorticoids. Massive intake of licorice conducts to similar manifestations. The glycyrrhizinic acid, which is a compound of licorice, inhibits the enzyme 11ß-hydroxysteroid dehydrogenase which allows to metabolize cortisol in cortisone. Thus, licorice permits cortisone to behave as a real mineralocorticoid leading to increase in urinary potassium excretion. AHT with hypokalemia, elevated kaliuresis, and low reninism can be due to mutations in genes encoding this enzyme. This is the case of "glucocorticoid-remediable aldosteronism." Congenital adrenal hyperplasia conducts to a loss of the 11ß-hydroxylase function which is responsible of the production of corticosterone, a precursor of aldosterone, by the glomerular zone of adrenal glands. The resulting blockade of aldosterone synthesis conducts to an increased synthesis of ACTH due to the overstimulation of the reticular zone of adrenal glands. The clinical presentation is an AHT associated with signs of virilization and low plasma levels of renin, aldosterone, and cortisol. The paraneoplastic Cushing's syndrome induces an overproduction of cortisol which leads to clinical signs of mineralocorticoids. The Liddle's syndrome is an acquired gene abnormality which consists in the activation of the renal epithelial sodium channel (ENaC). The resulting effect is the reabsorption of sodium associated with the potassium excretion (amiloride-like effect). This syndrome is present in children or teenagers and consists in AHT with urinary sodium reabsorption and low plasma levels of renin and aldosterone.
  - Renal hypokalemias without AHT: in these situations, chloruresis is also elevated (> 20 meq/L). These hypokalemias are mostly induced by renal pathologies and iatrogenic causes. A more precise diagnosis can be approached thanks to the presence of the association of hypokalemia with metabolic acidosis or alkalosis. Renal pathologies associated with metabolic alkalosis are caused by congenital tubulopathies with sodium losses among the collecting duct. They are usually diagnosed in adult patients with clinical manifestations of secondary hyperaldosteronism. On a pathophysiological point of view, Gitelman's syndrome consists in an inactivation of the gene encoding the NaCl thiazide-sensible cotransporter on the distal tubule, while Barter's syndrome corresponds to the inactivation of the gene encoding the type B chloride furosemide-sensible channel on the loop of Henle [77]. Gitelman's

syndrome associates preferentially hypomagnesemia and hypocalcemia, whereas Barter's syndrome associates hypercalcemia and normal magnesemia. Hypokalemias caused by loop diuretics and thiazides are the most common iatrogenic causes of hypokalemias [2, 51]. The severity of hypokalemia is dose-dependent and duration-of-treatment-dependent. Furosemide inhibits NKCC2 which is located in the ascending limb of the loop of Henle and in turn blocks sodium and potassium reabsorption: furosemide is natriuretic, kaliuretic, and diuretic. On the other hand, thiazides block chloride channels in the distal tubule. The presence of a metabolic acidosis suggests a treatment by acetazolamide (carbonic anhydrase inhibitor) or the diagnosis of renal tubular acidosis (RTA) type 1 (proximal) or type 2 (distal). RTA type 2 is characterized by an increased renal potassium excretion in response to the excessive load of sodium which is delivered in the tubule. In RTA type 1, sodium reabsorption through sodium channels of the apical membrane is compensated electrically by a simultaneous increase in potassium excretion.

- Other causes of hypokalemias due to renal losses: regardless of their causes, all osmotic polyurias can increase kaliuresis by increasing the distal urinary flow—hyperglycemia, mannitol infusions, and high doses of penicillin. Amphotericin B enables to induce real hypokalemias by stimulating urinary potassium excretion through the collecting duct [3]. Hypomagnesemia favors renal losses of potassium and may induce arrhythmias such as "torsades de pointes." At last, hypokalemias caused by renal removal therapies remain frequent and have been reported to be observed in more than 50% of patients [33, 78–80].

3.5.3 Treatments

The treatment of hypokalemia consists primarily of treating the specific cause (not developed in this chapter). Symptomatic treatment depends on the severity of hypokalemia and the related clinical and ECG manifestations, and an empirical approach remains common. Apart from hypokalemias resulting from transfers that are commonly transitory, the sole treatment consists of providing a supplementation [9, 71, 76, 81]. The consensual rule is to promote potassium intake orally over intravenously to provide a progressive elevation of plasma potassium level while decreasing side effects of the treatment [5, 46]. In all cases, iatrogenic causes must be stopped, and simultaneous treatments of favoring factors (hypomagnesemia) are needed. Patients presenting a mild asymptomatic hypokalemia require a simple oral supplementation by KCl (Diffu-K®, capsules of 8 mmoles; or Kaléorid®, tablets of 13.4 mmoles). Urgent treatment is needed in patients with symptomatic and ECG signs of hypokalemia. In this situation, potassium must be administered intravenously using chloride or gluconate potassium (various concentration of 7.46%, 10%, 15%, and 20%) with a dose of 1–2 g in 3–4 h. Life-threatening treatment required in case of arrhythmia is based on the intravenous infusion of potassium at a dose of 1–1.5 g per hour, without exceeding 2 g per hour. Additional doses can be administered until kalemia reaches 4 mmol/L. Despite the risk of vascular necrosis, such high doses can be infused through peripheral venous in case of absolute emergency. In other situations, infusion of potassium through a central venous is preferable. Intravenous magnesium sulfate at a dose of 5 g over 30 min is required in severe hypokalemia. At last, it is essential to monitor regularly ECG and plasma potassium levels.

Conclusion

Potassium is the second most abundant cation of total body. It plays major various physiological functions, especially the maintenance of the resting membrane potential which controls neuromuscular excitability thanks to the steady state of [Ki]/[Ke] ratio. There are two systems for controlling potassium homeostasis. The internal balance consists to maintain the asymmetric distribution of potassium between the intra- and the extracellular volume in order to maintain the potential of membrane. This phenomenon provides a short-term regulation of potassium. The external balance of potassium is essentially governed by the kidney. Aldosterone is the major hormonal mechanisms that regulate urinary potassium excretion. Only severe (profound or acute) dyskalemias can induce severe and life-threatening cardiovascular complications. Iatrogenic drug-related dyskalemias are very frequent as well as those induced by transfers. Hyperkalemias caused by inappropriate renal reabsorption can be observed in patients suffering renal insufficiency, hypovolemia, or primary and secondary hypoaldosteronism. The therapeutic strategy to manage hyperkalemia depends on its severity. Besides the emergent treatment, additional intermediate- and long-term treatments are needed to prolong the normalization of plasma potassium level. Hypokalemias can be caused by excessive intestinal or renal losses (hyperaldosteronisms). The symptomatic treatment of hypokalemia is based on a substitution preferentially administered orally when possible. In all cases, treating the underlying cause remains the most efficient and obligatory curative therapy of dyskalemias.

References

1. Perrone RD, Alexander EA (1994) Regulation of extrarenal potassium metabolism. In: Narins RG (ed) Maxwell & Kleeman's clinical disorders of fluid and electrolyte metabolism. Mc Graw Hill, New York, pp 129–145
2. Clausen T (2010) Hormonal and pharmacological modification of plasma potassium homeostasis. Fundam Clin Pharmacol 24:595–605
3. Buckley MS, Leblanc JM, Cawley MJ (2010) Electrolyte disturbances associated with commonly prescribed medications in the intensive care unit. Crit Care Med 38(suppl 6):S253–S264
4. Weisberg LS (2008) Management of severe hyperkalemia. Crit Care Med 36:3246–3251
5. Alfonzo AV, Isles C, Geddes C, Deighan C (2006) Potassium disorders-clinical spectrum and emergency management. Resuscitation 70:10–25
6. Gennari FJ (2002) Disorders of potassium homeostasis: hypokalemia and hyperkalemia. Crit Care Clin 18:273–288
7. Ichai C (2010) Dyskaliémies. In: Lehot JJ, Arvieux CC (eds) Réanimation et urgences. Spinger, Paris, pp 171–177

8. Guidon C (2011) Dyskaliémies de l'adulte. In: Encycl Med Chir Anesthésie-Réanimation, vol 36-860-A. Elsevier, Paris, p 15
9. Viera AJ, Wouk N (2015) Potassium disorders: hypokalemia and hyperkalemia. Am Fam Physician 92:487–495
10. Kovesdy CP (2015) Management of hyperkalemia: an update for the internist. Am J Med 128:1281–1287
11. Brown RS (1986) Extrarenal potassium homeostasis. Kidney Int 30:116–127
12. Weiner ID, Linus S, Wingo CS (2014) Disorders of potassium metabolism. In: Freehally J, Johnson RJ, Floege J, eds. Comprehensive clinical nephrology. St Louis (5th ed), Saunders: 118p
13. Mount DB, Zandi-Nejad K (2012) Disorders of potassium balance. In: Taal MW, Chertow GM, Marsden PA, Brenner BM (eds) The kidney, 9th edn. Elsevier, Philadelphia, pp 640–688
14. Gennari FJ (2011) Pathophysiology of metabolic alkalosis: a new classification based on the centrality of stimulated collecting duct ion transport. Am J Kidney Dis 58:626–636
15. Perez GO, Oster JR, Vaamonde CA (1981) Serum potassium concentration in academic states. Nephron 27:233–243
16. Magner PO, Robinson L, Halperin RM et al (1988) The plasma potassium concentration in metabolic acidosis: a re-evaluation. Am J Kidney Dis 11:220–224
17. Adrogué HJ, Madias NE (1981) Changes in plasma potassium concentration during acute acid-base disturbances. Am J Med 71:456–467
18. McDonough AA, Thompson CB, Youn JH (2002) Skeletal muscle regulates extracellular potassium. Am J Phys 282:F967–F974
19. Mount DB, Yu ASL (2007) Transport of inorganic solutes: sodium, chloride, potassium, magnesium, calcium, phosphorus. In: Brenner B (ed) Brenner and Rector's the kidney, 8th edn. Saunders, Philadelphia, pp 181–183
20. Malnic G, Giebisch G, Muto S, Wang W, Bailey MA, Satlin LM (2013) Regulation of K^+ excretion. In: Alpern RJ, Caplan MJ, Moe OW (eds) Seldin and Giebisch's kidney: physiology and pathophysiology. Academic, London, pp 1659–1716
21. Gurmz ML, Rabinowitz L, Wingo CS (2015) An integrated view of potassium homeostasis. N Engl J Med 373:60–72
22. Terker AS, Zhang C, McCormick JA et al (2015) Potassium modulates electrolyte balance and blood pressure through effects on distal cell voltage and chloride. Cell Metab 21:39–50
23. Ellison DH, Terker AS, Gamba G (2016) Potassium and its discontents: new insight, new treatments. J Am Soc Nephrol 27:981–989
24. Youn JH (2013) Gut sensing of K intake and its role in potassium homeostasis. Semin Nephrol 33:248–256
25. Juurlink DN, Mamdani MM, Lee DS et al (2004) Rates of hyperkalemia after publication of the randomized Aldactone evaluation study. N Engl J Med 351:543–551
26. Moore ML, Bailery RR (1989) Hyperkalaemia in patients in hospital. N Z Med J 102:557–558
27. Paice B, Gray JM, McBride D et al (1983) Hyperkalaemia in patients in hospital. Br Med J 286:1189–1192
28. Shemer J, Modan M, Ezra D, Cabili S (1983) Incidence of hyperkalemia in hospitalized patients. Isr J Med Sci 19:659–661
29. Ahmed J, Weisberg LS (2001) Hyperkalemia in dialysis patients. Semin Dial 14:348–356
30. Evans KJ, Greenberg A (2005) Hyperkalemia: a review. J Intensive Care Med 20:272–290
31. Acker CG, Johnson JP, Palevsky PM, Greenberg A (1998) Hyperkalemia in hospitalized patients: causes, adequacy of treatment, and results of an attempt to improve physician compliance with published therapy guidelines. Arch Intern Med 158:917–924
32. Sarafidis PA, Blacklock R, Wood E et al (2012) Prevalence and factors associated with hyperkalemia in predialysis patients followed in a low-clearance clinic. Clin J Am Soc Nephrol 7:1234–1241
33. Sedlacek M, Schoolwerth AC, Remillard BD (2006) Electrolytes disturbances in the intensive care unit. Semin Dialysis 19:496–501
34. McMahon GL, Mendu ML, Christopher KB (2012) Association between hyperkalemia at critical care initiation and mortality. Intensive Care Med 38:1834–1842

35. An JN, Lee JP, Jeon HJ et al (2012) Severe hyperkalemia requiring hospitalization: predictors of mortality. Crit Care 16:R225
36. Ponce SP, Jennongs AE, Madias NE et al (1985) Drug-induced hyperkalemia. Medicine 64:357–370
37. Aslam S, Friedman EA, Ifudu O (2002) Electrocardiography is unreliable in detecting potentially lethal hyperkalaemia in haemodialysis patients. Nephrol Dial Transplant 17:1639–1642
38. Crop MJ, Hoorn EJ, Lindemans J, Zietse R (2007) Hypokalaemia and subsequent hyperkalaemia in hospitalized patients. Nephrol Dial Transplant 22:3471–3477
39. Nyirenda MJ, Tang JI, Padfield PL, Seckl JR (2009) Hyperkalaemia. BMJ 339:b4114
40. Hoskote SS, Joshi SR, Ghosh AK (2008) Disorders of potassium homeostasis: pathophysiology and management. J Assoc Physicians India 56:685–693
41. Schaefer TJ, Wolford RW (2005) Disorders of potassium. Emerg Med Clin North Am 23:723–747
42. Pepin J, Shields C (2012) Advances in diagnosis and management of hypokalemic and hyperkalemic emergencies. Emerg Med Pract 14:1–17
43. Palmer BF, Clegg DJ (2015) Hyperkalemia. JAMA 314:2405–2406
44. Montague BT, Ouellette JR, Buller GK (2008) Retrospective review of the frequency of ECG changes in hyperkalemia. Clin J Am Soc Nephrol 3:324–330
45. Freeman K, Feldamn JA, Mitchell P et al (2008) Effects of presentation and electrocardiogram on time to treatment of hyperkalemia. Acad Emerg Med 15:239–249
46. Rose BD, Rennke HG (1995) Anomalies du bilan potassique. Chapitre 7. In: Physiopathologie des affections rénales et des désordres hydroélectrolytiques. L'essentiel. Pradel, Paris. 188–212
47. Ethier JH, Kamel KS, Magner PO, Lemann J Jr, Halperin ML (1990) The transtubular potassium concentration in patients with hypokalemia and hyperkalemia. Am J Kidney Dis 15:309–315
48. Berrebi R, Orban JC, Levraut J, Grimaud D, Ichai C (2009) Secondary hyperkalaemic acute flaccid tetraplegia. Ann Fr Anesth Reanim 28:381–383
49. Perazella MA (2000) Drug-induced hyperkalemia: old culprits and new offenders. Am J Med 190:307–314
50. Indermitte J, Burkolter SQ, Drewe J et al (2007) Risk factors associated with a high velocity of the development if hyperkalaemia in hospitalised patients. Drug Saf 30:71–80
51. Gennari FJ (1998) Hypokalaemia. N Engl J Med 339:451–458
52. Strivens E, Siddiqi A, Fluck R, Hutton A, Bell D (1996) Hyperkalaemic cardiac arrest: may occur secondary to misuse of diuretics and potassium supplements. Br Med J 313:693
53. Bosch X, Poch E, Grau JM (2009) Rhabdomyolysis and acute kidney injury. N Engl J Med 361:62–72
54. Martyn JAJ, Richtsfeld M (2006) Succinylcholine-induced hyperkalemia in acquired pathologic states. Anesthesiology 104:158–6940
55. Gronert GA, Theye RA (1975) Pathophysiology of hyperkalemia induced by succinylcholine. Anesthesiology 43:89–99
56. Faridi AB, Weisberg LS (2008) Acid-base, electrolytes and metabolic abnormalities. In: Parillo JE, Dellinger RP (eds) Critical care medicine: principles of diagnosis and management in adults, 3rd edn. Elsevier, Philadelphia, pp 1203–1243
57. Oster J, Singer I, Fishman L (1995) Heparin-induced aldosterone suppression and hyperkalemia. Am J Med 98:575–586
58. Canova CR, Fischler MP, Reinhart WH (1997) Effect of low-molecular weight heparin on serum potassium. Lancet 349:1447–1448
59. Elliott MJ, Ronksley PE, Clase CM, Ahmed SB, Hemmelgarn BR (2010) Management of patients with acute hyperkalemia. CMAJ 182:1631–1635
60. Sterns RH, Grieff M, Bernstein PL (2016) Treatment of hyperkalemia: something old, something new. Kidney Int 89:546–554
61. Mahoney BA, Smith WAD, Lo D, Tsoi K, Tonelli M, Clase C (2005) Emergency interventions for hyperkalaemia. Cochrane Data Base Syst Rev 2:CD 003235

62. Allon M, Takeshian A, Shanklin N (1993) Effect of insulin-plus-glucose infusion with or without epinephrine on fasting hyperkalemia. Kidney Int 43:212–217
63. Harel Z, Kamel KS (2016) Optimal dose and method of administration of intravenous insulin in the management of emergency hyperkalemia: a systematic review. PLoS One 11:e0154963
64. Nair S, Thomas E, Pearson SB et al (2005) A randomized controlled trial to assess the optimal dose and effect of nebulized albuterol in acute exacerbations of COPD. Chest 128:48–54
65. Chaitman M, Dixit D, Bridgeman MB (2016) Potassium-binding agents for the clinical mangement of hyperkalemia. PT 41:43–50
66. Mistry M, Shea A, Giguère P, Nguyen ML (2016) Evaluation of sodium polystyrene sulfonate dosing strategies in the inpatient management of hyperkalemia. Ann Pharmacother 50:455–462
67. Allon M (1995) Hyperkalemia in end-stage renal disease: mechanisms and management. J Am Soc Nephrol 6:1134–1142
68. Putcha N, Allon M (2007) Management of hyperkalemia in dialysis patients. Semin Dial 20:431–439
69. Evans K, Reddan DN, Szczech LA (2004) Nondialytic management of hyperkalemia and pulmonary edema among end-stage renal disease patients: an evaluation of the evidence. Semin Dial 17:22–29
70. Kamel SK, Wei C (2003) Controversial issues in the treatment of hyperkalaemia. Nephrol Dial Transplant 18:2215–2218
71. Cohn JN, Kowey PR, Whelton PK et al (2000) New guidelines for potassium replacement in clinical practice. Arch Intern Med 160:2429–2436
72. MacDonald JE, Struthers AD (2004) What is the optimal serum potassium level in cardiovascular patients? Nephrol Dial Transplant 43:155–611
73. Emmett M (2000) Non-dialytic treatment of acute hyperkalaemia in the dialysis patients. Semin Dial 13:279–280
74. Sacchetti A, Stuccio N, Panebianco P, Torres M (1999) Haemodialysis for treatment of renal failure emergencies. Am J Emerg Med 17:305–307
75. ECC Committee, sub-committees and task forces of the American Heart Association (2005) American Heart Association guidelines for cardiopulmonary resuscitation and emergency cardiovascular care. Part 10.1: life-threatening electrolyte abnormalities. Circulation 112 (suppl 24): IV121–IV125
76. Weir MR, Espaillat R (2015) Clinical perspectives on the rationale for potassium supplementation. Postgrad Med 127:539–548
77. Favre G, Orban JC, Ichai C (2009) Syndrome de Gitelman et syndrome de Bartter classique. In: Leone M (ed) Maladies rares en réanimation. Spinger, Paris, pp 277–280
78. Fall P, Szerlip HM (2010) Continuous renal replacement therapy: cause and treatment of electrolyte complications. Semin Dialysis 23:581–585
79. The renal replacement therapy study investigators (2009) Intensity of continuous renal-replacement therapy in critically ill patients. N Engl J Med 361:1627–1638
80. The VA/NIH acute renal failure trial network (2009) Intensity of renal support in critically ill patients with acute kidney injury. N Engl J Med 359:7–20
81. Paltiel O, Salakhov E, Ronen I (2001) Management of severe hypokalaemia in hospitalised patients. Arch Intern Med 161:1089–1095

Phosphate and Calcium Disorders

4

Carole Ichai

4.1 Introduction

Calcium and phosphate metabolisms are closely connected. Body function of calcium is double: the divalent cation form plays a major role in various cell functions. The association of calcium with phosphate induces the formation of hydroxyapatite crystals which provide the rigidity of bones. Independently of bone and calcium, phosphorus exerts several essential cell functions. The ionized form represents the major intracellular buffer. Phosphate and calcium homeostasis is essentially controlled by three hormones (parathormone, vitamin D, and calcitonin) which exert their effect on three targeted organs: bone tissue and intestinal and renal tubular cells. This chapter is focused on body distribution of calcium and phosphorus and their control. Clinical manifestations, diagnosis, and symptomatic treatments of phosphate and calcium disorders are reviewed.

4.2 Calcium in the Body

4.2.1 Body Distribution

The total amount of body calcium represents 1–1.3 kg in adults. The skeleton is the reservoir of calcium as 99% is stored in skeletal tissue and the remaining 1% in soft tissues (10 g) and extracellular fluids [1–4] (Fig. 4.1).

C. Ichai
Intensive Care Unit, Pasteur 2 Hospital, 30 Voie Romaine, 06001 Nice, Cédex 1, France

IRCAN (INSERM U1081, CNRS UMR 7284), University Hospital of Nice, Nice, France
e-mail: ichai@unice.fr

C. Ichai et al. (eds.), *Metabolic Disorders and Critically Ill Patients*,
http://doi.org/10.1007/978-3-319-64010-5_4

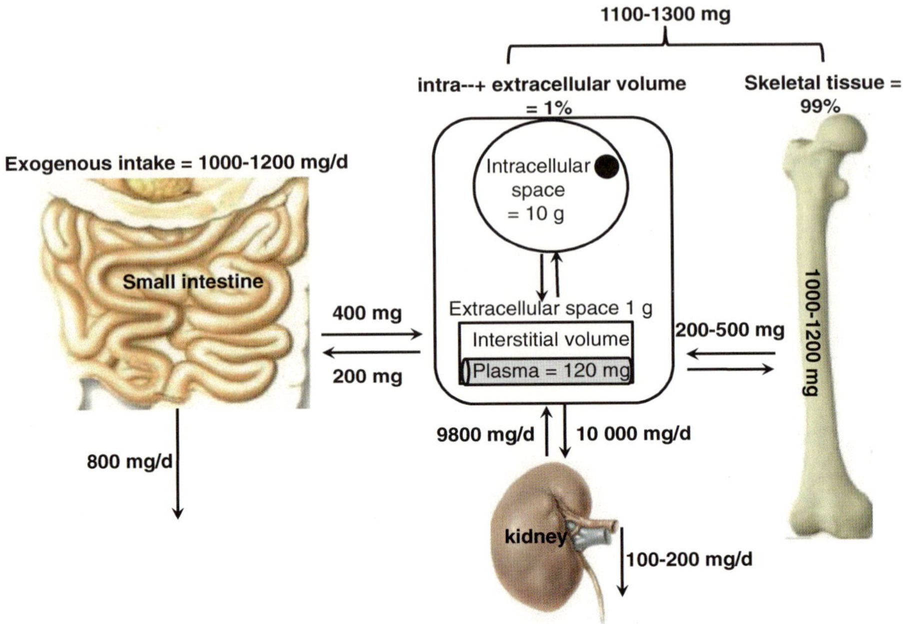

Fig. 4.1 Body calcium distribution and balance in a healthy adult. Daily exogenous intake of calcium represents 1000–2000 mg, among which approximately 400 mg are absorbed by the small intestine. The equilibrium of calcium balance is reached, thanks to an equivalent amount excreted in the feces and the urines (respectively, 800 mg and 100–200 mg daily). Calcium continuously exchanges between all body compartments, especially between the skeletal tissue and the extra- and intracellular spaces. 1 mmol of calcium = 40 mg of calcium

4.2.1.1 Skeletal Calcium

In bones, calcium is present for 69% in an inorganic form among which more than 90% are hydroxyapatite crystals and the remaining part is calcium carbonate crystals. Approximately 22% of calcium in the bone is present in an organic form with 90% being collagen, and the remaining 10% enters in the composition of structural proteins such as proteoglycans and glycoproteins. Only 200–500 mg of this calcium which is located at the surface of the bone is freely exchangeable with the extracellular compartment and allows the process of mineralization of the organic matrix of bone (see paragraph "skeletal metabolism").

4.2.1.2 Extracellular Calcium

Extracellular calcium is distributed almost in an equivalent concentration between the interstitial and plasma volume. Normal total serum calcium concentration (calcemia) is 8.8–10.4 mg/dL (2.2–2.6 mmol/L). It breaks down in diffusible into the cells and filtrated at the glomerulus (60%) and nondiffusible (40%) calcium (Fig. 4.2) [1–3, 5]:

- *Ultrafilterable blood calcium* includes ionized and complexed calcium. Ionized calcium (iCa) represents the most abundant form: 50% of total serum

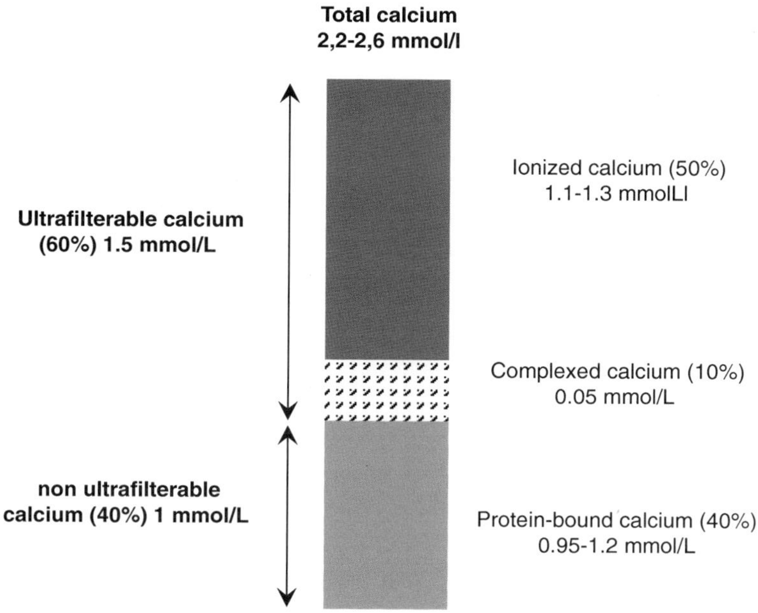

Fig. 4.2 Distribution of total plasma calcium. Total plasma calcium is distributed for 60% in ultrafilterable calcium (50% as an ionized form and 10% as a complexed form) and for 40% in protein-bound non-ultrafilterable form

calcium and 85% of the diffusible serum calcium. iCa varies according to the serum calcium concentration, pH, protidemia, and polyvalent anions: acidosis decreases the protein bound leading in turn to increase the proportion of the ionized form, whereas alkalosis and elevated serum anions concentration reduce it. The ionized component of calcium is qualitatively the most important as it represents the active biologic form. It is therefore the regulated component that maintains calcium homeostasis. Complexed calcium which is linked to counterions such as phosphate, bicarbonate ($CaHCO_4^{2-}$), sulfate, and citrate ions represents 10% of serum calcium and 15% of ultrafilterable calcium.

- *Non-ultrafilterable blood calcium* accounts for 40% of total calcemia and is bound to plasma protein. Eighty percent is bound to albumin and the remaining 20% to globulins (alpha-, ß-, and γ-globulins). Therefore, it is essential to take into account serum albumin concentration to interpret total calcemia: in case of hypoalbuminemia, calcemia decreases and conversely, but the ionized form remains unchanged and consequently without any clinical impact. Total calcemia can be corrected by taking into account albuminemia, using the following formula: $Ca_{corrected}$ (mM) = $Ca_{measured} - 0.025 \times$ (albuminemia – 40 [g/L]).

4.2.1.3 Intracellular Calcium

The intracellular concentration of calcium is approximately 0.1 μmol/L. Calcium is stored in cell membranes, sarcoplasmic and endoplasmic reticulums, and mitochondria. Thanks to active transporters, a flux of calcium ions allows to maintain gradient of concentration between mitochondria, cytosol, and the extracellular fluid, with rapid exchanges between these three compartments [1–3]. Therefore, the intracellular concentration of calcium depends at the same time of the influx, the efflux, and the mitochondrial and sarcoplasmic reticulum storage of calcium. Calcium enters passively in the cells, thanks to transmembrane voltage-dependent calcium channels which create an electrochemical gradient. The efflux of calcium must be performed against this gradient and consequently requires energy which is provided by ATP issued from the Ca^{2+}-ATPase pump or from the Na^{+} gradient promoted by the Na^{+}/Ca^{2+}exchanger. Intracellular calcium plays a major role of second messenger involved in multiple intracellular pathways for message transmission.

4.2.2 Calcium Balance

4.2.2.1 Needs and Supply

Exogenous calcium intake represents approximately 1 g/day in adults. Daily needs vary according to age and physiological modifications (pregnancy, menopause) and reach 400–1000 mg/day in adults (1000 mg/day in children and pregnant women). Considering the obligatory digestive losses, a minimal dietary intake of 10 mg/kg/day (0.25 mmol/kg/day) is needed to maintain an equilibrium between the entry and the output of calcium in adults (Fig. 4.1). The gastrointestinal absorption of calcium is performed essentially in the proximal digestive tract including the duodenum, the jejunum, and ileum [1, 2, 4, 6]. The major part of absorbed calcium comes from intestinal secretions (800 mg). Its proportion varies according to the intake, between 10 and 15% with a normal calcium diet, without high limit due to a passive diffusion. Therefore, an oral intake of 1 g calcium will be associated with an excretion of approximately 800 mg in the feces. The absorbed dietary calcium enters in the extracellular fluid and is further incorporated into the skeleton. Calcium reabsorption is performed by a transcellular pathway through the cell. It crosses the apical microvillar membranes of enterocytes, thanks to calcium epithelial channels which are "transient receptor potential vanilloid" (TRPV) 5 and 6. Inside the enterocyte, calcium binds to calbindin proteins allowing to move calcium to the basal membrane and to protect the cell from the toxic effect of high calcium concentrations. The efflux of calcium from the basolateral membrane toward blood is mainly performed by two systems: a Ca^{2+}-ATPase pump which shows a decreasing activity along the small intestine and a Na^{+}/Ca^{2+} exchanger (NCX1) which is activated by the Na^{+}-K^{+} ATPase pump (Fig. 4.3). A paracellular pathway allows a passive calcium reabsorption through "tight junctions" whose opening/closing is controlled by some proteins (claudins, occludins) that are synthetized by adjacent cells [5]. Calcium

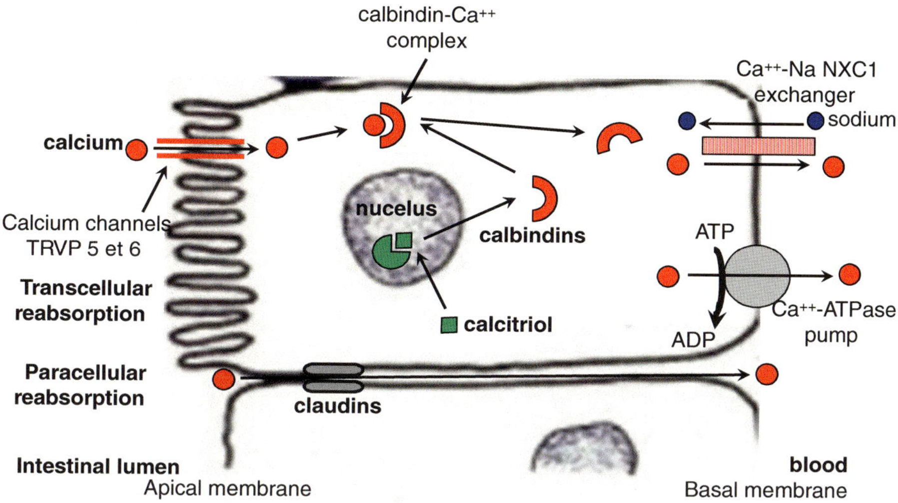

Fig. 4.3 Mechanisms of intestinal calcium reabsorption. This reabsorption is performed by two mechanisms: The first one is an active transcellular reabsorption; calcium enters into the intestinal epithelial cells along the microvilli, thanks to transmembrane calcium epithelial channels, the "transient receptor potential vanilloid or TRVP." Intracellular calcium bounds then to proteins, the calbindins, to create a calcium-calbindin complex which allows the transport of calcium to the basal membrane. The extrusion of calcium through the basal membrane is performed, thanks to a sodium-calcium exchanger (NXC-1) or a Na-K-ATPase pump. This phenomenon is activated by calcitriol. The second one is a passive paracellular reabsorption: calcium crosses tight junctions using claudins, structural protein membranes, which conduct to open the pathway

intestinal absorption is stimulated by 1,25-dihydroxycholecalciferol (1,25$(OH)_2D_3$ or calcitriol) the active form of vitamin D, parathormone (PTH), and growth and gonadal hormones. On contrary, it is inhibited by corticoids, thyroxin, calcitonin (CT), and age [7, 8].

4.2.2.2 Calcium Excretion

Calcium losses are essentially performed by the kidney, less by the intestinal tract, and for a very small amount by skin. The amount of calcium eliminated by the intestinal tract represents the sum of the non-absorbed dietary intake and the calcium issued from the secretions of saliva, gastric juice, bile, and pancreatic juice. This represents a quantity of approximately 800 mg/day (Fig. 4.1). The kidney is the most important organ involved in calcium homeostasis. It regulates urinary calcium excretion, thanks to the metabolization of the inactive into the active form of vitamin D [1, 3, 9]. Around 10 g of free calcium is filtered in the glomerulus per day, and 98% of it is reabsorbed, leading to a final urinary excretion of 100–200 mg/day. Sixty to 70% of calcium is reabsorbed in the proximal convoluted tubule, 20% in the ascending limb of the loop of Henle, 5–10% in the distal convoluted tubule under the control of PTH, and 5% in the collecting tube [3, 10, 11]. Mechanisms responsible for the transfer of calcium in the kidney are similar to those existing in the intestinal tract (Fig. 4.4). The absorption of calcium in the proximal convoluted tubule and the loop of Henle is performed for 80% by passive diffusion (paracellular and transcellular pathways). This phenomenon is favored by an electrochemical force which is produced by both the Na-K- 2Cl (NKCC2) cotransporter of the apical membrane and the potassium channel "renal outer medullary potassium, ROMK" which is the limiting parameter. Na^+ and Cl^- which in turn accumulate in the cell are therefore reabsorbed through the basal membrane, thanks to the Na-K-ATPase pump and chloride channels. The passive paracellular transport of calcium becomes possible, thanks to the positive potential of the membrane. On the proximal convoluted tubule, such a passive paracellular reabsorption is also modulated by calcium receptors (CaSR) which are located on basal membranes. The activation of CaSR stimulates the expression of some constitutive proteins of calcium channels (claudins) of paracellular tight junctions. This phenomenon closes these channels and inhibits the passive reabsorption of calcium. Ten to 15% of calcium is actively reabsorbed in the proximal convoluted tubule and the thick ascending limb of the loop of Henle (Fig. 4.4A). On the distal convoluted tubule, calcium is actively reabsorbed against an electrochemical gradient. This phenomenon is produced by three successive steps: apical

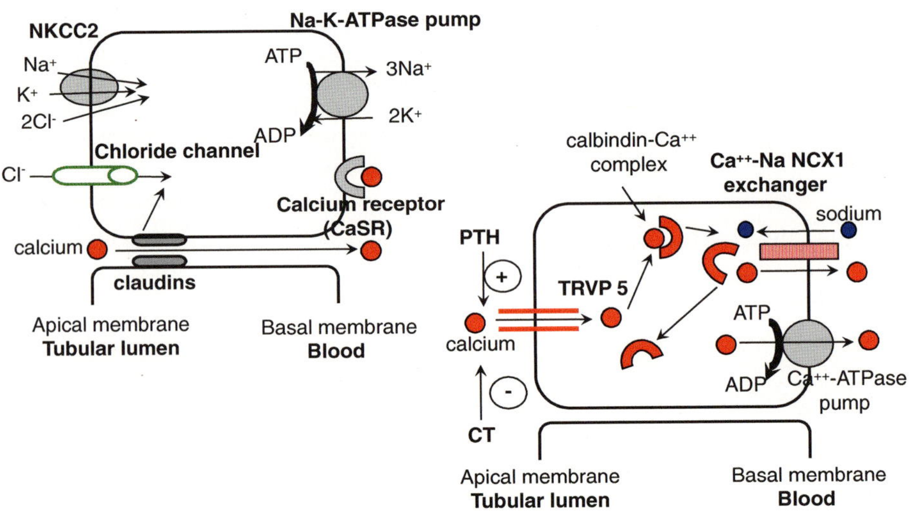

Fig. 4.4 Mechanisms of renal calcium reabsorption. A: *Reabsorption in the ascending limb of the loop of Henle.* Calcium reabsorption is essentially performed passively through the paracellular tight junctions pathway, thanks to claudins which are activated by the calcium-sensing receptors (CaSR) located in the basolateral membrane, leading to open the pathway. Calcium reabsorption can be performed also by sodium-potassium, NKCC2 cotransporters and by chloride channels located in the apical membrane, thanks to an electrogenic gradient which favors the calcium transport. B: *Reabsorption in the distal convoluted tubule.* Transient receptor potential vanilloid 5, TRVP5, which is located in the apical membrane of renal epithelial cells, allows the calcium intracellular reabsorption; the intracytosolic transport needs the formation of calcium-calbindins complexes; the extrusion of calcium is performed in the basolateral membrane using the sodium-calcium NXC1 exchanger and the Ca^{++}-ATPase pump

transmembrane reabsorption through the epithelial calcium channels TRVP 5, intracytosolic calcium diffusion induced by binding with calbindin proteins, and then calcium extrusion through the basal membrane by the sodium-calcium NCX1 exchanger and the calcium-ATPase transporter (Fig. 4.4B). Parathormone (PTH) and active vitamin D stimulate calcium reabsorption on the thick ascending limb of the loop of Henle and above all on the distal convoluted tubule, whereas calcitonin inhibits it. Urinary excretion varies according to the sex (more elevated in male) and the circadian rhythm.

4.2.3 Biological Functions of Body Calcium

Calcium is implicated in many cell functions: muscular excitability-contractility coupling; automatic cardiac contractility; neurotransmission; endocrine and exocrine secretion of hormones; gene expression; mitotic division; integrity, permeability, and stability of cell membranes; and second messenger of various signal transduction pathways. Moreover, this cation is essential for activating multiple calcium-dependent enzymatic reactions, including the coagulation cascade [1, 3, 12]. At last, calcium plays a major role in determining the skeletal structure and bone mineralization.

4.3 Phosphorus in the Body

4.3.1 Phosphorus Distribution

Phosphorus is an essential component of skeleton and the most abundant intracellular anion. The total amount of body phosphorus represents 600–800 g in an adult of 70 kg. Phosphorus is present in two forms: organic and inorganic [3, 4, 13]. Phosphates, the inorganic forms, are bound to proteins or complexed to other ions such as calcium ($CaHPO_4$) and magnesium ($MgHPO_4$) or free as orthophosphates (H_3PO_4, $H_2PO_4^-$, HPO_4^{2-}). Most of phosphorus, approximately 85% (550–600 g), is present in skeleton as hydroxyapatite (Fig. 4.5) [4, 11–14]. The remaining 15% is distributed among extraskeletal sites, essentially in the cells of soft tissues, as lipids, proteins, and nucleic acids components. The extracellular compartment is less than 1% of total body phosphorus. Plasma phosphorus amount represents 120 mg which are distributed for 2/3 as organic phosphorus such as phospholipids (85 mg) and the remaining 1/3 as phosphates. Ten percent of plasma phosphates are bound to proteins and therefore non-ultrafilterable. The other 90% exists as a diffusible ionized form (Fig. 4.6). Because of its pK (6.8), blood phosphate presents in two forms of orthophosphates, $H_2PO_4^-$ and HPO_4^{2-}. When plasma pH is normal, the divalent form HPO_4^{2-} is two times greater than the monovalent one. The determination of serum phosphorus concentration relates only to the inorganic fraction and is therefore serum phosphate or phosphatemia. It is commonly accepted that 1 mmol of phosphate is equivalent to 320 mg. The normal serum phosphate concentration is comprised between 0.8 and 1.15 mmol/L. This concentration is physiologically

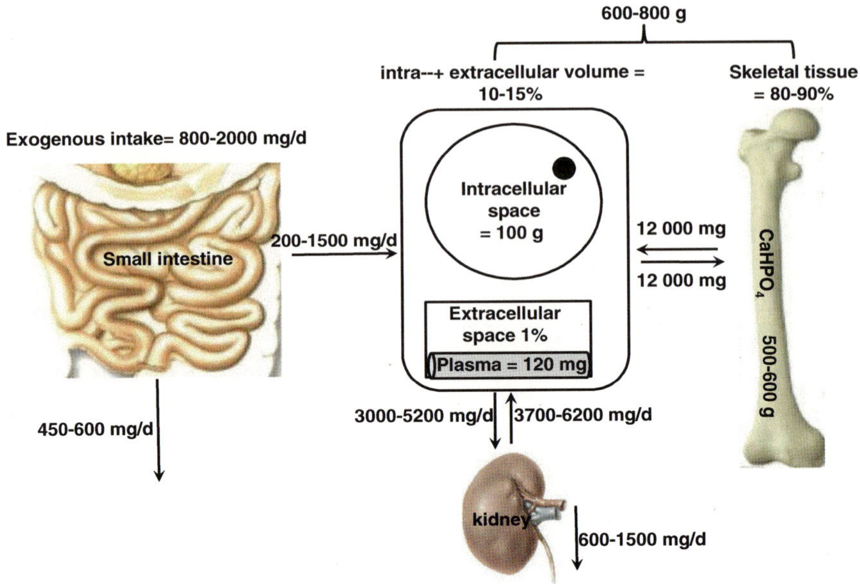

Fig. 4.5 Body phosphorus distribution and balance in a healthy adult. Daily exogenous intake of phosphate represents approximately 800–2000 mg among which 200–1500 mg is absorbed in the grelic intestine. Phosphate homeostasis is reached, thanks to an equivalent renal excretion of 600–1500 mg. Phosphate exchanges continuously between the different body compartments, especially the skeletal tissue and the intra- and extracellular spaces. 1 mmol of phosphate = 320 mg of phosphate

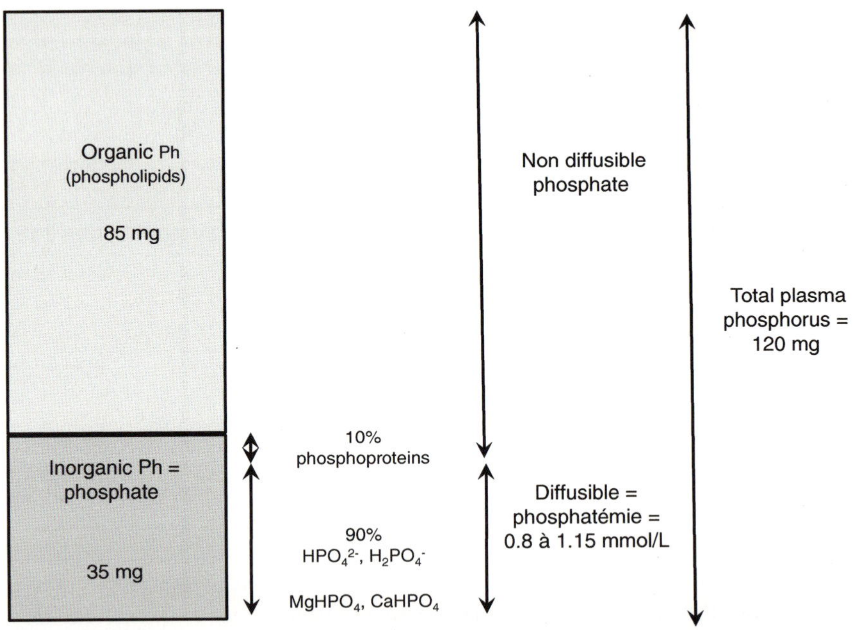

Fig. 4.6 Distribution of total plasma phosphorus. Total plasma phosphorus is distributed for 66% in organic phosphorus which is bound to lipids and for 34% in inorganic phosphorus, i.e., phosphate. Among plasma phosphate, 90% represents the ionized diffusible form

higher in infants and children and then decreases over the life. Other factors that enable to induce variations in phosphatemia are the circadian cycle (higher concentration between 8 am and 8 pm), food intakes, and acute transports between the extra- and the intracellular spaces.

4.3.2 Phosphate Transporters

All movements of phosphate between the different body compartments are performed, thanks to transporters: intestinal reabsorption toward the plasma, transports between the extra- and the intracellular fluids, transports between the skeleton and the intracellular fluid, and renal excretion-reabsorption [13–21]. These systems are transepithelial proteins which are located on the apical renal brush border membrane and which associate a sodium-phosphate (Na/Pi) cotransport. In the same time, sodium transmembrane gradient is maintained, thanks to the Na-K-ATPase pump. Three types of phosphate membrane transporters are described (Table 4.1) [17, 19]. Type 1, called NPT1, is a nonspecific anion transporter of phosphate. NPT1 is expressed in the apical side of cells from the proximal convoluted tubule of kidneys and liver. Its role in the phosphorus balance is not clearly established. Type 3 cotransporters present in two forms: phosphate 1 and 2 sodium-dependent transporters, called PiT1 and PiT2, respectively (Fig. 4.7). These proteins are largely expressed in many tissues which show a high affinity for phosphate. This suggests their preferential role in controlling the amount of intracellular phosphate, rather than in the global regulation of phosphorus homeostasis. These transporters might be involved in the pathophysiology of vascular or tissue calcifications.

Table 4.1 Characteristics of major phosphate cotransporters

Cotransporter	Location	Characteristics	Effects on phosphate
Type 1			
NPT1	Proximal convoluted tubular cells	Nonspecific anion transport	Probably low
Type 2			
NPT2a	Proximal convoluted tubular cells	Strong affinity for phosphate, saturable $3\ Na^+/1\ HPO_4^{2-}$	Regulation of renal phosphate reabsorption (target of PTH and FGF-23)
NPT2b	Lung, small intestine	$2\ Na^+/1\ H_2PO_4^-$	Regulation of intestinal phosphate absorption
NPT2c	Proximal convoluted tubular cells	$2\ Na^+/1\ H_2PO_4^-$	Decrease with age
Type 3			
PiT1 PiT2	Large expression in numerous tissues	Strong affinity for phosphate	Intracellular amount of phosphate, extraskeletal calcifications

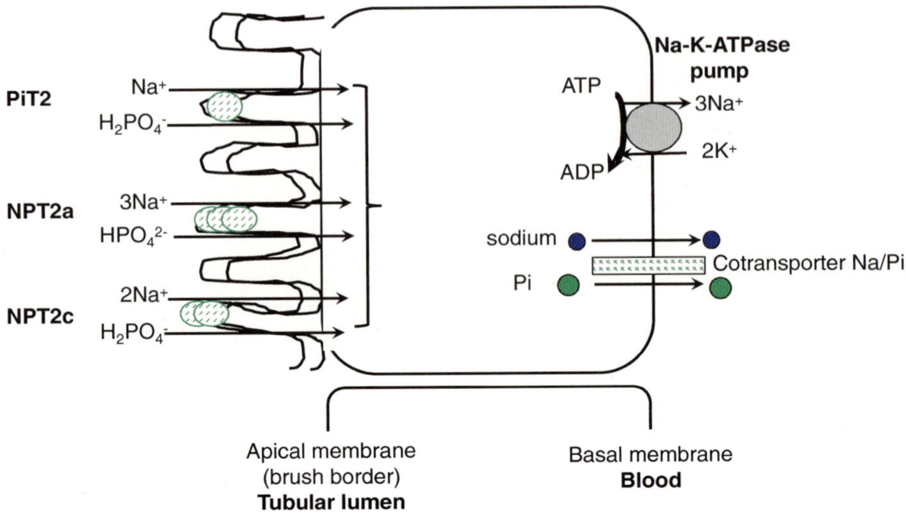

Fig. 4.7 Schematic representation of major phosphate cotransporters in tubular renal cells. Sodium-phosphate NPT2a and NPT2c (and incidentally PiT2) cotransporters are responsible for phosphate movements across renal cells. Their activation requires to be expressed on the brush border of tubular cells located on the apical side. The entry of sodium in the cell is possible, thanks to a persistent transmembrane gradient of sodium which is created by the Na-K-ATPase pump located in the basal membrane (and may be other Na/Pi cotransporters)

Type 2 cotransporters are expressed as three isoforms: NPT2a, NPT2b, and NPT2c. NPT2b is largely expressed in the lungs and small intestine [3, 6, 18, 19]. It plays a substantial role in phosphate reabsorption by these organs and induces an electroneutral transport of two Na^+ with one HPO_4^{2-}. Its renal expression remains minor, explaining that in case of genetic mutations, tissue calcifications (pulmonary) may be present without any abnormality in phosphatemia. NTP2a and NTP2c have a similar affinity for phosphate. They are exclusively expressed on the brush border membranes of the proximal convoluted tubule cells. Both forms assure an electrogenic transport, but their characteristics differ. NTP2a is characterized by a cotransport of three Na^+ with one HPO_4^{2-}. They are saturable so that there is a maximal threshold of phosphate reabsorption by the kidney (TmPi). Therefore, the number of NPT2 determines the capacity of proximal renal reabsorption of phosphate. If TmPi exceeds this threshold, phosphaturia will appear and will increase linearly with hyperphosphatemia. NPT2c cotransport associates two Na^+ with one HPO_4^{2-} and is therefore neutral electrogenic transport. Their expression decreases with age. On the basal side of the membrane, the transport of phosphate remains unclear and is probably associated with the Na-K-ATPase pump or an anion/phosphate type 3 cotransporter (PiT).

4.3.3 Phosphate Balance

There are many exchanges and movements of phosphate between the different body compartments. More than 3000 mg per week of skeletal phosphate is exchanged with the extra- and the intracellular spaces. These exchanges are performed at a slower rate than those between the intra- and the extracellular compartments. Therefore, phosphatemia is not always well correlated with the total body phosphate amount. Several factors activate phosphate transmembrane transports. By this way, they control the internal balance of phosphate, leading to modifications in intracellular and plasma concentrations. Insulin, glucose, variations in pH, and catecholamines activate the entry of phosphate in the cells leading to hypophosphatemia. Plasma phosphate follows three pathways: entry in the intracellular pool, component of the skeletal and soft tissues, and excretion mainly performed by the kidney [2, 4]. Despite its very low concentration in plasma (only 1% of its total amount in the body), phosphatemia is closely regulated to maintain a normal value which is essential to exert all of its cellular, structural (skeleton, membranes), and muscular functions.

The external balance of phosphate is physiologically equilibrated in healthy adults (Fig. 4.5). Needs represent approximately 1000 mg/day (800–2000 mg/day) and are essentially provided by the daily dietary intake. Approximately 65–75% of phosphate contained in food is absorbed in the small intestine (mainly jejunum) and is mediated by the NTP2b membrane transporters which are located on the apical and the basal sides of enterocytes. There are two routes for this phenomenon: a passive diffusion which is proportional to the digestive supply and an active sodium cotransport which requires energy [1, 3]. This active reabsorption is favored by a concomitant low absorption of phosphate issued from diet and by calcitriol. On the other hand, excessive intake of calcium and magnesium decreases the enteral reabsorption of phosphate. The kidney plays the major role in regulating the external balance of phosphorus [3, 10, 17]. In physiological situation, renal excretion of phosphate equals its intestinal absorption and consequently maintains serum phosphate concentration in a normal range [9, 21]. Approximately 5000 mg/day (3000–5200 mg/day) of phosphate unbound to proteins is filtered in the glomerulus. Eighty to 85% of this filtered load occurs within the proximal convoluted tubule leading to a net urinary excretion of phosphate of 600–1500 mg/day. Three types of transporters are involved in this reabsorption: NTP2a (electrogenic), NTP2c (neutral), and the PiT2 (electrogenic) (Fig. 4.7) [3, 22]. Renal proximal reabsorption is saturable (TmPi) and active requiring energy. Therefore, the amount of phosphate which is excreted by the kidney depends on serum phosphate concentration and on glomerular filtration rate (GFR) [11, 13, 14, 22]. TmPi/DFG ratio (mmol/L or mg/L) represents the threshold of phosphatemia below which all the filtered phosphate is reabsorbed and above which it is totally excreted. The normal value of TmPi/DFG ratio is approximately 0.70 mmol/L. This parameter allows to distinguish renal from extrarenal causes of phosphatemia disorders [11].

4.3.4 Biological Functions of Body Phosphate

Phosphate is among the most abundant anion of body [1, 4]. It is one of the components of nucleic acids and of membrane lipids (phospholipids). It is involved in the protein transduction pathways and in many enzymatic and coenzymatic activities.

It is also a major component of ATP energetic substrates (ADP and AMP). Phosphate is needed for glycolysis, gluconeogenesis, and ammoniogenesis and influences hemoglobin dissociation by regulating the concentration of 2,3-diphosphoglycerate (2,3-DPG). Finally, ionized phosphate is the major intracellular buffer (pK = 7.21).

4.4 Regulation of Phosphate and Calcium Homeostasis

Regulation of phosphate and calcium metabolism is performed, thanks to three major organs: kidneys, digestive tract, and skeleton. The regulation is based on the control of calcium and phosphate cotransporters functioning which is under the influence of extrinsic and intrinsic hormonal and gene factors.

4.4.1 Hormonal Regulation

The hormonal control of calcium and phosphate homeostasis is the critical regulating mechanism [2, 3, 12, 21]. Besides the very classical vitamin D, PTH, and calcitonin, more recent data have emphasized the implication of additional hormones such as fibroblast growth factor 23 (FGF-23) and other phosphatonins which act to tightly control phosphate range. All of these hormones exert their effects on targeted kidneys, digestive tract, and skeleton. The integrated and concomitant action on these three organs allows to provide a permanent control of calcium and phosphate metabolism (Table 4.2). This led to emphasize the concept of the hormonal regulation by the skeleton-intestinal tract-kidney axis (Figs. 4.8 and 4.9) [2, 3, 10].

4.4.1.1 Hypercalcemic Hormones

- *Vitamin D3* or cholecalciferol is a steroid that is produced endogenously in the skin. It is synthetized from the metabolite 7-dehydrocholesterol which is produced by the skin from cholesterol to become 25(OH)D_3 under the influence of ultraviolet radiations (UVB). This metabolite represents the major circulating form of vitamin D, and therefore its serum concentration is the most accurate indicator of the body storage of vitamin D. To become active, vitamin D3 requires further metabolism which consists of two successive hydroxylations. The first one is performed in the liver, thanks to the 25-hydroxylase leading to the production of calciferol or 25(OH)D_3. This hormonal form serves as paracrine/autocrine function in skin, immune cells, and intestinal epithelium, but it is essentially converted in the proximal renal tubule by the 1-α hydroxylase. This second hydroxylation conducts to the production of the major hormonal active form of vitamin D, the 1,25$(OH)_2D_3$ or 1,25-dihydroxycalciferol or calcitriol. This production is closely regulated through the renal 1-α hydroxylase activity by PTH, FGF-23, calcemia, and phosphatemia. The production of calcitriol is stimulated by a low serum concentration of vitamin D, hypocalcemia, hypophosphatemia, and a poor diet in phosphate [1–3]. Most of vitamin D and its metabolites are carried in the blood bound to vitamin D binding protein (DBP) and albumin. The

Table 4.2 Mechanisms of action and effects of major hormones responsible for calcium and phosphate metabolism

	Intestinal tract	Bone tissue	Kidney
Active vitamin D (1,25-dihydroxycalciferol = calcitriol) = hypercalcemic and hyperphosphatemic hormone			
Effects	• **Increased calcium and phosphate reabsorption**	• Indirect increased bone resorption (*via* PTH) • Reduction in bone mineralization	• *Increased renal reabsorption of calcium and phosphate*
Targets	**Duodenum, proximal jejunum**	• Osteoblasts • Osteoclasts	• *Distal convoluted tubule and collecting tube*
Parathormone (PTH): hypercalcemic and hypophosphatemic hormone			
Effects	• *Indirect increased* calcium and phosphate *reabsorption (via vitamin D)*	• Increased bone resorption	• **Increased calcium renal reabsorption**
Targets	*Duodenum, proximal jejunum*	• Osteoblasts	• **Distal (calcium) and proximal convoluted tubule (phosphate)** • Collecting tube, proximal convoluted tubule, and ascending limb of the loop of Henle
Calcitonin = hypocalcemic and hypophosphatemic hormone			
Effects		• Reduction of bone resorption	• **Inhibition of renal phosphate reabsorption** • Reduction of calcium renal reabsorption
Targets		• Osteoclasts	• **Distal and proximal convoluted tubule and collecting tube (phosphate)** • Distal and proximal convoluted tubule and collecting tube (calcium)
Phosphatonin FGF-23 = hypophosphatemic hormone			
Effects		• *Indirect increased bone demineralization (via vitamin D)*	• **Inhibition of renal phosphate reabsorption**
Targets		• *Osteoclasts*	• **Proximal convoluted tubule**

Bold text indicate the most important location and effects of the hormones

free substrate only enters in most tissues [23]. A second form of vitamin D, the vitamin D2, is also available and is issued from an exogenous diet intake and comes from the ergocalciferol which is produced by ultraviolet radiations of plants. Approximately 75% of the ingested exogenous vitamin D (cholecalciferol and ergocalciferol) is absorbed by the small intestine in the presence of biliary salts and is subsequently carried by chylomicrons in the lymphatic system

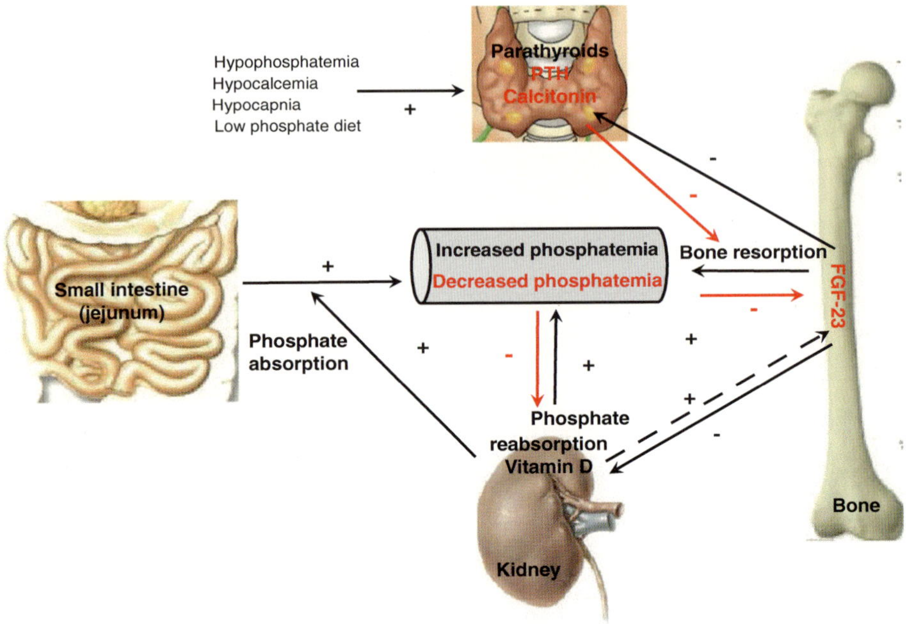

Fig. 4.8 Regulation of phosphatemia via the intestine-bone-kidney axis. Active vitamin D exerts a global hyperphosphatemic effect. It stimulates phosphate intestinal (in the jejunum) absorption and phosphate release from bone by a permissive action on parathormone (PTH) and inhibits its tubular renal excretion. The synthesis of PTH induced essentially by hypocalcemia exerts globally a hypophosphatemic effect: it promotes phosphate renal excretion (phosphaturia) as a result of an increased action of the renal 1α-hydroxylase which induces an activation of vitamin D and bone resorption and essentially inhibits proximal tubular phosphate reabsorption. FGF-23 which is synthetized in the skeletal tissue exerts a global hypophosphatemic effect. FGF-23 which is released in response to hyperphosphatemia or to an increase in vitamin D strongly inhibits phosphate renal reabsorption and indirectly intestinal absorption by reducing vitamin D synthesis (inhibition of renal 1α-hydroxylase). FGF-23 also inhibits PTH release which in turn allows to control phosphatemia

and finally in blood. Half-life of calcitriol is approximately 5 h. It is catabolized by a 24-hydroxylase enzyme, inactivated in calcitroic acid by liver glucurono-conjugation, and eliminated essentially in the biliary tract. Vitamin D need in healthy situations is 600–800 IU, and blood concentration is 20–30 ng/mL.

Globally, vitamin D provides a hypercalcemic and hyperphosphatemic effect. This is the principal hormone that stimulates calcium and phosphate intestinal absorption by modifying the structure and functions of enterocytes which are responsible at last of the calcium and phosphate cotransporters. Vitamin D exerts its effects after binding to its receptor (VDR) which is located in the nucleus and present on various tissues. The intranuclear binding of vitamin D activates a transduction pathway which conducts to the effects on the targeted organs [24]. Vitamin D increases the intestinal absorption of calcium (essentially in the proximal portion of the small

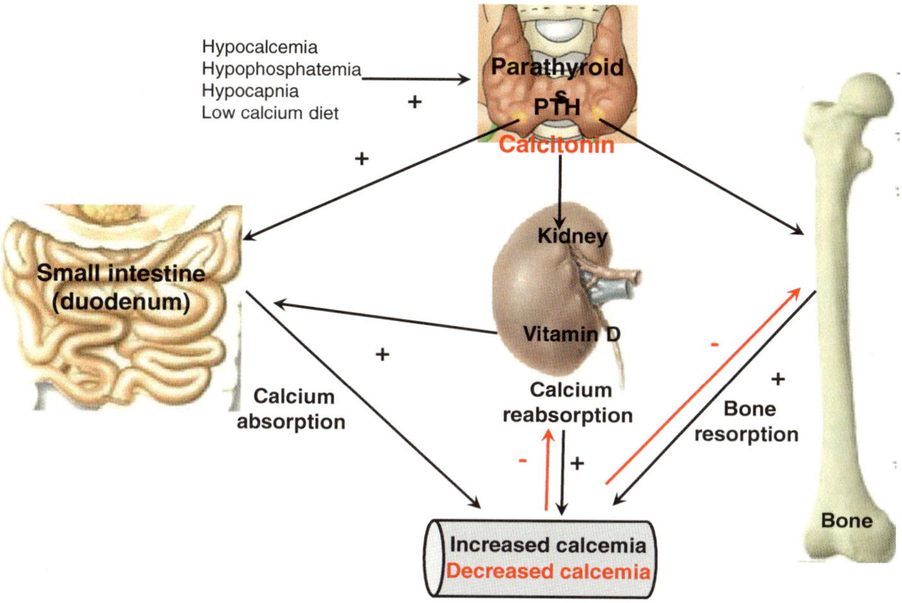

Fig. 4.9 Regulation of calcemia via the intestine-bone-kidney axis. Active vitamin D exerts a global hypercalcemic effect. It stimulates calcium intestinal (duodenum) absorption and indirectly calcium release from bone resorption by a permissive action on parathormone (PTH). Vitamin D also stimulates the renal proximal tubule reabsorption of calcium, but this phenomenon is minor in the control of calcemia homeostasis. Calcitonin is the physiological antagonist hormone of PTH. It exerts a global hypocalcemic effect by reducing calcium release from bone and by increasing calcium renal reabsorption (increased calciuria)

intestine) by activating rapidly and directly the expression of the TVRP 5 and 6, present in the brush border of the intestinal cells. Vitamin D also elevates slowly this intestinal absorption of calcium by increasing the synthesis of intracellular proteins that transport calcium, the calbindins D (Fig. 4.3) [6]. The intestinal paracellular absorption of calcium is also stimulated by vitamin D. However, the digestive absorption of calcium is only efficient if the amount of ingested vitamin D is sufficient. Vitamin D activates the absorption of phosphate essentially in the duodenum and the jejunum by stimulating the transmembrane cotransporters NPT2b. On bones, it favors mineral resorption by activating osteoclasts and indirectly by exerting a permissive effect on PTH, the final effect being a release of calcium and phosphate from bones [24]. This increases also the production of collagen by osteoblasts and the production of carboxy-glutamic which favors the skeleton mineralization, thanks to a greater intestinal reabsorption of calcium. Its role for regulating calcium and phosphate is important and can also lead sometime to bone mineralization [24, 25]. The role of vitamin D on bone is finally to maintain skeletal homeostasis against modifications of phosphate and calcium balance. Vitamin D stimulates the active transcellular reabsorption of calcium and phosphate in the renal distal tubule, but this action remains minor to regulate the metabolism of phosphate and calcium (Table 4.3):

Table 4.3 Most important parameters enabled to modify renal reabsorption of calcium and phosphate

Increase in renal reabsorption	Reduction in renal reabsorption
Calcium	
• Parathormone • Calcitriol (vitamin D) • Hypocalcemia • Hypovolemia • Metabolic alkalosis • Thiazide diuretics	• Hypercalcemia • Hypervolemia • Metabolic acidosis • Loop diuretics • Growth hormone (GH)
Phosphate	
• Low vitamin D or phosphate diet • Vitamin D • Hypophosphatemia • Thyroid hormones • Metabolic alkalosis	• Parathormone • Calcitonin • Phosphatonins (FGF23) • Rich-phosphate diet • Glucocorticoids, estrogens • Metabolic acidosis • Deficit in potassium • Dopamine

FGF-23 fibroblast growth factor 23

- *Parathormone (PTH)* is an 84-amino acid peptide which is initially synthetized by the parathyroid glands as an inactive prehormone (115 amino acids) and released further as the active hormonal form. Its half-life is 4 min, and it is metabolized in inactive peptides and eliminated by kidneys and biliary secretion. PTH release from parathyroid glands is regulated by serum calcium concentration through a transcriptional and a non-transcriptional pathway; hypocalcemia stimulates PTH secretion. In parathyroid cells, variations in calcemia are detected by membrane calcium-sensing receptors (CaSR) which transmit the message to modify the synthesis of PTH. Acute hypocalcemia is responsible for a very rapid response within some minutes, whereas prolonged hypocalcemia increases the mass of the gland [17, 26]. Hypercalcemia and 1,25-dihydroxyvitamin D exert a negative feedback on PTH and activate its metabolization. Other parameters also enable to stimulate this secretion such as glucocorticoids, estrogens, hyperkalemia, and hypomagnesemia. PTH is the most important regulator of calcium homeostasis [3, 7, 8]. PTH exerts its effects by binding to its receptor which is a transmembrane glycoprotein located on the basolateral membrane. The PTH-PTH-R1 complex activates successive mechanisms of transduction including the activation of cAMP, C phospholipase/C and A protein kinases synthesis. PTH is the major hormone allowing to control renal excretion of calcium by reducing its clearance: in presence of PTH, the reabsorption of calcium increases in the collecting tube, the ascending limb of the loop of Henle, and the proximal convoluted tubule (Fig. 4.4; Table 4.3). In the same time, phosphate reabsorption in the proximal convoluted tubule is reduced. The mechanism by which phosphate is excreted by kidney is based on the action of NPT2a and secondarily NPT2c cotransporters (Fig. 4.7). To work correctly, these NPT2s require to be located and expressed on the brush border of tubular cells [17, 18]. Besides the presence

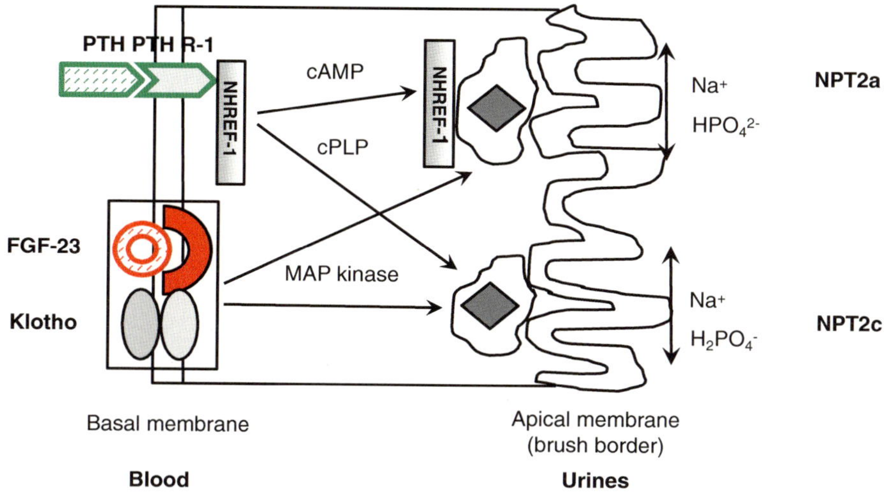

Fig. 4.10 Mechanisms of action of parathormone (PTH) and fibroblast growth factor 23 (FGF-23) on phosphate cotransporters in the proximal renal tubules. PTH and FGF-23 activate phosphaturia by inhibiting the action of NPT2a and NPT2c cotransporters, thanks to their internalization from the brush border membrane to subapical intracytoplasmic vesicles. PTH binds to its receptor. The PTH-PTH-R1 complex activates transduction messages: phospholipase and C protein kinase pathways deactivate NPT2c; cAMP and A protein kinases pathways deactivate NPT2a. This last effect needs a bind to another cofactor, the sodium-hydrogene-exchanger 1 (NHERF-1) allowing a partial bind to the PTH-PTH-R1 complex, and also to NPT2a. To exert its phosphaturic action, FGF-23 requires to be associated with its cofactor Klotho in a complex formed by the association of FGF-23-FGF-23 receptor with Klotho-Klotho-receptor. This large complex activates a MAP kinase signaling pathway which in turn deactivates NPT2a and NPT2c

of PTH, the preferential location of NPT2 on the renal brush border membrane (active form for reabsorption) or conversely inside vesicles of the apical submembrane (inactive form for reabsorption) needs the presence of another factor, the sodium-hydrogen-1 exchanger (NHERF-1). After binding to the PTH-R1 receptor and to NPT2a cotransporter, NHERF-1 inactivates phosphate renal reabsorption which is promoted by NPT2a and by NPT2c, thanks to the activation of C phospholipase (Fig. 4.10). In bone tissue, PTH stimulates osteoclasts to mobilize calcium and phosphate. PTH also increases indirectly the intestinal reabsorption of phosphate and calcium by stimulating the 1-α hydroxylase which allows the active synthesis of calcitriol in the renal proximal convoluted tubule. Considering all of these effects, PTH acts as a hypercalcemic and hypophosphatemic hormone and is still the major hormone that regulates calcium metabolism, while its role in phosphate metabolism is less important.

- *Parathyroid hormone-related peptide (PTHrP)* are proteins of approximately 150 amino acids issued from the hydrolysis of a prehormone by convertases. They are synthetized by various normal or tumoral tissues: bone, cartilage, smooth muscle, breast, skin, and parathyroid gland [12, 27]. They provide their effect after binding to the PTH receptors, but they have a paracrine action. The effects of PTHrP on kidneys and the skeleton are similar to those observed with PTH, i.e., hypercalcemia. When PTHrP is secreted in large amount by malignant tumors, an abnormal hypercalcemia develops due to the excessive skeleton resorption which is related to the activation of PTH receptors located on the osteoblasts.

4.4.1.2 Hypocalcemic Hormone: Calcitonin

Calcitonin (CT) is a 32-amino acid polypeptide with a half-life of less than 15 min. Its secretion by the parafollicular cells of the thyroid is regulated essentially by iCa: an increase in serum calcium concentration stimulates its secretion and conversely. Other molecules can stimulate CT secretion: catecholamines via their ß-adrenergic effect, glucagon, gastrin, and magnesium which act by increasing the concentration of cAMP of parafollicular cells. CT is a hypocalcemic and hypophosphatemic hormone because of its decreasing effect on the skeletal catabolism and its stimulating effect of phosphate excretion by kidneys (Table 4.2) [1, 2, 4, 7]. This is the sole hormone that acts directly on the osteoblast by favoring an important but transitory binding of calcium on bone; in the same time, CT reduces bone resorption. These effects lead to a reduction in calcium release from bone and in turn to hypocalcemia. CT represents the physiological antagonist of PTH. Hypophosphatemic effects of CT result from comparable mechanisms on bone catabolism. CT increases urinary excretion of calcium and phosphate, but these effects remain minor compared to the skeleton effect.

4.4.1.3 Hypophosphatemic Hormones: Phosphatonins

Real hypophosphatemias related to an excessive phosphaturia without any hyperparathyroidisms are reported in tumoral pathologies with osteomalacia. These observations strongly support that apart PTH, other factors exert a phosphaturic effect. Since more than 10 years, phosphaturic hormones, called phosphatonins, have been identified in patients presenting renal losses of phosphate. The most common is the fibroblast growth factor 23 (FGF-23) [13, 15, 20, 28]. This hormone formed by 252 amino acids is synthetized by osteoblasts and osteoclasts when phosphatemia, calcitriol, or oral ingestion of phosphate increase. To exert its phosphaturic and hypophosphatemic effects, FGF-23 needs a double bond with its FGF-R1 receptor which is located in the basal membrane of distal convoluted tubule cells and with its protein cofactor Klotho. A FGF-23-Klotho-FGF-R1 complex creates (Fig. 4.10) [13, 17, 28]. This complex triggers a MAP kinase-dependent transduction which induces a reduction in the expression of NPT2A and NPT2c and at a lower level of PiT2 of the brush border of proximal tubular cells [19, 20]. FGF-23 also stimulates bone demineralization and inhibits the synthesis of calcitriol by decreasing the activity of the renal 1-α hydroxylase. In the absence of the cofactor Klotho, FGF-23 is unable to regulate phosphatemia and vitamin D metabolism. FGF-23 inhibits also directly the secretion of PTH and its synthesis by parathyroids. In summary, FGF-23 is really a major hormone that regulates phosphate metabolism with an integrated action on the kidney-bone-intestinal axis (Table 4.2; Fig. 4.9) [13, 15, 20].

4.4.1.4 Other Hormones

Other hormonal factors can regulate calcium and phosphate balances (Table 4.3) [1–3, 7]:

- *Thyroid hormones*, in cooperation with vitamin D, favor calcium reabsorption in the small intestine and bone resorption leading to hypercalcemia. Therefore, hyperthyroidism may induce osteoporosis. Thyroid hormones can be also responsible for hyperphosphatemia by stimulating proximal tubular reabsorption of phosphate secondary to a transcriptional increased number of NPT2a cotransporters.
- *Glucocorticoids* have a low global impact on calcemia as they inhibit bone formation by binding to specific receptors which decrease the differentiation of osteoblast precursors while favoring bone resorption. On the other hand, glucocorticoids are hypophosphatemic because they decrease renal proximal tubular reabsorption of phosphate by reducing the synthesis and number of NPT2a cotransporters.
- *Estrogens* are implicated to maintain the skeletal mass. They reduce bone resorption by the osteoclasts and stimulate the secretion of CT and the synthesis of the active vitamin D. They provide hypophosphatemia because of a decrease in the NPT2a cotransporters of the renal proximal convoluted tubule.
- *Growth hormone* (GH) acts locally by controlling the growth factor called somatomedin C or insuline-like-1 growth factor (IGF-1) which enables to increase bone formation. Its action on phosphate and calcium metabolism remains limited to the bone remodeling. The hyperphosphatemic and hypocalcemic effect remains minor despite the stimulation of digestive and renal reabsorption of phosphate.

4.4.2 Nonhormonal Regulation

4.4.2.1 Calcemia, Phosphatemia, and Calcium and Phosphate Diet [3, 4]

High serum concentration of calcium and high oral intake of calcium increase renal calcium excretion by PTH-dependent and PTH-independent mechanisms. The independent one is related to the increased filtered calcium amount in the glomerulus, leading by a negative feedback to reduce renal tubular reabsorption of calcium. Hypocalcemia provides the inverse effects. Low serum concentration of phosphate and calcium and a poor diet of phosphate stimulate the intestinal and renal reabsorption of phosphate by increasing the number of NPT2 cotransporters on the brush border of proximal tubular cells [29]. A prolonged low oral intake of phosphate for 8 days increases the ADN transcriptional synthesis of NPT2. Conversely, a high exogenous load in phosphate, hyperphosphatemia, and hypercalcemia inhibit renal tubular phosphate reabsorption (Table 4.3).

4.4.2.2 Acid-base Disorders

Metabolic acidosis enables to induce hypocalcemia by increasing its renal excretion, independently of the PTH action. It stimulates phosphaturia aiming to buffer urines and correct metabolic acidosis. On contrary, metabolic alkalosis induces hypercalcemia and hyperphosphatemia (Table 4.3).

4.4.2.3 Volemia and Arterial Hypertension

Hypovolemia reduces renal excretion of calcium (sodium and chloride) as a result of regulating mechanisms of volemia, especially those induced by the renin-angiotensin-aldosterone system. Arterial hypertension decreases renal reabsorption of phosphate by reducing the number of NPT2a cotransporters (Table 4.3).

4.4.2.4 Drugs

Loop diuretics decrease renal reabsorption of calcium due to their inhibiting effect on the NKCC2 cotransporters located on the ascending limb of the loop of Henle. On contrary, thiazides provide a hypocalcemic effect. At last, dopamine stimulates renal excretion of phosphate by reducing the number of NPT2a cotransporters (Table 4.3).

4.5 Skeletal Metabolism

Skeleton ensures three major physiological functions: mechanic (locomotion), metabolic (calcium and phosphorus reservoir), and hematopoiesis. The bone tissue, which is the real reservoir of body, consists of an extracellular matrix. The latter is essentially made of an organic framework produced by bone cells (organic phase) on which phosphate and calcium crystals settle (mineral phase) [8, 25]. Bone mineral is present in two forms in the skeleton: cortical bone (80%), the major reservoir of calcium (850 g), and trabecular bone (spongy bone) located on the large exchanging surfaces with the plasma compartment. Bone which contains 99% of total body calcium is a dynamic tissue with permanent remodeling: approximately 1% of stored calcium can be rapidly mobilized to be exchanged with the extracellular space. It participates largely (jointly with the small intestine and the kidney) to control calcium and phosphate metabolism.

4.5.1 Organic Phase

The organic phase represents approximately 30% of the skeleton dry weight and is essentially composed of type 1 collagen (90%) which consists of an alpha peptide chain containing glycine, proline, hydroxyproline, lysine, hydroxylysine, and a fundamental substance made of mucoproteins, chondroitin, and hyaluronic acid sulfates. Hydroxyproline is eliminated by urines and appears as a good marker of bone resorption. The association of three alpha peptide chains constitutes a helicoidal heteropolymer, the tropocollagen, which forms fibrils containing calcium crystals in nucleus sites. The polymerization of these fibers leads to a first spatial conformation in beams followed by successive layers of lamellae and a concomitant formation of covalent intermolecular bond between collagen fibers. Non-collagenic proteins, including osteocalcin and phosphoproteins such as osteonectin, insert calcified collagen. These proteins are secreted by the osteoblasts and are predominantly involved in calcium homeostasis and in osteogenesis [1, 5].

4.5.2 Mineral Phase

The mineral phase is mostly constituted by hydroxyapatite crystals which are composed of calcium and phosphate [$Ca_{10}(PO_4)_6(OH)_2$] [1]. All of these crystals represent an important surface of ion exchanges with the extracellular compartment. Therefore, the skeleton constitutes the reservoir of body calcium, which is available according to the modifications in the extracellular composition (formation or dissolving of hydroxyapatite crystals), thanks to the activation of osteoclasts.

4.5.3 Cells

The skeleton alternates bone within basic multicellular units. These structural units are composed of two populations of cells with opposite activities aiming to perform bone remodeling: osteoclasts and osteoblasts. Osteoclasts, issued from monocytes-macrophages, induce bone resorption by destructing the extracellular matrix of calcium [2]. The activity of osteoclasts, measured by hydroxyprolinuria, is the fundamental phenomenon of bone resorption: it acts both on skeletal growth and repair and on the regulation of calcium-phosphate metabolism. Osteoblasts issued from the conjonctive stroma of bone marrow synthetize type 1 collagen and non-collagenic proteins of the extracellular matrix. During the mineral phase, they initiate the deposition of calcium crystals (apatite crystals) in the nucleus sites of tropocollagen fibrils. The action of osteoblasts is reflected by the serum concentration of alkaline phosphatases.

4.5.4 Regulation of Bone Homeostasis

The equilibrium between the formation and the resorption of bone allows the regulation of skeletal remodeling. This constant remodeling is controlled by a hormonal regulation which is dependent of the action of PTH, vitamin D, and prostaglandin E_2 on osteoblasts and by a nonhormonal regulation. During resorption, osteoclasts secrete H^+ protons and lysosomial enzymes; this conducts to the development of Howship's lacunas in the trabecular bone and Harvers channels in the cortical bone. Monocytes and macrophages complete this resorption by digesting residues and release growth factors. During the formation phase, osteoblasts produce new bone tissue.

The hormonal regulation of bone and cartilage is dependent on the PTH-vitamin D axis, calcitonin, estrogens, and glucocorticoids. Calcitonin inhibits transitory skeletal resorption by reducing the proliferation and maturation of osteoclasts *via* cAMP. PTH and estrogens are involved in the differentiation of osteoclasts by acting on osteoblasts: indeed, these cells express a ligand on their surface, the RANK-L (*receptor activator of nuclear factor* x*B ligand*), and secrete a glycoprotein, the osteoprotegerin [2, 30]. The OPG/RANK-L ratio is essential for regulating this metabolism. Estrogens increase this ratio leading in turn to activate osteoblasts and finally bone formation. PTH reduces this ratio, activates osteoclasts, thanks to cytokines secreted by osteoblasts, and inhibits the synthesis of bone collagen. At last, it favors renal activation of $1,25(OH)_2D_3$. Vitamin D stimulates the synthesis of the matrix, alkaline phosphatases, bone proteins (among which osteocalcin), and the fusion of osteoclasts. It has also an indirect effect on skeletal cells by inhibiting the proliferation of T-cells and the production of cytokine IL2. Glucocorticoids have a complex effect on osteoblasts by decreasing their multiplication as a result of the reduction of IGF-1 synthesis, by increasing the effect of PTH on osteoblasts, and by reducing the synthesis of various cytokines. The global effect of glucocorticoids on bone is rather the consequence of a decrease in protein synthesis and in the intestinal absorption of calcium.

The nonhormonal regulation involves various factors such as age, weight loss, physical inactivity, bed rest or prolonged immobilization, zero gravity (reduction of the skeletal mass), and serum concentration in inorganic phosphate (increase in formation and decrease in resorption in case of elevated concentration). Bone accretion is favored by a local elevation of calcium and phosphate amount. Conversely, in situations associated with low intake of calcium (postmenopausal period), bone calcium mobilization increases and bone calcium pool decreases (osteoporosis). The mobilization of skeletal calcium is evaluated by measuring calcium/urinary creatinine ratio (normal <15 μg/mg) and hydroxyproline/creatinine ratio (normal <25 μg/mg). At last, many local factors (prostaglandins, cytokines, growth factor) modulate the activity of osteoclasts and osteoblasts of bones.

4.6 Calcium Disorders: Definitions and Clinical Presentations

4.6.1 Hypocalcemia

4.6.1.1 Definition and Epidemiology

Total hypocalcemia is defined by a serum concentration level < 2.2 mmol/L (<8.8 mg/dL). Because only iCa is the active biological form, hypocalcemia is considered mostly by this concentration and is defined by a serum level < 1.1 mmol/L (4.4 mg/dL). It is considered to be mild between 0.9 and 1.1 mmol/L (3.6–4.4 mg/dL) and severe below 0.9 mmol/L (<3.6 mg/dL) [31]. In all cases, it is important to eliminate false hypocalcemia by correcting total calcemia with albuminemia. The frequency of hypocalcemia in emergency departments and ICUs highly varies from

18 to 88%, depending on the threshold considered and on the type of patients [32–35]. In a retrospective trial performed in the emergency department and including a total of 8270 patients, hypocalcemia was found in 29.6% of patients [36]. Mild hypocalcemia has been reported to be very frequent in ICU patients, up to 90% of patients, while severe hypocalcemia was uncommon occurring in 2–3% of them [37]. Hypocalcemia is independently associated with an increased mortality (HR = 2) and an increased morbidity (longer in-ICU and in-hospital stay, higher severity of patients) [31, 36, 37]. There is a negative relationship between the frequency of hypocalcemia and the severity of critically ill patients, especially for severe hypocalcemia. Mortality rate increases with the severity of critically ill patients: 22%, 40.4%, and 53.9% with an APACHE score < 10, between 10 and 19 and >19, respectively [32]. However, the real impact of hypocalcemia on mortality is not demonstrated and remains debated. Steele et al. [31] support this as they showed that 55.2% of critically ill patients presented hypocalcemia on admission; among them only 6.2% were severe and showed longer ICU stay without any difference in mortality rate. Most of these patients normalized their calcemia within 4 days. Mortality was higher in those who failed to correct their serum calcium concentration. In ICU, hypocalcemia results from multifactorial causes: impaired calcium homeostasis due essentially to vitamin D deficiency or secondary hypoparathyroidism, inflammation and sepsis, and iatrogenic origin related to medication or technique side effects (catecholamines, blood transfusion, regional citrate anticoagulation) [38–40].

4.6.1.2 Clinical Manifestations

Hypocalcemia-related symptoms are nonspecific. Clinical presentation of hypocalcemia depends on the severity, duration, and rate of development of hypocalcemia [41–43]. Chronic mild hypocalcemia is usually asymptomatic or pauci-symptomatic and well tolerated. The diagnosis is therefore incidentally discovered on laboratory findings. Most signs are sneaky and include:

- Neurologic signs: seizures, paresthesias, headache, anxiety, cognitive and neuropsychiatric dysfunctions, impaired vision, confusion, central irritability, extrapyramidal signs, abnormal movements (Parkinson syndrome)
- Ectodermal signs: dry skin, brittle nails, alopecia, dental abnormalities, psoriasis, atopic eczema
- Respiratory and gastrointestinal signs: laryngospasm, bronchospasm, epigastric pain, dysphagia, biliary colic, all of them being caused by smooth muscle dysfunction

Acute and severe hypocalcemias are usually symptomatic and a life-threatening condition which requires an emergent treatment. Clinical symptoms are characterized by neuromuscular and cardiovascular signs as follow:

- Neuromuscular manifestations: neuromuscular irritability expressed by tetany, Chvostek or Trousseau sign, muscle weakness and cramps

- Cardiovascular manifestations: dyspnea, edema, syncopes, hypotension, palpitations, congestive heart failure, dysrhythmias such as prolonged corrected QT interval (exacerbated by hypomagnesemia)

4.6.2 Hypercalcemia

4.6.2.1 Definition and Epidemiology

Hypercalcemia is defined by a total calcium serum concentration level > 2.65 mmol/L (>10.6 mg/dL). However, it is also important to eliminate false hypercalcemia related to changes in albuminemia, and at least calcemia must be corrected taking into account albuminemia. Be aware of falsely elevated calcemia observed in case of hyperalbuminemia and conversely of false total hypercalcemia due to low serum albumin levels. Therefore it is strongly suggested to measure directly iCa which is considered to be elevated if >1.3 mmol/L (>5.3 md/dL). Severe hypercalcemia is defined by a serum level of total calcium >3 mmol/L (>12 mg/dL). Hypercalcemia remains an uncommon disorder in emergency situations. Sauter et al. [36] have reported that only 2% of patients admitted at the emergency department presented hypercalcemia. In this population, hypercalcemia was found to be an independent risk factor for mortality, but the role of hypercalcemia is not proved as hypercalcemia was frequently associated with cancer. The prevalence of hypercalcemia in ICU depends on the threshold and the severity of the disorder: from 8% in medicosurgical critically ill patients (iCa >1.27 mmol/L) [44] to 15% in surgical critically ill patients (iCa >1.33) [45]. In both studies, there was no difference in mortality rate between patients with normo- and hypercalcemia. Recently, Egi et al. [37] confirmed that hypercalcemia was uncommon in medicosurgical ICU (2–3% of patients). Severe hypercalcemia (iCa >1.4 mmol/L) was found in 0.24% of them and was only found as an independent risk factor of mortality.

4.6.2.2 Clinical Manifestations

Symptoms of hypercalcemia are not specific and can be associated with the causal disorder. The presence of clinical manifestations depends on the rapidity of the onset and the severity of hypercalcemia. Hypercalcemia impacts essentially on four organ systems: neuromuscular and psychiatric, gastrointestinal, cardiovascular, and renal functions, leading to the famous mnemotechnic sentence "bones—stones—groans, and psychic moans" [5, 12, 41, 46].

Acute and rapid hypercalcemia is commonly symptomatic and is manifested by:

- Neurocognitive manifestations: depression, confusion, stupor, insomnia, headache, seizures, altered mental status, coma
- Gastrointestinal manifestations: anorexia, nausea, vomitings, pancreatitis, epigastric pain,
- Cardiovascular manifestations: shortened QT interval (due to a decrease in the potential of action), ventricular fibrillation, ST segment abnormalities, first degree atrioventricular block, bradycardia
- Renal manifestations: nephrogenic diabetes insipidus with polyuria (hypercalciuria) responsible for volume depletion and intracellular dehydration, distal renal tubular acidosis

Chronic hypercalcemia presents frequently with insipidus signs or is incidentally discovered on a laboratory exam. Clinical presentation includes:

- Neurocognitive manifestations: memory loss, fatigue, leukoencephalopathy, behavioral disturbances, weakness, bone and muscle pains, fractures, arthralgia
- Gastrointestinal manifestations: dyspepsia, constipation
- Cardiovascular: arterial hypertension, valvular calcifications
- Renal manifestations: nephrolithiasis, nephrocalcinosis (due to hypercalciuria), chronic renal failure

4.7 Phosphate Disorders: Definitions and Clinical Presentations

4.7.1 Hypophosphatemia

4.7.1.1 Definition and Epidemiology

Hypophosphatemia is defined by a serum concentration < 0.65 mmol/L (<25 mg/L). It is considered as moderate between 0.32 and 0.65 mmol/L and as severe below 0.32 mmol/L [4, 11, 47, 48]. The incidence or prevalence of such disorders is highly variable, depending on the cause of hypophosphatemia and on the type of patient. Mean prevalence of moderate in-hospital hypophosphatemia is between 2.2 and 3.1% and is 0.2–0.4% for severe hypophosphatemias [13, 49, 50]. The incidence in ICU varies from 17.3 to 67% in critically ill surgical patients [51] and from 6 to 75% in critically ill medical patients [52–54]. Hypophosphatemia occurs within the first days caused in 80% of ICU patients by renal losses, especially in patients with unaltered renal function [55]. Such a high variability is probably due to the threshold of serum phosphate level considered as abnormally low: an incidence of 100% has been reported in the literature in the postoperative period of hepatic surgery [56] or after renutrition in ICU [57, 58] when hypophosphatemia is defined by a threshold below 0.80 mmol/L. The risk of hypophosphatemia also increases in some pathologies such as diabetic ketoacidosis [59] and sepsis [60], in the postoperative period of hepatic or cardiac surgery [51, 56], in trauma patients [52], or during continuous renal replacement therapies [61–63]. Hypophosphatemia is associated with an increased risk of morbi-mortality. In case of severe hypophosphatemia, mortality risk is multiplied by 4–8 [51, 60, 64].

4.7.1.2 Clinical Manifestations

Hypophosphatemia does not obligatorily indicate a reduction in total body level of phosphate. Therefore, clinical signs are not always correlated with the severity of hypophosphatemia. Nevertheless, muscular and respiratory clinical symptoms are only present in case of severe hypophosphatemia ≤0.5 mmol/L. Neurological and cardiovascular manifestations occur only when phosphatemia is ≤0.3 mmol/L [47–50]. All of these signs are favored by special underlying conditions such as chronic alcoholism, undernutrition, cancer, or severe digestive dysfunctions [65, 66]. Sepsis and postoperative period represent the most frequent acute situations which favor this disorder [51, 56, 60, 67]. The impact on all organs is the consequence of energy modifications induced by hypophosphatemia. Several mechanisms may be implicated (the decrease in the synthesis of intracellular ATP, the elevation of hemoglobin affinity for oxygen, the impaired glycolysis caused by the reduced activity of glyceraldehyde phosphate dehydrogenase enzyme (GAPDH) which needs the presence of phosphate as a cofactor):

- *Neuromuscular manifestations*: they include muscular weakness, proximal myopathies, or myalgias. Rhabdomyolysis may occur in case of severe hypophosphatemia, especially when the disorder develops rapidly in patients with a chronic preexisting depletion of phosphate [68].
- *Neurologic manifestations*: central and peripheral neurological signs can be present including paresthesia, peripheral polyneuropathy, hyporeflexia, confusion, seizures, coma, and Wernicke encephalopathy or centropontine myelinolysis [67, 68].
- *Respiratory manifestations*: respiratory insufficiency or failure is caused by the dysfunction of respiratory muscles, especially the diaphragmatic function [69]. This muscular impairment is worsened by the shift of the curve of hemoglobin dissociation toward the left which results in a reduction of oxygen delivery to tissues.
- *Cardiovascular manifestations*: severe hypophosphatemia is responsible for an impairment in myocardial contractility which may conduct to a real cardiac failure requiring an inotropic support [68]. These signs disappear totally with the normalization of phosphatemia. Various rhythm abnormalities such as ventricular fibrillation or tachycardia or ventricular extrasystoles have been also reported.
- *Renal lithiasis*: the increased urinary phosphate excretion favors the formation of calcium phosphate (hydroxyapatite) and calcium oxalate crystals in the kidneys. This phenomenon needs the concomitant urinary excretion of both phosphate and calcium (calciuria). The latter is induced by vitamin D which is stimulated by hypophosphatemia, leading in turn to increase the intestinal reabsorption of calcium and therefore calciuria [18, 47].
- *Bone demineralization*: this disorder is characterized by hypophosphatemia associated with a normal serum concentration of vitamin D or resistance to vitamin D. Indeed, phosphate is needed for osteoblasts differentiation and skeletal calcification.
- *Other manifestations*: hypophosphatemia can be responsible for hematologic abnormalities such as hemolytic anemia, reduced red blood cell deformability, alterations in thrombocyte and leukocyte functions, and abnormalities in phagocytic functions and in chemotactism, which might explain a greater susceptibility for sepsis. Metabolic modifications such as insulin resistance or proximal renal tubular acidosis are possible. Severe and prolonged hypophosphatemia impacts on bones: due to an increased skeletal resorption, demineralization with osteomalacia or bone deformities can develop. These signs are associated with a bone resorption of both calcium and magnesium which is manifested by hypercalicuria and hypermagnesiuria.

4.7.2 Hyperphosphatemia

4.7.2.1 Definition and Epidemiology

Hyperphosphatemia is defined by a serum concentration > 1.15 mmol/L (>35 mg/L). Hyperphosphatemia is an independent risk factor of an increased morbi-mortality [70–73]. Hyperphosphatemia is not very frequent in ICU, the two most common causes being chronic renal insufficiency or acute kidney injury and the specific tumor lysis syndrome.

4.7.2.2 Clinical Manifestations

Clinical signs of hyperphosphatemia are caused by the simultaneous association with hypocalcemia. Therefore, neuromuscular signs include tetany and calcifications of soft tissues or vessels due to extraskeletal deposits of calcium phosphate crystals. Hyperphosphatemia can also be complicated by renal insufficiency.

4.8 Diagnosis of Calcium and Phosphate Disorders

As calcium and phosphate homeostasis are closely linked in most pathologies, we propose to present causes which associate calcium and phosphate disturbances followed by those with isolated phosphate or calcium abnormalities. The determination of the causes of dyscalcemias and dysphosphatemias needs a careful history, a detailed drug history, and physical examination of the patient. Total calcemia abnormality must be confirmed by measuring albuminemia and determining corrected calcemia to eliminate pseudodyscalcemias (see previous chapter). Additional biological measurements must include ionized calcium measurement, creatininemia, and magnesemia. When dyscalcemia is confirmed, PTH level and if necessary vitamin D measurement will strongly orientate the etiologic diagnosis.

Dyscalcemias can be caused by three mechanisms: (1) an abnormal intestinal reabsorption, (2) an abnormal renal reabsorption, and (3) an abnormal bone resorption. In some cases, dyscalcemia is caused by an association of two or three of these mechanisms. Dysphosphatemias can be the consequence of three mechanisms [47, 48, 50]: (1) an abnormal intestinal reabsorption, (2) an abnormal renal reabsorption, and (3) a transcellular shift or an internal redistribution of the inorganic phosphate. Most of the two first mechanisms associate dysphosphatemias and dyscalcemias, while transcellular shift is responsible for only phosphatemia disorders.

4.8.1 Causes of Hypercalcemia and Dysphosphatemia

It is classical to distinguish parathyroid hormone (PTH)-dependent hypercalcemias from those that are PTH independent (Table 4.4) [1, 5, 12, 38, 41].

Table 4.4 Major causes of hypercalcemia

Causes of hypercalcemia (>2.8 mmol/L)	
Causes	Associated disorders
Caused by an increase in renal reabsorption	
• PTH dependent related to hyperparathyroidism	
• Sporadic: adenoma, hyperplasia, parathyroid carcinoma, ectopic PTH production • Familial hyperparathyroidism: multiple endocrine neoplasia type 1 and 2, other genetic mutations • Tertiary hyperparathyroidism: chronic kidney disease, familial hypocalciuric hypercalcemia, phosphate treatment of hypophosphatemic rickets, or osteomalacia	• **Elevated or "inappropriately elevated" PTH concentration** in the setting of high/normal calcemia • Associated with **hypophosphatemia** and normal vitamin D concentration
• PTH independent	
• Elevated PTHrP production: malignancy, endocrine disorders (thyrotoxicosis, adrenal deficiency, pheochromocytoma, VIPoma), lithium • Genetic abnormalities: hereditary (familial tumoral calcinosis) or acquired (Fanconi's syndrome, mutation on PTH-R1) • Medications (estrogens, thiazides, theophylline), metabolic alkalosis, hypovolemia	• **Normal or low PTH concentration** • Associated with **hyperphosphatemia** • Associated with **hyperphosphatemia** • Associated with **normophosphatemia**
Caused by an increase in intestinal reabsorption	
• Vitamin D intoxication • Non-infectious granulomatous disorders: sarcoidosis, Wegener's syndrome • Infectious granulomatous disorders: tuberculosis, histoplasmosis	• **Normal PTH concentration** • Associated with **hyperphosphatemia** and elevated vitamin D concentration
Caused by an increase in bone resorption	
• Prolonged immobilization • Osteolytic metastasis • Cell lysis: lymphomas, neuroleptic malignant syndrome	• **Normal PTH concentration** • Associated with **hyperphosphatemia**
Other causes	
• Paget's disease • Vitamin A intoxication, rich-calcium diet	

PTH parathormone, *PTH-R1* PTH receptor
Bold text indicate the most important location and effects of the hormones

4.8.1.1 PTH-Dependent Hypercalcemias

They are characterized by an elevated or an inappropriately high level of PTH caused by hyperparathyroidism which means that PTH level is "normal" in the setting of elevated calcemia. Hypercalcemia is the consequence of an increased renal calcium reabsorption. All of them are associated with hypophosphatemia which is caused by an increased renal excretion (reduced TmPi/GFR). Both metabolic changes are induced by an inappropriate PTH release. Hyperparathyroidism can be observed in three situations [5, 38, 41]:

- *Primary sporadic hyperparathyroidism*: this endocrine disorder is characterized by an autonomous abnormal production of PTH by the parathyroid glands. This is the most common cause of hypercalcemia. The prevalence is of 0.1–1% in a general population with a higher incidence in patients aged 50 years or older and in female (risk multiplied by 2–3). In most patients (80%), hypercalcemia is asymptomatic and is discovered incidentally on laboratory tests. Some of them present signs of chronic mild symptoms of hypercalcemia: renal manifestations including nephrolithiasis or nephrocalcinosis with hypercalciuria occur in up to 20% of patients; bone disease occurs in 2% of patients and is expressed by osteoporosis, osteopenia, and in the major form osteitis fibrosa cystica. Hypercalcemic hyperparathyroidism crisis is currently very rare [46]. In 90–95% of cases, primary hyperparathyroidism is caused by an abnormal sporadic excessive PTH release caused by a solitary or double adenomas (80–90%), multiglandular hyperplasia (10–15%), or rarely parathyroid carcinoma or ectopic PTH production.
- *Primary familial hyperparathyroidism*: they represent 5% of primary hyperparathyroidisms caused by multiple endocrine neoplasia (MEN) type 1 or 2 (autosomal dominant diseases) which are observed during neoplasia of thyroid, adrenal, and parathyroid glands or other genetic disorders.
- *Tertiary hyperparathyroidism*: they occur as the consequence of the evolution of a secondary hyperparathyroidism with an evolution toward an autonomic overproduction of PTH by hyperplasic parathyroid glands associated with an absence of negative feedback in the presence of hypercalcemia. Tertiary hyperparathyroidism is observed in patients with chronic kidney disease (patient on hemodialysis), those treated by phosphate for hypophosphatemia for rickets or osteomalacia, or those presenting a familial hypocalciuric hypercalcemia. The latter disease is an autosomal dominant pathology caused by a mutation that inactivates CasR mutation gene.
- *Lithium-related hypercalcemia* is classified in PTH-dependent hyperparathyroidism probably caused by an abnormal low threshold of PTH release, but the exact mechanism remains unclear.

4.8.1.2 PTH-Independent Hypercalcemias

They are characterized by a normal or low PTH production and serum concentration. Depending on the cause, hypercalcemia can be associated with hypo-, normo-, or hyperphosphatemia [1, 5, 12, 38]. The mechanism of hypercalcemia depends also on the cause as it can be due mainly to an increased intestinal reabsorption or an increased bone resorption. Besides hyperparathyroidism, malignancy is the second most common cause of hypercalcemia that may occur in up to 44% of patients with cancer and concerns 90% of patients hospitalized for hypercalcemia [2, 5, 12, 38].

In this context, hypercalcemia can result from various mechanisms that lead to an elevation in calcium renal reabsorption or in bone resorption or in excessive vitamin D activity. Patients with hypercalcemia caused by malignancy are usually symptomatic because calcium levels are higher and develop more rapidly than in other causes:

- *Conditions with elevated PTHrP*: PTHrP is a polypeptide produced by normal and malignant tissues. It represents the major humoral mediator of cancer-related hypercalcemia accounting for 80% of this disturbance in this context. PTH production is normal or low. PTHrP increases calcemia by two mechanisms: an activation of osteoclasts and in turn bone resorption and a stimulation of calcium renal reabsorption. PTHrP-related hypercalcemia is observed in solid tissue cancers such as urinary tract, breast, ovarian, and lung cancers, non-Hodgkin's lymphomas, and leukemias. Elevated PTHrP can be caused by some endocrine disorders: thyrotoxicosis, adrenal insufficiency, pheochromocytoma, VIPoma, etc. In all of these situations, hypercalcemia is associated with hyperphosphatemia.
- *Bone osteolysis*: in these situations hypercalcemia is associated with hypercalciuria and hyperphosphatemia which is due to an intracellular transport. Caused by metastasis, bone resorption accounts for approximately 20% of malignancy-related hypercalcemia. Most of the cases are related to breast cancer and multiple myeloma. An excessive bone resorption can be present in case of prolonged immobilization, cell lysis (lymphoma), and neuroleptic malignant syndrome. Paget's disease is characterized by an elevated bone resorption caused by an autonomous multiplication and activity of osteoclasts and osteoblasts [74]. PTH and vitamin D levels are normal, while total serum alkaline phosphate concentration increases, indicating the importance of bone resorption. This disease occurs in patients from 50 years old and increases with age (10% of patients at 90 years). The common clinical presentation consists of pain on bones, joints, and muscle which developed over many years and skeletal deformity mostly located on the femur. Radiologic exam shows area of osteolysis and osteosclerosis.
- *Genetic abnormalities*: depending on the gene mutation, hypercalcemia can be associated with hyperphosphatemia or hypophosphatemia caused essentially by a decreased (reduced TmPi/GFR) or an increased renal reabsorption (elevated TmPi/GFR). PTH level is normal and calcitriol is elevated [13, 75, 76] (Table 4.4). The two most common hereditary mutations responsible for hypercalcemia and hyperphosphatemia are the familial tumoral calcinosis and the hyperostosis hyperphosphatemic syndrome which is manifested by soft tissue calcifications (shoulder, knee, hip). Phosphaturia and calciuria are low. These diseases are rare and occur preferentially in black young people. They are related to a recessive autonomic gene mutation encoding for FGF-23 or N-acetylgalactosaminyltransferase 3 (GALNT-3), the latter being implicated in the FGF-23 synthesis and stability. In both cases, active FGF-23 serum

concentration is low (or normal), while its inactive C-terminal fraction is strongly high. Hypercalcemia associated with hypophosphatemia can be caused by acquired genetic mutations. Among them, Fanconi's syndrome manifests fatigability, bone pains, osteomalacia, osteoporosis, and kidney lithisasis. Hypophosphatemia and hypercalcemia are associated with hypercalciuric hypokalemia, glucose and amino acid urine excretion, proteinuria, hyperuricemia, and type 2 renal tubular acidosis. This syndrome can be congenital and induce rickets and a severe stunting in children. It can be also acquired and caused by medications such as tenofir, biphosphonates, tetracyclines, or heavy metals, but the most common acquired causes are myelomas or monoclonal gammapathies. Acquired disorders which associate hypercalcemia and hypophosphatemia due to an increased renal reabsorption can be observed in genetic mutations encoding for calcium responsive receptors (CaSR) [13, 16, 75–77] or mutations of PTH-R1 (Jansen syndrome, metaphyseal chondrodysplasia). Other causes of hypercalcemia and hypophosphatemia with a normal PTH level result from gene mutations responsible for various syndromes present in children. In these situations, FGF-23 serum concentration allows to distinguish genetic mutations of Na/Pi cotransporters from those of other hormones or exchangers. Inactivating mutations of NPT2a and NPT2c cotransporters alter directly renal phosphate reabsorption, whereas those of NERF-1 favor phosphaturia caused by the action of PTH on the proximal tubule. In both cases, FGF-23 concentration is normal.

- *Conditions with excessive vitamin D production*: the excess of vitamin D results in an increased intestinal reabsorption of calcium and phosphate associated with an increased bone resorption leading to hypercalcemia and hyper- or normophosphatemia (if the elevation in renal excretion is sufficient). Some cancers, especially lymphomas and ovarian cancers can be associated with an ectopic activity of 1-α-hydroxylase and vitamin D. Granulomatous disorders induce an excessive production of vitamin D by extrarenal mononuclear cells. This can be caused by noninfectious granulomatous disorders such as sarcoidosis and Wegener's syndrome as well as infectious ones such as tuberculosis and histoplasmosis.
- *Medications*: thiazides associated with hypovolemia favor proximal convoluted tubule reabsorption leading to a reduction in calciuria, metabolic alkalosis, and estrogen. In these cases hypercalcemia is present without relevant phosphate disorders.

4.8.2 Causes of Hypocalcemia and Dysphosphatemia

Hypocalcemias are also classified according to PTH levels. Therefore, PTH-dependent hypocalcemia are characterized by a low or inappropriately low PTH production (= normal in the setting of hypocalcemia) (Table 4.5). PTH-independent hypocalcemia is characterized by a normal or high PTH serum concentration [2, 78].

Table 4.5 Major causes of hypocalcemia

Causes of hypocalcemia (<2.2 mmol/L)	
Causes	Associated disorders
Caused by a decrease in renal reabsorption	
• PTH dependent • Primary hypoparathyroidism: accidentally (postoperative, postradiation), autoimmune, genetic disorders (PTH, CaSR mutation, activating mutations) • Reversible impairment in PTH secretion or action: dysmagnesemia, metabolic acidosis, hypervolemia, loop diuretics, rhabdomyolysis, multiple endocrine syndrome deficiency	• **Low or "inappropriately low" PTH concentration** in the setting of low/normal calcemia • Associated with **hyperphosphatemia** and normal vitamin D concentration • Associated with **hypophosphatemia** and normal vitamin D concentration
Caused by a decrease in renal/intestinal reabsorption	
• PTH independent • Secondary hyperparathyroidism caused by renal insufficiency • Genetic mutations: NPT2, NHERF-1, FGF-23 • Vitamin D resistance, rickets (increased phosphaturia) • Pseudohypoparathyroidism (resistance to PTH) • Bone metastasis • Rhabdomyolysis (favored by acute kidney injury)	• **"Inappropriately elevated" PTH concentration** • Associated with **hypophosphatemia** and elevated vitamin D concentration • Associated with **hyperphosphatemia**
Other causes	
• Hyperaldosteronism • Rich-sodium diet	

PTH parathormone, *FGF-23* fibroblast growth factor 23, *NHERF-1* sodium-hydrogen exchanger 1, *NPT2* cotransport sodium-phosphate type 2
Bold text indicate the most important location and effects of the hormones

4.8.2.1 PTH-Dependent Hypocalcemias

In these situations hypocalcemia is associated with hyperphosphatemia which results from the reduction of phosphate renal excretion caused by the low concentration in PTH (increased TmPi and normal GFR) [41, 43, 78]:

- *Primary hypoparathyroidism*: this disorder most commonly occurs accidentally after parathyroidectomy, after neck surgery for thyroidectomy (0.5–6.6% of cases), or postradiation [79]. It can be also the result of an acquired or inherited autoimmune destruction of parathyroid glands, either isolated (38% of cases) or in the context of a multiple endocrine deficiency syndrome or rarely in parathyroid cancer (40% of cases). Clinical symptoms indicate hypocalcemia such as tetany. Hypocalcemia is related to the decrease in intestinal calcium reabsorption and bone resorption. Hyperphosphatemia which is due to an increased renal reabsorption is associated with a normal or low level of vitamin D and a normal level of alkaline phosphatase and PTH. Hyperthyroidism and acromegaly present as hypoparathyroidism with a moderate hyperphosphatemia.
- *Hypoparathyroidism caused by acquired genetic mutation*: these are familial isolated hypoparathyroidisms, dominant or recessive autosomal hypoparathyroidisms which are caused by genetic mutations encoding either for PTH or for the "glial cell missing B" (GCMB), a protein that plays a role in the development of

parathyroid glands, or for CaSR activating mutation (only dominant). All of them are characterized by hypocalcemia and hyperphosphatemia with a low or normal PTH level.

- *Hypoparathyroidism caused by metabolic disease*: these disorders are caused by mitochondrial gene defects and include various pathologies in infants.
- *Conditions associated with an impairment in PTH secretion or action*: in these situations hypocalcemia is usually associated with a normal or low phosphatemia which results from a reduction in renal reabsorption. Such disorders can be observed in case of metabolic acidosis, hypomagnesemia, hypervolemia, and rhabdomyolysis or may be drug induced (loop diuretics).

4.8.2.2 PTH-Independent Hypocalcemias

In these situations hypocalcemia, PTH, and phosphate serum concentration are elevated or normal/low, depending on the cause of the disorder. PTH serum concentration is elevated [43]:

- *Pseudohypoparathyroidism*: this disorder is defined by a genetic resistance of tissues to PTH. Therefore, hypocalcemia is associated with hyperphosphatemia, both resulting from a reduction in calcium and phosphate renal reabsorption caused by the inefficiency of PTH. Vitamin D serum concentration is normal or low. Clinical manifestations are commonly characterized by morphologic modifications such as a circular face, short neck and phalanges, and sometimes skin calcifications. Depending on the response to a PTH test (which consists to administer PTH), it is possible to distinguish two types: PTH administration in type I induces a reduction in phosphaturia and urinary cyclic AMP, while in type II it increases them.
- *Secondary hyperparathyroidism*: such a disorder occurs commonly in the setting of chronic kidney disease. Hypocalcemia is associated at the beginning with hypophosphatemia and later with hyperphosphatemia which is mostly caused by renal function impairment (normal TmPi and reduced GFR) and vitamin D deficit [43, 80]. These acquired metabolic abnormalities during chronic renal insufficiency have been reported to be risk factor of morbi-mortality [81–89]. Renal function worsening leads to more severe hyperparathyroidism with clinical signs. Skeletal manifestations associated with frequent fractures (risk x 4) and generalized osteodystrophy are associated with soft tissue and vascular calcifications which worsen leading to coronaropathies and renal dysfunction. At the beginning, the decrease in phosphate renal excretion is counterbalanced by an elevation in FGF-23 production and release caused by the decrease in phosphaturia [28]. This phenomenon, by inhibiting the renal 1- α -hydroxylase, reduces calcitriol concentration and therefore phosphate intestinal reabsorption. All of these phenomenons induce at least the secondary hyperparathyroidism and renal osteodystrophy [16, 18, 28, 83, 85, 90, 91]. Until GFR remains >30 mL/min, phosphatemia does not elevate [21]. Below this threshold, the compensatory mechanisms become insufficient, and despite the phosphaturic effect of FGF-23, the loss in nephrons conducts to hyperphosphatemia. Despite a low diet in phosphate and dialysis, phosphate balance becomes positive. When renal dysfunction is severe requiring dialysis, the secondary hyper-

parathyroidism becomes refractory and resistant to vitamin D and calcium administration. Another cause of secondary hypoparathyroidism is vitamin D deficiency or resistance, and hypocalcemia is associated with normo- or hypophosphatemia caused by a decreased in intestinal reabsorption.

- *Tumor lysis syndrome (TLS)*: this entity associates hypocalcemia with hyperphosphatemia and hyperkalemia caused by the shift of intracellular material to the extracellular compartment. Extracellular potassium and phosphate occur because of a coexisting kidney dysfunction which limits their excretion [92]. This syndrome occurs rarely spontaneously in severe hematologic malignancies or more frequently triggered by chemotherapy during solid cancers. TLS is associated with a high risk of mortality when associated with acute kidney injury. Urate nephropathy is a classical manifestation caused by the precipitation of uric acid crystals in the renal tubules. Hyperphosphatemia resulting from its release of cells chelates with calcium explaining hypocalcemia and calcium-phosphate salt deposition on tissues.
- *Other causes*: rhabdomyolysis enables to induce hypocalcemia and hyperphosphatemia which is favored by acute kidney injury, bone metastasis, and hyperaldosteronism [93].

4.8.3 Causes of Dyscalcemia Without Phosphate Disorders (Table 4.6)

- Hypercalcemias: vitamin A or vitamin D intoxication can be responsible for hypercalcemia with normophosphatemia in case of renal insufficiency which reduces calcium renal excretion. Milk-alkali syndrome, rich-calcium diet, and Burnett syndrome can lead to comparable disorders.
- Hypocalcemias: poor-calcium diet, calcium malabsorption, end-stage liver disease, vitamin D-dependent rickets

Table 4.6 Major causes of isolated dyscalcemias and dysphosphatemias

Causes of isolated dyscalcemias	
Hypercalcemia	*Hypocalcemia*
• Rich-calcium diet • Burnett syndrome, milk-alkali syndrome	• Poor-calcium diet, malabsorption • End-stage liver diseases • Vitamin D-dependent rickets
Causes of isolated dysphosphatemias	
Hyperphosphatemia	*Hypophosphatemia*
• By increased intestinal absorption: rich-phosphate diet, laxatives • Cell transport: rhabdomyolysis, cell lysis (lymphomas, leukemias, tumor lysis syndrome), respiratory acidosis	• By decreased intestinal absorption: poor-phosphate diet, vomitings, diarrhea, steatorrhea, antacids • Cell transport: glucose-insulin, catecholamines, glucagon, ß2-agonists, steroids, undernutrition, malabsorption, chronic alcoholism, acute leukemias, lymphomas, respiratory alkalosis • By increased renal losses: renal replacement therapy, metabolic acidosis, genetic mutations (see Table 4.7)

4.8.4 Causes of Dysphosphatemia Without Calcium Disorders (Table 4.6)

4.8.4.1 Hyperphosphatemias

Most common causes of isolated hyperphosphatemia are secondary to phosphate transport from cell to the extracellular space such as in case of rhabdomyolysis, cell lysis (TLS), respiratory acidosis, rich-phosphate diet, or laxative treatment.

4.8.4.2 Hypophosphatemias

They are due to various mechanisms (cell transport and excessive phosphaturia):

- *Transport-related hypophosphatemias:* hypophosphatemias due to redistribution are very common and caused by numerous treatments: glucose-insulin (comparable effect on potassium), catecholamines, glucagon, ß2-agonists, steroids, chronic undernutrition or malabsorption, chronic alcoholism, acute leukemia, and lymphomas. Refeeding syndrome is a major cause of acute symptomatic hypophosphatemia and various metabolic disorders in critically ill patients [58, 94–100]. The mechanism of its development is essentially the rapid and important carbohydrates load in chronic underfed patients with a preexisting catabolic global metabolism. Active renutrition reverses the metabolism which becomes acutely anabolic, leading to increase glycogen and protein synthesis, lipogenesis, gluconeogenesis, and glycolysis. All of these modifications require a high level of energy (ATP) which cannot be provided to cells. As a consequence, hypokalemia, hypophosphatemia, hypomagnesemia, and ATP and thiamine deficits lead to multiple organ failure. Patients at risk of refeeding syndrome are well defined: anorexia nervosa, chronic alcoholism, oncology, postoperative period, elderly patients, chronic malnutrition, and long-term users of antacids or diuretics. The risk of refeeding syndrome is present when body mass index (BMI) is low (<16 g/m^2) or in patients with unintentional rapid weight loss (>10–15% within 3–6 months), very little nutrition for more than 10 days, and preexisting potassium, phosphate, and magnesium depletions. Clinical signs of refeeding syndrome include neurological (consciousness impairment, encephalopathy, coma, seizures), muscular (weakness, myopathy), respiratory failure, and cardiovascular (ventricular arrhythmias) manifestations. Approximately 0.2–2% of patients present a severe hypophosphatemia. The best treatment is preventive based on a progressive increase in nutritional supply.
- *Hypophosphatemias caused by excessive phosphaturia:* acute hypophosphatemia is a common and major metabolic complication of continuous renal replacement therapy. The risk increases when the hemodialysis or hemofiltration dose elevates (efficiency of the technique) with a frequency that can reach up to 60% of patients [61, 62, 98]. Preventive supplementation enables to maintain normophosphatemia in these patients. Besides this iatrogenic cause, it has been reported that hypophosphatemia occurs in 24% of critically ill patients within the first 3 days of ICU stay, especially when renal function is preserved [55]. In 80% of these situations, hypophosphatemia is caused by an increased renal phosphate

Table 4.7 Major syndromes with hypophosphatemia induced by gene mutations

Syndrome	Genetic mutation
Normal serum concentration of FGF-23	
– Hypophosphatemia with renal lithiasis and bone demineralization	– NPT2a, NPT2c – NHERF-1
Elevated serum concentration of FGF-23	
– X-linked hypophosphatemia (XLH) – Autosomal dominant hypophosphatemia rickets (ADHR) – Autosomal recessive hypophosphatemia rickets (ADHR) McCune-Albright syndrome (fibrous dysplasia)	– PHEX – FGF-23 – DMP-1 – GNAS

FGF-23 fibroblast growth factor 23, hormone synthetized by bone tissue which inhibits renal reabsorption of phosphate
NHERF-1 sodium-hydrogen exchanger-1, cofactor which bounds to FGF-23 and to sodium-phosphate NPT2a cotransporter required to obtain the phosphaturic action of FGF-23
PHEX phosphate regulating gene with homology to endopeptidase on the X chromosome, protein which activates the expression of FGF-23 and inhibits bone mineralization
DMP-1 dentin matrix protein-1, protein produced by osteoblasts
GNAS guanine nucleotide-binding protein

excretion which cannot be explained by common reasons (normal PTH, PTHrP, FGF-23, and calcitonin serum concentrations). The exact mechanisms that lead to this excessive phosphaturia remain unclear. Hyperphosphaturic hypophosphatemias can be the consequence of various activating gene mutations encoding for FGF-23 synthesis or other proteins implicated in renal phosphate exchanges. These syndromes usually manifest bone deformities, osteomalacia, and sometimes soft tissue calcifications. In all cases, hypophosphatemia is associated with an increased FGF-23 serum concentration, normocalcemia, and normal serum concentration of PTH and vitamin D (Table 4.7) [13, 77]. In these cases, hypophosphatemia is associated with normal calcemia.

- *Hypophosphatemias caused by low-phosphate intestinal absorption:* this can be observed in cases of low-phosphate diet, vomitings, diarrhea, and steatorrhea or induced by antacids.

4.9 Treatment of Calcium and Phosphate Disorders

The specific treatment of the underlying cause of dyscalcemia and dysphosphatemia is always required but will not be detailed in this chapter. We will focus on the non-specific symptomatic management of these disorders. Regardless the type of disorder, the treatment depends on the severity, rapidity, and symptoms of calcium and phosphate disorders. An emergent treatment is needed in case of life-threatening symptoms aiming to normalize the trouble and its consequences.

4.9.1 Treatment of Hypercalcemia

The main risk of hypercalcemia is cardiovascular, including severe arrhythmias and hypotension or shock related to hypovolemia because hypercalcemia inhibits renal sodium reabsorption. The aggressive treatment must be considered in case of severe hypercalcemia (>3–3.5 mmol/L or >12–14 mg/dL) [5, 46]. The first-line therapy aims to lower hypercalcemia by restoring euvolemia and correcting dehydration. Fluid resuscitation is nonspecific and must be conducted as usual with a close hemodynamic and biological monitoring in an intensive care unit. Cristalloids (such as 0.9% NaCl) are usually prescribed with a posology of 200–300 mL/h. The subsequent reduction in calcemia results from the increased calciuria that is favored by two phenomenons: the increased GFR caused by the normalization of volemia increased the load of calcium filtered in the glomerulus and the increased load of sodium increases calciuresis at the distal nephron. Such a therapy enables to reduce hypercalcemia by 0.4–0.6 mmol/L (1.6–2.4 mg/dL). Diuretic loops may be combined with saline infusion but always after having restored normovolemia. The decrease in calcemia is caused by an elevation in calcium renal excretion caused by a blockage of its reabsorption in the ascending limb of the loop of Henle. The administration can be orally or intravenously, depending on the severity of hypercalcemia and on the condition of the patient. The dose is approximately 40–80 mg/day, the best approach being to adapt it by titration based on the response of the patient. Thiazide diuretics are contraindicated in severe hypercalcemia.

The treatment aiming to reduce or inhibit calcium release caused by bone resorption is the first-line therapy of malignant-related hypercalcemia unless contraindicated and associated with fluid resuscitation. Biphosphonates block osteoclasts causing bone resorption by promoting their apoptosis. Such class of drug is efficient to reduce only hypercalcemias caused by cancer but not by other causes. Intravenous biphosphonates are favored because they are better tolerated than oral which causes nausea and vomitings. Such a strategy is approved by the US Food and Drug Administration (FDA) in this indication. Both molecules essentially prescribed are pamidronate (Aredia®) and zoledronate (Reclast®, Zometa®). Pamidronate is prescribed at a dose of 60–90 mg per day but must be infused in 4 h. It has the advantage to need no change of dose in case of renal dysfunction. Zoledronate is prescribed at a dose of 4 mg infused in 15 min and then 8 mg per day. Its efficiency seems to be higher and more rapid to reduce calcemia than pamidronate in this indication, but the dose must be adapted in case of renal dysfunction. For this class of drug, the peak of calcium decrease is observed at 4 days. Calcitonin decreases calcemia by both an increased renal excretion and a reduction in osteoclastic bone resorption. This therapy is safe and has a rapid onset of action. However, its beneficial effect is only moderate and transitory due to a tachyphylaxis within 48 h (down regulation of its receptors). Therefore, calcitonin must be considered to be successful only in combination with biphosphonates, as temporizing and facilitating agents. The dose is 6–8 UI/kg intravenously in saline during 4 h.

Recent approach for treating severe hypercalcemia seems to suggest less aggressive fluid resuscitation and diuretic and to favor biphosphonates and calcitonin [99]. Glucocorticoids are indicated in some myelomas and lymphomas at a posology of 200–300 mg intravenously for 3–5 days and must be associated with the administration of oral vitamin D. Finally, renal removal therapy remains the most efficient symptomatic therapy in case of emergent treatment in patients with renal failure or if other treatments are contraindicated.

4.9.2 Treatment of Hypocalcemia

The main risk of hypocalcemia is cardiovascular including severe arrhythmias and hypotension [42]. Cardiac monitoring and rapid determination of ionized calcium are needed [100]. Acute symptomatic hypocalcemia is a life-threatening condition which requires an emergent intravenous supplementation. This can be performed using calcium gluconate or chloride with comparable efficiency. The difference is the concentration in calcium as 10 mL of calcium gluconate contains 91 mg of calcium, while 10 mL of calcium chloride contains 184 mg of calcium. The infusion is performed within 10 min (10–20 mL) followed by a continuous infusion of 0.5–2 mg/kg/h if necessary [101]. Usually calcium gluconate is preferred on calcium chloride which can be responsible for venous necrosis. The risk of arrhythmias is present in case of a too rapid intravenous administration. If needed, magnesium supplementation must be associated. The switch to an oral calcium supplementation is recommended as soon as possible. Only chronic hypocalcemia can be treated with oral calcium ingestion and vitamin D. Calcium carbonate is prescribed orally (Calcidia®, Eucalcic®, etc.). Both non-active and active vitamin D can be administered orally. Among non-active vitamin D, it can be vitamin D3 (cholecalciferol, Uvedose®) or vitamin D2 (ergocalciferol, Sterogyl® or calcifediol, Dedrogyl®).

4.9.3 Treatment of Hyperphosphatemia

The preventive treatment is based on a decrease in phosphate load in diet associated with a close monitoring of phosphatemia, especially in chronic renal insufficiency. In case of hyperphosphatemia caused by cell lysis, the prevention is based on an appropriate hydration and a treatment with allopurinol. For a long time, hyperphosphatemia caused by chronic renal insufficiency was treated by vitamin D or analogues or by antiparathormone drugs [80, 94]. Recent data found that the treatment of hyperphosphatemia is more important than that of hyperparathyroidism [102]. Aluminum phosphate binding therapies are now largely abandoned due to their toxicity. Calcium digestive phosphate binders are more efficient, leading to use them preferentially [103–105]. They are commercialized in several forms. Calcium binders are used as calcium carbonate (Calcidia®, Eucalcic®, Os-Cal®, Caltrate®) or calcium acetate (PhosLo®, Eliphos®) at the dose of 500–1200 mg/day. Anion exchange resins (sevelamer 800 mg/day) have similar effects as compared with previous phosphate binders. Lanthanum carbonate (Fosrenol®) does not contain calcium or aluminum but seems to produce more side effects (250 per 1000 mg/day) [103–105]. Magnesium phosphate binders (Gaviscon®) can worsen a hypermagnesemia in these patients and are not recommended as a first therapeutic strategy. In summary, current recommendations for hyperphosphatemia in chronic renal insufficient patients include a low-phosphate diet, calcium phosphate binders, and an exogenous calcium supplementation (200 mg/day). If such a treatment failed, magnesium binders can be considered as an alternative strategy associated with a regular monitoring of serum magnesium concentration. Due to their high cost and the absence of any superior efficiency, sevelamer and lanthanum cannot be recommended as a first-line therapeutic strategy. In all cases, the goal is to normalize serum phosphate concentration.

4.9.4 Treatment of Hypophosphatemia

Prevention of hypophosphatemia in alcoholic or underfed patients or during the refeeding syndrome is needed using a daily oral supplementation of approximately 1–2 g/day (32 à 64 mmol) [49]. In case of renutrition, the appropriate phosphate/kcal ratio is of 300 mg for 1000 kcal. Antacid oral absorption without food is also a preventive measure. Milk ingestion has the advantage to provide both phosphate and calcium which allows to prevent tetany.

A curative supplementation is only indicated in case of symptomatic hypophosphatemia associated with phosphate depletion. An oral supplementation is preferred in case of moderate hypophosphatemia aiming to decrease the occurrence of treatment-related complications [5, 16, 49, 106]. A dose of 2.5–3.5 g/day (80–100 mmol/day) in two or three times of manganese glycerophosphate (Phosphore Alko®) or glucose-1-phosphate-disodique (Phocytan®) is suggested. The intravenous infusion is indicated only in case of symptomatic severe hypophosphatemias <0.35 mmol/L. Complications such as diarrhea, hypocalcemia, arterial hypotension, metabolic acidosis, or renal failure can be observed in case of a too rapid or too important supplementation. To our knowledge, there is no real randomized study that evaluated the most appropriate time and modality for phosphate supplementation in severe hypophosphatemia in ICU. Moreover, the efficiency of phosphate supplementation is not really demonstrated in term of morbi-mortality of such patients. Nevertheless, several studies have evaluated the efficiency and safety of various protocols of phosphate supplementation in ICU [107–110]. Monopotasium and monosodium phosphate can be prescribed. The dose of infusion is safe from 5 to 20 mmol/h. In case of hyperkalemia, monosodium phosphate must be chosen. Formulas are usually inadequate, and the response to supplementation is not related to the administered amount of phosphate which remains unpredictable in ICU [109]. Therefore, it is necessary to monitor frequently phosphatemia in these situations.

Conclusion

Calcium and phosphate metabolism are closely connected. The regulation of calcium and phosphate metabolism is essentially under a hormonal control including vitamin D, parathormone and calcitonin, and FGF-23 for phosphate. The targeted organs are kidneys, digestive tract, and bones which work in total connection. This conducts to an integrated regulation by the digestive-kidney-bone axis. Both calcium and phosphate play a major role in various cell functions and in bone metabolism. Both shift continuously between the different body compartments. Dyscalcemias are classified in PTH-dependent and PTH-independent causes. Most frequent causes of hypercalcemias are hyperparathyroidism (primary and pseudohyperparathroidism) and malignancy-related hypercalcemia.

Major causes of hypocalcemias are hypoparathyroidism and secondary hyperparathyroidism. Hypophosphatemias in ICU patients are usually caused by cell transfers or iatrogenic renal losses (renal replacement therapy) without sufficient supplementation. Hyperphosphatemia is frequently caused by renal insufficiency. Only severe and rapid dyscalcemias and dysphosphatemias need an emergent treatment.

References

1. Bourdeau JE, Attie MF (1994) Calcium metabolism. In: Narins RG (ed) Clinical disorders of fluid and electrolyte metabolism. McGraw Hill Inc, New York, pp 243–306
2. Shaker JL, Deftos L (2000) Calcium and phosphate homeostasis. In: De Groot LJ, Beck-Peccoz P, Chrousos G, Chrousos G, Dungan K, Grossman A, Hershman JM, Koch C, McLachlan R, New M, Rebar R, Singer F, Vinik A, Weickert MO (eds) Endotext [internet]. South Darmount (MA): MD Text.com, Inc 2000- update 2014 Apr 11
3. Blaine J, Chonchol M, Levi M (2015) Renal control of calcium, phosphate, and magnesium homeostasis. Clin J Am Soc Nephrol 10:1257–1272
4. Taylor JG, Bushinsky DA (2009) Calcium and phosphorus homeostasis. Blood Purif 27:387–394
5. Goltzman D (2015) Hypercalcemia. In: De Groot LJ, Beck-Peccoz P, Chrousos G, Chrousos G, Dungan K, Grossman A, Hershman JM, Koch C, McLachlan R, New M, Rebar R, Singer F, Vinik A, and Weickert MO (eds) Endotext [internet]. South Darmount (MA). MD Text. com: Inc 2000- update 2015 Apr 12
6. Diaz de Barbosa G, Guizzardi S, Tolosa de Talamani N (2015) Molecular aspects of intestinal calcium absorption. World J Gastroenterol 21:7142–7154
7. Brown EM (2001) Physiology of calcium homeostasis. In: Bilezikian JP, Marcus R, Levine A (eds.). The parathyroids. 2nd ed. Chapter 10: 167–182
8. Nissenson RA, Juppner H (2013) Parathyroid hormone. In: Rosen CJ ed. Primer on the metabolic bone diseases and disorders of mineral metabolism. 8th ed. Chapter 26: 208–214
9. Kurakawa K (1994) The kidney and calcium homeostasis. Kidney Int 44:S97–105
10. Suki WN, Lederer ED, Rouse D (2002) Renal transport of calcium, magnesium, and phosphate. In: Brenner BM (ed) The kidney. Saunders, Philadelphia, pp 520–574
11. Magyar CE, Friedman PA (2002) Renal regulation of calcium, phosphate and magnesium. In: DuBose TD, Hamm LL (eds) Acid-base and electrolyte disorders: a companion to Brenner's and Rector's the kidney. Saunders, Philadelphia, pp 435–452
12. Mirrakhimov AE (2015) Hypercalcemia of malignancy: an update on pathogenesis and management. N Am J Med Sci 7:483–493
13. Lee R, Weber TJ (2010) Disorders of phosphorus homeostasis. Curr Opin Endocrinol Diabetes Obes 17:561–571
14. Delanaye P, Krzesinski JM (2005) News about phosphorus metabolism. Rev Med Liege 60:1889–1897
15. Marks J, Debnam ES, Unwin RJ (2010) Phosphate homeostasis and the renal-gastrointestinal axis. Am J Physiol Renal Physiol 299:F285–F296
16. Razzaque M, Lanske B (2007) The emerging role of the fibroblast growth factor-23-klotho axis in renal regulation of phosphate homeostasis. J Endocrinol 194:1–10
17. Murer H, Forster I, Hilfiker H et al (1998) Cellular/molecular control of renal Na/Pi-cotransport. Kidney Int 65(suppl):S2–10
18. Prié HD, Urena Torres P, Friedlander G (2009) Fibroblast Growth Factor 23-Klotho: a new axis of phosphate balance. Med Sci 25:489–495
19. Segawa H, Onitsuka A, Furutani J et al (2009) Npt2a and Npt2c in mice play distinct and synergistic roles in inorganic phosphate metabolism and skeletal development. Am J Physiol Renal Physiol 297:F671–F678

20. Tomoe Y, Segawa H, Shiozawa K et al (2010) Phosphaturic action of fibroblast growth factor 23 in Npt2 null mice. Am J Physiol Renal Physiol 298:F1341–F1350
21. Hruska KA (2002) Hypophosphatemia and hyperphosphatemia. In: DuBose TD, Hamm LL (eds) Acid-base and electrolyte disorders: a companion to Brenner's and Rector's the kidney. Saunders, Philadelphia, pp 489–512
22. Biber J (1989) Cellular aspects of proximal tubular phosphate reabsorption. Kidney Int 36:360–365
23. Bickle D (2014) Vitamin D: production, metabolism, and mechanisms of action. In: De Groot LJ, Beck-Peccoz P, Chrousos G, Chrousos G, Dungan K, Grossman A, Hershman JM, Koch C, McLachlan R, New M, Rebar R, Singer F, Vinik A, and Weickert MO (eds) Endotext [internet]. South Darmount (MA). MD Text.com: Inc 2000- update 2014 Apr 11
24. Carmeliet G, Dermauw V, Bouillon R (2015) Vitamine D signalling in calcium and bone homeostasis: a delicate balance. Best Practice Res Clin Endocrinol Metab 29:621–631
25. Quarles LD (2008) Endocrine functions of bone in mineral metabolism regulation. J Clin Invest 118:3820–3828
26. Thakker RV (2015) The calcium-sensing receptor: and its involvement in parathyroid pathology. Ann Endocrinol 76:81–83
27. Goldner W (2016) Cancer-related hypercalcemia. J Oncol Pract 12:426–432
28. Nakai K, Komaba H, Fukagawa M (2010) New insights into the role of fibroblast growth factor 23 in chronic kidney disease. J Nephrol 23:619–625
29. Ritthaler T, Traebert M, Lötscher M, Biber J, Murer H, Kaissling B (1999) Effects of phosphate intake on dstribution of type I Na/Pi cotransporter mRNA in rat kidney. Kidney Int 55:976–983
30. Hofbauer LC, Khosla S, Dunstan CR et al (2000) The roles of osteoprotegerin and osteoprotegerin ligand in paracrine regulation of bone resorption. J Bone Miner Res 15:2–12
31. Steele T, Kolamunnage-Dona R, Downey C, Cheng-Hock T, Welters I (2013) Assessement and clinical course of hypocalcemia in critically illness. Crit Care 17:R106
32. Iqbal M, Rehmani R, Hijazi M, Abdulaziz A, Kashif S (2011) Hypocalcemia in Saudi intensive care unit. Ann Thor Med 3:57–59
33. Hastbacka J, Pettila V (2003) Prevalence and predictive value of ionized hypocalcemia among critically ill patients. Acta Anesthesiol Scand 47:1264–1269
34. Zivin JR, Gooley T, Zager RA et al (2001) Hypocalcemia: a pervasive metabolic abnormality in the critically ill. Am J Kidney Dis 37:689–698
35. Zaloga GP (1992) Hypocalcemia in critically il patients. Crit Care Med 20:251–262
36. Sauter TC, Lindner G, Ahmad SS et al (2015) Calcium disorders in the emergency department: independent risk factors for mortality. PLoS One 10:e0132788
37. Egi M, Kim I, Nichol A et al (2011) Ionized calcium concentration and outcome in critically ill patients. Crit Care Med 39:314–321
38. Kelly A, Levine MA (2013) Hypocalcemia in the critically ill patient. J Intensive Care Med 28:166–177
39. Amrein K, Sourij H, Holl A, Wagner G et al (2011) Short-term effects of high-dose oral vitamin D3 in critically ill vitamin D deficient patients: a randomized, double-blind, placebo-controlled pilot study. Crit Care 15:R104
40. Akhnoundi A, Sing B, Vela M et al (2015) Incidence of adverse events during continuous renal replacement therapy. Blood Purif 39:339–336
41. Michels TC, Kelly KM (2013) Parathyroid disorders. Am Fam Physician 88:249–257
42. Schafer AL, Shoback DM (2016) Hypocalcemia: diagnosis and treatment. In: De Groot LJ, Beck-Peccoz P, Chrousos G, Chrousos G, Dungan K, Grossman A, Hershman JM, Koch C, McLachlan R, New M, Rebar R, Singer F, Vinik A, and Weickert MO (eds) Endotext [internet]. South Darmount, MA. MD Text.com: Inc 2000- update 2016 January 3
43. Hendy GN, Cole DEC, Bastepe M (2011) Hypoparathyroidism and pseudohypoparathyroidism. In: De Groot LJ, Beck-Peccoz P, Chrousos G, Chrousos G, Dungan K, Grossman A, Hershman JM, Koch C, McLachlan R, New M, Rebar R, Singer F, Vinik A, and Weickert MO (eds) Endotext [internet]. South Darmount (MA). MD Text.com: Inc 2000- update 2011 Aug 1

44. Zaloga GP, Chernow B, Cook D et al (1985) Assessment of calcium homeostasis in the critically ill surgical patient. The diagnosis pitfalls of the Mc-Lean-Hastings nomogram. Ann Surg 202:587–594
45. Forster J, Querusio L, Burchard KW et al (1985) Hypercalcemia in critically ill surgical patients. Ann Surg 202:512–518
46. Ahmad S, Kuraganti G, Steenkamp D (2015) Hypercalcemic crisis: a clinical review. Am J Med 128:239–245
47. Yanagawa N, Nakhoul F, Kurokawa K, Lee DBN (1994) Physiology of phosphorus metabolism. In: Narins RG (ed) Clinical disorders of fluid and electrolyte metabolism. Mac Graw Hill, New York, pp 307–372
48. Gaasbeek A, Meinders AE (2005) Hypophosphatemia: an update on its etiology and treatment. Am J Med 118:1094–1101
49. Geerse DA, Bindels AJ, Kuiper MA, Roos AN, Spronk PE, Schultz MJ (2010) Treatment of hypophosphatemia in the intensive care unit: a review. Crit Care 14:R147
50. Amanzadeh J, Reilly RF Jr (2006) Hypophosphatemia: an evidence-based approach to its clinical consequences and management. Nat Clin Pract Nephrol 2:136–148
51. Cohen J, Kogan A, Sahar G, Lev S, Vidne B, Singer P (2004) Hypophosphatemia following open heart surgery: incidence and consequences. Eur J Cardiothorac Surg 26:306–310
52. Polderman KH, Bloemers FW, Peerdeman SM, Girbes AR (2000) Hypomagnesemia and hypophosphatemia at admission in patients with severe head injury. Crit Care Med 28:2022–2025
53. Kruse JA, Al-Douahji M, Carlson RW (1992) Hypophosphatemia in critically ill patients: incidence and associations. Crit Care Med 20:s107
54. Sedlacek M, Schoolwerth AC, Remillard BD (2006) Electrolytes disturbances in the intensive care unit. Sem Dialysis 19:496–501
55. Bech A, Blanc M, Telting D, de Boer H (2013) Incidence and aetiology of renal phosphate loss in patients with hypophosphatemia in the intensive care unit. Intensive Care Med 39:185–191
56. Salem RR, Tray K (2005) Hepatic resection-related hypophosphatemia is of renal origin as manifested by isolated hyperphosphaturia. Ann Surg 241:343–348
57. Marik PE, Bedigian MK (1996) Refeeding hypophosphatemia in critically ill patients in an intensive care unit. A prospective study. Arch Surg 131:1043–1047
58. Gentile MG, Manna GM (2012) Refeeding hypophosphatemia in malnutrition patients: prevention and treatment. Clin Nutr 31:429
59. Ravenscroft AJ, Valentine JM, Knappett PA (1999) Severe hypophosphatemia and insulin resistance in diabetic ketoacidosis. Anaesthesia 54:198
60. Shor R, Halabe A, Rishver S et al (2006) Severe hypophosphatemia in sepsis as a mortality predictor. Ann Clin Lab Sci 36:67–72
61. The VA/NIH Acute Renal Failure Trial Network (2008) Intensity of renal support in critically ill patients with acute kidney injury. N Engl J Med 359:7–20
62. The Renal Replacement Therapy Study Investigators (2009) Intensity of continuous renal-replacement therapy in critically ill patients. N Engl J Med 361:1627–1638
63. Fall P, Szerlip HM (2010) Continuous renal replacement therapy: cause and treatment of electrolyte complications. Semin Dial 23:581–585
64. Hoffman M, Zemlin AE, Meyer WP, Erasmus RT (2008) Hypophosphataemia at a large academic hospital in South Africa. J Clin Pathol 61:1104–1107
65. Singhal PC, Kumar A, Desroches L, Gibbons N, Mattana J (1992) Prevalence and predictors of rhabdomyolysis in patients with hypophosphatemia. Am J Med 92:458–464
66. Falcone N, Compagnoni A, Meschini C, Perrone C, Nappo A (2004) Central pontine myelinolysis induced by hypophosphatemia following Wernicke's encephalopthy. Neurol Sci 24:407–410
67. Schwartz A, Gurman G, Cohen G et al (2002) Association between hypophosphatemia and cardiac arrhythmias in the early stages of sepsis. Eur J Intern Med 13:434

68. Minisola S, Pepe J, Piemonte S, Cipriani C (2015) The diagnosis and management of hypercalcemia. BMJ 350:h2723
69. Gravelyn TR, Brophy N, Siegert C, Peters-Golden M (1988) Hypophosphatemia-associated respiratory muscle weakness in a general inpatient population. Am J Med 84:870–876
70. Kestenbaum B, Sampson JN, Rudser KD et al (2005) Serum phosphate levels and mortality risk among people with chronic kidney disease. J Am Soc Nephrol 16:520–528
71. Connolly GM, Cunningham R, McNamee PT, Young IS, Maxwell AP (2009) Elevated serum phosphate predicts mortality in renal transplant recipients. Transplantation 87:1040–1044
72. Dhingra R, Sullivan LM, Fox CS et al (2007) Relations of serum phosphorus and calcium levels to the incidence of cardiovascular disease in the community. Arch Intern Med 167:879–885
73. Tonelli M, Curhan G, Pfeffer M et al (2009) Relation between alkaline phosphatase, serum phosphate, and all-cause of cardiovascular mortality. Circulation 120:1784–1792
74. Singer F (2016) Paget's disease of bone. In: De Groot LJ, Beck-Peccoz P, Chrousos G, Chrousos G, Dungan K, Grossman A, Hershman JM, Koch C, McLachlan R, New M, Rebar R, Singer F, Vinik A, and Weickert MO (eds) Endotext [internet]. South Darmount (MA). MD Text.com: Inc 2000- update 2016 January 8
75. Levtchenko E, Schoeber J, Jaeken J (2010) Genetic disorders of renal phosphate transport. N Engl J Med 363:2399–2409
76. Prié D, Friedlander G (2010) Genetic disorders of renal phosphate transport. N Engl J Med 362:2399–2409
77. Prié D, Ravery V, Boccon-Gibod L, Friedlander G (2001) Frequency of renal phosphate leak among with calcium nephrolithiasis. Kidney Int 60:272–276
78. Hendy GN, Canaff L (2016) Calcium-sensing receptor, proinflammatory cytokines and calcium homeostasis. Sem Cell Dev Biol 49:37–43
79. Kakava K, Tournis S, Papadakis G et al (2016) Postsurgical hypoparathyroidism: a systematic review. In Vivo 30:171–179
80. Qazi RA, Martin KJ (2010) Vitamin D in kidney disease: pathophysiology and the utility of treatment. Endocrinol Metab Clin N Am 39:355–363
81. Goodman WG (2005) Calcium and phosphorus metabolism in patients who have chronic kidney disease. Med Clin North Am 89:631–647
82. London G, Coyne D, Hruska K, Malluche HH, Martin KJ (2010) The new kidney disease: improving global outcomes (KDIGO) guidelines - expert clinical focus on bone and vascular calcification. Clin Nephrol 74:423–432
83. Spasovski G, Massy Z, Vanholder R (2009) Phosphate metabolism in chronic kidney disease: from pathophysiology to clinical management. Semin Dial 22:357–362
84. Covic A, Kothawala P, Bernal M, Robbins S, Challan A, Goldsmith D (2009) Systematic review of the evidence underlying the association between mineral metabolism disturbances and risk of all-cause mortality, cardiovascular mortality and cardiovascular events in chronic kidney disease. Nephrol Dial Transplant 24:1506–1523
85. Gutierrez OM, Januzzi JL, Isakowa T et al (2009) Fibroblast growth factor 23 and left ventricular hypertrophy in chronic kidney disease. Circulation 119:2545–2552
86. Parker BD, Schugers LJ, Brandenburg VM et al (2010) The associations of fibroblast growth factor 23 and uncarboxylated matrix Gia protein with mortality in coronary artery disease: the heart and soul study. Ann Intern Med 152:640–648
87. Felsenfeld AJ, Levine BS, Rodriguez M (2015) Pathophysiology of calcium, phosphorus and magnesium dysregulation in chronic kidney disease. Semin Dial 28:564–577
88. Gutierrez OM, Mannstadt M, Isakova T et al (2008) Fibroblast growth factor 23 and mortality among patients undergoing hemodialysis. N Engl J Med 359:584–592
89. Jean G, Terrat JC, Vanel T et al (2009) High levels of serum fibroblast growth factor (FGF)-23 are associated with increased mortality in long haemodialysis patients. Nephrol Dial Transplant 24:2792–2797

90. Moe S, Drüeke T, Cunningham J, Goodman W et al (2006) Definition, evaluation and classification of renal osteodystrophy: a position statement from Kidney Disease: Improving Global Outcomes (KDIGO). Kidney Int 69:1945–1953
91. Mason MA, Shepler BM (2010) Evaluation of morbidity and mortality data related to cardiovascular calcification from calcium-containing phosphate binder use in patients undergoing hemodialysis. Pharmacotherapy 30:741–748
92. Wilson FP, Berns JS (2014) Tumor lysis syndrome: new challenges and recent advances. Adv Chronic Kidney Dis 21:18–26
93. Higaki M, Tanemoto M, Shiraishi T, Taniguchi K, Fujigaki Y, Uchida S (2015) Acute kidney injury facilitates hypocalcemia by exacerbating the hyperphosphatemic effect of muscle damage in rhabdomyolysis. Nephron 131:11–16
94. Byrnes MC, Stangenes J (2011) Refeeding in the ICU: an adult and pediatric problem. Curr Opin Clin Nutr Metab Care 14:186–192
95. Mehanna HM, Moledina J, Travis J (2008) Refeeding syndrome: what it is, and how to prevent and treat it. BMJ 336:1495–1498
96. Marinella MA (2005) Refeeding syndrome and hypophosphatemia. J Intensive Care Med 20:155–159
97. Nutrition Support in Adults: oral nutrition support, enteral tube feeding and parenteral nutrition; Clinical guidelines CG32; National Institute for Health and Clinical Excellence: London, UK, 2006
98. Morabito S, Pistolesi V, Tritapepe L et al (2013) Continuous venovenous hemodiafiltration with a low citrate dose regional anticoagulation protocol and a phosphate-containing solution: effects on acid-base status and phosphate supplementation needs. BMC Nephrol 14:232
99. Maier JD, Levine SN (2015) Hypercalcemia in the intensive care unit: a review of pathophysiology, diagnosis, and modern therapy. J Intensive Care Med 30:235–252
100. Aberegg SK (2016) Ionized calcium in the ICU: should it be measured and corrected? Chest 149:846–855
101. Forsythe RM, Wessel CB, Billiar TR, Angus DC, Rosengart MR (2008) Parenteral calcium for intensive care unit patients. Cochrane Database Syst Rev 5:CD006163
102. Melamed ML, Buttar RS, Coco M (2016) CKD-mineral bone disorder in stage 4 and 5 CKD: what we know today? Adv Chronic Kidney Dis 23:262–269
103. Tonelli M, Pannu N, Manns B (2010) Oral phosphate binders in patients with kidney failure. N Engl J Med 362:1312–1324
104. Kandula P, Dobre M, Schold JD, Schreiber MJ Jr, Mehrotra R, Navaneethan SD (2010) Vitamin D suplementation in chronic kidney disease: a systematic review and meta-analysis of observational studies and randomized controlled trials. Clin J Am Soc Nephrol 6:50–62
105. Navaneethan SD, Palmer SC, Craig JC, Elder GJ, Strippoli GF (2009) Benefits and harms of phosphate binders in CKD: a systematic review of randomized controlled trials. Am J Kidney Dis 54:619–637
106. Kraft MD, Btaiche IF, Sacks GS, Kudsk KA (2005) Treatment of electrolytes disorders in adult patients in the intensive care unit. Am J Health Syst Pharm 62:1663–1682
107. Brown KA, Dickerson RN, Morgan LM, Alexander KH, Minard G, Brown RO (2006) A new graduated dosing regimen for phosphorus replacement in patients receiving nutrition support. J Parenter Enter Nutr 30:209–214
108. Taylor BE, Huey WY, Buchman TG, Boyle WA, Coopersmith CM (2004) Treatment of hypophosphatemia using a protocol based on patient weight and serum phosphorus level in a surgical intensive care unit. J Am Coll Surg 198:198–204
109. Charron T, Bernard F, Shrobik Y, Simoneau N, Gagnon N, Leblanc M (2003) Intravenous phosphate in the intensive care unit: more aggressive repletion regimens for moderate and severe hypophosphatemia. Intensive Care Med 29:1273–1278
110. Bech A, Blans M, Raaijmakers M, Mulkens C, Telting D, de Boer H (2013) Hypophosphatemia on the intensive care unit: individualized phosphate replacement based on serum levels and distribution volume. J Crit Care 28:838–843

Part II

Acid-Base Disorders

Interpretation of Acid-Base Disorders

5

Hervé Quintard, Jean-Christophe Orban, and Carole Ichai

5.1 Introduction

The definition of an acid or a base varies largely according to the context. From a physiological point of view, an acid or an alkaline solution is characterized by its capacity to release or conversely to consume them. This chapter will review most of the pathophysiological concepts of acid-base equilibrium and the mechanisms which are involved in its regulation. The history of the patient, the context, and clinical signs are essential to diagnose an acid-base disorder. However, the final interpretation of an acid-base disorder is based on biological data issued from blood samples tools which allow to move on step by step.

5.2 Acid-Base: Fundamental Notions

5.2.1 Definitions

Since the beginning of the twentieth century, many definitions have been proposed. All of them are right, but depends on the context. Therefore, in cooking, acid defines a taste. For a chemist, the definition of an acid is based on the movements of electrons, whereas a physiologist takes into account protons H^+ production [1–3]. In 1987, Arrhenius defines an acid as a substance that enables to produce H^+ ions by dissolving in water. On contrary, a base dissolves in water by releasing hydroxyl

H. Quintard • J-C. Orban
Intensive Care Unit, Pasteur 2 Hospital, 30 Voie Romaine, 06001 Nice, Cédex 1, France

C. Ichai (✉)
Intensive Care Unit, Pasteur 2 Hospital, 30 Voie Romaine, 06001 Nice, Cédex 1, France

IRCAN (INSERM U1081, CNRS UMR 7284), University of Nice, Nice, France
e-mail: ichai@unice.fr

C. Ichai et al. (eds.), *Metabolic Disorders and Critically Ill Patients*,
http://doi.org/10.1007/978-3-319-64010-5_5

OH^- ions. But, this definition is limited to aqueous solutions and excludes nonaqueous acids (or bases) such as CO_2. A half-century later, Bronsted and Lowry (1923) proposed a close definition in which an acid is a donor of protons and conversely. As a consequence of its dissociation in a solution, an acid AH produces an H^+ with its conjugated anion A^-. In the same time, Lewis gave a unique chemical definition which allows to include CO_2, by defining an acid as a substance enabled to accept electrons and conversely for a base.

All of these definitions are totally appropriate from a chemical point of view and available also for plasma which can generate protons and hydroxyl ions from plasma water as follows:

$H_2O \longleftrightarrow H^+ + OH^-$. Nevertheless, none allows to give a physiological point of view. During the 1920s, Van Slyke underlined the implication of electrolytes in the pH equilibrium [4]. An acid can be therefore defined as a substance that releases cations or uptakes anions and conversely for a base. This concept has been taken over in the 1980s by P. Stewart to interpret variations in pH [5]. As a consequence, we must distinguish acid solution for which $[H^+]$ concentration is higher than that of $[OH^-]$, from the acid substance that produces H^+ ions or binds with OH^- ions.

The proton H^+ alone does not exist and is always combined with a cation. Its concentration in physiological compartment is very low. However, due to its small size, it provides a high capacity to produce electric charges. By binding to proteins, it induces modifications of their structure and consequently their activity (e.g., enzymes). The pH is a logarithmic expression of $[H^+]$ concentration of the solution. The mathematical relationship between both is given by the following formula: $pH = \log_{10}(1/[H^+])$ or $[H^+] = 10^{-pH}$

Thus, small changes in pH enable to express high variations in $[H^+]$.

5.2.2 Relations Between pH, Acid, and Base

The pH of a solution finally expresses a chemical potential of protons which indicates the gain or the loss of hydrogen. For practical reasons, $[H^+]$ concentration of a solution is always expressed by the pH. Indeed, pH is easily and directly measured (measurement of an electrical potential difference) by a specific device, a "pH meter." From a mathematical point of view, pH is the ratio between a non-dissociated acid (AH) and its dissociated form in an anion salt (A^-), the degree of dissociation being determined by the constant of dissociation Ka: $Ka = ([H^+] \,.\, [A^-]) / [HA]$. When translated in pH, the formula becomes: $pH = pKa + \log_{10}([A^-] / [AH])$ [1–3, 6–8]. If we consider the plasma and the bicarbonate-carbonic acid buffer system, we get the well-known Henderson-Hasselbalch equation, $pH = 6{,}10 + \log_{10}([HCO_3^-] / [\alpha PCO_2])$,

6,10 being the plasma pKa, α the CO_2 solubility coefficient, and PCO_2 that reflects carbonic acid according to $H^+ + HCO_3^- \underset{\text{spontaneous}}{\leftrightarrow} H_2CO_3 \underset{\text{carbonic anhydrase}}{\leftrightarrow} CO_2 + H_2O$.

However, plasma pH can be expressed by taking into account not only the bicarbonate buffer but also all other acids present in the plasma with their own constant of dissociation (Table 5.1).

Table 5.1 Most important plasma acids and their constant of dissociation, pKa

Plasma acids	pKa
Strong acids	
Lactate	3.7–3.9
Sulfate	0.3–2.0
Pyruvate	2.3–2.5
Acetoacetate	3.6
ß-Hydroxybutyrate	4.3
Succinate	5.2–5.6
Citrate	1.7–6.4
Ammonia (NH_4^+)	9.2–9.3
Weak acids	
Bicarbonate	6.0–6.4
Phosphate	6.7–6.8
Albuminate	7.6

5.3 Pathophysiological Concepts of Acid-Base Equilibrium

5.3.1 Henderson-Hasselbalch Concept

Close to the definition of Bronsted and Lowry, both physiologists Henderson and Hasselbalch focused their concept on the sole role of plasma bicarbonate and its relationship with plasma strong acids. In this approach, changes in plasma pH result from changes in plasma bicarbonates (metabolic disorder) or in partial pressure in carbon dioxide ($PaCO_2$) (respiratory disorder) [6–14]. This concept was the most popular during the first half of the twentieth century. The Henderson-Hasselbalch equation is mathematically always valid, but it considers only the bicarbonate buffer system and ignores numerous parameters that are involved in acid-base balance:

- The nonvolatile buffers such as albumin, globulin, phosphate, and citrate, all presents also in plasma
- The role of weak acids (albuminate, phosphate)
- The obligatory mathematical relationship between bicarbonate-carbonic acid and carbon dioxide (PCO_2)

5.3.2 Base Excess (BE) Concept of Siggaard-Andersen

During the1950s, Siggaard-Andersen proposed to use a very pragmatic and global evaluation of acid-base disorders (ABD). Therefore, the concept of BE was developed as the amount of strong acid (or base) (in meq/L) that must be added to the oxygenated blood sample to return to pH 7.40 while maintaining a PCO_2 of 40 mmHg and a temperature of 37 °C [3, 9–14]. If plasma pH is of 7.40 associated with a PCO_2 of 40 mmHg, BE will be equal to zero. If compared with Henderson-Hasselbalch equation, BE is free of PCO_2 variations. Therefore, BE allows to simply evaluate the global load of plasma acid or base while taking into account all extracellular nonvolatile buffers. Thanks to nomograms (based on the Van Slyke equation), BE is directly calculated by blood gas analyzers [4]. Despite all of these advantages, BE presents some limitations too [2]. The most important is that this parameter remains calculated from in vitro measurements which do not take into account:

- Physiological changes in $PaCO_2$ usually induced in case of metabolic ABD (= respiratory response).
- The in vivo continuity of plasma with the interstitial fluid that has less buffer capacity, leading to overestimate BE. To minimize this problem, it has been proposed to calculate the standard base excess (SBE) which considers a theoretical hemoglobin concentration of 5 g/L that would correspond to a similar buffer capacity in both fluids.

Nevertheless, SBE remains a global measurement that does not permit to distinguish the variations of strong and weak acids. SBE provides a global evaluation of the degree of plasma acidity (or alkalinity) but is totally inadequate to determine precisely the initial mechanism of the disorder from its compensation.

5.3.3 Stewart's Concept

At the end of the 1970s, P. Stewart proposed a physicochemical approach which is close to that of Arrhenius and Van Slyke. In this concept, plasma pH variations are generated by modifications in the level of water dissociation. Therefore, a substance is an acid because it increases water dissociation (by elevating H^+ production or its bound with OH^-) and conversely for a base [5, 8–10, 15–18]. In the plasma, water dissociation, i.e., H^+ concentration, is determined by three simultaneous principles of physical chemistry laws:

- Electroneutrality whereby total plasma-positive charges are equal to the negative ones.
- Conservation of mass in which every substance present in an aqueous solution remains constant. If we consider the example of a weak acid, the formula is: $[HA] + [A^-] = [Atot]$.
- Equilibrium of electrolyte dissociation. The degree of electrolyte dissociation in an aqueous solution depends on the dissociation constant K. Strong ions are characterized by a pK which is far from pH, in such a way that the ions are almost completely dissociated. Therefore, due to its very low pK (3.9), the strong anion lactate is exclusively dissociated in plasma and lactic acid cannot be pres-

ent. By definition, weak acids are characterized by a pK close to plasma pH, and consequently they are partly dissociated according to the plasma pH: the more plasma pH is taken away from pK, the more the dissociated form is high. Regardless, the approach, pH can be accurately calculated according to the Henderson-Hasselbalch equation: $pH = pKa + \log_{10} ([A^-] / [Atot] - [A^-])$.

In the Stewart approach, changes in plasma pH can only be determined by changes of one (or more) of the following three independent variables [15, 19–21]:

- The difference of charges between plasma strong cations and anions, called the strong ion difference (SID)
- $PaCO_2$, an essential variable which is the sole opened buffer system thanks to the ventilation
- The total weak acid concentration (Atot)

Due to its mathematical dependency, variation in bicarbonate cannot be the mechanism responsible of change in pH, but simply the consequence of modifications of one (or several) independent mentioned variables. Strong ions can be produced or eliminated, but weak ions H^+ and OH^- are generated or consumed depending on plasma water dissociation. An elevation in chloride concentration $[Cl^-]$ increases plasma water dissociation and consequently generates $[H^+]$ ions; conversely an elevation in sodium concentration $[Na^+]$ reduces plasma water dissociation and binds to $[H^+]$ ions.

5.4 Body Acid-Base Equilibrium

5.4.1 Regulation of pH: Fundamental Notions

The higher body acid load is generated by CO_2 and represents approximately 15–20,000 mEq/day. Daily lactate production is approximately of 1500 mEq. In the presence of oxygen (aerobic condition), it enters the Krebs cycle to be finally metabolized in the phosphorylative oxidation pathway, leading to a production of H_2O and CO_2, a consequent acid load of 4500 mEq/day. Most of the nonvolatile acid load is issued from the protein metabolism which represents 100–150 mEq/day. The total production of $[H^+]$ ions is of 15–25,000 mEq/day. Plasma pH remains usually stable thanks to various regulating systems that are characterized by variable efficiency and delay of initiation. Buffer systems are couples of non-dissociated/dissociated molecules which enable to uptake or release protons in a close system. Therefore, changes in the dissociation of the buffer will minimize changes in pH value. Volatile buffers are defined by their ability to be excreted by the lung (CO_2) and nonvolatile ones by their ability to be excreted by the kidney. Their efficiency is higher with weak acids and their dissociated anion salts (e.g., the couple H_2CO_3/HCO_3^-) and their pK is close to pH. Their nature and concentration vary according to organs and their localization [2, 6, 8, 19, 22]. While bicarbonate/CO_2 represents a crucial buffer system in an open system, weak acids participate in approximately 93% of the pH regulation in a closed system. This explains why during metabolic ABD, pH regulation is very rapidly initiated thanks to modifications in ventilation. On the other hand, in case of respiratory ABD, the first line of regulation is rapidly performed by nonvolatile weak acids (proteins) before the activation of the longer but more efficient mechanisms based on a renal excretion of strong ions. Moreover, it is important to underline that the metabolization of H_2CO_3 in CO_2+ H_2O is not spontaneous, but requires the carbonic anhydrase enzyme activity, which is variable according to type of tissue (and cells) and to their environment.

5.4.2 Regulation of Plasma and Interstitial pH

The major extracellular buffer (interstitial and plasma) is the couple bicarbonate/carbonic acid. At pH 7.40 (40 nanomoles of H^+), there is 6800 mmol of bicarbonates (HCO_3^-) and 340 mmol of CO_2 for 1 mmol of carbonic acid (H_2CO_3). Therefore, in physiological values, the ratio HCO_3^-/CO_2 is maintained approximately to 20/1. Despite its unfavorable pKa (6.1), this buffer is essential because it represents the sole opening system which allows a real excretion of CO_2 by the lung. Other nonvolatile plasma buffers are weak acids too and include proteins and phosphate (pKa = 6.8). Red blood cells contain a special buffer system, the couple hemoglobin/hemoglobinate which is characterized by pKa of 6.8 (Table 5.2).

The interstitial pH is similar to the plasma one, but it characterizes by its poor concentration in proteins (weak acids). Both fluids show very close electrolyte concentrations, i.e., in strong ions, thanks to their passive exchanges across the cell membrane (Table 5.3).

Table 5.2 Mathematical relationship between pH and plasma buffers

$pH = pKa + \log_{10}$ [A^- Anion / AH Acid]
Plasma
Strong acid
$pH = 3.9 + \log_{10}$ [lactate$^-$ / lactic acid]
Weak acids
$pH = 6.10 + \log_{10}$ [HCO_3^- / (0.03 × $PaCO_2$)]
$pH = 7.60 + \log_{10}$ [albuminate$^-$ / albumin)]
$pH = 6.80 + \log_{10}$ [HPO_4^{2-} / HPO_4^-]
$pH = 6.80 + \log_{10}$ [proteinate$^-$ / protein]
Red blood cell
$pH = 6.80 + \log_{10}$ [hemoglobinate$^-$ / hemoglobin]

Ka plasma constant of dissociation

Table 5.3 Acid-base equilibrium and electrolyte composition of most body volumes

	Extracellular volume			
	Arterial plasma	Interstitial volume	Red blood cell	Intracellular volume
pH	7.40	7.40	7.20	7
H^+ (nEq/L)	41	42	64	100
OH^- (μEq/L)	1.1	1.1	0.69	0.43
PCO_2 (mmHg)	40	50	40	50
HCO_3^- (mEq/L)	25	31	15	46
Na^+ (mEq/L)	143	137	19	10
K^+ (mEq/L)	4	3	9.5	155
Mg^{++} (mEq/L)	2	2	5	10
Ca^{++} (mEq/L)	1	1	–	–
Cl^- (mEq/L)	107	111	10	10
Atot (mEq/L)	20	–	60	200
SID (mEq/L)	42	31	57	130

Atot total amount of plasma weak acids, *SID* strong ion difference

5.4.3 Regulation of Cell pH

Cell pH varies from 6.2 to 7.2 according to the cells [2, 6, 8, 22]. Moreover, inside cells, pH varies also according to the various structures, from eight for mitochondrias to five lysosomes. Cell pH modulates many intracellular processes, such as enzymatic reactions, regulation of energy potential (ATP/ADP), activity of pumps, and channels. Thus, the regulation of this pH is essential to maintain cell volume and some molecules in their ionized form. Proteins/proteinates represent the major cytoplasmic buffer of the cell. Due to its high membrane diffusibility, CO_2 which is produced by the cell is continuously excreted toward the extracellular fluids, then eliminated by the lung allowing to prevent an intracellular acidosis. On the other hand, any elevation in extracellular CO_2 concentration (respiratory acidosis) may conduct to an intracellular acidosis because of its passive entry in the cell. The regulation of cell pH is also dependent of changes in SID, as a result of transmembrane movements of strong ions. These latter are performed by cotransporters or exchangers which are activated by pumps or through channels.

5.4.4 Regulation of Body pH and Exchanges Between Fluids

Besides the buffer systems, several organs are involved in the plasma acid-base regulation (Fig. 5.1). The lung plays a major role by excreting very rapidly almost the volatile acid CO_2. This phenomenon (VCO_2) depends on three parameters that are producing CO_2, alveolar ventilation (AV), and cardiac output (CO), (VCO_2) = AV × (k × $PaCO_2$), k being the conversion factor of a pressure into a volume. In physiological conditions, produced CO_2 is equal to VCO_2 in order to maintain a VCO_2 of approximately 40 mmHg. This equilibrium can be broken in case of

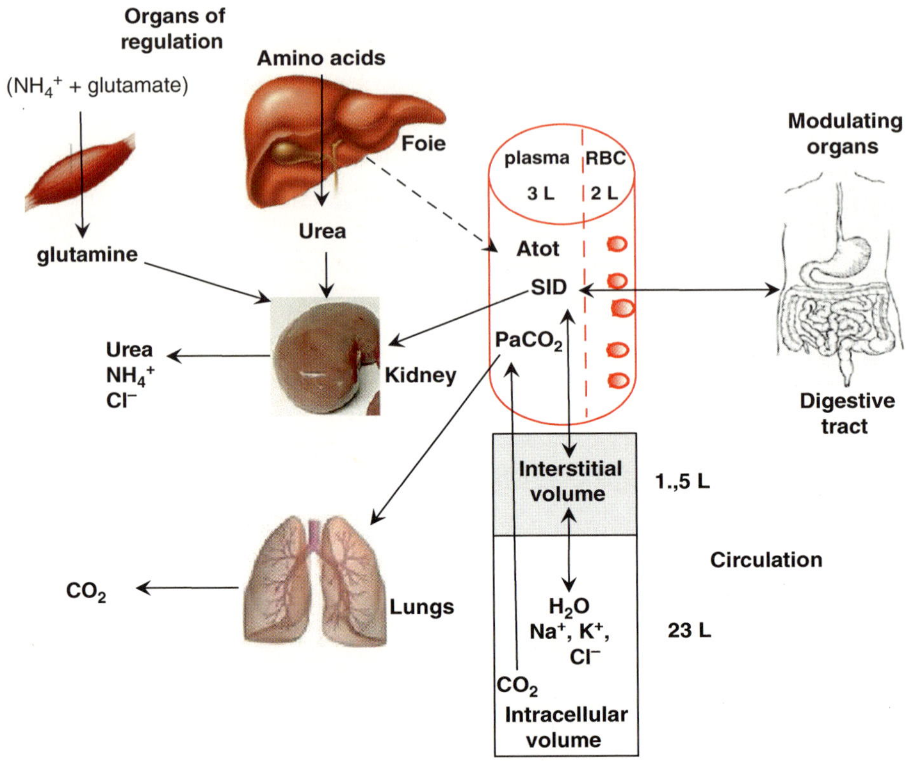

Fig. 5.1 Parameters and principal organs involved in total body acid-base equilibrium. *SID* strong ion difference, *Atot* total amount of plasma weak acids. The pH value differs among organs. Each of them enables to regulate immediately its pH thanks to buffer systems. All of them are strongly connected due to continuous transmembrane exchanges. Plasma pH regulation is performed thanks to two major organs: the lung (elimination or retention of PCO_2 via the alveolar ventilation) and the kidney (by SID variations and urea/glutamine excretion that are produced by the liver/the muscles)

changes in ventilation or of cardiac output: VCO_2 increases and $PaCO_2$ decreases if AV or CO elevates, and conversely. Because CO_2 is highly diffusible through the membranes, acute respiratory modifications will have a major impact on the plasma pH (and on body pH).

Kidneys are involved in plasma acid-base equilibrium via their role in the determination of plasma concentrations in strong ions [1, 2, 8, 22–24]. The phenomenon of chloride excretion-reabsorption represents the major mechanism of regulation. In case of acidosis caused by a reduction of SID, the kidney filtrates and excretes Cl^-, leading to a reduction of urinary SID and pH too, and in turn a re-increase in plasma SID and pH, and conversely. Because Na^+ plays a fundamental role in maintaining cell volume, this is not the major ion involved in the acid-base regulation performed by the kidney. The classical titrable urinary acidity which is defined as the urinary excretion of protons, finally, only reflects the higher urinary excretion of strong anions than that of strong cations. Urea, usually considered as a urinary buffer, plays a minor role in plasma pH regulation. Its high urinary concentration contributes to increase that of protons, but its very low plasma concentration cannot induce relevant effect on SID and on plasma pH. At last, ammoniac (NH_4^+) renal excretion which is issued from glutamine, couples with Cl^-, and induces in turn an alkalinizing effect. The liver (and in a less proportion muscles) plays an indirect role by modulating various metabolic pathways [25, 26]. It produces an acidifying effect by producing CO_2 from lipids and carbohydrate oxidations. The metabolism of organic acids such as ketone bodies, lactate, or citrate conducts to an elevation of SID and in turn of pH. The amino acid metabolism may lead to a production of urea or glutamine. The kidney requires glutamine to produce NH_4^+.

The digestive tractus is also largely involved in body acid-base equilibrium thanks to its capacity to eliminate or reuptake high amount of strong ions contained in digestive fluids. The movements of fluids and electrolytes depend on the part of the intestinal tractus [2]. In the stomach, plasma chloride is secreted in the gastric fluid, then reuptaked in the grelic tube, leading finally to a neutral exchange for pH. However, in case of abundant vomitings, the persistent chloride losses induce a metabolic alkalosis which is related to the increase of SID. The grelic tube is a major site of Na^+ and Cl^- reabsorption. The colic tube is mainly involved in the excretion of Na^+ and K^+ in feces, leading to decreased plasma SID. Therefore, abundant diarrhea can be responsible for the development of metabolic acidosis.

In summary: intracellular pH is more acid than the plasma one. Inside the cell, pH varies according to the structure and the localization. These differences are due to the various amounts of strong ions and nonvolatile buffers such as weak acids (proteins) (Table 5.3). Plasma pH is the only parameter that is routinely used in clinical practice because it is directly and rapidly measured by a pH meter. Therefore, considering only plasma pH to approach the global body acid-base equilibrium is finally a simplified way, but it remains the only one possible at bedside. Because of the constant exchanges of ions between the different compartments, any modification in the amount of strong ions or of buffers in one of them may change the acid-base status of the other. Plasma pH depends on three

independent variables, i.e. ,SID, $PaCO_2$, and weak acid concentrations. The lung strongly and quickly regulates plasma pH via the volatile buffer CO_2. Because CO_2 is highly diffusible through cell membranes, the lung plays a major role in the regulation of intracellular pH. The kidney acts slowly by modifying strong ion concentrations and in turn SID (Fig. 5.1). For these reasons, acute respiratory changes impact rapidly and deeply to the plasma as well as interstitial and intracellular pH, whereas chronic respiratory changes offer enough time to the kidney to initiate its regulation. On contrary, metabolic ABD related to plasma SID or Atot variations induce immediate changes of alveolar ventilation, leading to control plasma CO_2; this is the classical ventilatory response (inappropriately called compensation). Finally, the digestive tube can modulate plasma pH by modifying plasma SID and inducing ABD in severe digestive diseases. The liver appears as a modulator organ that enables to produce CO_2 issued from carbohydrate and lipid metabolism and glutamine and urea issued from amino acid metabolism. Its impact on weak acids (albumin production) remains minor (Fig. 5.1).

5.5 Which Tools to Interpret Acid-Base Disorders?

The diagnosis of ABD must begin by questions to build the patient's history associated with a clinical examination. However, biological data are essential and mostly issued from blood gas analysis and electrolyte measurements performed simultaneously in arterial blood (Table 5.4).

5.5.1 Blood Gas Analysis [15, 19, 27–29]

Arterial blood gas analysis is only required in the presence of suggestive clinical or biological signs. The sample should avoid pain and anxiety that could cause hyperventilation [6, 30]. Bubbles must be eliminated and the syringe tip closed rapidly. Measurements must be performed as soon as possible in order to stop the

Table 5.4 Tools required for the diagnosis of an acid-base disorder (normal values)

Measured parameters	
Common tools	*Additional tools*
– Arterial blood gas analysis . pH (7.40 ± 2) . $PaCO_2$ (40 ± 4 mmHg) . Calculated HCO_3^- (24 ± 2 mmol/L)	
– Plasma electrolyte concentration . Total CO_2 (26 ± 2 mmol/L) . Na^+ (140 ± 2 mmol/L); K^+ (3.5 ± 0.5 mmol/L) . Cl^- (105 ± 2 mmol/L)	– Phosphorus (0.8–1.2 mmol/L) – Albumin (40 g/L)
	– Urinary pH and osmolarity – Urinary electrolyte concentration (Na^+, K^+, Cl^-)
Calculated parameters	
– AG = $Na^+ - (Cl^- + HCO_3^-)$ = 12 ± 2 mEq/L	. Base excess (0 mEq/L) . Standard base excess (0 mEq/L)
– Corrected AG = calculated AG + 0.25 × (40 – measured albumin [g/L])	– aSID = ($Na^+ + K^+ + Ca^{++} + Mg^{++}$) – ($Cl^-$ + lactate$^-$) = 40 ± 2 mEq/L – eSID = [HCO_3^-] + [albumin (g/L) × (0.123 × pH – 0.631)] + phosphorus (mEq/L) × (0.309 × pH – 0.469)] = 40 ± 2 mEq/L – SIG = aSID – eSID = 2 ± 2 mEq/L

AG plasma anion gap, *aSID* apparent difference between strong ions (apparent strong ion difference), *eSID* effective difference between strong ions (effective strong ion difference), *SIG* strong ion gap metabolism of red blood cells. Plasma pH is accurately measured by an electrode of glass, while $PaCO_2$ is performed using a microelectrode and reaches a percentage error of 10%. Normal plasma pH and $PaCO_2$ are 7.40 ± 2 and 40 ± 2 mmHg, respectively. Blood gas analysis provides also the value of calculated bicarbonates (HCO_3^-c) from the Henderson-Hasselbalch equation, using measured pH and $PaCO_2$. The normal value of HCO_3^-c is 24 ± 2 mmHg. BE and SBE are also calculated with those data.

5.5.2 Plasma Electrolyte Concentration [15, 19, 27–29]

Measurements must be performed simultaneously on the same arterial blood sample [6, 10, 17, 30]. The following parameters are provided and must be considered:

. *Total arterial CO_2 (TCO_2)*: the sole measurement of plasma HCO_3^- is technically impossible because bicarbonate (dissociated form) is unstable and constantly in equilibrium with carbonic acid and CO_2. Therefore, measured plasma "bicarbonates" are really that of TCO_2 which represents the sum of real plasma dissociated bicarbonates (HCO_3^-), carbonic acid (H_2CO_3), and CO_2 gas concentrations. The normal value is slightly higher than the calculated one using blood gas analysis and is of 26 ± 2 mmHg.

. *Chloremia*: chloride is the major plasma strong anion and it is an essential parameter for diagnosing ABD. However, in case of dysnatremia, chloremia may vary independently of ABD [31, 32]. Usually, in this situation, changes in chloremia are proportional to those of natremia. Such proportionality can be demontrated by calculating the Cl/Na ratio which is normally equal to 0.75 or by calculating the corrected chloride using the following formula: corrCl = measured Cl × 140 / Na = 105 mEq/L.

. *Kalemia*: this parameter is not really needed to diagnose ABD, but rather useful to establish the cause of the trouble [33]. Kalemia is not obligatory inversely related to changes in pH [34]. Indeed, acidosis caused by the accumulation of organic acids does not induce hyperkalemia, because the organic anion freely enters into the cell accompanied with a concomitant entry of protons that allow to maintain electroneutrality independently from transmembrane shifts of K^+. In these situations, hyperkalemia must conduct to research another cause than acidosis to explain hyperkalemia: insulinopenia, renal insufficiency, or hyperglycemia. In hyperchloremic acidosis, because chloride cannot enter into the cell, an efflux of potassium from the cell to the interstitium is needed to maintain electroneutrality. Respiratory acidosis does not induce changes in kalemia [34]. At least, hypokalemia is frequently present during hypochloremic alkalosis.

. *Natremia*: sodium is the most abundant strong cation of plasma. Therefore, natremia is required to diagnose ABD, especially when using the Stewart concept. It is also an essential parameter required to calculate plasma anion gap (see infra).

. *Albuminate and phosphate*: both essential plasma weak acids represent approximately 78% and 20%, respectively, of the negative plasma charges. According to the Stewart model, an increase in one of these parameters (the third independent variable) is responsible of a metabolic acidosis and conversely [35, 36]. Figge et al. [35] have shown that at pH = 7.40, proteinates exert a negative charge of 12 mEq/L.

. *Other parameters*: calcium, magnesium, and lactate are strong ions which enter in the SID calculation. Their measurement, even not always routinely performed, must be done (as well as albumin dosage) in critically ill patients suffering of severe and complex ABD.

5.5.3 Urinary Parameters [15, 19, 27–29]

. *Urinary pH*: this reflects the urinary degree of acidification, in the absence of urine infection [37]. This is essentially useful to establish the cause of some metabolic acidosis and a very important marker used to monitor the efficiency of the treatment of some metabolic alkalosis.

. *Urinary electrolytes*: the measurement of sodium, potassium, and chloride urinary concentration is essential to evaluate the renal response in case of an ABD, allowing to orientate the etiology of the disorder.

All of these measurements can be performed on a small urine sample, "the urine spot" [37]. Nevertheless, such data must be cautiously interpreted in case of prior treatment by diuretics or water and sodium loads. In all cases, these samples should be performed before any treatment that may modify the results.

5.5.4 Calculations

. *Plasma anion gap (AG)* [6, 15, 27–30, 38–46]

Anion gap is based on the plasma electroneutrality principle whereby the sum of positive charges (cations) is equal to that of negative charges (anions). AG is finally the artificial result of the calculation, because the usual dosage of Na^+, K^+, Cl^-, and HCO_3^- ions is not known in all other ions which are also implicated in unmeasured cations such as $Ca^{++}$and Mg^{++} and unmeasured anions such as proteinates, sulfates, phosphates, and other organic acids (Fig. 5.2). AG which reflects the presence of unmeasured anions can be easily calculated at bedside using the following formula [27–30, 39]: $AG\ (mEq/L) = Na^+ - (Cl^- + HCO_3^-) = 12 \pm 2$ mEq/L.

This parameter is frequently used as a marker of metabolic acidosis when using the classical Henderson-Hasselbalch approach. This allows to distinguish metabolic acidosis with a high AG ("organic" metabolic acidosis) from those with a normal AG and hyperchloremia ("mineral" metabolic acidosis) (Fig. 5.3). However, AG has some limitations [8, 35, 36, 38–41, 47]. Hypoalbuminemia, which is present in more than 50% of critically ill patients, is the major cause of AG decrease. Therefore, for a constant value of pH, a 10 g/L decrease in albumin induces an AG decrease of approximately 2.5 mEq/L. To address this error, Figge et al. [36] have proposed to correct the AG calculation by taking into account albuminemia as follows:

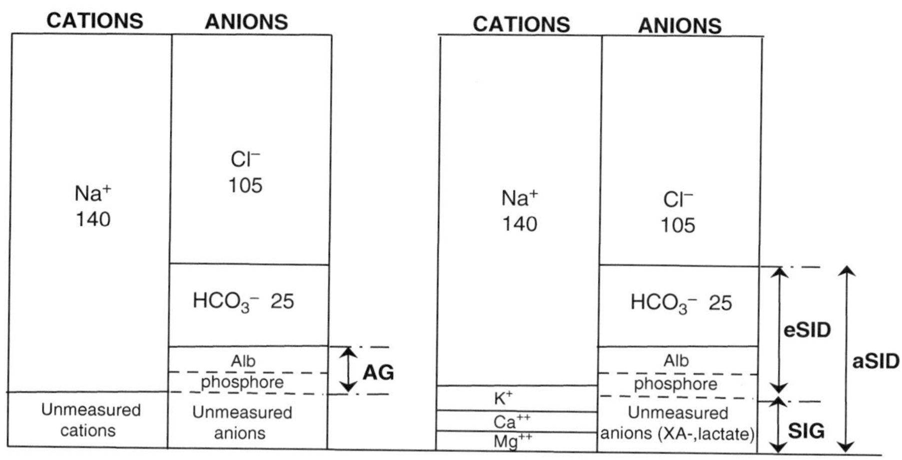

Fig. 5.2 Schema of positive and negative plasma charges allowing to calculate plasma anion gap (AG), apparent strong ion difference (aSID), effective strong ion difference (eSID), and strong ion gap (SIG). *Alb* albuminate, *Ph* phosphate. Unmeasured cations include essentially Ca^{++} and Mg^{++}; SID is always positive and normally equal to 40 ± 4 mEq/L. The difference between aSID and eSID is the SIG (normal value = 2 ± 2 mEq/L) and increases in case of excessive anions. AG is constituted by both unmeasured strong and weak anions. AG (normal value = 12 ± 2 mEq/L) increases in case of high concentration of plasma organic acids (lactate, ketone bodies)

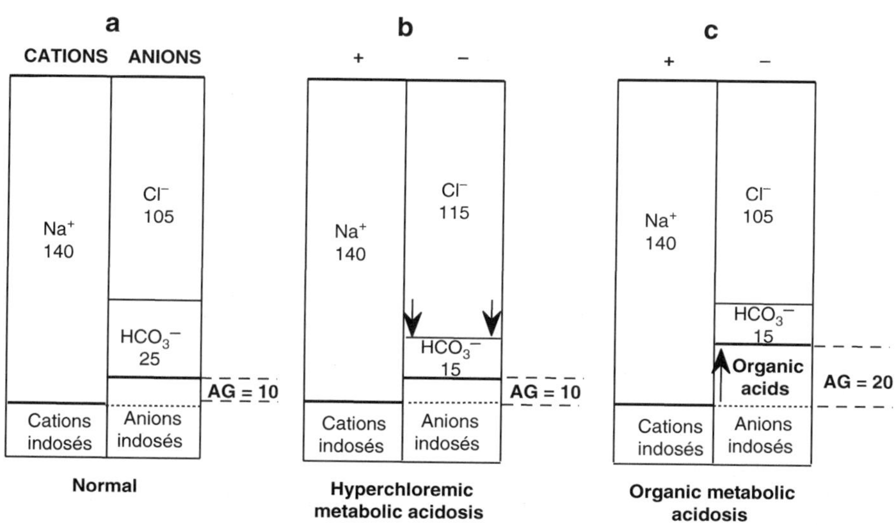

Fig. 5.3 Schema representing the two classes of metabolic acidosis according to Henderson-Hasselbalch method. (**a**) Normal situation: anon gap (AG) corresponds to the difference between all unmeasured anions and cations. (**b**) In mineral metabolic acidosis, each excessive HCl releases H^+ ions which is buffered by one HCO_3^- and one Cl^-; AG is therefore normal. (**c**) In organic metabolic acidosis, each excessive organic anion releases one H^+ ion which is buffered by one HCO_3^- ion and one dissociated acid$^+$ (anion); AG is therefore elevated >12 mmol/L

$$\text{Corrected cAG}\left(\text{mEq/L}\right) = \text{AG} + 0.25 \times (\text{normal albumin} - \text{measured albumin}\left(\text{g/L}\right)$$
$$= \text{AG} + 0.25\left(40 - \text{measured albumin}\right)$$

Nevertheless, such a correction is not always sufficient to eliminate the limitations of AG determination [42]. Any change in natremia, if not associated with a proportional change in chloremia, can modify AG independently of organic acid concentrations.

. *Base excess (BE), standard base excess (SBE)* [6, 15, 27–30, 38–46]

BE is calculated taking into account bicarbonate as the major extracellular buffer and hemoglobin which is the major red blood cell buffer (Table 5.4). BE and SBE are calculated using arterial blood gas analysis according to the following formulas: BE (mEq/L) = [(HCO_3^-) − 24.4 + (2.3 × Hb + 7.7) × (pH − 7.4)] × 1–0.023 × Hb] (mEq/L), Hb in mmol/L; SBE = 0.9287 × [([(HCO_3^-) − 24 + 14.83 × (pH − 7.4)].

. *Strong ion difference (SID)* [5, 12, 15, 17, 21, 22, 43, 44, 47]

SID can be calculated using two formulas. Taking into account plasma electroneutrality, the effective SID (eSID) is the sum of bicarbonate anion with both major plasma weak anions represented by albuminate and phosphate (Fig. 5.2): eSID (mEq/L) = HCO_3^- + albuminate$^-$ + phosphate$^-$. HCO_3^- concentration is calculated considering parameters of arterial blood gas analysis using Henderson-Hasselbalch equation. Albuminate$^-$ and phosphate$^-$ (Atot) are calculated considering their respective pK and pH. These parameters allow finally to calculate the eSID according to the following formula [2, 5, 15, 19, 48]:

$$\text{eSID}\left(\text{mEq/L}\right) = \left[\text{HCO}_3^-\right] + \left[\text{albuminemia}\left(\text{g/L}\right) \times \left(0.123 \times \text{pH} - 0.631\right)\right]$$
$$+ \text{phosphoremia}\left(\text{mEq/L}\right) \times \left(0.309 \times \text{pH} - 0.469\right)] = 40 \pm 2\,\text{mEq/L}$$

However, using this formula in daily clinical practice remains limited, and the calculation of the apparent SID (aSID) is easier and more practical at bedside:

$$\text{aSID}\left(\text{mEq/L}\right) = \left[\text{Na}^+ + \text{K}^+ + \text{Ca}^{++} + \text{Mg}^{++}\right] - \left[\text{Cl}^- + \text{lactate}^-\right] = 40 \pm 2\,\text{mEq/L}$$

Normal values of SID in a healthy human show large ranges, with extreme values from SID of 35 to 54 mEq/L [17, 20, 45]. The reduction in SID indicates the presence of an acidosis which is related to an accumulation in strong acids or to a decrease in cations (especially Na^+) and conversely [45].

. *Strong ion gap (SIG)* [5, 15, 35, 44, 49]

The unmeasured strong anions (XA^-) can be quantified by the calculation of the SIG which is the difference between all unmeasured strong cations and anions, according to the following formula: SIG (mEq/L) = aSID − eSID. In normal situations, SIG is of zero, but because of the presence of some low concentrated strong cations and anions which are not considered in the simplified calculation of aSID, SIG is physiologically slightly positive.

5.6 Definition and Pathophysiological Classification of Acid-Base Disorders

5.6.1 Identification and Classification of ABD

The biological tools required to diagnose an ABD are summarized in Table 5.4. The four successive stages that allow a practical identification of ABD are summarized in Fig. 5.4 [7, 17, 19, 27, 28, 30, 46].

(1) Validation of blood gas analysis: arterial blood gas analysis might be interpreted only if calculated bicarbonates ($cHCO_3^-$) do not differ of more than 2–3 mmol/L from measured bicarbonates (TCO_2) on arterial electrolyte determination [17]. A discrepancy between these two values indicates usually a technical error and must conduct to repeat measurements.

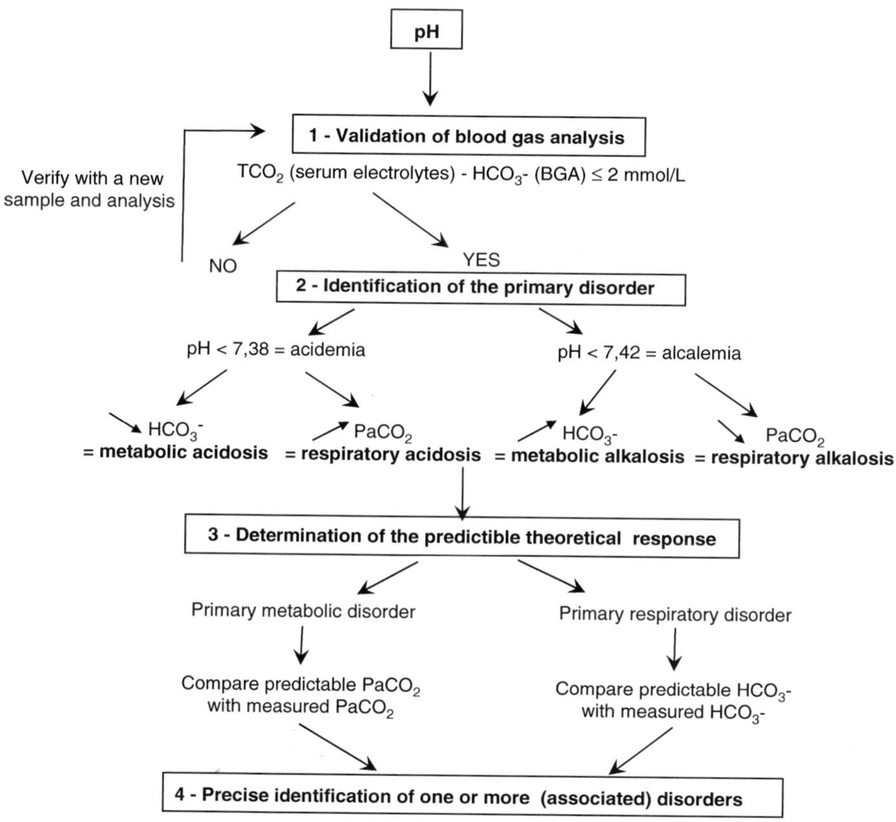

Fig. 5.4 Algorithm including the four successive steps required to interpret an acid-base disorder. *BGA* blood gas analysis, *TCO₂* total CO_2

(2) Identification of the primary ABD: stricto sensu, acidemia (alkalemia) might be distinguished from acidosis (alkalosis). Acidemia and alkalemia indicate a value of pH, in other words a concentration in protons: acidemia is defined by a pH <7.38 and alkalemia by a pH >7.42 [6, 17]. On the other hand, acidosis is a pathophysiological process which is responsible for an increase in plasma proton concentration and conversely. This latter definition indicates the causal processes and is not obligatory associated with a change of pH in the same direction (as in complex ABD). Nevertheless, in current practice, acidemia (alkalemia) and acidosis (alkalosis) are merged. A primary metabolic disorder is defined by a variation in plasma bicarbonates, whereas a respiratory one is induced by a primary change in $PaCO_2$.

(3) Evaluation of the predictable secondary response to the primary trouble: every primary ABD activates mechanisms of regulation which are able to minimize pH modifications, but never enable to normalize totally pH. This response, sometimes inappropriately referred to as "compensation," is highly reproducible from statistical models which were determined according to a linear regression [6, 22, 29]. In case of a primary metabolic disorder, the predictable response is a respiratory one which is immediate and based on $PaCO_2$ variations. In case of respiratory primary disorders, the predictable response is performed by the kidney. Its delay is longer (minimum of 12 h), and its degree depends on the speed of development of the respiratory trouble. Therefore, acute respiratory ABD must be distinguished from the chronic ones. Theoretical predictable responses are characterized by their mechanisms, their delay of initiation, and their limits (Table 5.5). A normal value of pH associated with an abnormal $PaCO_2$ or plasma bicarbonate concentration always indicates the presence of two or three associated disorders.

(4) Precise determination of the disorder(s): a simple (or pure) metabolic (respiratory) disorder is characterized by a variation in plasma bicarbonates (variation in

Table 5.5 Characteristics of predictable responses to primary acid-base disorders (ABD)

Primary ABD	Degree of response	Delay	Limits
Metabolic disorders			
– Acidosis (↘ HCO_3^-)	– ↘ $PaCO_2$ = 1.3 × ↘ HCO_3^-	– 12–24 h	– $PaCO_2$ = 10 mmHg
– Alkalosis (↗ HCO_3^-)	– ↗ $PaCO_2$ = 0.6 × ↗ HCO_3^-	– 24–36 h	– $PaCO_2$ = 55 mmHg
Respiratory disorders			
– Acidosis (↗ $PaCO_2$)			
. Acute	– ↗ 10 mmHg $PaCO_2$ = ↗ 1 mEq/L HCO_3^-	– 5–10 min	– HCO_3^- = 30 mEq/L
. Chronic	– ↗ 10 mmHg $PaCO_2$ = ↗ 3.5 mEq/L HCO_3^-	– 72–96 h	– HCO_3^- = 45 mEq/L
– Alkalosis (↘ $PaCO_2$)			
. Acute	– ↘ 10 mmHg $PaCO_2$ = ↘ 2 mEq/L HCO_3^-	– 5–10 min	– HCO_3^- = 18 mEq/L
. Chronic	– ↘ 10 mmHg $PaCO_2$ = ↘ 5 mEq/L HCO_3^-	– 48–72 h	– HCO_3^- = 14 mEq/L

$PaCO_2$) without any other additional disorder, i.e., with a theoretical predictable respiratory (kidney) response equal to that measured in the patient. Mixed ABD are defined by the association of both metabolic and respiratory ABD in the same direction or by the association of two or three ABD, some of them being in inverse direction. Because variations in $PaCO_2$ induced by changes in ventilation are the sole causes of respiratory ABD, the patient can present only one respiratory trouble. Therefore, the most complex ABD may associate a maximum of three disorders: metabolic acidosis and alkalosis with one respiratory trouble (acidosis or alkalosis). The diagnosis of a mixed association of metabolic acidosis and alkalosis can be performed by comparing the variation of bicarbonate with the chloremia and/or AG or SID one [17, 48, 50, 51].

5.6.2 Pathophysiology of Acid-Base Disorders

Metabolic disorders [17, 23, 30, 52, 53]

According to the classical Henderson-Hasselbalch approach, the decrease in pH is caused by the reduction in plasma bicarbonates which is secondary to the accumulation of H^+ ions. These modifications may result from the accumulation of organic acids (lactate, ketone bodies) or chloride (mineral acidosis) or from bicarbonate losses (digestive or renal) [6, 27, 28]. In the Stewart concept, metabolic acidosis results from a shift on the right of plasma water dissociation which induces an elevation in plasma H^+ concentration. This shift can be generated by a reduction in SID or an increase in plasma weak acid concentration (Atot). The decrease in SID can result from hyperchloremia, a high strong anion concentration (lactate, ketone bodies, or other unmeasured anions XA^-), or a low strong cation concentration (essentially Na^+) [2, 3, 5, 7, 8, 23, 50, 54–56]. In this last situation, plasma and chloride concentrations decrease proportionally and result in a higher reduction in sodium amount than of chloride. The final result is a decrease in SID. The inverse processes explain the development of metabolic alkalosis.

Respiratory disorders [17, 23, 30, 52, 53, 57]

Regardless the approach that is used, Henderson-Hasselbalch or Stewart, $PaCO_2$ is the independent variable responsible for the respiratory ABD.

5.6.3 Diagnosis of Acid-Base Disorders

Metabolic acidosis

In all cases, metabolic acidosis is diagnosed on the association of low values of pH, plasma bicarbonates, and $PaCO_2$, the latter being the predictable respiratory response which tends to return pH close to the normal value [17, 58, 59]. However, in case of severe and profound metabolic acidosis, the magnitude of the respiratory response is limited: below a pH of 6.90, $PaCO_2$ does not continue to decrease but on contrary tends to re-elevate.

According to the Henderson-Hasselbalch approach, the decrease in plasma bicarbonates induced by the accumulation of H^+ ions is responsible for the reduction in pH. It is therefore classical to precise the diagnosis by calculating the AG [6, 8, 27–29, 38, 46]. The AG is based on plasma electroneutrality principle whereby all positive (cations) and negative (anions) charges are equal (Fig. 5.2). AG allows to detect the presence in plasma of unmeasured anions such as sulfates, phosphates, and other organic acids that are not currently measured blood samples. Using this parameter, it is possible to distinguish high AG (organic) metabolic acidosis from those with a normal AG and hyperchloremia (mineral) (Fig. 5.3). However, the AG determination has limitations and must be interpreted with caution, because albumin is its major component leading to modify its value [8, 35, 36, 38, 39, 47, 60]. Indeed, hypoalbuminemia is the most frequent cause of reduction of AG: at a constant pH, a reduction of 10 g/L of albumin is associated with a reduction of approximately 2.5 mEq/L of AG. The calculation of the corrected AG (cAG) can minimize this error [36]. Chloremia must be interpreted by considering simultaneously sodium changes thanks to the chloremia/natremia ratio or to the corrected chloremia [31, 32].

According to the Stewart approach, the decrease in pH can be induced by a decrease in SID and/or an increase in weak acids, both being responsible of the decrease in plasma bicarbonates which is obligatory to maintain electroneutrality (bicarbonate plays its role of buffer) [5, 9, 17, 18, 21, 43, 44, 47, 54]. Therefore, a reduction in SID responsible for an acidosis may be secondary to an excess in strong organic or nonorganic acids (chloride, Cl^-) or to a decrease in cations and conversely [2, 8, 15, 45, 57]. The magnitude of unmeasured strong anion accumulation can be estimated by calculating the "strong ion gap" or SIG [5, 15, 21, 40, 49, 51]. The prognostic value of SID compared with that of AG remains controversial [5, 16, 40, 41, 49, 58, 61, 62].

Metabolic alkalosis

In all cases, metabolic acidosis is characterized by high values of pH, plasma bicarbonates, and $PaCO_2$, the latter being the predictable respiratory response which tends to return pH close to the normal value [6, 8, 27, 28, 63–65]. However, the respiratory response is autolimited by the concomitant induced hypoxemia.

According to the Henderson-Hasselbalch approach, the elevation of plasma bicarbonates is the primary cause of the elevation of pH. In hypochloremic alkalosis or "chloride-depletion metabolic alkalosis," the mechanism of alkalosis is the loss of nonvolatile protons, which can be initiated by the digestive tractus or by the kidney. These losses are associated with a concomitant loss of chloride, which explains the presence of hypochloremia, and usually a loss of potassium to which explains the presence of hypokalemia. An exogenous (usually iatrogenic) overload of bicarbonate may also induce a chloride-depletion metabolic alkalosis. Chloride nondepleted metabolic alkalosis is caused by a renal reabsorption of bicarbonates.

According to the Stewart approach, chloride-depleted metabolic alkalosis is caused by the decrease of chloremia which is proportionally higher than that of natremia and thus conducts to increase SID and finally pH. Chloride losses may be initiated by the digestive tractus or the kidney. Metabolic alkalosis may also result

Table 5.6 Classification of most primary acid-base disorders (ABD) according to the Henderson-Hasselbalch and Stewart concepts

	Metabolic ABD		*Respiratory ABD*
Henderson-Hasselbalch concept			
	pH	HCO_3^-	$PaCO_2$
– Acidosis	↘	↘	↗
	. Elevated anion gap		
	. Hyperchloremia		
– Alkalosis	↗	↗	↘
Stewart concept			
	SID	Atot	$PaCO_2$
– Acidosis	↘	↗	↗
	. Hyperchloremia	. ↗ Albuminate	
	. Hyponatremia	. ↗ Phosphate	
	. ↗ XA^- (± ↗ SIG)		
– Alkalosis	↗	↘	↘
	. Hypochloremia	. ↘ Albuminate	
	. Hypernatremia		

SID strong ion difference, *Atot* total weak acids, *XA^-* unmeasured strong ions, *SIG* strong ion gap

from an elevation in natremia which is more often iatrogenic related to an excessive exogenous intake of sodium bicarbonate and is responsible for an increased SID [8, 9, 18, 19]. The same mechanism is involved in the metabolic alkalosis which is currently considered to be related to volume depletion. Indeed, there is no volume depletion but an increased SID secondary to hypernatremia. Nondepleted chloride metabolic alkalosis is generated by renal reabsorption of sodium associated with an elevation of SID. At last, the elevation of pH can be due to a reduction in weak acids, essentially in hypoalbuminemia.

In summary: Table 5.6 summarizes the classification and causes of ABD according to Henderson-Hasselbalch or Stewart concepts. It is important to highlight that ABD that are generated by dysnatremia are not identified in the classical Henderson-Hasselbalch approach.

Conclusion

The pH of a solution represents its degree of acidity (or alkalinity). In the body, it is variable among organs and structures. Only plasma pH is easily available in clinical practice thanks to a rapid measurement by a pH meter. Plasma pH is closely regulated thanks to buffer systems and to the elimination (or uptake) of CO_2 by the lung and of electrolytes by the kidney.

The classical Henderson-Hasselbalch approach is based on the analysis of plasma pH, $PaCO_2$, bicarbonates, and AG, which allows to interpret acid-base disorders. This approach remains the most routinely used at bedside. The Stewart concept is based on the analysis of three independent variables that are $PaCO_2$, the strong ion difference (SID), and the plasma concentration of weak acids (albuminate and phosphate). This approach appears less easy for a daily practice and requires to understand some physical principles. However, in critically ill patients with complex acid-base disorders, this is the sole way to analyze exactly the disorder and its real cause(s). Such an approach is particularly useful in case of hypoalbuminemia and hypernatremia which generate metabolic alkalosis. Such an association which is totally ignored by the Henderson-Hasselbalch concept may blunt or minimize the severity of a concomitant metabolic acidosis and conduct to errors in diagnosis and treatment. In these cases, it is essential to measure plasma lactate, albumin concentrations, as well as other required parameters which are necessary to calculate the SID.

References

1. Hasan A (2009) Handbook of blood gas/acid-base interpretation. Springer Verlag, London, 361 p
2. Kellum J, Elbers PWG (2009) Stewart's textbook of acid-base. Lulu Enterprises, Amsterdam, Netherlands, 501 p
3. Story DA (2004) Bench -to-bedside review: a brief history of clinical acid-base. Crit Care 8:253–258
4. Siggaard-Andersen O (1977) The Van Slyke equation. Scand J Clin Lab Invest 37(suppl):15–20
5. Stewart PA (1978) Independent and dependent variables of acid-base control. Resp Physiol 33:9–26
6. Narins RG, Kupin W, Faber MD, Goodkin DA, Dunfee DP (1995) Pathophysiology, classification, and therapy of acid-base disturbances. In: Arieff AI, DeFronzo RA (eds) Fluid, electrolyte and acid-base disorders. Churchill Livingstone, New York, pp 105–198
7. Spital A, Garella S (1998) Pathophysiology of metabolic acid-base disturbances in patients with critical illness. In: Ronco C, Bellomo R (eds) Critical care nephrology. Kluwer Academic Publisher, Dordrecht, pp 327–344
8. Madger S (1998) Pathophysiology of metabolic acid-base disturbances in patients with critical illness. In: Ronco C, Bellomo R (eds) Critical care nephrology. Kluwer Academic Publisher, Dordrecht, pp 279–296
9. Gomez H, Kellum JA (2015) Understanding acid-base disorders. Crit Care Clin 31:849–860
10. Ayers P, Dixon C, Mays A (2015) Acid-base disorders: learning the basics. Nutr Clin Pract 30:14–20
11. Siggaard-Andersen O, Fogh-Andersen N (1995) Base excess or buffer base (strong ion difference) as a measure of non-respiratory acid-base disturbance. Acta Anaesthesiol Scand 39(suppl 107):123–128
12. Schilchtig R (1997) [Base excess] vs [strong ion difference]: which is more helpful? Adv Exp Med Biol 411:91–95
13. Kofstad J (2001) Base excess: a historical review- has the calculation of base excess been more standardised the last 20 years? Clin Chim Acta 307:193–195
14. Story DA, Morimatsu H, Bellomo R (2004) Strong ions, weak acids and base excess: a simplified Fencl-Stewart approach to clinical acid-base disorders. Br J Anaesth 92:54–60
15. Gunnerson KJ, Kellum JA (2003) Acid-base and electrolyte analysis in critically ill patients: are we ready for the new millennium? Curr Opin Crit Care 9:468–473
16. Kaplan LJ, Frangos S (2005) Clinical review: acid-base abnormalities in the intensive care unit. Crit Care 9:198–203
17. Quintard H, Hubert S, Ichai C (2007) Qu'apporte le modèle de Stewart à l'interprétation des troubles de l'équilibre acide base? Ann Fr Anesth Réanim 26:423–433
18. Ring T, Kellum JA (2016) Strong relationships in acid-base chemistry - Modeling protons based on predictable concentrations of strong ions, total weak acid concentrations, and PCO_2. PLoS One 11:e0162872

19. Kellum JA (2000) Determinants of blood pH in health and disease. Crit Care 4:6–14
20. Story DA, Poustie S, Bellomo R (2001) Quantitative physical chemistry analysis of acid-base disorders in critically ill patients. Anaesthesia 56:530–535
21. Gunnerson K (2005) Clinical review: the meaning of acid-base abnormalities in the intensive care unit. Part I - Epidemiology. Crit Care 9:508–515
22. Leblanc M, Kellum JA (1998) Biochemical and biophysical principles of hydrogen ion regulation. In: Ronco C, Bellomo R (eds) Critical care nephrology. Kluwer Academic Publisher, Dordrecht, pp 261–277
23. Moviat M, van Haren F, van der Hoeven H (2003) Conventional or physicochemical approach in intensive care unit patients with metabolic acidosis. Crit Care 7:R41–R46
24. Soriano JR (2002) Renal tubular acidosis; the clinical entity. J Am Soc Nephrol 13:2160–2168
25. Cohen RD (1995) The liver and acid-base regulation. In: Arieff AI, DeFronzo F (eds) Fluid, electrolyte and acid-base disorders, 2nd edn. Churchill Livingstone, New York, pp 777–790
26. Haussinger D, Gerok W (1985) Hepatic urea synthesis and pH regulation: role of CO_2, HCO_3, pH and the activity of carbonic anhydrase. Eur J Biochem 152:381–386
27. Adrogue H, Madias NE (1998) Medical progress: management of life-threatening acid-base disorders: first of two parts. N Engl J Med 338:26–34
28. Gluck SL (1998) Acid-base. Lancet 352:474–479
29. Kraut JA, Madias NE (2001) Approach to patients with acid-base disorders. Respir Care 46:392–403
30. Narins RG (1994) Acid-base disorders: definitions and introductory concepts. In: Maxwell MH, Kleeman CR, Narins RG (eds) Clinical disorders of fluid and electrolyte metabolism, 5th edn. Mac Graw Hill, New York, pp 755–767
31. Funk GC, Doberer D, Heinze G, Madi C, Holzinger U, Schneeweiss B (2004) Changes of serum chloride and metabolic acid-base state in critically illness. Anaesthesia 59:1111–1115
32. Durward A, Skellett S, Mayer A, Taylor D, Tibby SM, Murdoch IA (2001) The value of chloride:sodium ratio in differentiating the aetiology of metabolic acidosis. Intensive Care Med 27:223–254
33. Wiseman AC, Linas S (2005) Disorders of potassium and acid-base balance. Am J Kidney Dis 45:941–949
34. Magner PO, Robinson L, Halperin RM, Zettle R, Halperin ML (1988) The plasma potassium concentration in metabolic acidosis: a re-evaluation. Am J Kidney Dis 11:220–224
35. Figge J, Rossing TH, Fencl V (1991) The role of serum proteins in acid-base equilibria. J Lab Clin Med 117:453–467
36. Figge J, Jabor A, Kazda A, Fencl V (1998) Anion gap and hypoalbuminemia. Crit Care Med 26:1807–1810
37. Fumeaux Z, Stoermann-Chopard C (2005) Le spot urinaire: utilité et pièges à éviter. Rev Med Suisse 1:557–561
38. Reilly RF, Anderson RJ (1998) Interpreting the anion gap. Crit Care Med 26:1771–1772
39. Moe OW, Fuster D (2003) Clinical acid-base pathophysiology: disorders of plasma anion gap. Best Pract Res Clin Endocrinol Metab 17:559–574
40. Story DA, Poustie S, Bellomo R (2002) Estimating unmeasured anions in critically ill patients: anion gap, base deficit, and strong ion gap. Anesthesia 57:1109–1114
41. Emmett M (2006) Anion-gap interpretation: the old and the new. Nat Clin Pract 2:4–8
42. Dinh CH, Grandinetti A, Joffe A et al (2006) Correcting the anion gap for hypoalbuminemia does not improve detection of hyperlactatemia. Emerg Med J 23:627–632
43. Wilkes P (1998) Hypoproteinemia, strong ion difference and acid-base status in critically ill patients. J Appl Physiol 84:1740–1748
44. Kellum JA (2007) Disorders of acid-base balance. Crit Care Med 35:2630–2636
45. Story DA, Morimatsu H, Bellomo R (2006) Hyperchloremic acidosis in the critically ill: one of the strong-ion acidoses? Anesth Analg 103:144–148
46. Berend K, de Vries APJ, Gans ROB (2014) Physiological approach to assessment of acid-base disturbances. New Engl J Med 371:1434–1445
47. Corey HE (2005) Bench-to-bedside review: fundamental principles of acid-base physiology. Crit Care 9:184–192

48. Adrogue HJ, Madias NE (1995) Mixed acid-base disorders. In: Jacobson HR, Striker GE, Klarh S (eds) The principles and practice of nephrology, 2nd edn. Mosby-Year Book, St Louis, pp 953–962
49. Kellum JA, Kramer DJ, Pinsky MR (1995) Strong ion gap: a methodology for exploring unexplained anions. J Crit Care 10:51–55
50. Emmett M, Narins RG (1994) Mixed acid-base disorders. In: Maxwell MH, Kleeman CR, Narins RG (eds) Clinical disorders of fluid and electrolyte metabolism, 5th edn. Mac Graw Hill, New York, pp 991–1007
51. Fall PJ (2000) A stepwise approach to acid-base disorders. Practical patient evaluation for metabolic acidosis and other conditions. Postgrad Med 107:75–82
52. Fencl V, Jabor A, Kazda A, Figge J (2000) Diagnosis of metabolic acid-base disturbances in critically ill patients. Am J Resp Crit Care Med 162:2246–2251
53. Sirker AA, Rhodes A, Grounds RM, Benett ED (2002) Acid-base physiology: the "traditional" and the "modern" approaches. Anaesthesia 57:348–356
54. Story DA, Tosolini A, Bellomo R, Leblanc M, Bragantini L, Ronco C (2005) Plasma acid-base changes in chronic renal failure: a Stewart analysis. Int J Artif Organs 28:961–965
55. Constable PD (2003) Hyperchloremic acidosis: the classic example of strong ion acidosis. Anesth Analg 96:919–922
56. Ichai C, Levraut J (2003) Hyperchloremic metabolic acidosis and fluid resuscitation. Crit Care & Shock 6:31–39
57. Gattinoni L, Lissoni A (1998) Pathophysiology and diagnosis of respiratory acid-base disturbances in patients with critical illness. In: Ronco C, Bellomo R (eds) Critical Care Nephrology. Kluwer Academic Publisher, Dordrecht, pp 297–311
58. Gauthier PM, Szerlip HM (2002) Metabolic acidosis in the intensive care unit. Crit Care Clin 18:289–308
59. Narins RG, Krishna GG, Yeel J, Ikemiyashiro D, Schmidt RJ (1994) The metabolic acidosis. In: Maxwell MH, Kleeman CR, Narins RG (eds) Clinical disorders of fluid and electrolyte metabolism, 5th edn. Mac Graw Hill, New York, pp 769–825
60. Levraut J, Bounatirou T, Ichai C, Ciais JF, Jambou P, Grimaud D (1997) Reliability of anion gap as an indicator of blood lactate level in critically ill patients. Intensive Care Med 23:417–422
61. Cusack RJ, Rhodes A, Lochhead P et al (2002) The strong ion gap does not have prognostic value in critically ill patients in a mixed medical/surgical adult ICU. Intensive Care Med 28:864–869
62. Rocktaeschel J, Morimatsu H, Uchino S et al (2003) Unmeasured anions in critically ill patients: can they predict mortality? Crit Care Med 31:2131–2134
63. Galla JH (1995) Metabolic alkalosis. In: Arieff AI, DeFronzo F (eds) Fluid, electrolyte and acid-base disorders, 2nd edn. Churchill Livingston, New York, pp 199–221
64. Sabatini S (1996) The cellular basis of metabolic alkalosis. Kidney Int 49:906–917
65. Ichai C, Verdier JF, Grimaud D (1997) Les alcaloses. In: Société Française d'Anesthésie et de Réanimation ed. Conférence d'actualisation. Elsevier, Paris, pp 499–521

Acidosis: Diagnosis and Treatment

6

Hervé Quintard and Carole Ichai

6.1 Introduction

Acidosis is characterized by a decrease in plasma pH. The first chapter will focus on the pathophysiological principles responsible for the development of an acidosis. Clinical signs of an acidosis are not specific, and the diagnosis is based on the context, on the history, and finally on the biological abnormalities. Metabolic acidosis (MA) must be distinguished from respiratory acidosis (RA) because causes and treatment are totally different. The treatment of acidosis will be developed in the last chapter.

6.2 Pathophysiology of Acidosis

Stricto sensu, the term "acidemia" refers to a low plasma pH ($<7.38 \pm 2$) [1]. On the other hand, acidosis defines a pathophysiological process which induces an increase in plasma proton concentration ($[H^+]$) (expressed by a decrease in pH) [1–5]. Indeed, a complex acid-base disorder can associate both acidosis and alkalosis, the final resulting value of pH depending on the severity of each disorder. In practical, both acidemia and acidosis are routinely merged and only acidosis is routinely used.

The pathophysiology of MA differs according to the concept used for their interpretation. In the traditional Henderson-Hasselbalch approach, the decrease in pH is caused by an excess of plasma protons issued from an organic or a mineral acid or

H. Quintard
Intensive Care Unit, Hôpital Pasteur 2, 30 Voie Romaine, 06001 Nice, Cedex 1, France

C. Ichai (✉)
Intensive Care Unit, Hôpital Pasteur 2, 30 Voie Romaine, 06001 Nice, Cedex 1, France

IRCAN (INSERM U1081, CNRS UMR 7284), University Hospital of Nice, Nice, France
e-mail: ichai@unice.fr

C. Ichai et al. (eds.), *Metabolic Disorders and Critically Ill Patients*,
http://doi.org/10.1007/978-3-319-64010-5_6

by a loss of plasma bicarbonates [1, 2, 4]. The Stewart concept which considers all of the involved parameters but not only bicarbonates attributes the decline in pH to a greater dissociation of plasma water leading to elevate plasma proton concentration according to the following relation: $H_2O \Leftrightarrow H^+ + OH^-$. Two independent major parameters may impact this degree of dissociation and in turn the plasma pH: the strong ion difference (SID) which is the difference between the strong cations and anions and the amount of weak acids (cf Chap. 5). Any decrease in plasma SID, whether resulting from a decreased strong cations (Na^+) or an increased strong anions (Cl^-, lactate$^-$, ketone bodies$^-$), induces a decrease in pH and bicarbonate concentration. Any increase in weak acids (albuminate) will lead to comparable consequences [6–8]. Finally, irrespective of its mechanism, MA is characterized by a low pH and plasma bicarbonates concentration and can be calculated by the mathematical Henderson-Hasselbalch equation: $pH = 6{,}10 + \log [HCO_3^-]/0.03 \times PaCO_2$ (6.1 being the constant half-dissociation pKa of plasma bicarbonate, 0.03 being the solubility coefficient of CO_2). The secondary adaptative respiratory response (inappropriately called "compensation") consists in hyperventilation for increasing CO_2 removal, aiming to attenuate the decrease in plasma pH. In simple MA (isolated disorder), the magnitude of the secondary respiratory response can be calculated and is considered as the expected (or predictable) $PaCO_2$ (Table 6.1). However, it must be underlined that such an answer never enables to normalize completely the pH.

Regardless the pathophysiological approach, RA is always initiated by an elevation of $PaCO_2$ [6–9]. The normal daily endogenous production of CO_2 represents 15–20,000 meq/d, which comes essentially from protein metabolism. The lung is the major organ that enables to remove CO_2 (volatile anion). Therefore, an efficient alveolar ventilation associated with an appropriate hemodynamic status is needed to maintain a constant level of $PaCO_2$. It is important to distinguish acute from chronic RA which conducts to different clinical, biological signs and has different causes. Acute RA is associated with a slight to a moderate secondary renal response due to the short delay for the kidney to develop and exert it completely; in this situation, the predictable response can be evaluated as follows: any increase of $PaCO_2$ by 10 mmHg induces a 1 meq/L increase of HCO_3^- (Table 6.1). In chronic RA, the

Table 6.1 Characteristics of predictable responses in case of simple metabolic and respiratory acidosis

Primary acidosis	Level of response	Delay	Limits
Metabolic disorders			
– Acidosis ($\searrow HCO_3^-$)	– $\searrow PaCO_2 = 1.3 \times \searrow HCO_3^-$	– 12–24 h	– $PaCO_2 = 10$ mmHg
Respiratory disorders			
– Acidosis ($\nearrow PaCO_2$)			
• Acute	– $\nearrow$ 10 mmHg $PaCO_2$ = $\nearrow$ 1 $meq.L^{-1}$ HCO_3^-	– 5–10 min	– $HCO_3^- = 30$ meq/L
• Chronic	– $\nearrow$ 10 mmHg $PaCO_2$ = $\nearrow$ 3.5 $meq.L^{-1}$ HCO_3^-	– 72–96 h	– $HCO_3^- = 45$ meq/L

secondary renal response can develop completely to reach a steady-state level, and an increase of 10 mmHg of $PaCO_2$ induces a 3.5 meq/L elevation of HCO_3^- (Table 6.1). This increase in plasma bicarbonate concentration is usually associated with a simultaneous urinary excretion of chloride which induces an alkalosis: this is the classical metabolic alkalosis associated with chronic RA. In all cases, the sole expected renal response cannot normalize totally the decrease in pH. A normal plasma pH in the presence of an abnormal value of $PaCO_2$ or HCO_3^- has to make evoke a mixed acid-base disorder (association of 2–3 disorders).

6.3 Diagnosis of Metabolic Acidosis

The diagnosis of MA can only be confirmed with certainty using biological data. However, questioning on the history and on the underlying comorbidities associated with a clinical exam remains an essential step for the diagnosis.

6.3.1 Questioning: Clinical Signs

The first step of acidosis diagnosis consists in a careful clinical evaluation. Questions must precise the context and the possible absorption of toxic or drugs that may orientate the diagnosis. Clinical signs are not specific and present only in severe MA [1, 4, 6, 9]. Cardiovascular manifestations include arrhythmias, collapse, or shock. Neurological signs can be slight to severe: headache, obtundation, confusion, seizures, or coma. A skeletal muscle weakness can be present due to the reduction in intracytoplasmic ionized calcium. Acidosis can also manifest by gastrointestinal symptoms such as nausea, vomitings, and diarrhea. Hyperventilation as the secondary response to MA manifests as regular, wide, and deep respiratory cycles. Patients with controlled ventilation can become unsynchronized from the ventilator. Acidosis causes pulmonary vasoconstriction and a shift of the hemoglobin dissociation curve on the right, favoring in turn tissues O_2 delivery. Prolonged MA (as in chronic renal insufficiency) has metabolic consequences: increased protein catabolism, insulin resistance, modifications of calcium metabolism, hyperparathyroidism with osteodystrophy, abnormal secretion of thyroid, and growth hormones.

6.3.2 Biological Signs

The diagnosis with certainty is based on measured and calculated parameters issued from arterial samples to perform simultaneously blood gas analysis and electrolytes measurements. The absolute criteria for diagnosing MA are the association of both a low pH and bicarbonate concentration (and a negative standard base excess, SBE) and a decrease in $PaCO_2$ (respiratory response) [1, 3, 6]. MA is the sole disorder (pure or simple MA) if the measured $PaCO_2$ is equal to the predictable one and if no additional metabolic alkalosis is associated. MA is a part of a mixed acid-base disorder when the secondary renal response differs from what would be expected [1]. RA is associated with a primary MA when actual $PaCO_2$ exceeds predictable $PaCO_2$; respiratory alkalosis is associated with a primary MA when actual $PaCO_2$ is lower than the predictable one.

6.3.3 Etiologic Diagnosis

MA is commonly classified according to the value of the anion gap (AG) and of serum chloride concentration [1, 3]. The AG is based on plasma electroneutrality which indicates that the sum of cations is equal to that of anions. The AG reflects the presence of unmeasured anions and is calculated according to the following formula: $AG = Na^+ - (Cl^- + HCO_3^-) = 8–12$ meq/L [5, 8]. Therefore, there are two groups of MA, those with an elevated AG and those with a normal AG and hyperchloremia (Tables 6.2 and 6.3, Fig. 6.1). The elevated unmeasured anion concentration is responsible for the increase in AG which is associated with the decrease in pH and bicarbonates. MA caused by hyperchloremia (classical mineral acidosis) or by bicarbonate loss does not induce any changes in the AG value. However, the AG tool may be imprecise and inaccurate, especially in critically ill patients with complex acid-base disorders. Indeed, the weak anion albuminate represents a major component of the AG; therefore, its variation may lead to misinterpretation of acid-base disorders [1, 2, 10, 11]. For a constant pH, a 10 g/L variation of albumin modifies the AG of approximately 2.5 meq/L. To minimize this problem, Figge et al. [10] have proposed to calculate the corrected AG according to the following formula: cAG (meq/L) = AG + 0.25 (40 − actual Alb). However, this correction is not always sufficient to avoid this pitfall because nonproportional between variations of strong cations (Na^+) and strong anions (Cl^-) can also modify AG values [11, 12].

Table 6.2 Classification of acidosis according to the Henderson-Hasselbalch and Stewart concepts

Metabolic acidosis		Respiratory acidosis
Henderson-Hasselbalch concept		
pH	HCO_3^-	$PaCO_2$
↘	↘	↗
• High anion gap		
• Hyperchloremia		
Stewart concept		
SID	Weak acids	$PaCO_2$
↘	↗	↗
• Hyperchloremia	• ↗ Albuminate	
• Hyponatremia	• ↗ Phosphate	
• ↗ XA^- (± ↗ SIG)		

SID strong ion difference, *XA^-* unmeasured strong acids, *SIG* strong ion gap

Table 6.3 Classification of metabolic acidosis according to the anion gap (AG)

High AG metabolic acidosis
– *Caused by organic acid production*
• Hyperlactatemia
• Ketone bodies: diabetic ketoacidosis, fast ketoacidosis
– *Caused by a decreased renal excretion of organic acids: acute renal failure*
• Hyperphosphatemia, hypersulfatemia
– *Caused by an exogenous toxic anion poisoning*
• Salicylates
• Methanol, ethylene glycol
• Paraldehyde
Normal AG metabolic acidosis
– *Renal origin*
• Renal tubular acidosis
• Hyperparathyroidism
• Hypoaldosteronism
• Neoplasia
– *Gastrointestinal origin*
• Diarrhea
• Grelic/pancreatic draining or fistula drainage
– *Dilutional acidosis = hyponatremia*
– *Exogenous intake (iatrogenic or overdoses)*
• NH_4Cl, $CaCl_2$, $MgCl_2$
• Parenteral nutrition
• Inhibitors of carbonic anhydrase
• Bile acid sequestrant (cholestyramine)

Based on the Stewart approach, MA can be caused by a decreased SID or by an increased amount of weak acids (Table 6.2). The decrease in SID can be the consequence of three abnormalities [7]:

- A decrease of the difference between the major nonorganic (nonmetabolizable) extracellular strong cation (Na^+) and strong anion (Cl^-). Due to their low plasma concentration, magnesium (Mg^{++}), calcium (Ca^{++}), and potassium (K^+) cannot induce relevant modifications of SID and in turn of pH [1, 2].
- An increase of organic strong anions (lactate, ketone bodies).
- The presence of abnormal exogenous strong anions such as toxic or drugs.

The presence of organic (exogenous or endogenous) strong anions will be detected by calculating the "strong ion gap" (SIG) given by the following formula: SIG (meq/L) = apparent SID – effective SID (Table 6.4). It is not unusual to observe some associations between these abnormalities [7, 13]. The sole slight or moderate increase in weak anions (sulfate, phosphate) cannot really modify the pH because as compared to previous parameters, this absolute amount is negligeable [2]. All calculations needed for the diagnosis are summarized in Table 6.5 and Fig. 6.2.

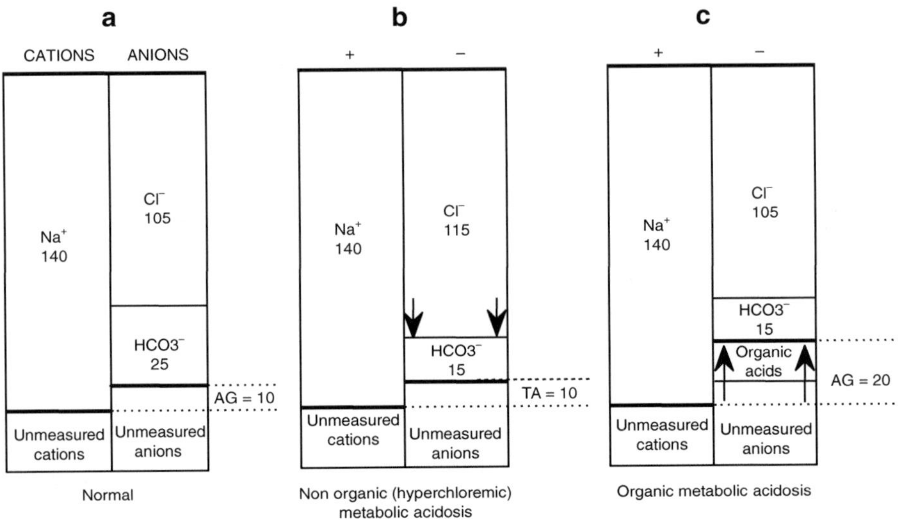

Fig. 6.1 Schematic representation of the two categories of metabolic acidosis according to the variation in anion gap (AG). (**a**) Normal situation: AG represents the difference between all unmeasured anions and cations present in plasma. (**b**) Mineral hyperchloremic metabolic acidosis: each excessive molecule Cl^- releases a proton H^+ which is buffered by one HCO_3^- to maintain electroneutrality; chloride Cl^- is elevated, and as it enters in the calculation of AG, this latter remains normal <12 mmol/L. (**c**) Organic metabolic acidosis: each excessive strong anion releases a proton H^+ which is buffered by one HCO_3^- to maintain electroneutrality; the remaining strong dissociated anion does not enter in the calculation of AG leading to a high AG >12 mmol/L

Table 6.4 Classification of metabolic acidosis according to plasma strong ion gap (SIG) and urinary strong ion difference (SID)

High SIG metabolic acidosis	Normal SIG metabolic acidosis
Endogenous anions	*Urinary SID > 0 = renal causes*
• Lactate • Ketone bodies	• Renal tubular acidosis
Exogenous anions	*Urinary SID < 0 = extrarenal causes*
• Salicylate • Methanol, ethylene glycol, paraldehyde	• Gastrointestinal losses: diarrhea, grelic/pancreatic draining, uretero-digestive anastomosis, neobladder • Iatrogenic: parenteral nutrition, unbalanced solutions infusion • Anion exchange resins (bile acid sequestrant)
Unmeasured anions	
• Intermediate substrates of the Krebs cycle (produced during sepsis, renal or liver insufficiency/failure): pyroglutamate, formate, oxalate, glycolate, etc.	

Several studies have reported that the Stewart method allows to identify more acid-base disorders, especially in case of mixed disorders and more precisely their mechanisms in intensive care unit when compared with the traditional approach [14–16]. Indeed, an acid-base disorder has been identified in 14% additional patients with the Stewart approach as compared to the Henderson-Hasselbalch one [16].

Table 6.5 Formulas required for the etiologic diagnosis of metabolic acidosis

– AG = $Na^+ - (Cl^- + HCO_3^-)$ = 8–12 mEq/L or = $(Na^+ + K^+) - (Cl^- + HCO_3^-)$ = 8–17 mEq/L
– Corrected AG = calculated AG + 0.25 × (40 – measured albumin [g/L])
• Standard base excess = 0.9287 × [HCO_3^- – 24.4 + 14.83 × (pH – 7.4)] = 0 mEq/L
– SIDa = $(Na^+ + K^+ + Ca^{++} + Mg^{++}) - (Cl^- + lactate^-)$ = 40 ± 2 mEq/L
– SIDe = [HCO_3^-] + [albumin (g/L) × (0.123 × pH – 0.631)] + phosphate (mEq/L) × (0.309 × pH – 0.469)] = 40 ± 2 mEq/L
– SIG = SIDa – SIDe = 2–6 mEq/L
– Urinary SID = (urinary Na + urinary K) – urinary Cl

AG plasma anion gap, *SIDa* apparent strong ion difference, *SIDe* effective strong ion difference, *SIG* strong ion gap

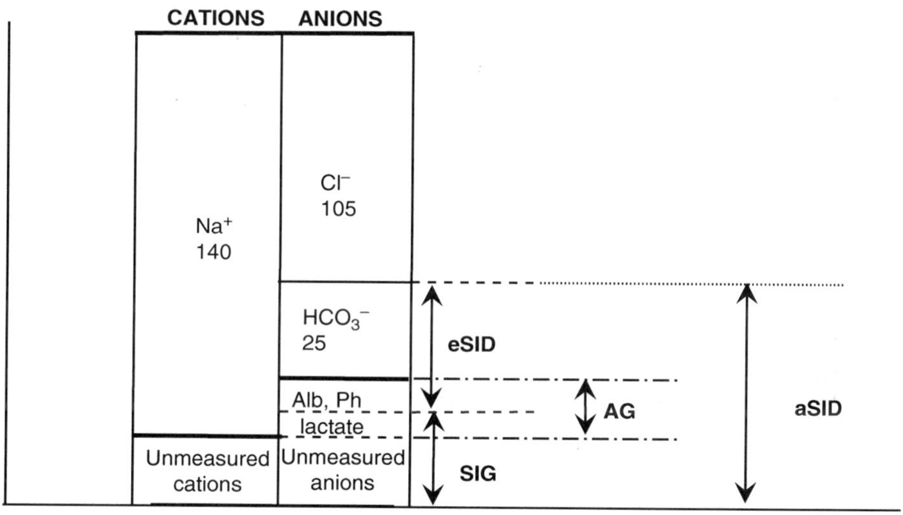

Fig. 6.2 Representation of plasma positive and negative charges. Unmeasured cations include Ca^{++} and Mg^{++}; SID is always positive, with a normal value of 40 meq/L. The normal difference between eSID and aSID (SIG) is of 0–5 meq/L, but increases if unmeasured strong anions accumulate. AG is also composed by unmeasured strong anions by also of weak acids such as albuminate and phosphate. Normal AG value is approximately 12 meq/L; it elevates in case of accumulation of organic acids (lactate, ketone bodies). *AG* plasma anion gap, *aSID* apparent strong ion difference, *eSID* effective strong ion difference, *SIG* strong ion gap, *Alb* albuminate, *Ph* phosphates

Recently, Szrama et al. [14] confirmed that critically ill patients with sepsis suffered from mixed acid-base disorders. Hypoalbuminemia was present in 100% of patients, and despite a normal standard base excess, patients presented acid-base abnormalities: hyperlactatemia, hyperchloremia, and a high SIG were observed in 21.3%, 98.4%, and 13.9%, respectively. On the other hand, acidosis (SBE < -2) was associated with hyperlactatemia in 35% and hyperchloremia in 96.9% of cases, and alkalosis (SBE $> +2$) was associated with hyperlactatemia in 18.4% and hyperchloremia in 88% of cases.

6.3.3.1 High SIG Metabolic Acidosis

Metabolic Acidosis Caused by Hyperlactatemia (see Chap. 8)

This represents one of the major causes of MA in intensive care unit, as it is observed in approximately 2/3 of patients [7, 11, 17]. Lactic acidosis is commonly defined as a metabolic acidosis associated with an elevated serum lactate concentration ≥ 5 mmol/L. However, hyperlactatemia is not obligatory associated with acidosis [12, 18]. Lactate is a strong organic (metabolizable) anion and is included in the group of MA with an elevated AG and cAG. However, the low precision of these two parameters forces us to measure lactatemia to confirm the diagnosis [7, 12]. According to the Stewart concept, an acidosis with hyperlactatemia is characterized by a low SID associated with a high SIG. In 1976, Cohen and Wood classified MA with hyperlactatemia into two groups according to the presence or not of an impairment of tissue oxygenation. Nevertheless, this classification proves to be inaccurate, as hyperlactatemia is caused by various disorders which associates aerobic and anaerobic metabolism such as observed during sepsis [1, 7]. In these situations, an increased lactate/pyruvate ratio can only confirm that hyperlactatemia is caused by an anaerobic metabolism [7]. But in clinical practice, the measurement of serum pyruvate concentration is difficult and not routinely available because such a measurement is long and requires to be performed rapidly as pyruvate is very labile.

Metabolic Acidosis Caused by Ketoacidosis

Diabetic ketoacidosis (DKA) is one of the acute metabolic complications of diabetes. Since more than 15 years, the mortality rate reaches less than 5%, thanks to an improved medical management [11, 19–21]. DKA is related to the accumulation in plasma of ketone bodies (acetone, acetoacetate, ß-hydroxybutyrate), all strong organic anions which are issued from an enhanced ß-oxidation of free fatty acids due to insulin deficiency and excessive concentration in counter-regulatory hormones. DKA is classically described as a pure MA with an elevated AG associated with hyperglycemia. However, it is preferred to characterize it by a decreased SID and an increased SIG which reflects the presence of excessive amount of strong organic anions (in this case ketone bodies). The determination of serum ketone bodies (ketonemia) is long and leads to perform an indirect but rapid detection in urines (ketonuria). Usually, polyuria caused by hyperglycemia induces an acute renal failure which is responsible for an accumulation of weak acids (sulfate, phosphate) that worsen MA. In the early period, the decrease in renal excretion of ketone bodies is associated with a concomitant increase in urinary chloride excretion in order to maintain urine electroneutrality. This phenomenon may cause a slight metabolic alkalosis associated with the MA. This hypochloremic metabolic alkalosis is aggravated by frequent vomitings [21]. Therefore, acid-base disorders of DKA are rarely a simple isolated organic MA. During the treatment of DKA, the development of hyperchloremia is frequently observed and is caused by two phenomenons: a high exogenous intake of chloride related to unbalanced crystalloids infused for vascular expansion and the improvement of renal function which allows to eliminate ketone bodies in urines in return to chloride reuptake. Therefore, during the improvement of DKA, the early organic MA is progressively replaced by a hyperchloremic MA. The diagnosis of DKA is usually easy, based on the history, the context, and the classical Küssmaul polypnea. The efficacy of treatment is based on the decreased rate of hyperglycemia and on the decrease of ketone body production which is monitored by ketonuria. It must be underlined that ketone body determination by urine dipsticks uses a nitroprusside reagent which reacts only with acetoacetate (and acetone). When ketonemia is strongly high, the thermodynamic reaction favors the production of ß-hydroxybutyrate from acetoacetate and conversely [22]. This explains the discordant results between ketonuria and ketonemia (and the evaluation of DKA severity). When the patient's condition improves and ketonemia decreases, the common trap is to observe a paradoxical re-increase of ketonuria which simply indicates the inverse preferential thermodynamic metabolism of ß-hydroxybutyrate in acetoacetate. Capillary measurement of ketonemia has been advocated, using point of care devices, which presents the advantage to be rapid, in real time and available at bedside. However, values from these devices, even with the most recent generation, remain not precise and dependent on the staff training. Finally, recommendations on the method for measuring ketone body production (in plasma, capillary, or urine) for the diagnosis of DKA and its severity and monitoring its resolution remain debated [22].

The prolonged fast which is physiologically accompanied by insulinopenia and hyperglucagonemia can also stimulate ketone body production leading to the classical fast ketoacidosis, with comparable acid-base disorders as in diabetic patients.

Metabolic Acidosis Caused by Toxic Intake

In these situations, MA is also caused by the accumulation of strong anions and is characterized by a high AG or a decreased SID with an increased SIG. These strong anions are usually issued from drug or toxic catabolism (salicylate, pyroglutamate, formate, oxalate, and glycolate) [23].

Acetylsalicylate overdose associates MA with a predominant respiratory alkalosis due to the stimulation of respiratory centers by salicylate. Therefore, pH is frequently alkaline, especially within the first hours and in less severe situations [1, 2]. The association of consciousness disorders with MA with high AG/SIG in the context of poisoning must orientate to an intake of methanol or ethylene glycol. This diagnosis is strongly evoked in case of an elevated osmolar gap (measured plasma osmolarity − calculated plasma osmolarity [>10 mosm/L]). A direct measurement of serum concentration of these two toxics can confirm the diagnosis. The oxidation of methylene in formate and formaldehyde may cause blindness due to a direct toxicity on the optic nerve. The ethylene glycol poisoning can manifest by neurological disorders, cardiovascular collapse, and liver and renal failures. Its catabolism in oxalate and formate is responsible for the decreased SID and the increased SIG.

In critically ill patients, SIG is frequently elevated, independently of any abnormal excessive amount of lactate, ketone bodies, or toxics. The elevated SIG indicates the presence of unknown strong anions which seems to be intermediate substrates issued from the Krebs cycle [23].

Metabolic Acidosis Caused by Renal Insufficiency

MA during renal insufficiency has been classically attributed to an abnormal excretion of protons and bicarbonates reabsorption [1, 2]. But this pathophysiological point of view ignores totally the dependency of bicarbonates and protons and the role of other factors implicated in acid-base equilibrium. The kidney plays a major role in this equilibrium because of its involvement in plasma-urine electrolytes exchanges which modulate plasma and urine SIDs [2, 7]. The three strong ions mostly implicated in these phenomenons are Na^+ cation (and secondarily K^+) and Cl^- anion. Therefore, if Na^+ losses are superior to Cl^- ones, urinary SID and pH will increase while plasma SID and pH will decrease [7]. The excretion of Cl^- would be the principal mechanism of plasma pH regulation by the kidney. The kidney must excreted chloride anions without excreting concomitantly Na^+ or K^+, leading to acidify urines and in turn, to alkalinize plasma pH. For preserving electroneutrality, the cation that accompanies Cl^- in urines is ammoniac NH_4^+ which comes from nitrogenous metabolism.

During renal insufficiency, the mechanisms of MA are complex, multiple, and depending on the length of the disease [3, 4, 7, 24]. At the early phase of renal insufficiency, hyperchloremia is the major cause of the decreased SID and thus of the decreased pH [25]. Acidosis is therefore a MA with a low SID but a normal SIG (and a normal AG). In severe, end-stage, and terminal renal insufficiency, renal excretion of strong anions is impaired and may be responsible for more than 50% of MA with a low SID and a high SIG (and AG). In acute renal failure, the accumulation of sulfates and phosphates in plasma associated with hypocalcemia can be implicated in the development of MA with an elevated SIG. On the other hand, all these acidifying factors are frequently counterbalanced by hypoalbuminemia and hyperkalemia which cause alkalinization, leading finally to a slight-to-moderate MA.

6.3.3.2 Normal SIG Metabolic Acidosis

They are caused by solely changes in electrolyte concentrations which induce a decrease in plasma SID, due to a decrease in cations or an increase in anions or the association of both. Therefore, these MA are characterized by an increase in chloride/sodium ratio (>0.75) because of an absolute excess of chloride or a relative excess caused by a loss of sodium while SIG is normal. A recent retrospective study has evaluated the participation of chloride in MA associated with a low SID using three parameters: Na/Cl ratio, the base excess chloride (BEcl = $Na^+ - Cl^- - 32$), and the nonlactate SID (nlSID) [$(Na^+ + K^+ + Ca^{++} + Mg^{++}) - Cl^-$] [20]. One thousand sixty-nine critically ill patients were included; a high nlSID was present in 16.3% of patients and was independently associated with an increased mortality. The classification between a renal and a nonrenal cause is confirmed by the calculation of urinary SIG according to the following formula: uSIG (meq/L) = $(uNa^+ - uK^+) - uCl^-$ (Table 6.5) [7].

Metabolic Acidosis Caused by Renal Tubular Acidosis

These disorders are due to tubular function abnormalities while glomerular filtration rate is not impaired [6, 7, 26, 27]. Irrespective of the type of the tubular acidosis,

MA is caused by hyperchloremia with a decrease in SID, but a normal SIG associated with a positive urinary SIG. All tubular acidosis are characterized by abnormalities of electrolytes channels or transporters that induce finally a greater renal reabsorption of chloride and sodium reabsorption, leading to an elevation of the urine SID and a reduction of the plasma SID and pH.

In the renal distal tubular acidosis (type 1), disorders are essentially caused by abnormalities of intercalated cells of the collecting tube. Abnormalities are located on cells of proximal convoluted tubule in proximal tubular acidosis (type 2). Type 4 renal tubular acidosis (pseudohypoaldosteronism type 2) induces various metabolic abnormalities which are characterized by a hyperchloremic MA associated with arterial hypertension and hyperkalemia [6, 7]. This acidosis is due to multiple abnormalities of channels which are located on cells of distal convoluted tubule and collecting tube and which are involved in Na^+, K^+, and Cl^- movements and in kinase transporters.

Metabolic Acidosis Caused by Digestive Losses

The intestinal losses due to diarrhea or grelic/pancreatic draining induce MA because the gastrointestinal tube reuptakes sodium and chloride in an equal amount, leading finally to decrease plasma SID. This is a hyperchloremic MA with a low SID and a normal SIG, but the urinary SIG is negative indicating an appropriate response of the kidney (Table 6.5). Patients with a new bladder issued from the digestive tube develop a similar type of acidosis because accumulated urines in the colon undergo a comparable reuptake of both Na^+ and Cl^-.

Metabolic Acidosis Caused by Fluids

The infusion of large volume of solutions for vascular expansion can induce complex acid-base disorders which are different according to their composition. The composition, i.e., concentration in cations and anions of most solutions, is summarized in Table 6.6. One of the most common acid-base disorders is hyperchloremic MA [28]. Considering the Henderson-Hasselbalch approach, these hyperchloremic acidoses are induced by a decrease in plasma bicarbonates, leading to a dilutional acidosis. However, several studies failed to confirm the presence of any change in plasma volume or of hemodilution [29]. The accurate explanation of the mechanism of this disorder is given by the Stewart method which attributes acidosis to a decrease in SID by two phenomenons. First, the infusion of hypotonic solution induces a reduction of Na^+ which is proportionally greater than that of Cl^-, leading to a decrease in SID and in turn in pH: the classical dilutional acidosis is finally an acidosis caused by hyponatremia (not proportional to hypochloremia). But the most frequent and severe disorder is an inorganic MA due to hyperchloremia which is provoked by the infusion of solutions rich in chloride, called "unbalanced" solutions [4, 7, 8, 14, 25, 30, 31]. The best "balanced" solutions are those with a SID of approximately 24 meq/L [32–34]. Crystalloids such as saline ("normal" 0.9% NaCl or hypertonic) are characterized by a SID equal to zero, as sodium concentration equals chloride concentration, explaining their acidifying effect [35]. In the same time, they have also an alkalinizing effect because they induce a dilutional

Table 6.6 Classification of intravenous solutions in "unbalanced" and "balanced" according to their qualitative and quantitative composition

Solutions	Na^+ (meq/L)	K^+ (meq/L)	Cl^- (meq/L)	Other anions (meq/L)	Osmolarity (mosm/L)	In vivo SID (meq/L)
Crystalloids						
• *Unbalanced*						
NaCl 0.9%	154	0	154	–	308	–
NaCl 3%	510	0	510	–	1026	–
NaCl 7.5%	1275	0	1275	–	2395	–
• *Balanced*						
Ringer's lactate	130	4	108	Lactate (27.6)	277	27
Ringer's acetate	132	4	110	Acetate [28]	277	27
Acetate gluconate (Plasma-Lyte®)	140	5	98	Acetate [26] Gluconate [22]	294	50
Acetate malate (Isofundin®)	145	4	127	Acetate [23] Malate [5]	304	27
Colloids						
• *Unbalanced*						
Hydroxyethyl starch (Voluven®)	154	0	154	–	308	–
Albumin	154	0	154	–	308	–
• *Balanced*						
Hydroxyethyl starch (Tetraspan®)	140	4	118	Acetate [23] Malate [5]	297	29
Hydroxyethyl starch (Hextend®)	143	3	124	–	307	28
Gelatins 4% (Plasmion®)	154	0	120	–	307	32
Gelatins 3% (Gelofusine®)	150	0	100	–	284	56

albuminemia (they do not contain albumin). The resulting effect is still an acidification related to hyperchloremia. Balanced solution must add some strong anions to reach electroneutrality. Various anions are present in such commercialized solutions, depending on the laboratory: lactate, acetate, malate, gluconate, and citrate. The metabolization of these anions can then induce an alkalotic rebound due to a re-increase of SID. The impact of colloids such as hydroxyethyl starch or dextrans on the acid-base status depends on the SID of the solvent. Gelatins and albumin are proteins and weak acids and induce a slight acidosis [36]. But the negative charges of these proteins must conduct to increase the solvent SID, leading to minimize the acidifying effect. The "SAFE" study has shown that in clinical practice, vascular expansion with 0.9% NaCl or 4% albumin induces the same degree of MA, with a progressive normalization within the 5 following days [37]. Red blood cell transfusion has an alkalinizing effect which is caused by both the dilution of plasma albumin and the presence of sodium citrate. Indeed when citrate is metabolized, sodium cation remains in plasma and requires an elevation of bicarbonates to reach electroneutrality. At last the SID increases and the plasma too. However, in case of liver failure, citrate anion accumulates and produces MA with an increased SIG (and AG) in association with ionized hypocalcemia.

Numerous studies conducted in the perioperative period confirm the relationship between the infusion of unbalanced solutions and hyperchloremic MA [30, 35, 38, 39]. In an experimental model of mice with hemorrhagic shock, vascular expansion was performed using iso- or hypertonic saline. All animals developed hyperchloremic MA within the first 5 min, but MA was more pronounced with hypertonic saline crystalloids [38]. Scheingraber et al. [29] compared isotonic saline versus Ringer's lactate aiming to perform vascular expansion during gynecologic surgery. These authors found that only patients receiving isotonic saline developed hyperchloremic MA. An observational prospective study including various types of surgery has shown that patients developed MA with a decrease in SID without increase in AG, which confirms the role of chloride in the development of such a disorder [35]. On the other hand, no change in plasma volume was detected within the study period, leading to eliminate any dilution to explain the decrease in plasma bicarbonates. A double-blind randomized controlled study has compared the effect of two solutions used for the priming of extracorporeal circuit during cardiac surgery: one group received unbalanced solutions vs one group receiving balanced solutions containing acetate and gluconate [36]. While plasma bicarbonates and albumin decreased initially in the same proportion in both groups, a sustained hyperchloremic MA with a decreased SID was observed only in the group receiving unbalanced solutions. In the balanced group, chloremia and SID remained normal, but the pH and bicarbonates decreased initially as indicated by the increase in AG and SIG. These results are explained by the presence of strong anions contained in the balanced solution (acetate, gluconate). The acid-base equilibrium normalizes further when these strong anions are metabolized. Globally, the severity of acidosis is correlated to the excessive level of chloride, the volume, and the speed of infusion. When renal function is normal, hyperchloremic acidosis is often transitory. In intensive care unit, hyperchloremic acidosis is frequent, present in 60–98% of patients [3, 14]. In a canine model of endotoxinic shock, Kellum et al. [30] have shown that vascular expansion with isotonic saline was associated with MA due in 1/3 of cases to hyperchloremia.

All these data questioned on the real clinical risk and the risk of inappropriate treatment in case of hyperchloremic MA. During the intraoperative period, acidosis might be interpreted as a persisting hemodynamic instability due to hypovolemia, leading to an additional inappropriate vascular expansion with unbalanced crystalloids with a worsening hyperchloremic acidosis. Therefore, it is essential to distinguish iatrogenic hyperchloremic acidosis from hyperlactatemic acidosis caused by cell deficit energy. Moreover, hypoalbuminemia secondary to dilution can blunt the usual biological markers of acidosis by minimizing the decrease in plasma pH and bicarbonates.

The second question is the real clinical impact of such disorders. Until now, there is no double-blind randomized controlled study that confirms definitively the deleterious effect of hyperchloremic acidosis. Nevertheless, since several years, some data report real deleterious effects of hyperchloremia on numerous organ functions [40]. Hyperchloremic MA has been reported to induce renal dysfunction in healthy volunteers. The experimental infusion of chloride in the renal artery induced a sustained vasoconstriction [41]. These effects are due to a tubular reabsorption of chloride and are aggravated by a previous depletion in sodium. These effects would be closely correlated to the amount of chloride delivered to the kidney but independent from that of sodium. Clinical studies are still contradictory [35, 42–44]. Some of them have found that 0.9% NaCl infusion was associated with decrease and delayed urine output as compared with balanced solutions [44]. In a recent randomized, double-blind crossover study, the infusion of 0.9% NaCl in healthy volunteers was associated with a decrease in urine output and a decrease in mean renal artery flow velocity and in renal cortical perfusion as compared with Plasma-Lyte® infusion [42]. A randomized controlled study in patients with kidney graft has reported that isotonic saline infusion was associated with hyperchloremic MA and hyperkalemia as compared with Ringer's lactate infusion [45]. Some data underline the relationship between hyperchloremia and hematological and coagulation abnormalities during elective abdominal aortic surgery [35]. The dilution of blood with 0.9% NaCl induces coagulation impairment with platelet dysfunction and thromboelastogram abnormalities in the perioperative period [46]. Hyperchloremia is also associated with some impairment in digestive functions leading to an increase in postoperative nausea and vomitings and an increase in feeding intolerance in critically ill patients with enteral nutrition [44, 47, 48]. Some experimental studies report also that hyperchloremic acidosis increases proinflammatory phenomenons by stimulating IL6, IL10, and TNF release [49]. These effects seem to be independent from the pH as for a comparable pH; MA caused by hyperlactatemia does produce inverse effects, i.e., anti-inflammatory effects [50]. In the septic rats, the infusion of balanced solutions prevents the development of MA and prolonged their survival compared with NaCl infusion [39]. A recent large randomized trial designed in crossover has compared the effects of balanced (Plasma-Lyte®) vs unbalanced (0.9% saline) solutions in critically ill patients. More than 100 patients were included in each group, and there was no difference in term of both risk of acute kidney injury and mortality rate between groups. However, these results must be interpreted cautiously, as various patients were included and not severe (ICU mortality rate was 6–7%), the mean volume of infusion was very low (approximately 2 L in 4 days), and chloremia was not measured [43]. Therefore, despite the large number of patients, in nonsevere critically ill patients requiring low volume of vascular expansion, balanced crystalloids do not reduce the risk of acute kidney injury nor the mortality rate as compared with unbalanced crystalloids. Based on two recent studies, potential beneficial effects of large volume of fluid resuscitation by balanced crystalloids must be still considered. In a retrospective propensity-matched cohort study analyzing 53,448 critically ill adults with sepsis, Raghunathan et al. [51] have reported that in-hospital rate was lower in the group receiving balanced solutions as compared to the group receiving saline, while the rate of acute renal failure was similar in both groups. A recent meta-analysis included 21 studies (observational and randomized) and 6253 patients [52]. The results show that high-chloride fluids did not modify mortality but was weakly associated with a higher risk of acute kidney injury.

6.4 Diagnosis of Respiratory Acidosis

6.4.1 Clinical Signs [1, 9]

Acute hypercapnia induces arterial hypertension with an increased cardiac output and cerebral blood flow. Acute RA is associated with an elevated release of catecholamines, glucocorticoids, renin, aldosterone, and antidiuretic hormones leading to water and sodium retention. The more the development of hypercapnia is rapid, the more the neurological signs are severe: nausea, vomitings, confusion, obtundation, coma, seizures, etc.

Clinical manifestations of chronic hypercapnia are those of a chronic pulmonary heart with arterial hypertension. Ventricular and supraventricular arrhythmias are essentially caused by hypoxia and electrolytes abnormalities and not really related to a cardiomyopathy. Except in case of an acute worsening, chronic RA induces few central neurologic symptoms.

6.4.2 Biological Signs

Hypercapnia is the cause of the low pH. The expected secondary renal response depends on the speed of hypercapnia development, acute or chronic (Table 6.1). Hypoxemia is due to alveolar hypoventilation. During acute RA, serum concentrations of Na^{+}, K^{+}, and AG do no modify, except in case of the presence of an additional disorder such as MA. During chronic RA, serum concentrations of Na^{+}, K^{+}, and AG are normal because the increase in HCO_3^- is counterbalanced by a proportional decrease in Cl^- ($\Delta HCO_3^- = \Delta\ Cl^-$).

6.4.3 Etiologic Diagnosis [1, 9]

6.4.3.1 Acute Respiratory Acidosis

Most frequent causes of acute RA in anesthesia and intensive care unit are a decompensation of a preexisting chronic pulmonary disease, an airway obstruction, and a severe bronchospasm (Table 6.7). Only severe pulmonary edema is accompanied by acute RA. During anesthesia, RA is possible if minute ventilation on the ventilator is not sufficient or in case of airway obstruction, of pneumothorax or an abnormality in the ventilator circuit. Permissive hypercapnia is particular and decided as one of measures included in the therapeutic strategy of acute respiratory distress syndrome. Such a disorder does not induce deleterious effects until $PaCO_2$ is $\leq$60 mmHg [9].

Table 6.7 Major causes of respiratory acidosis (nonexhaustive list)

Acute respiratory acidosis	Acute respiratory acidosis
Airway obstruction	
Aspiration pneumonia, laryngospasm, severe bronchospasm, obstruction of superior airway	Chronic obstructive bronchopneumopathy
Inhibition of respiratory centers	
General anesthesia, sedative drugs, traumatic brain injury, stroke	Sedative drug chronic overdose, Pickwickian syndrome, brain tumor
Cardiovascular failure	
Cardiac arrest, severe pulmonary edema	
Neuromuscular deficits	
Botulism, tetanus, hypokalemia, Guillain-Barré syndrome, myasthenia crisis, toxics (neuromuscular blockers, organophosphorus)	Poliomyelitis, amyotrophic lateral sclerosis, multiple sclerosis, myopathies, diaphragmatic paralysis, myxedema
Thoracopulmonary injuries	
Pneumothorax, hemothorax, severe pneumonia, acute respiratory distress syndrome	Kyphoscoliosis, pulmonary fibrosis, obesity, hydrothorax, ascitis, diaphragmatic function impairment
Controlled ventilation	
Iatrogenic hypoventilation, permissive hypercapnia	

6.4.3.2 Chronic Respiratory Acidosis

They are observed mostly in patients with obstructive pulmonary disease, rarely in restrictive pathologies (Table 6.7). In clinical practice, it may be difficult to determine the part of acute from chronic RA. The clinical history only enables to precise this point.

6.5 Treatment of Acidosis

The treatment of the cause is necessary and frequently sufficient, but will not be detailed in this chapter. The symptomatic treatment which consists to alkalinize the pH is still strongly debated due to contradictory data.

6.5.1 The Buffer Solutions

6.5.1.1 Sodium Bicarbonate (SB)

Due to its reaction $NaHCO_3^- + H^+ \Leftrightarrow Na^+ + H_2O + CO_2$, SB is eliminated finally into CO_2 and leaves only the strong cation Na^+ in plasma. The consequence is an elevation of SID which induces in turn an increase in plasma pH. Therefore, SB is really an efficient alkalinizing solution [53, 54]. In many experimental and observational clinical studies, such an effect is accompanied by an improvement in hemodynamic parameters. However, the causality between this benefit and the correction of acidosis is not clearly established, and this effect might be the consequence of an improvement in vascular expansion due to the sole sodium of the solution. In this point of view, SB appears as an interesting solution for vascular expansion. Indeed, BS infusion in septic pigs [55] and in patients with severe sepsis [56] improved significantly hemodynamics.

6.5.1.2 Carbicarb®

This solution is an equimolar association of bicarbonate and sodium carbonate which reacts with water as follow: $Na_2HCO_3^- + H_2O + CO_2 \Leftrightarrow 2HCO_3^- + 2Na^-$ [50]. This composition allows to produce less CO_2 than SB. However, this theoretical advantage has never been demonstrated in experimental nor in clinical studies. This solution is not available in France.

6.5.1.3 Tham® (Tris(hydroxymethyl)aminomethane)

This is also a synthetic buffer which allows to alkalinize with a lower production of CO_2 than SB, according to the following reaction: Tham + H_2O + CO_2 $\Leftrightarrow$ HCO_3^- + Tham-Na^+. Its theoretical advantage is to cross easily cell membranes, to enter the cell, and to exert an intracellular buffering effect. But, it has also numerous side effects such as vasodilation, hyperkalemia, hypoglycemia, and vascular necrosis. As underlined for Carbicarb®, it has never been demonstrated that Tham® is a better buffer than SB, and clinical data remain limited.

6.5.1.4 Renal Removal Therapy

Renal removal therapy using SB as a buffer remains the most elegant method to increase pH, especially in case of renal failure. Such a technic allows to increase plasma pH by reducing SID by several mechanisms: removal of organic and inorganic anions (sulfate, phosphate), increased serum sodium concentration caused by SB contained in dialysate, and filtration solutions [57, 58].

6.5.2 Which Arguments to Treat Acidosis?

The treatment of acidosis using SB remains strongly debated: is severity of acidosis due to the low level of pH or to its underlying cause? Does any alkalinizing treatment using SB improve the patient's prognosis?

6.5.2.1 Acidosis: Friend or Foe?

The impact of a low pH on the prognosis of patients is clearly more dependent on the underlying cause of acidosis than on the level of pH. In a retrospective study, Gunnerson et al. [59] have shown that in critically ill patients, in-hospital mortality was higher in acidosis caused by hyperlactatemia than in those induced by other excessive strong anions or hyperchloremia. In this study, hyperphosphatemia and hyperlactatemia were independent parameters of a poor prognosis, while the pH value did not. A recent study supports such results showing that mortality rate was less than the expected one and was dependent on the reason of acidosis in patients presenting severe acidosis (pH <7) on admission [60]. These data strongly support that the alkalinization to normalize a low pH is not logical.

Data concerning the administration of SB are contradictory and stimulate the debate. Nevertheless, considering the pathophysiological mechanisms allows to explain these contradictions. Indeed, it is not surprising to observe different effects in metabolic and respiratory acidosis or between MA as a consequence of cell energy failure and as cell suffering of hyperchloremia.

Acidosis: A Foe

Numerous deleterious effects have been attributed to acute MA. Cardiovascular disorders and myocardial depression are the most frequently described in experimental model of isolated heart or in animals [61]. In these studies, these effects were reversed by the infusion of SB. Other studies report arrhythmias, vasodilation counterbalanced by a stimulation of the sympathetic system, and an impaired response to catecholamines [62, 63]. However, the interpretation of these data must be careful due to numerous methodological bias (no control group, extreme level of acidosis pH <7 in normal conditions of oxygenation). On the other hand, myocardial depression with pH >7 was not confirmed [63]. During hemorrhagic shock, MA is classically considered to worsen shock and coagulation abnormalities by decreasing fibrinogen and platelets. But, alkalization using SB is not able to normalize coagulation [64]. The consequences of acute RA remain debated [65–67]. Jaber et al. [65] showed in a porcine model that hypercapnia enables to reduce diaphragm contractility in a sustained manner with a delayed recovery. In ventilated rats with hypercapnia, Caples et al. [66] have found that SB or Tham® administration decreased pulmonary injury. In a model of myocardial ischemia-reperfusion, preconditioning with hypercapnia reduced the volume of infarction [67].

Chronic acidosis (metabolic and respiratory) can cause hormonal abnormalities, osteodystrophy with ionized hypocalcemia, or muscle weakness.

Acidosis: A Friend

Acidosis brakes glycolysis by an inhibition of phosphofructokinase (PFK). It is also responsible for a shift on the right of the dissociation hemoglobin curve, which facilitates the release of O_2 from hemoglobin for tissues. Such modifications can easily be considered as an adaptative goal aiming to facilitate cell functions in case of energy failure. Indeed, acidosis facilitates oxygen supply to hypoxic cells, and by braking glycolysis, it allows to fight against early energy storage exhaustion.

The beneficial effects of acidosis in hypoxic conditions or ischemia-reperfusion are largely reported on various experimental models. During ischemia-reperfusion, myocardial, endothelial cells and cerebral function are improved in acidotic conditions [68–71]. In similar conditions, acidosis protects cells from necrosis and apoptosis, regardless, the tissue (myocardium, hepatocytes, or neurons) [69–71]. The most likely mechanism of these protective effects would be an intracellular acidification (pHi) which could trigger a preconditioning [69] or a postconditioning process [70]. On contrary, other authors have reported proapoptotic effects on ex vivo myocytes but out of hypoxic conditions [72].

Sodium Bicarbonate: Balance Benefit/Risk

Most randomized controlled studies failed to demonstrate any benefit of the administration of SB in organic MA. During DKA, even in case of severe-extreme low pH, the alkalinization using SB increases pH, but does not normalize more rapidly glycemia or ketonemia nor improve myocardial function and mortality [19]. Indeed, some studies describe even deleterious effects such as a reduction in tissue oxygenation [73]. No beneficial effect has been demonstrated in randomized controlled studies in patients with shock and lactic acidosis despite the correction of acidosis by SB [53]. No benefit of SB administration has been demonstrated also for cardiac arrest, except if prolonged for more than 10 min [74, 75]. This result seems to be logical as acidosis in the early period following cardiac arrest is essentially a respiratory acidosis, and, therefore, the best treatment is to improve ventilation and to restore a spontaneous circulation.

To our knowledge, no randomized study has been performed to evaluate the efficiency of SB in patients presenting hyperchloremic MA. Treat these acidosis when chronic (as observed in chronic renal insufficiency) might be logical to fight against some side effects related to acidosis such as muscle weakness, osteodystrophia, and hormonal abnormalities. In this case, renal removal therapy remains the best treatment. The alkalinization of acute inorganic MA caused by digestive diseases is a matter of convictions because no objective data exists. If considering the Henderson-Hasselbalch pathophysiology among which acidosis is caused by bicarbonate losses, an exogenous replacement of these losses by SB seems appropriate. If referring to the Stewart approach, the treatment of acidosis should aim to correct plasma SID. Therefore, SB may reach this objective, thanks to the administration of Na^+ without Cl^-, but other balanced crystalloids such as sodium lactate will have similar alkalinizing effects [76].

Some experimental data found that hyperchloremia independently from acidosis, induces deleterious effects, which may represent an argument to prevent hyperchloremia. Indeed, for a long time, numerous pathological processes such as cell edema and arterial hypertension were attributed exclusively to an excess of sodium. However, recent data confirm the deleterious effects of high concentration of chloride which were underestimated. For example, the classical sodium-dependent arterial hypertension induced in uninephrectomized rats does not develop with the exclusive administration of sodium without chloride (bicarbonate or citrate sodium) or with the exclusive administration of chloride without sodium (ammonium chloride) [77]. Chloride channels which are membrane proteins allow to underline the major role of chloride in numerous pathophysiological processes, including the regulation of cell volume, transepithelial exchanges of fluids, muscle contraction, and neuroexcitability [78]. Nowadays, five groups of chloride channels are described in mammals. Among them, some are cyclic-AMP-dependent phosphorylation, while others are activated by calcium-, GABA-, or glycine-activating chloride channels. The most studied are the volume-regulatory channels (VRC) which depend on the membrane potential and the voltage-gated chloride channel (ClC). The distribution, the nature, and the role of each are summarized in a review [78]. Chloride exchanges are performed by cotransporters with other anions or cations. Most studied are the Na^+/Cl^- (NCC), K^+/Cl^- (KCC), and $Na^+/K^+/Cl^-$ (NKCC) [79, 80]. NCC and NKCC facilitate the entry of sodium, potassium, and chloride in cells and are inhibited by the increase in intracellular chloride concentration. KCC favors the extrusion of potassium and chloride from cells and are stimulated by the reduction in intracellular chloride concentration. Voltage-dependent channels, type ClC-3, seem to be preferentially involved in volume cell regulation, cell multiplication, and apoptosis [81]. The role of chloride cotransporters has been particularly highlighted in the central nervous system and its disorders. Neurons intracellular concentration of chloride regulates neuronal excitability by mediating the GABAergic neurotransmission, thanks to GABA-activating gated chloride channels. This parameter is also involved in the regulation of cell volume caused by osmolar variations or ischemic injury [82]. Plasma hypertonicity activates NKCC 1 cotransporter which enhances the cell concentration in Na^+, K^+, and Cl^- (active osmotic molecules) leading to the regulatory volume increase (RVI). Indeed, cerebral shrinkage caused by plasma hypertonicity is reduced. Plasma hypotonicity activates KCC 3 which extrudes K^+ and Cl^- from the cell; this represents the well-known regulatory volume decrease (RVD) which minimizes cerebral edema [82, 83]. Cerebral ischemia induces cell changes in electrolyte concentrations and metabolism that are characterized by an accumulation of Na^+, Ca^{++}, and Cl^- inside and of K^+ outside cells. These phenomenons are observed in brain cells (neurons, astrocytes, and endothelial cells of the cerebrospinal barrier) and conduct to the development of cerebral edema which may cause brain death [79, 80, 84]. Pond et al. [80] have shown that the inhibition of NKCC 1 and KCC 2 cotransporters by furosemide or bumetanide enabled to restore ATP storage and to reduce neurons injury in human undergoing ischemia-reperfusion without glucose supply. In a model of focal ischemia-reperfusion, NKCC $1^{-/-}$ knockout mice presented with a 30–45% decrease in cerebral infarction area and edema compared with the wild NKCC $1^{+/+}$ control ones [84]. Neuronal cultures issued from NKCC $1^{-/-}$ mice showed a significant reduction of both cell death rate and Na^+ entry in the cell compared with NKCC $1^{+/+}$ cultures. The inhibition of NKCC 1 transporter by bumetanide is responsible for protective phenomenon on neurons and astrocytes: cerebral edema is associated with an intracellular accumulation of Na^+ and Cl^- while K^+ extracellular concentration is high. NKCC 1 transporter activation is also closely linked with neuronal and astrocyte excitotoxicity [79, 85]. All neurological injury (stroke, traumatic brain injury, epilepsy) triggers cerebral excitotoxicity which manifests by glutamate release and cerebral edema [83, 86]. The activation of N-Methyl-D-Aspartate (NMDA) receptors by glutamate favors the entry of chloride in the cells by opening both GABA-gated and volume-sensitive chloride channels. In case of persistent activation, cerebral edema develops followed by cell necrosis. On contrary, glutamate reuptake and disappearance facilitates chloride and potassium extrusion from the cell by activating same volume-sensitive chloride and potassium channels [85]. These data underline inverse effects of these channels according to the presence or not of excitotoxicity.

Considering these data, preventing hyperchloremia seems to be justified and suggests to favor the infusion of balanced solutions for large volume expansion. However, such a benefit has to be further demonstrated in clinical practice

Beside potential beneficial effects, SB may induce deleterious effects. Among them, intracellular hypercapnic acidosis is commonly reported. Due to its high solubility, CO_2 which is produced by SB metabolism enters the cell and is responsible for a "paradoxical" acidosis. This phenomenon has been shown experimentally in vitro [70] and in patients too [53]. But, this phenomenon depends on conditions; intracellular acidosis does not occur in opened systems, i.e., if CO_2 can be eliminated by the lung or cells are in a fluid which contains buffers [87, 92]. In practical, most relevant side effects are a decrease in ionized calcium, hypernatremia, hyperosmolarity, sodium and water overload, and hypokalemia. Using iso- or hypotonic SB by continuous slow infusion without bolus enables to minimize or prevent these complications.

6.5.3 Which Clinical Indications of BS Alkalinization?

MA caused by the accumulation of strong anions must be distinguished from that caused by inorganic anions (Cl, Na). Organic MA requires essentially the treatment of the underlying cause; the metabolism of organic anions conducts to normalize concomitantly plasma SID and pH without any need of SB infusion. Therefore, DKA does not require BS alkalinization; even acidosis is severe [19]. The etiologic treatment by hydration and insulin restores the metabolism of carbon hydrates. Ketone body metabolization and urinary excretion induced by rehydration manifest by the simultaneous disappearance of ketonemia and acidosis. For the same reasons, it is not logical to alkalinize acidosis caused hyperlactatemia during shock [88]. In this situation, acidosis caused by changes in cell metabolism reflects energy impairment which may be considered as an adaptative response and in this view probably not treated, at least when transitory. The best treatment remains to restore an appropriate hemodynamic and oxygenation of tissues. Lactate metabolism conducts to correct spontaneously pH without need for any alkalinization. During septic shock, the indication of BS alkalinization remains debated due to controversial data. In a retrospective uncontrolled trial, El-Solh et al. [89] reported that BS infusion (0.2 mmol/kg/h) in 72 patients in septic shock with a pH <7.3 shortened time for respiratory weaning and for in-ICU length of stay. Nevertheless, such a treatment failed to restore shortly hemodynamics or to decrease the mortality rate. Based on two clinical randomized studies [53], the Surviving Sepsis Campaign does recommend to perform BS alkalinization only in case of severe acidosis with a pH <7.15; in septic shock with a pH ≥ 7.15, BS administration is not recommended [90]. Other authors advocate BS alkalinization only for lower pH <7 [88].

BS alkalinization is only recommended during cardiac arrest prolonged over 10 min or in case of associated hyperkalemia or of tricyclic antidepressant overdose or of preexisting acidosis. In this situation, normalization of pH requires before all to restore an efficient ventilation and circulation as acidosis is mostly a respiratory one. When cardiac arrest is prolonged and if spontaneous circulation activity is not restored, BS administration is possible [91].

During inorganic MA, the indication of BS infusion remains debated. In this case, acidosis is the primary disorder which is imposed to the cell caused by electrolyte modifications of the SID and which might exert potential deleterious effects on cell functions. Therefore, in these situations, BS administration is suggested if the pH is <7.20 [75]. But this strategy remains only symptomatic and the treatment of the cause is still the most appropriate. If considering the possible deleterious effects of hyperchloremia, a preventive attitude based on a preferential infusion of balanced solutions in case of large volume expansion appears to be the favorite.

Acute RA does not justify any exogenous administration of SB, especially if ventilation or circulation is impaired. In this situation, SB would worsen CO_2 release and accumulation in tissues and blood. Nevertheless, some studies report that BS infusion during acidosis caused by permissive hypercapnia decreases alveolar injury and improves systemic and regional circulations [66]. In practice, the threshold tolerated of acidosis induced by permissive hypercapnia is of 7.15–7.20 pH below which BS administration might be justified.

The reasons for alkalinizing chronic acidosis are completely different. As chronic renal insufficiency represents the major cause of chronic acidosis, BS is supplied with dialysis sessions. Chronic RA is usually not severe due to a complete secondary renal response that increases plasma bicarbonates and creates metabolic alkalosis. In this context, BS infusion is not justified. In case of artificial ventilation, acetazolamide might facilitate the reduction of plasma bicarbonates and the respiratory weaning.

Conclusion

Metabolic acidoses are frequent in intensive care units. They can be caused by an elevation in strong anions (lactate, ketone bodies) which represents the organic metabolic acidosis. Those resulting from disequilibrium between strong nonorganic cations and anions (mostly sodium and chloride) are called mineral or nonorganic metabolic acidosis. The diagnosis of metabolic acidosis is essentially based on arterial blood gases and electrolyte concentrations. It is essential to determine the cause in order to administer the etiologic treatment which is clearly the most appropriate. The benefit of a symptomatic alkalinization with sodium bicarbonate remains strongly debated and depends on both severity and cause of the trouble. Among respiratory acidosis, it is important to distinguish acute from chronic disorders, because causes and treatment are fundamentally different.

References

1. Berend K, de Vries APJ, Gans ROB (2014) Physiological approach to assessment of acid-base disturbances. New Engl J Med 371:1434–1445
2. Madger S (1998) Pathophysiology of metabolic acid-base disturbances in patients with critical illness. In: Ronco C, Bellomo R (eds) Critical care nephrology. Kluwer Academic Publisher, Dordrecht, pp 279–296

3. Kraut JA, Madias NE (2010) Metabolic acidosis: pathophysiology, diagnosis and management. Nat Rev Nephrol 6:274–278
4. Fencl V, Jabor A, Kazda A, Figge J (2000) Diagnosis of metabolic acid-base disturbances in critically ill patients. Am J Resp Crit Care Med 162:2246–2251
5. Kaplan LJ, Frangos S (2005) Clinical review: acid-base abnormalities in the intensive care unit. Crit Care 9:198–203
6. Stewart PA (1978) Independent and dependent variables of acid-base control. Resp Physioi 33:9–26
7. Kellum J, Elbers PWG (2009) Stewart's textbook of acid-base. Lulu Enterprises, Amsterdam, Netherlands, 501 p
8. Quintard H, Hubert S, Ichai C (2007) Qu'apporte le modèle de Stewart à l'interprétation des troubles de l'équilibre acide base? Ann Fr Anesth Réanim 26:423–433
9. Gattinoni L, Lissoni A (1998) Pathophysiology and diagnosis of respiratory acid-base disturbances in patients with critical illness. In: Ronco C, Bellomo R (eds) Critical care nephrology. Kluwer Academic Publisher, Dordrecht, pp 297–326
10. Figge J, Jabor A, Kazda A, Fencl V (1998) Anion gap and hypoalbuminemia. Crit Care Med 26:1807–1810
11. Kraut JA, Madias NE (2007) Serum anion gap: its uses and limitations in clinical medicine. Clin J Am Soc Nephrol 2:162–174
12. Dinh CH, Grandinetti A, Joffe A et al (2006) Correcting the anion gap for hypoalbuminemia does not improve detection of hyperlactatemia. Emerg Med J 23:627–632
13. Kellum JA, Kramer DJ, Pinsky MR (1995) Strong ion gap: a methodology for exploring unexplained anions. J Crit Care 10:51–55
14. Szrama J, Smuszkiewicz P (2016) An acid-base disorders analysis with the use of the Stewart approach in patients with sepsis treated in an intensive care unit. Anaesth Intensive Ther 48:181–184
15. Doberer D, Funk GC, Kirchner K, Schneeweiss B (2009) A critique of Stewart's approach: the chemical mechanism of dilutional acidosis. Intensive Care Med 35:2173–2180
16. Dubin A, Menises MM, Masevicius FD et al (2007) Comparison of three different methods of evaluation of metabolic acid base disorders. Crit Care Med 35:1264–1270
17. Orban JC, Leverve X, Ichai C (2010) Lactate: le substrat énergétique de demain. Réanimation 19:384–392
18. Levraut J, Bounatirou T, Ichai C, Ciais JF, Jambou P, Grimaud D (1997) Reliability of anion gap as an indicator of blood lactate level in critically ill patients. Intensive Care Med 23:417–422
19. Kraut JA, Kurtz I (2005) Metabolic acidosis of CKD: diagnosis, clinical characteristics, and treatment. Am J Kidney Dis 45:978–993
20. Gucyetmez B, Atalan HK (2016) Non-lactate strong ion difference: a clearer picture. J Anesth 30:391–396
21. Orban JC, Lena D, Bonciu M, Grimaud D, Ichai C (2007) Complications métaboliques aiguës du diabète. Urgence pratique 83:13–17
22. Misra S, Oliver NS (2015) Utility of ketone measurement in the prevention, diagnosis and management of diabetic ketoacidosis. Diabet Med 32:14–23
23. Forni LG, McKinnon W, Hilton PJ (2006) Unmeasured anions in metabolic acidosis: unravelling the mystery. Crit Care 10:220–224
24. Rocktäschel J, Morimatsu H, Uchino S et al (2003) Acid-base status of critically ill patients with acute renal failure: analysis based on Stewart-Figge methodology. Crit Care 7:R60–R66
25. Story DA, Morimatsu H, Bellomo R (2006) Hyperchloremic acidosis in the critically ill: one of the strong-ion acidoses? Anesth Analg 103:144–148
26. Karet FE (2009) Mechanisms in hyperkalemic renal tubular acidosis. J Am Soc Nephrol 20:251–254
27. Laing CM, Unwin RJ (2006) Renal tubular acidosis. J Nephrol 19(suppl 9):S46–S52
28. Reddy S, Weinberg L, Young P (2016) Crystalloid fluid therapy. Crit Care 20:59
29. Scheingraber S, Rehm M, Sehmisch C, Finsterer U (1999) Rapid saline infusion produces hyperchloremic acidosis in patients undergoing gynecologic surgery. Anesthesiology 90:1265–1270

30. Kellum JA, Bellomo R, Kramer DJ, Pinsky MR (1998) Etiology of metabolic acidosis during saline resuscitation in endotoxemia. Shock 9:364–368
31. Ichai C, Levraut J (2003) Hyperchloremic metabolic acidosis and fluid resuscitation. Crit Care & Shock 6:31–39
32. Langer T, Santini A, Scotti E, Van Regenmortel N, Malbrain MLNG, Caironi P (2015) Intravenous balanced solutions: from physiology to clinical evidence. Anaesth Intensive Ther 47:s77–s88
33. Morgan TJ (2014) The ideal crystalloid—What is "balanced"? Curr Opin Crit Care 19:299–307
34. McDermid RC, Raghunathan K, Romanovsky A, Shaw AD, Bagshaw SM (2014) Controversies in fluid therapy: type, dose and toxicity. World J Crit Care Med 3:24–33
35. Waters JH, Gottlieb A, Schoenwald P, Popovich MJ, Sprung J, Nelson DR (2001) Normal saline versus lactated ringer's solution for intraoperative fluid management in patients undergoing abdominal aortic aneurysm repair: an outcome study. Anesth Analg 93:817–822
36. Liskaser FJ, Bellomo R, Hayhoe M et al (2000) Role of pump prime in the etiology and pathogenesis of cardiopulmonary bypass-associated acidosis. Anesthesiology 93:1170–1173
37. Bellomo R, Morimatsu H, French C et al (2006) The effects of saline or albumin resuscitation on acid-base status and serum electrolytes. Crit Care Med 34:2891–2897
38. Moon PF, Kramer GC (1995) Hypertonic saline-dextran resuscitation for hemorrhagic shock induces transient mixed acidosis. Crit Care Med 23:323–331
39. Kellum JA (2002) Fluid resuscitation and hyperchloremic acidosis in experimental sepsis: improved short-term survival and acid-base balance with Hextend compared with saline. Crit Care Med 30:300–305
40. Lobo DN, Awad S (2014) Should chloride-rich crystalloids remain the mainstay of fluid resuscitation to prevent "pre-renal" acute kidney injury?: con. Kidney Int 86:1096–1105
41. Wilcox CS (1983) Regulation of renal blood flow by plasma chloride. J Clin Invest 71:726–735
42. Chowdhury AH, Cox EF, Francis ST, Lobo DN (2012) A randomized, controlled, double-blind cross over study on the effects of 2-L infusions of NaCl 0.9% saline and Plasma-Lyte® 48 on renal blood flow velocity and renal cortical tissue perfusion in healthy volunteers. Ann Surg 256:18–24
43. Young P, Bailey M, Beasley R et al (2015) Effect of buffered crystalloid solution vs saline on acute kidney injury among patients in the intensive care unit. The SPLIT randomized clinical trial. JAMA 314:1701–1710
44. Wilkes NJ, Wool R, Mutch M et al (2001) The effects of balanced versus saline-based hetastarch and crystalloid solutions on acid-base and electrolyte status and gastric mucosal perfusion in elderly surgical patients. Anesth Analg 93:811–816
45. O'Malley CM, Frumento RJ, Hardy MA et al (2005) A randomized, double-blind comparison of lactated Ringer's solution and 0.9% NaCl during renal transplantation. Anesth Analg 100:1518–1524
46. Martin G, Bennett-Guerrero E, Wakeling H et al (2002) A prospective, randomized comparison of thromboelastography coagulation profile in patients receiving lactated Ringer's solution, 6% hetastarch in a balanced-saline vehicle, or 6% hetastarch in saline during major surgery. J Cardiothorac Vasc Anesth 16:441–446
47. Moretti EW, Robertson KM, El-Moalem H, Gan TJ (2003) Intraoperative colloid administration reduces postoperative outcomes compared with crystalloid administration. Anesth Analg 96:611–617
48. Reddy S, Bailey M, Beasley R et al (2016) Effect of saline 0.9% or Plasma-Lyte 148 therapy on feeding intolerance in patients receiving nasogastric enteral nutrition. Crit Care Resusc 18:198–204
49. Kellum JA, Song M, Venkataraman R (2004) Effects of hyperchloremic acidosis on arterial pressure and circulating inflammatory molecules in experimental sepsis. Chest 125:243–248
50. Kellum JA, Song M, Li J (2004) Lactic, and hydrochloric acids induce different patterns of inflammatory response in LPS-stimulated RAW 264.7 cells. Am J Physiol Regul Integr Comp Physiol 286:R686–R692

51. Raghunathan K, Shaw A, Nathanson B et al (2014) Association between the choice of IV crystalloid and in-hospital mortality among critically ill adults with sepsis. Crit Care Med 42:1585–1591
52. Krajewski ML, Raghunathan K, Paluszkiewicz SM, Schermer CR, Shaw AD (2015) Meta-analysis of high- *versus* low-chloride content in perioperative and critical care fluid resuscitation. Br J Surg 102:24–36
53. Cooper DJ, Walley KR, Wiggs BR, Russel JA (1990) Bicarbonate does not improve hemodynamics in critically ill patients who have lactic acidosis: a prospective, controlled clinical study. Ann Intern Med 112:492–498
54. Gehlbach BK, Schmidt GA (2004) Bench-to-bedside review: treating acid-base abnormalities in the intensive care unit—the role of buffers. Crit Care 8:259–265
55. Duburcq T, Favory R, Matthieu D et al (2014) Hypertonic sodium lactate improves fluid balance and hemodynamics in porcine endotoxic shock. Crit Care 18:467
56. Fang ZX, Li YF, Zhou XQ et al (2008) Effects of resuscitation with crystalloid fluids on cardiac function in patients with severe sepsis. BMC Infect Dis 8:50
57. Rocktäschel J, Morimatsu H, Uchino S, Ronco C, Bellomo R (2003) Impact of continuous veno-venous hemofiltration on acid-base balance. Int J Artif Organs 26:19–25
58. Naka T, Bellomo R (2004) Bench-to-bedside review: treating acid-base abnormalities in the intensive care unit—the role of renal replacement therapy. Crit Care 8:108–114
59. Gunnerson KJ, Saul M, He S, Kellum JA (2006) Lactate versus non-lactate metabolic acidosis: a retrospective outcome evaluation of critically ill patients. Crit Care 10:R22
60. Allyn J, Vaudroux D, Jabot J et al (2016) Prognosis of patients presenting extreme acidosis (pH <7) on admission to intensive care unit. J Crit Care 31:243–248
61. Orchard C, Cingolani H (1994) Acidosis and arrhythmias in cardiac muscle. Cardiovasc Res 28:1312–1319
62. Barton M, Lake CR, Rainey TG, Chernow B (1982) Is catecholamine release pH mediated? Crit Care Med 10:751–753
63. Huang YG, Wong KC, Yip WH, McJames SW, Pace N (1995) Cardiovascular response to graded doses of three catecholamines during lactic and hydrochloric acidosis in dogs. Br J Anaesth 74:583–590
64. Martini WZ (2009) Coagulopathy by hypothermia and acidosis: mechanisms of thrombin generation and fibrinogen availability. J Trauma 67:202–208
65. Jaber S, Jung B, Sebbane M et al (2008) Alteration of the piglet diaphragm contractility in vivo and its recovery after acute hypercapnia. Anesthesiology 108:651–658
66. Caples SM, Rasmussen DL, Lee WY, Wolfert MZ, Hubmayr RD (2009) Impact of buffering hypercapnic acidosis on cell wounding in ventilator-injured rat lungs. Am J Physiol Lung Cell Mol Physiol 296:L140–L144
67. Luo H, Chang Y, Cai H, Wang D, Guo Q (2008) The effect of hypercapnic acidosis preconditioning on rabbit myocardium. J Huazhong Univ Sci Technolog Med Sci 28:706–710
68. López D, Rodríguez-Sinovas A, Agulló L, Inserte J, Cabestrero A, García-Dorado D (2008) Acidic reoxygenation protects against endothelial dysfunction in rat aortic rings submitted to simulated ischemia. Am J Physiol Heart Circ Physiol 295:H2409–H2401
69. Flacke JP, Kumar S, Kostin S, Reusch HP, Ladilov Y (2009) Acidic preconditioning protects endothelial cells against apoptosis through p38- and Akt-dependent Bcl-xL overexpression. Apoptosis 14:90–96
70. Cohen MV, Yang XM, Downey JM (2007) The pH hypothesis of postconditioning: staccato reintroduces oxygen and perpetuates myocardial acidosis. Circulation 115:1895–1903
71. Inserte J, Barba I, Hernando V et al (2008) Effect of acidic reperfusion on prolongation of intracellular acidosis and myocardial salvage. Cardiovasc Res 77:782–790
72. Thatte HS, Rhee JH, Zagarins SE et al (2004) Acidosis-induced apoptosis in human and porcine heart. Ann Thorac Surg 77:1376–1383
73. Viallon A, Zeni F, Lafond P et al (1999) Does bicarbonate therapy improve the management of severe diabetic ketoacidosis? Crit Care Med 27:2690–2693

74. Vukmir RB (2006) Sodium bicarbonate improves outcome in prolonged prehospital cardiac arrest. Am J Emerg 24:156–161
75. Castaing Y, Bengler C, Delafosse B et al (1998) Correction de l'acidose métabolique en réanimation. XIXè Conférence de Consensus en Réanimation et Médecine. Réanim Urg 8:426–432
76. Leverve XM, Boon C, Hakim T, Anwar M, Siregar E, Mustafa I (2008) Half-molar sodium-lactate has a beneficial effect in patients after coronary artery bypass grafting. Intensive Care Med 34:1796–1803
77. Kotchen TA (2005) Contributions of sodium and chloride to NaCl-induced hypertension. Hypertension 45:849–850
78. Verkman AS, Galietta LJV (2009) Chloride channels as drugs targets. Nature 8:153–171
79. Beck J, Lenart B, Kintner DB, Sun D (2003) Na-K-Cl cotransporter contributes to glutamate-mediated excitotoxicity. J Neurosci 23:5061–5068
80. Pond BB, Galeffi F, Ahrens R, Schwartz-Bloom RD (2004) Chloride transport inhibitors influence recovery from oxygen-glucose deprivation-induced cellular injury in adult hippocampus. Neuropharmacology 47:253–262
81. Sardini A (2007) Cell volume homeostasis: the role of volume-sensitive chloride channels. Adv Mol Cell Biol 38:199–214
82. Kahle KT, Staley KJ, Nahed BV et al (2008) Roles of the cation-chloride cotransporters in neurological disease. Nature Clin Pract 4:490–503
83. O'Donnell ME, Duong V, Suvatne J, Foroutan S, Johnson DM (2005) Arginine vasopressin stimulation of cerebral microvascular endothelial cell Na-K-Cl cotransporter activity is V1 receptor and [Ca] dependent. Am J Physiol Cell Physiol 289:C283–C292
84. Chen H, Luo J, Kintner DB, Shull GE, Sun D (2005) Na+-dependent chloride transporter (NKCC1) -null mice exhibit less gray and whiter matter damage after focal cerebral ischemia. J Cereb Blood Flow Metab 25:54–66
85. Inoue H, Okada Y (2007) Roles of volume-sensitive chloride channel in excitotoxic neuronal injury. J Neurosci 27:1445–1455
86. Su G, Kintner DB, Flagella M, Shull GE, Sun D (2002) Astrocytes from Na^+-K^+-Cl^- cotransporter-null mice exhibit absence of swelling and decrease in EEA release. Am J Physiol Cell Physiol 282:C1147–C1160
87. Levraut J, Giunti C, Ciebiera JP et al (2001) Initial effect of sodium bicarbonate on intracellular pH depends on the extracellular nonbicarbonate buffering capacity. Crit Care Med 29:1033–1039
88. Boyd JH, Walley KR (2008) Is there a role for sodium bicarbonate in treating lactic acidosis from shock? Curr Opin Crit Care 14:379–383
89. El-Solh AA, Abou Jaoude P, Porhomayon J (2010) Bicarbonate therapy in the treatment of septic shock: a second look. Intern Emerg Med 5:341–347
90. Dellinger RP, Lévy MM, Carlet JM et al (2008) Surviving sepsis campaign: international guidelines for management of severe sepsis and septic shock: 2008. Intensive Care Med 34:17–60
91. Morrison LJ, Deakin CD, Morley PT et al (2010) Advanced life support chapter collaborators. Part 8: advanced life support: 2010 International consensus on cardiopulmonary resuscitation and emergency cardiovascular care science with treatment recommendations. Circulation 122:213–247
92. Ritter JM, Doktor HS, Benjamin N (1990) Paradoxical effect of bicarbonate on cytoplasmic pH. Lancet 10:1243–1246

Alkalosis: Diagnosis and Treatment

7

Jean-Christophe Orban and Carole Ichai

7.1 Introduction

Despite its frequency, alkalosis has not been largely studied. The pathophysiology of metabolic alkalosis is rather complex: generating factors cause the trouble, but its maintenance requires the presence of sustained factors. The classical Henderson-Hasselbalch theory is more and more replaced by the Stewart concept for interpreting metabolic alkalosis. The treatment of metabolic alkalosis is based on the simultaneous normalization of the generating and maintaining factors. Respiratory alkalosis is classified into acute and chronic disorders and is caused by alveolar hyperventilation due to central nervous system abnormalities or tissue hypoxia.

7.2 Metabolic Alkalosis

7.2.1 Definition and Epidemiology

Metabolic alkalosis is defined by a primary increase of plasma bicarbonates >28 mmol/L associated with an increased pH > 7.45. The predictable secondary response consists in hypoventilation aiming to increase $PaCO_2$ and in turn reach a pH close from normalization [1–6]. A respiratory response is associated to this disorder (increase of 0.6–1.2 mmHg of carbon dioxide per mmol of bicarbonate) [7, 8]. The incidence of such a disorder varies largely according to the period and the method of diagnosis. Old data reported an incidence higher than 50–60% in patients who experienced abdominal (gastric) surgery [9]. However, due to the reduction of

J-C. Orban (✉) • C. Ichai
Intensive Care Unit, Hôpital Pasteur 2, 30 Voie Romaine, 06001 Nice, Cédex 1, France

IRCAN (INSERM U1081, CNRS UMR 7284), University Hospital of Nice, Nice, France
e-mail: orban.jc@chu-nice.fr

C. Ichai et al. (eds.), *Metabolic Disorders and Critically Ill Patients*,
http://doi.org/10.1007/978-3-319-64010-5_7

this specific type of patients associated with an improved postoperative management (reducing gastric aspiration), a decrease in metabolic alkalosis related to gastric losses seems probable. On the other hand, based on the recent interpretation using the Stewart concept, recent data highlight that metabolic alkalosis is very frequent in ICU [10–12]. Using the Henderson-Hasselbalch method, the incidence of this disorder in general ICU is close to 5%, whereas it culminates at 85% using Stewart concept which considers hypoalbuminemia as a major cause of metabolic alkalosis [13–15]. In a large retrospective cohort of critically ill patients, metabolic alkalosis was reported to be present in approximately 30% of them and was caused by multiple usual factors such as diuretics and hypokalemia [11]. While metabolic acidosis is mainly present on admission and within the first day, metabolic alkalosis develops within the first 3–4 days of hospitalization in intensive care unit (ICU) [10]. Indeed, metabolic alkalosis is not frequently present as a pure disorder but essentially as a part of mixed acid-base disorder [13–15]. In these situations, the diagnosis of metabolic alkalosis can be totally ignored when considering only pH and bicarbonates which can be closed for normal values in 15–30% of patients. In fact, the large incidence of hypoalbuminemia present in 75–100% of patients masks the presence of metabolic acidosis.

Few studies reported that metabolic alkalosis is associated with an increased morbi-mortality [11, 16, 17]. For some of them, there was a linear relationship between pH values and mortality [5]: a pH value >7.60 was associated with a 50% increased mortality rate. Harmful effects and increased morbidity [11, 16] were also reported. The causality between this metabolic disorder and morbi-mortality is not proved and might reflect severity of the disease. However, a recent clinical study showed that an increase of 5 meq/L of bicarbonates increased independently mortality (OR = 1.21), and these results were observed regardless of the cause of metabolic alkalosis [11]. But mortality (19%) was lower than that reported previously.

7.2.2 Pathophysiology

The pathophysiology of respiratory alkalosis is solely caused by a decreased $PaCO_2$. The pathophysiology of metabolic alkalosis varies according to the methodology of acid-base disorder interpretation. In the traditional Henderson-Hasselbalch approach, the increase in pH is caused by a loss of plasma nonvolatile protons (by the kidney or the digestive tractus) or by an increase of plasma bicarbonates due to an iatrogenic exogenous overload or a renal reabsorption [3–6]. Considering the Stewart model, the increase of pH results from a lower dissociation of water according to the following relation: $H_2O \Longleftrightarrow H^+ + OH^-$. Two independent variables can modify the magnitude of water dissociation and cause in turn changes in plasma pH: the strong ion difference (SID), which is the difference between strong cations and anions, and the weak acid mass (see specific chapter on acid-base disorders) [14, 18–20]. An elevation of plasma SID, resulting from an increase of strong cations (sodium) or a decrease of strong anions (chloride), leads to elevate plasma bicarbonates for maintaining electroneutrality and in turn pH. A reduction of weak acids (albuminate) conducts also to an elevation in pH and plasma bicarbonates. Finally, regardless of the model used, metabolic alkalosis is biologically characterized by an increased plasma pH and bicarbonate and mathematically obeys to the Henderson-Hasselbalch equation: $pH = 6.10 + \log [HCO_3^-]/0{,}03 \times PaCO_2$ (6.1 is plasma bicarbonate pKa and 0.03 is CO_2 coefficient of solubility). The predictable secondary response to a primary metabolic alkalosis consists in a respiratory response which is characterized by hypoventilation aiming to diminish CO_2 elimination to damper plasma pH increase.

Metabolic alkalosis is a special acid-base disorder which is characterized by its evolution in three phases: generation (the cause), maintenance, and correction [21–23]. When plasma bicarbonates increase sharply (regardless of the cause exogenously or endogenously), a normal kidney enables to excrete large amounts of bicarbonates, and theoretically metabolic alkalosis should not persist despite the factors responsible for the generation of the trouble. Therefore, the occurrence and persistence of metabolic alkalosis require the presence of both mechanisms of generation and maintenance. Indeed, metabolic alkalosis can persist despite the normalization of generating factors until maintaining factors are present.

7.2.2.1 Generation

Metabolic alkalosis is classified into two groups depending essentially on chloremia: "chloride-depletion" (or chloride-responsive) and "non-chloride-depletion" or "potassium-depletion" metabolic alkalosis (chloride resistant) (Table 7.1). According to the Henderson-Hasselbalch model, chloride-depletion metabolic alkalosis is caused by a loss of proton (accompanied with chloride). This type of metabolic alkalosis is called "ion exchange," as any loss of protons results in a secondary production of equimolar amount of bicarbonate secondary to intracellular dissociation of carbonic acid [24, 25]: $CO_2 + H_2O \leftrightarrow H_2CO_3 \leftrightarrow H^+$ + bicarbonate. This loss of protons will be in the form of H^+Cl^- or ammonium. Non-depletion chloride metabolic alkalosis is caused by an elevation of bicarbonate (caused by excessive exogenous intake or excessive renal reabsorption) with a normal amount of chloride. Based on the Stewart concept, chloride-depletion metabolic alkalosis is caused by the higher chloride loss than that of natremia and thus conducts to increase SID and finally pH. Chloride losses may be initiated by the digestive tractus or the kidney. Metabolic alkalosis may also result from an elevation in natremia which is more often iatrogenic related to an excessive exogenous intake of sodium bicarbonate and is responsible for an increased SID [14, 18–20]. The same mechanism is involved in the metabolic alkalosis which is currently considered to be related to volume depletion. Indeed, there is no volume depletion but an increased SID secondary to hypernatremia. All mineralocorticoid excess cause non-depletion chloride metabolic alkalosis by generating renal reabsorption of sodium associated with potassium excretion and finally an elevation of SID [26]. These metabolic alkaloses are characterized by potassium depletion. At last, the elevation of pH can be due to a reduction in weak acids, essentially in hypoalbuminemia (Table 7.1).

Table 7.1 Generation and main causes of metabolic alkalosis

Generation	Main causes
Elevation of the strong ion difference due to chloride losses	
– Gastrointestinal tract	– Vomiting, gastric suction – Villous adenoma, congenital chloridorrhea
– Kidney Increase of tubular flux and chloride loss	– Chloruretic diuretics
Increase of negative charge in the tubular lumen	– Penicillin, carbenicillin, sulfate
Hypercapnia	– Correction of chronic hypercapnia without salt diet
Low chloride diet, hypercalcemia, hypoparathyroidism	
Elevation of the strong ion difference due to sodium load	
– Intracellular transfer	– Hypokalemia
– Exogenous alkali overload by sodium: bicarbonate, acetate, lactate, citrate	– Excessive alkalinization of acidosis – Overnutrition, transfusions, – Antacids, milk-alkali syndrome
– Hypovolemia with hypernatremia	
– Renal sodium reabsorption due to mineralocorticoid excess	– Hyperreninism: contraction of extracellular volume, low magnesium – Primary mineralocorticoid excess: primary and secondary hyperaldosteronism, Cushing syndrome
Reduction of weak acids	
– Hypoalbuminemia	– Dilution – Denutrition, cirrhosis, – Renal losses (nephrotic syndrome)

7.2.2.2 Maintenance

The kidney is always responsible of sustained metabolic alkalosis maintenance due to tubular reabsorption of chloride with sodium or ammoniac excretion: this is the well-known "paradoxical aciduria." This phenomenon characterizes the maintenance phase and explains why metabolic alkalosis persists despite the disappearance of the causal factor responsible for the generation of the disorder. In chloride-responsive metabolic alkalosis, this paradoxical aciduria which appears a priori as inappropriate is rather appropriate [24]. Indeed, renal excretion of bicarbonate is necessarily accompanied by a urinary excretion of equimolar Na^+ and K^+ to maintain electroneutrality. This could lead to a contraction of the extracellular volume and severe hypokalemia. Thus, the paradoxical aciduria in chloride-responsive metabolic alkalosis should be considered as an expected renal response, aiming to prevent hypovolemia and hypokalemia. This phenomenon could also provide a protection toward an acidotic rebound during HCl reabsorption.

Several factors are reported as responsible for the maintenance of metabolic alkalosis, in full or in combination. Their mechanisms of action are based on an increased renal reabsorption of bicarbonate or chloride, depending on the acid-base approach (Table 7.2). The decline in glomerular filtration of sodium and chloride

Table 7.2 Major maintenance factors of metabolic alkalosis

1. Decreased glomerular filtration
2. Decrease of extracellular volume (stimulation of tubular reabsorption of sodium bicarbonate)
3. Hypokalemia Decreased glomerular filtration Increased tubular reabsorption of sodium bicarbonate
4. Hypochloremia Decreased glomerular filtration Increased proton or sodium excretion in medullar duct
5. Passive bicarbonate backflow
6. Aldosterone (increase of sodium excretion in the medullary duct independent of protons)
7. Continuous acid loss
8. Continuous bicarbonate load

represents another factor favoring the maintenance of metabolic alkalosis in patients with hypovolemia or renal failure [1, 27]. Hypochloremia decreases glomerular filtration rate and reabsorption of sodium bicarbonate. In addition, it increases renin and aldosterone.

7.2.2.3 Correction

In chloride-responsive metabolic alkalosis, correction will appear with the normalization of both generating and maintaining factors by targeting a normalization of body chloride (and potassium) amounts: chloremia rises, while bicarbonatemia decreases in the same manner, so that the pH normalizes. In urine, simultaneous sodium excretion and chloride reabsorption reappear, and urinary pH increases above 6. The disappearance of "paradoxical aciduria" is the marker of the correction of maintaining factors which is essential to correct metabolic alkalosis. The correction of chloride-resistant metabolic alkalosis is based primarily on the normalization of potassium levels and plasma concentrations of mineralocorticoids.

7.2.3 Diagnosis

The diagnosis of metabolic acidosis requires to evaluate the history of the patients, its comorbidities, and its treatment. Because clinical manifestations are not specific, their presence needs to eliminate other reasons for symptoms. The diagnosis of metabolic alkalosis is confirmed on biological signs.

7.2.3.1 Clinical Signs

Clinical manifestations and their severity depend on the magnitude of alkalemia and respiratory response [28]. The reduction of cerebral blood flow induced by alkalemia is primarily responsible for neurological disorders. Predictable respiratory response leads to alveolar hypoventilation with hypoxia and hypercapnia. Some signs are related to the cause of metabolic alkalosis: hypokalemia, hypophosphatemia, etc. Metabolic alkalosis may be completely asymptomatic with only clinical signs due to the cause of the trouble (hypertension, vomiting, etc.).

Neuromuscular Signs

Alkalosis is responsible for a decrease in cerebral blood flow and glucose cerebral metabolic rate [29]. Manifestations of the central nervous system disorders can be apathy, confusion, weakness, seizures, or rarely encephalopathy with coma, especially in patients with hepatic impairment [30]. Some cases of psychosis have been reported presenting the problem of a differential diagnosis [31]. Neuromuscular signs are attributed to a decrease in plasma ionized calcium and potassium levels. This results in neuromuscular irritability with cramps, tetany, and more rarely Trousseau or Chvostek signs.

Cardiovascular Signs

These symptoms are not really related to alkalosis but rather attributed to hypoxia, hypophosphatemia, and decreased coronary blood flow [1]. Clinical manifestations can be heart failure, arterial hypotension, and especially arrhythmias such as atrial fibrillation, ventricular fibrillation, or torsade de pointes [32, 33]. These disorders resist generally to standard treatments and regress with the normalization of pH [1]. Likewise, metabolic alkalosis would be responsible for an increase of arrhythmias in patients treated with digitalis [34]. However, it is important to emphasize that hypokalemia which is often associated with metabolic alkalosis represents an additional factor of ventricular arrhythmia and worsens digitalis toxicity.

Respiratory Signs

Alveolar hypoventilation which represents the secondary predictable respiratory response is the main respiratory sign: an increase of 1 mmol/l of plasma bicarbonates induces an increase of 0.6–1 mmHg of $PaCO_2$ [1, 6–8]. The decrease in tidal volume and respiratory frequency leads to hypercapnia and tends to correct arterial pH. It is associated with hypoxemia, which is inversely correlated to hypercapnia [35, 36]. However, such a response is limited by the associated induced hypoxemia. In chronic respiratory failure patients, metabolic alkalosis may worsen hypoxemia, and alkalemia can compromise ventilator weaning. Hypoxemia can be explained both by a Bohr effect and worsening ventilation/perfusion abnormalities. This effect is more important in case of a preexisting chronic respiratory failure [37, 38].

7.2.3.2 Biological Signs

Plasma

- Metabolic alkalosis: Whether considering Henderson-Hasselbalch or Stewart approach, the diagnosis of metabolic alkalosis is based on an elevated pH > 7.45, a high concentration of plasma bicarbonate and hypercapnia. The disorder is pure if the actual respiratory response is close from the predictable one, that is, to say an increase of about 0.6–1.2 mmHg of $PaCO_2$ by increases of 1 mmol/L of bicarbonate. Correlation formulas between $PaCO_2$ and bicarbonate allow to determine the predictable respiratory response to the level of plasma bicarbonate (predicted $PaCO_2$) [35]. This relationship exists even in severe metabolic alkalosis with plasma bicarbonate >40 mmol/L. Pure nonfatal severe metabolic alkalosis has been reported with pH up to 7.87, plasma bicarbonate 87 mmol/L, and $PaCO_2$ 76 mmHg [39–41]. In these situations, hypercapnia limits pH increase but sustains the renal excretion of cations and hence bicarbonate reabsorption. If measured $PaCO_2$ is lower than expected, this means that respiratory alkalosis is superimposed leading to a mixed alkalosis which is characterized by a more severe alkalosis and a higher mortality [16]. A measured $PaCO_2$ higher than the expected one denotes that metabolic alkalosis is associated to a respiratory acidosis leading also to a mixed disorder. In this situation, the association of two opposite disorders leads to lower pH abnormalities or subnormal pH.

- Other biological disorders:
  - The plasma anion gap is typically normal in pure metabolic alkalosis as the increase of bicarbonate is counterbalanced by a reduction of chloride. However, it may be high in three situations [42]: (1) moderate hyperlactatemia secondary to the stimulation of phosphofructokinase enzyme by alkalosis and in turn activation of glycolysis [43], but the presence of a severe hyperlactatemia (> 5 mmol/L) must conduct to look for the presence of an associated metabolic acidosis; (2) association with a metabolic acidosis or overshoot alkalinization of a severe metabolic acidosis; and (3) increase of the negative charge of albumin secondary to alkalemia and volume contraction. The anion gap may be artificially modified by changes in pH, extracellular compartment volume, and/or weak acids (albumin, phosphorus). Therefore, some authors recommend calculating the strong ion difference (SID), which takes into account the strong and weak acids [43–46].
  - Tissue hypoxia is correlated with alveolar hypoventilation but the pathophysiology is multifactorial. The left shift of the dissociation curve of hemoglobin (Bohr effect) represents the first factor, i.e., an increase in the hemoglobin affinity for O_2 induced by alkalosis. The delivery of O_2 is also impaired by vasoconstriction and worsening of shunts, especially in the pulmonary circulation [37, 38]. However, these effects disappear after 6–8 h of alkalemia due to a lower intraerythrocyte amount of 2,3-diphosphoglycerate.
  - Electrolyte changes depend mainly on the cause of metabolic alkalosis. Hypochloremia is always present in chloride-responsive metabolic alkalosis and is usually associated with sodium depletion with or without hyponatremia [21, 47]. Hypokalemia is common, related either to intracellular transfer of potassium or urinary losses [48, 49]. Hypophosphatemia, hypomagnesemia, and decreased ionized calcium can also be found.

Urine

The most important elements are pH and urinary chloride.

- Urinary pH varies depending on the cause of metabolic alkalosis and its phase. During generation of a chloride-responsive disorder, pH is ≥6, corresponding to the renal excretion of bicarbonate. In all other situations, pH is <6, reflecting the paradoxical aciduria [24]. The elevation of urinary pH after aciduria reflects the correction of maintenance factors. In clinical practice, urinary pH is considered as a good and essential marker of treatment efficacy.

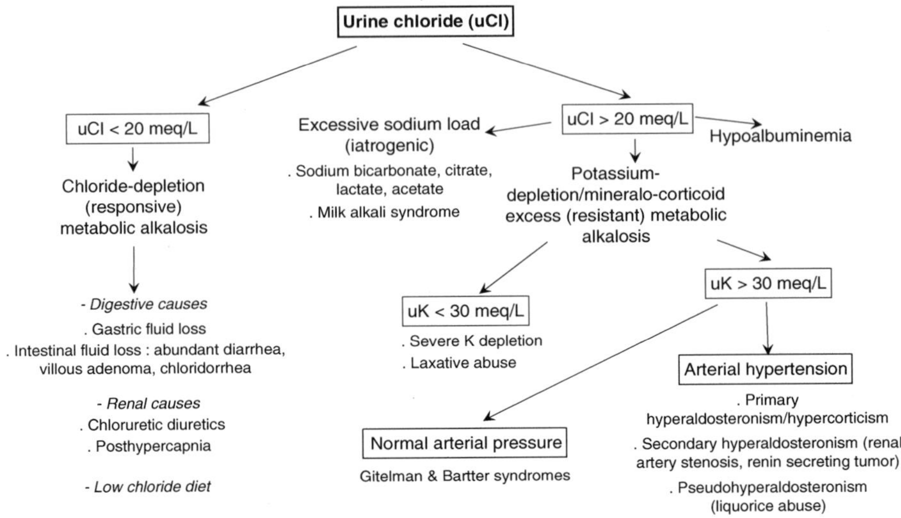

Fig. 7.1 Diagnosis algorithm of metabolic alkalosis based on urinary chloride

- Urinary chloride is the key for determining the causal diagnosis (Fig. 7.1). It allows to distinguish chloride-responsive metabolic alkalosis (low urine chloride concentration) from chloride-resistant disorders (low urine chloride concentration >20 mmol/L) [50].
- Urinary sodium and potassium are only secondary elements of etiological diagnosis.

7.2.4 Etiologies

In physiological conditions, chloride losses are located in the upper gastrointestinal tract, but rapidly reabsorbed in the small intestine, and finally no acid-base disorder develops. Finally, a cause of metabolic alkalosis explained only by the Stewart approach is hypoalbuminemia that reduces the total amount of weak acids. A diagnosis algorithm for metabolic alkalosis is summarized in Fig. 7.1.

7.2.4.1 Chloride-Depletion (or Responsive) Metabolic Alkalosis

Digestive Causes

Gastric juice contains a high concentration of HCl (H^+ 160–170 mmol/L, Cl^- 180 mmol/L), which is largely higher than in the plasma. Therefore, massive losses of gastric juice represent the most frequent cause of metabolic alkalosis [51]. The Henderson-Hasselbalch approach stipulates that metabolic alkalosis is caused by massive losses of proton and chloride in gastric juice which is coupled with an equimolar gain of bicarbonates (anion exchange alkalosis). This results in a high pH and chloride depletion. According to the Stewart approach, definitive losses of chloride caused by vomitings or gastric aspiration/drainage induce an increase of SID and thus a metabolic alkalosis. The magnitude of metabolic alkalosis therefore depends on the extent of HCl losses. Due to their low concentration in the gastric juice, sodium and potassium losses are usually low. Hypokalemia, often associated at this phase, results from urinary mandatory renal chloride reabsorption and secondary aldosteronism in cases of hypovolemia. At this phase of generation, urine sodium and potassium concentrations are high (>20 mmol/L), while urine chloride concentration is low (<10 mmol/L) leading to a high urine SID and a urinary pH > 6 [52–54].

Similarly, definitive losses of chloride in the intestine due to diarrheal states are also responsible for an increased SID and a metabolic alkalosis. The villous adenoma is responsible in 15–20% of cases of metabolic alkalosis due to considerable chloride losses. Congenital chloridorrhea is an autosomal recessive disease characterized by the inability of the intestine to reabsorb normally chloride at the apical membranes of ileum and colon epithelium.

Renal Causes

Metabolic alkalosis is explained by the same mechanisms as digestive metabolic alkalosis, but losses are located in urines. Using the Henderson-Hasselbalch concept, protons are excreted in the distal convoluted tubule (DCT) mainly in the form of ammonium or titratable acid [1, 21, 55]. In the Stewart concept, metabolic alkalosis is caused by urine chloride, sodium, and potassium losses (> 20 mmol/L), but chloride excretion is proportionally higher than the sodium one resulting in a reduction of urinary SID (urinary pH < 6) and an elevation on plasma SID. Such a metabolic alkalosis is caused essentially by the administration of chloruretic diuretics such as furosemide, bumetanide, and thiazide [55, 56]. Posthypercapnic state represents another cause of metabolic alkalosis which is observed in patients with chronic respiratory insufficiency. Indeed, respiratory acidosis triggers rapidly urinary chloride excretion (secondary predictable renal response) to reach a complete response within 24–48 h. A sudden correction of chronic hypercapnia (mechanical ventilation) does not reverse instantaneously this phenomenon leading to the development of a real metabolic alkalosis until chloride depletion is not corrected [56]. In these patients, metabolic alkalosis is exacerbated by diuretics that increase the chloride depletion and may cause potassium depletion, an additional factor of maintenance of the disorder.

Low Chloride Diet

This disorder has the same impact on acid-base equilibrium than excessive chloride losses. Therefore, a chloride-depletion metabolic alkalosis develops.

7.2.4.2 Non-chloride-Depletion (or Resistant) Metabolic Alkalosis

These disorders are less frequent. According to Henderson-Hasselbalch approach, the kidney is responsible for a loss of protons in the DCT and the collecting duct with concomitant reabsorption of bicarbonate. Considering the Stewart concept, metabolic alkalosis is caused by an increased renal reabsorption of sodium associated with potassium excretion which induces hypokalemia, hyperbicarbonatemia, and a high SID (Lindner). Therefore, these disorders are characterized by hypokalemia which is considered as the main factor of generation of metabolic alkalosis. Additional biological abnormalities are represented by normal or slightly lowered plasma chloride. In urine, sodium and chloride levels are high (>20 mmol/L) and pH < 6.5. Mineralocorticoid excess are the most frequent causes of these metabolic alkaloses. According to the urinary potassium concentration, two categories of metabolic alkalosis are described: those associated with a low urinary potassium excretion and those with a high urinary potassium excretion.

Resistant Metabolic Alkalosis with High Kaliuresis

Primary and Secondary Mineralocorticoid Excess

These situations are associated with arterial hypertension and a high urine potassium excretion (>30 mmol/L).

- Primary hyperaldosteronism or Conn's syndrome can be due to adenoma or carcinoma of the adrenal gland or adrenal hyperplasia [57]. The diagnosis is confirmed by the presence of high plasma aldosterone concentration, whereas plasma renin activity is low.
- Primary deoxycorticosterone excess in 11-β-hydroxylase and 17-α-hydroxylase deficiencies.
- Cushing syndrome due to adenoma, carcinoma, or adrenal hyperplasia is characterized by high plasma levels of renin and cortisol.
- Secondary hyperaldosteronism is biologically characterized by low plasma aldosterone levels and high plasma renin activity. They occur in two situations: (1) in malignant arterial hypertension with renal artery stenosis or renin-secreting tumor (normal cortisol levels) and (2) in pseudohyperaldosteronism caused by an excessive ingestion of licorice (containing glycyrrhizin which inhibits 11-β-hydroxysteroid dehydrogenase (high cortisol levels)) and more rarely in Liddle's syndrome (abnormality of tubular ion transport).

Congenital Tubulopathy

These disorders include Gitelman and Bartter syndrome which are characterized by a normal arterial pressure and biological disorders of secondary hyperaldosteronism such as metabolic alkalosis and hypokalemia. Urine potassium renal excretion is low. Symptoms are not specific and related to hypokalemia: muscle weakness, cramps, paresis/paralysis, extracellular dehydration, and cardiac arrhythmias. Both are autosomal recessive inheritance disease caused by gene mutations encoding for chloride channels. Hypomagnesemia and hypocalcemia are rather present in the Gitelman syndrome, while normomagnesemia and normocalcemia rather characterize the Bartter syndrome [58].

Resistant Metabolic Alkalosis with Low Kaliuresis

Severe isolated potassium depletion (rather than hypokalemia) and increase of the negative charge in the tubules, which can be generated by an overload of non-reabsorbable anions (laxative abuse), may generate and maintain metabolic alkalosis. They are characterized by low kaliuresis and normal arterial pressure.

7.2.4.3 Excessive Sodium Load

Considering the Henderson-Hasselbalch interpretation, sodium bicarbonate infusion results in an exogenous supply of bicarbonate which is the direct cause of metabolic alkalosis. But the Stewart approach considers that because bicarbonate is metabolized rapidly and sodium remains in plasma, plasma SID increases. In turn, bicarbonate increases to maintain plasma electroneutrality and metabolic alkalosis develops. All solutions which are composed by an association of sodium and an anion such as citrate, lactate, or acetate can cause metabolic alkalosis if the anion is metabolized [59–63]. The metabolizable anion enters the cell, while sodium remains in plasma leading to a high level of bicarbonate (the principal plasma buffer system) and a high pH. Therefore, the alkalinizing effect of these solutions is not really caused by the excessive production of bicarbonate but rather by the excessive unmetabolized sodium which conducts to SID" and the pH. The development of metabolic alkalosis during regional citrate anticoagulation in renal replacement therapy is the marker of an excessive dose of citrate and must conduct to stop at least temporarily citrate. Its incidence and its severity depend on the expertise of the team: up to 45% has been reported for this complication at the beginning of the technique [64]. But within time and a better technique and monitoring, this disorder reduced considerably [65], and most recent meta-analysis has reported that the frequency of metabolic alkalosis was similar using sodium citrate or heparin anticoagulation [66, 67]. It must be highlighted that if the anion is not metabolized due to a Krebs cycle or mitochondrial dysfunction such as during severe shock, the accumulation of strong anions is conducted to reduce SID, and a metabolic acidosis will develop.

In the milk-alkali syndrome, metabolic alkalosis is multifactorial [68]: vomiting, hypercalcemia, decreased glomerular filtration rate in relation with kidney dysfunction, and bicarbonate absorption (as calcium bicarbonates). Hyperphosphatemia and hypermagnesemia are associated to hypercalcemia.

7.2.4.4 Hypoalbuminemia

Only the Stewart approach allows to explain the development of metabolic alkalosis caused by hypoalbuminemia. Albumin is a weak acid and is an independent parameter implicated in the acid-base equilibrium. Its decrease causes a reduction in plasma water dissociation as a result of the respect of the conservation of mass, electroneutrality, and equilibrium electrolyte dissociation laws. In critically ill patients, the incidence of hypoalbuminemia is high (up to 90–100%), but very high pH is not frequently observed as hypoalbuminemia-related alkalosis is usually counteracted by additional causes of metabolic acidosis [13–15, 18, 69]. Such an association can be dangerous and lead to ignore the presence of concomitant severe metabolic acidosis.

7.2.5 Treatment

7.2.5.1 Principles

The treatment of metabolic alkalosis relies on the correction of both causes of generation and its maintenance mechanisms. The only correction of the cause will be insufficient without that of the maintenance factors [1, 47]. The correction of chloride-responsive metabolic alkalosis is based on the restoration of chloride amount in the body. The absolute need to associate Na (NaCl) and/or K (KCl) with chloride is still debated [47, 48]. Modern pathophysiological concepts of metabolic alkalosis show that it is certainly wrong to think about extracellular compartment abnormalities, regardless of concomitant changes in the intracellular one. It is difficult to separate chloride variations from those of sodium and potassium [70, 71]. The administration of NaCl in chloride-responsive metabolic alkalosis enables to correct both chloride depletion and hypovolemia. However, its exclusive administration could be inadequate, and studies suggest a systematic association of KCl [24, 70]. Indeed, NaCl alone can correct hyperbicarbonatemia, but cannot correct hypokalemia and associated intracellular acidosis. The treatment of chloride-resistant metabolic alkalosis is based essentially on the administration of KCl necessary to restore the potassium depletion and on the etiologic treatment.

7.2.5.2 Treatment Options

Chloride

- NaCl corrects chloride depletion, restores the extracellular volume, and improves glomerular filtration rate. Administered orally or preferentially intravenously, the first choice goes to isotonic NaCl (0.9%). The infusion of small volumes of hypertonic NaCl (3.6 or 7.2%) was proposed and appeared as effective as conventional treatment and safe [72].
- KCl corrects potassium depletion. This deficit may vary from 200 to 500 mmol for a bicarbonatemia between 30 and 40 mmol/L and from 600 to 1000 mmol for a bicarbonatemia between 40 and 50 mmol/L. Urinary potassium is not an accurate indicator of total body potassium. High kaliuria is present in persistent metabolic alkalosis or inadequately treated and does not necessarily reflect a restoration of total body potassium. The administration of KCl should not exceed 40 mmol/L and requires close monitoring of EKG and serum potassium.

Acidifying Agents

The intravenous administration of an acid salt or a metabolizable cation leads to a decrease of SID that causes a rapid decrease of pH value. The volume of distribution of bicarbonate in the body is approximately 50% of body weight. It is therefore possible to calculate the amount of proton needed to correct metabolic alkalosis from the formula: amount acid charge (mmol/L) = (measured bicarbonates × 25) × weight (kg) × 0.5. However, this estimation remains inaccurate because of a great interindividual variation of the volume of distribution (from 20 to 60% of body weight) and because formula is totally static and does not consider the evolution of the patient's condition [73]. This treatment should be reserved only for life-threatening metabolic alkalosis (pH ≥ 7.55) or symptomatic disorder (arrhythmias, coma). In all cases, it is unnecessary and even dangerous to normalize too quickly bicarbonate levels with a risk mixed acidosis (respiratory and metabolic), because of the slower pH change in cerebrospinal fluid compared to the blood. Administration of protons should induce a decrease of bicarbonates from about 8 to 12 mmol/L. Several agents are available:

- Ammonium, arginine, or lysine hydrochlorides: They are metabolized into urea and therefore contraindicated in patients with hepatic or renal failure [74, 75]. Ammonium hydrochloride may induce encephalopathy, and its administration requires a central line. Arginine hydrochloride can be administered on a peripheral vein; however, it can cause severe hyperkaliemia because arginine induces potassium efflux from cell independently of variations in pH, especially in patients with renal failure. Lysine hydrochloride can be administered orally. For practical reasons, especially the side effects, all of these solutions remain not currently prescribed.
- Hydrochloric acid: If administered, concentrations must range from 50 mmol to 500 mmol/L, knowing that the most used are those at 150 or 200 mmol/L [74, 75]. In the plasma, hydrochloric acid metabolizes as follows: $HCl + HCO_{3-} \leftrightarrow CO_2 + H_2O + Cl^-$. Water production diffuses homogeneously in all compartments without overloading intra- or extracellular compartment. Thus, unlike other acidifying agents, it can be used safely in patients with renal and hepatic failure or even in edematous states where NaCl is contraindicated [74]. Patients with chronic respiratory failure with respiratory acidosis could theoretically benefit for a treatment with hydrochloride acid, because HCl corrects $PaCO_2$ and improves PaO_2 [76]. In all cases, the infusion rate on a central line should not exceed 0.2 mmol/kg/h and an amount of 100–300 mmol per day [74–76]. However, ready commercialized solutions are not available, and its preparation must be performed by the hospital pharmacy.

Acetazolamide

This diuretic is an inhibitor of the carbonic anhydrase enzyme. The inhibition of bicarbonate reabsorption causes a bicarbonaturia but also a urinary loss of sodium, water, and potassium that may aggravate a preexisting depletion. Therefore, such a therapy is ineffective in hypovolemic patients but may be useful in edematous patients with normal glomerular flow. It is contraindicated in patients with hepatic and renal dysfunctions. The best indication is metabolic alkalosis occurring in posthypercapnic states. It is currently recommended to administer 250 mg of acetazolamide three or four times daily in short treatment. This can be simplified as a single intravenous administration of 500 mg that seems equivalent to four injections of 250 mg [77]. In chronic respiratory failure of patients with spontaneous breath, acetazolamide reduces $PaCO_2$ and plasma bicarbonate [78]. However, in chronic respiratory failure of patients under respiratory support, it was recently shown that acetazolamide had no effect on $PaCO_2$ or duration of weaning from the ventilator [79]. These results have been confirmed in a randomized controlled study showing no difference in duration of mechanical ventilation [80].

Dialysis

Dialysis is the most effective treatment allowing to normalize metabolic alkalosis, especially in cases of renal dysfunction [81, 82]. Different techniques can be used: peritoneal dialysis, hemodialysis, or continuous renal replacement therapy. Regardless of the technique, the basic principle relies on the administration of dialysis or substitutive solutions containing no or low bicarbonate concentration or even acid solutions.

7.3 Respiratory Alkalosis

Respiratory alkalosis is defined by a primary decrease in $PaCO_2$ which is responsible for an increased arterial pH > 7.45. Primary hypocapnia can result from an increased alveolar ventilation or a decrease in CO_2 production or a combination of both. The predictable secondary response consists in a reduction in plasma bicarbonate concentration, and its magnitude depends on the speed of development and the magnitude of hypocapnia.

7.3.1 Pathophysiology

Whether considering Henderson-Hasselbalch or Stewart approach, respiratory alkalosis is caused by the decrease in $PaCO_2$. The following decrease in plasma bicarbonate develops in to two steps. The first is rapid and performed by the intracellular buffers leading to minimize rapidly but temporarily the increase in pH. This adaptation is completed into 5–10 min. The second step is slow but sustained and consists in an increase in urinary SID (due to a reduction of chloride renal excretion/elevation of sodium renal excretion). This phenomenon explains why the magnitude for the predictable secondary metabolic response depends on the speed of development of respiratory alkalosis. Therefore, it is classical to distinguish acute from chronic respiratory alkalosis [83].

7.3.1.1 Acute Respiratory Alkalosis

As soon as respiratory alkalosis develops, protons cross the cell membrane to join the extracellular compartment and combine with plasma bicarbonate, leading to its decreased concentration. These protons are issued from various intracellular buffers (proteinates, phosphates, etc.) or from an increased production of lactate caused by an increased glycolysis which is stimulated by the alkalosis-related increased activity of phosphofructokinase.

7.3.1.2 Chronic Respiratory Alkalosis

A sustained hypocapnia induces a decrease in urine acidity which is due to an increase in urinary SID or a decrease of urine excretion of ammonium, both of them being responsible for an increase in plasma SID. This phenomenon takes approximately 48–72 h to develop completely (see chapter "Interpretation of Acid-Base Disorders"), and plasma bicarbonate decreases, on average, by approximately 5 meq/l for each 10 mmHg chronic decrease in $PaCO_2$.

7.3.2 Clinical Signs

Clinical manifestations frequently occur in the acute phase, but they are not specific.

7.3.2.1 Acute Respiratory Alkalosis [83]

Neurological Signs

They are essentially related to the reduction of cerebral blood flow which is caused by alkalosis ($PaCO_2$ between 15 and 20 mmHg induces a 45% reduction of cerebral blood flow): headache, mental confusion, or seizures. Such a phenomenon is also responsible for a decrease of intracranial and intraocular pressures. Other neurological manifestations consist in tingling or paresthesia in the extremities, Chvostek sign, etc., which are due to the associated biological disturbances: reduction in plasma ionized calcium concentration and hypophosphatemia.

Cardiovascular Signs

In severe respiratory alkalosis, acute hypocapnia can induce a decrease of cardiac output and of arterial pressure despite the elevation of peripheral resistances, especially in patients under general anesthesia and artificial ventilation [84]. Several mechanisms are proposed: increase in intrathoracic pressures, inhibition of reflex of tachycardia induced by hypocapnia, and decrease of coronary artery blood flow and of myocardial oxygen delivery [83].

7.3.2.2 Chronic Respiratory Alkalosis

They are usually asymptomatic, and initial manifestations usually disappear progressively within some days to weeks.

7.3.3 Biological Signs

The decrease of $PaCO_2$ leading to an increase of pH is associated with a decrease in plasma bicarbonate concentration with a variable magnitude. Plasma bicarbonate decreases, on average, by approximately 2 meq/L for each 10 mmHg acute decrease in $PaCO_2$ [83]. Chloremia is high and kalemia normal or more often low as well as ionized calcium concentration. In case of severe respiratory alkalosis, hypophosphatemia can be presented, due to a transfer of inorganic phosphates from plasma to the cells. This disorder seems to be commonly asymptomatic and does not require specific treatment. Hyperlactatemia is classical and is responsible of an increased plasma anion gap and a decrease of SID. During the initial phase of hypocapnia generation, urinary pH is often >7. In stable chronic hypocapnia, urinary pH is usually ≤ 6.

7.3.4 Etiologies

The major causes of respiratory alkalosis are summarized in Table 7.3. In critically ill patients or surgical patients under general anesthesia, the most frequent causes of

Table 7.3 Major causes of respiratory alkalosis

Central nervous system stimulation	
– Voluntary, pain, anxiety	
– Unintentional:	Central nervous system dysfunctions: traumatic brain injury, meningoencephalitis, brain tumor, subarachnoid hemorrhage, stroke, intracerebral hematoma Toxics (drugs): salicylates, nicotine, aminophylline, catecholamines, fever, sepsis, pregnancy, metabolic encephalopathies
Tissue hypoxia	
Reduction of FIO_2, high altitude, CO intoxication, severe anemia, severe circulatory failure, right-left shunt, ventilation/perfusion ratio disorder, pulmonary fibrosis, pneumonia	
Others	
Hemodialysis, inappropriate mechanical ventilation	

respiratory alkalosis are iatrogenic hyperventilation, especially, intraoperatively, hypoxia and cerebral edema (post-trauma, encephalopathy, etc.) [83].

7.3.5 Treatment

Respiratory alkalosis does not really require any symptomatic treatment. The appropriate management relies only on the correction of the underlying cause. Respiratory depressive drugs are rarely required. In patients with mechanical ventilation, hypocapnia can be normalized by decreasing minute ventilation or by increasing the pulmonary death space. In patients with spontaneous ventilation, the presence of a symptomatic hypocapnia caused by hypoxia must be verified and easily treated by oxygenotherapy.

Acknowledgments No conflict of interest

References

1. Laski LE, Sabatini S (2006) Metabolic alkalosis, bedside and bench. Sem Nephrol 26:404–421
2. Madger S (1998) Pathophysiology of metabolic acid-base disturbances in patients with critical illness. In: Ronco C, Bellomo R (eds) Critical care nephrology. Kluwer Academic Publisher, Dordrecht, pp 279–296
3. Adrogue H, Madias NE (1998) Medical progress: management of life-threatening acid-base disorders: first of two parts. N Engl J Med 338:26–34
4. Gluck SL (1998) Acid-base. Lancet 352:474–479
5. Ichai C, Verdier JF, Grimaud D (1997) Les alcaloses. In: Société Française d'Anesthésie et de Réanimation ed. Conférence d'actualisation. Elsevier, Paris, pp 499–521
6. Galla JH (2000) Metabolic alkalosis. J Am Soc Nephrol 11:369–375
7. Javaheri S, Shore NS, Rose B, Kazemi H (1982) Compensatory hypoventilation in metabolic alkalosis. Chest 81:296–301
8. Feldman M, Alvarez NM, Trevino M, Weinstein GL (2012) Respiratory compensation to a primary metabolic alkalosis in humans. Clin Nephrol 78:365–369

9. Okusawa S, Aikawa N, Abe O (1985) High incidence of postoperative metabolic alkalosis in surgical patients. Keio J Med 34:115–122
10. Maehle K, Haug B, Flaaten H, Nielsen EW (2014) Metabolic alkalosis is the most common acid-base disorder in ICU patients. Crit Care 18:420
11. Libório AB, Noritomi DT, Leite TT, de Melo Bezerra CT, de Faria ER, Kellum JA (2015) Increased serum bicarbonate in critically ill patients: a retrospective analysis. Intensive Care Med 41:479–486
12. Yunos MM, Kim B, Bellomo R et al (2011) The biochemical effects of restricting chloride-rich fluids in intensive care. Crit Care Med 39:2419–2424
13. Fencl V, Jabor A, Kazda A, Figge J (2000) Diagnosis of metabolic acid-base disturbances in critically ill patients. Am J Respir Crit Care Med 162:2246–2251
14. Stewart PA (1978) Independent and dependent variables of acid-base control. Resp Physiol 33:9–26
15. Dubin A, Menises MM, Masevicius FD et al (2007) Comparison of three methods of evaluation of metabolic acid-base disorders. Crit Care Med 35:1264–1270
16. Anderson LE, Henrich WL (1987) Alkalemia-associated morbidity and mortality in medical and surgical patient. South Med J 80:729–733
17. Majima HJ, Oberley TD, Furukawa K et al (1998) Prevention of mitochondrial injury by manganese superoxide dismutase reveals a primary mechanism for alkaline-induced cell death. J Biol Chem 273:8217–8224
18. Kellum J, Elbers PWG (2009) Stewart's textbook of acid-base. Lulu.com, New York, p 501
19. Gomez H, Kellum JA (2015) Understanding acid-base disorders. Crit Care Clin 31:849–860
20. Ring T, Kellum JA (2016) Strong relationships in acid-base chemistry - modeling protons based on predictable concentrations of strong ions, total weak acid concentrations, and PCO_2. PLoS One 11:e0162872
21. Rosen RA, Julian BA, Dubovsky EV, Galla JH, Luke RG (1988) On the mechanism by which chloride corrects metabolic alkalosis in man. Am J Med 84:449–457
22. Seldin DW, Rector FC (1972) The generation and maintenance of metabolic alkalosis. Kidney Int 1:306–321
23. Cogan MG, Liu FY, Berger BE, Sebastian A, Rector FC (1983) Metabolic alkalosis. Med Clin North America 67:903–915
24. Rubin SI, Sonnenberg B, Zettle R, Halperin ML (1994) Metabolic alkalosis mimicking the acute sequestration of HCl in rats: bucking the alkaline tide. Clin Invest Med 17:515–521
25. Galla JH, Gifford JD, Luke RG, Rome L (1991) Adaptations to chloride depletion alkalosis. Am J Phys 261:R771–R778
26. Vasconcelos DP, Souza LE, Libório AB (2013) Hypernatremic alkalosis or chloride depletion alkalosis. Intensive Care Med 39:1328–1329
27. Berger BE, Cogan MG, Sebastian A (1984) Reduced glomerular filtration and enhanced bicarbonate reabsorption maintain metabolic alkalosis in humans. Kidney Int 26:205–208
28. Finkle D, Dean RE (1981) Buffered hydrochloric acid: a modern method of treating metabolic alkalosis. Ann Surg 47:103–108
29. Schröck H, Kuschinsky W (1989) Cerebrospinal fluid ionic regulation, cerebral blood flow, and glucose use during chronic metabolic alkalosis. Am J Phys 257:H1220–H1227
30. Harrington JT (1984) Metabolic alkalosis. Kidney Int 26:88–97
31. Howard JS III (1993) The psychosis of metabolic alkalosis. Int Physiol Behav Sci 28:353–357
32. Horvat M, Tomsic M (1991) Torsades de pointes associates with combined severe metabolic and respiratory alkalosis. Clin Int Care 2:47–49
33. Nakane E, Kono T, Sasaki Y et al (2004) Gitelman's syndrome with exercise-induced ventricular tachycardia. Circ J 68:509–511
34. Brater DC, Morrelli HF (1981) Systemic alkalosis and digitalis related arrhythmias. Acta Med Scand 647:79–85
35. Shear L, Brandman IS (1973) Hypoxia and hypercapnia caused by respiratory compensation for metabolic alkalosis. Am Rev Resp Dis 107:836–841

36. Van Ypersele De Strihou C, Frans A (1973) The response to chronic metabolic alkalosis and acidosis in disease. Clin Sci Mol Med 45:439–448
37. Brimioulle S, Kahn RJ (1990) Effects of metabolic alkalosis on pulmonary gas exchange. Am Rev Resp Dis 141:1185–1189
38. Gordon JB, Martinez FR, Keller PA, Tod ML, Madden JA (1993) Differing effects of acute and prolonged alkalosis on hypoxic pulmonary vasoconstriction. Am Rev Resp Dis 148:1651–1656
39. Rama BN, Varghese J, Genova G, Kumar S (1993) Severe acute metabolic alkalosis. Nebraska Med J 2:151–154
40. Amundson DE, Diamant J (1994) Severe metabolic alkalosis. Transoesophageal Echocardiography 87:275–277
41. Lavie CJ, Crocker EF, Key KJ, Ferguson TG (1986) Marked hypochloremic metabolic alkalosis with severe compensatory hypoventilation. South Med J 79:1296–1299
42. Neary RH, Edward JD (1987) Metabolic alkalosis and hyperlactatemia. Br J Med 294:1462–1464
43. Hollidge-Horvat MG, Parolin ML, Wong D, Jones NL, Heigenhauser GJ (2000) Effect of induced metabolic alkalosis on human skeletal muscle metabolism during exercise. Am J Physiol Endocrinol Metab 278:E316–E329
44. Fencl V, Leith DE (1993) Stewart's quantitative acid-base chemistry: applications in biology and medicine. Resp Physiol 91:1–16
45. Kellum JA, Kraner DJ, Pinsky MR (1995) Strong ion gap: a methodology for exploring unexplained anions. J Crit Care 10:51–55
46. Jabor A, Kazda A (1995) Modelling of acid-base equilibria. Acta Anaesthesiol Scand 39:119–122
47. Norris SH, Kurtzman NA (1988) Does chloride play an independent role in the pathogenesis of metabolic alkalosis? Semin Nephrol 8:101–108
48. Hernandez RE, Schambelan M, Cogan MG, Colman J, Morris RC, Sebastian A (1987) Dietary NaCl determines severity of potassium depletion-induced metabolic alkalosis. Kidney Int 31:1356–1367
49. Jones JW, Sebastian A, Hulter HN (1982) Systemic and renal acid-base effects of chronic dietary potassium depletion in humans. Kidney Int 21:402–407
50. Mersin SS, Ramelli GP, Laux-End R, Bianchetti MG (1995) Urinary chloride excretion distinguishes between renal and extrarenal metabolic alkalosis. Em J Pediatr 154:979–982
51. Perez GO, Oster JR, Rogers A (1987) Acid-base disturbances in gastrointestinal diseases. Dig Dis Sci 32:1033–1042
52. Luke RG, Galla JH (1983) Chloride-depletion alkalosis with a normal extracellular fluid volume. Am J Phys 245:F419–F424
53. Galla JH, Bonduris DN, Luke RG (1987) Effects of chloride and extracellular fluid volume on bicarbonate reabsorption along the nephron in metabolic alkalosis in the rat. Reassessment of the classical hypothesis of the pathogenesis of metabolic alkalosis. J Clin Invest 80:41–50
54. Galla JH, Bonduris DN, Sanders PW, Luke RG (1984) Volume independent reductions in glomerular filtration rate in acute chloride depletion alkalosis in the rat: evidence for mediation by tubuloglomerular feed-back. J Clin Invest 74:2002–2008
55. Hroprot M, Fowler N, Halmark B, Giebisch G (1985) Tubular action of diuretics: distal effects on electrolyte transport and acidification. Kidney Int 28:477–483
56. Schwartz WB, Hays RM, Polak A, Haynie GD (1961) Effects of chronic hypercapnia on electrolyte and acid-base equilibrium II: recovery with special reference to the influence of chloride intake. J Clin Invest 40:1238–1249
57. Levi M (1990) Southwestern Internal Medicine Conference. Primary hyperaldosteronism. Am J Med Sci 300:189–196
58. Favre G, Orban JC, Ichai C (2014) The Gitelman and classical Bartter syndromes. In: Leone M, Martin C, Vincent JL (eds) Uncommon diseases in the ICU. Spinger, Paris, pp 199–203
59. Arieff AI (1991) Indications for use of bicarbonate in patient with metabolic alkalosis. Br J Med 67:165–177

60. Mustafa I, Leverve XM (2002) Metabolic and hemodynamic effects of hypertonic solutions: sodium-lactate versus sodium chloride infusion in postoperative patients. Shock 18:306–310
61. Ichai C, Armando G, Orban JC et al (2009) Sodium-lactate vs mannitol in the treatment of intracranial hypertensive episodes in severe traumatic brain-injured patients. Intensive Care Med 35:471–479
62. Ichai C, Payen JF, Orban JC et al (2013) Half-molar sodium lactate infusion to prevent intracranial hypertensive episodes in severe traumatic brain injured patients: a randomized controlled trial. Intensive Care Med 39:1413–1422
63. Lindner G, Schwarz C, Grüssing H, Kneidinger N, Fazekas A, Funk GC (2013) Rising serum sodium levels are associated with a concurrent development of metabolic alkalosis in critically ill patients. Intensive Care Med 39:399–405
64. Morgera S, Scholle C, Voss G et al (2004) Metabolic complications during regional citrate anticoagulation in continuous venovenous hemodialysis: single-center experience. Nephron Clin Pract 97:131–136
65. Morgera S, Schneider M, Slowinski T et al (2009) A safe citrate anticoagulation protocol with variable treatment efficacy and excellent control of the acid-base status. Crit Care Med 37:2018–2024
66. Bai M, Zhou M, He L et al (2016) Citrate versus heparin anticoagulation for continuous renal replacement therapy: an updated meta-analysis of RCTs. Intensive Care Med 41:2098–2110
67. Liu C, Mao Z, Kang H, Hu J, Zhou F (2016) Regional citrate versus heparin anticoagulation for continuous renal replacement therapy in critically ill patients: analysis of randomized controlled trials. Crit Care 20:144
68. Schuman CA, Jones HW (1985) The "milk-alkalosis" syndrome: two case reports with discussion of pathogenesis. Q J Med 55:119–122
69. Wilkes P (1998) Hypoproteinemia, strong ion difference and acid-base status in critically ill patients. J Appl Physiol 84:1740–1748
70. Scheich A, Donnelly S, Cheema-Dhadli S, Schweigert M, Vasuvattakul S, Halperin ML (1994) Does saline "correct" the abnormal mass balance in metabolic alkalosis associated with chloride depletion in the rat? Clin Invest Med 17:448–460
71. Wesson DE (1994) Combined K^+ and cl^- repletion corrects augmented H^+ secretion by distal tubules in chronic alkalosis. Am J Phys 266:F592–F603
72. Ward JL, Smith DF, Fubini SL, Grohn YT (1993) Comparison of 0.9, 3.6 and 7.2% NaCl for correction of experimentally induced hypochloremic hypokalemic metabolic alkalosis in sheep. Am J Vet Res 54:1160–1169
73. Bazilinski NG, Duner G, Ing TS (1987) Treatment of metabolic alkalosis in renal failure. Int J Artif Organs 10:284–286
74. Knutsen OH (1983) New method for administration of hydrochloric acid in metabolic alkalosis. Lancet 1:953–955
75. Brimioulle S, Vincent JL, Dufaye P, Berre J, Degaute JP, Kahn RJ (1985) Hydrochloric acid infusion for treatment of metabolic alkalosis: effects on acid-base balance and oxygenation. Crit Care Med 13:738–742
76. Brimioulle S, Berre J, Dufaye P, Vincent JL, Degaute JP, Kahn RJ (1989) Hydrochloric acid infusion for treatment of metabolic alkalosis associated with respiratory acidosis. Crit Care Med 17:232–236
77. Mazur JE, Devlin JW, Peters MJ, Jankowski MA, Iannuzzi MC, Zarowitz BJ (1999) Single versus multiple doses of acetazolamide for metabolic alkalosis in critically ill medical patients: a randomized, double-blind trial. Crit Care Med 27:1257–1261
78. Wagenaar M, Vos PJ, Heijdra YF, Teppema LJ, Folgering HT (2002) Combined treatment with acetazolamide and medroxyprogesterone in chronic obstructive pulmonary disease patients. Eur Respir J 20:1130–1137
79. Faisy C, Mokline A, Sanchez O, Tadié JM, Fagon JY (2010) Effectiveness of acetazolamide for reversal of metabolic alkalosis in weaning COPD patients from mechanical ventilation. Intensive Care Med 36:859–863

80. Faisy C, Meziani F, Planquette B et al (2016) Effect of acetazolamide vs placebo on duration of invasive mechanical ventilation among patients with chronic obstructive pulmonary disease: a randomized clinical trial. JAMA 315:480–488
81. Ponce P, Santana A, Vinhas J (1991) Treatment of severe metabolic alkalosis by "acid dialysis". Crit Care Med 19:583–585
82. Gerhardt RE, Koethe JD, Glickman JD, Ntoso KA, Hugo JP, Wolf CJ (1995) Acid dialysate correction of metabolic alkalosis in renal failure. Am J Kidney Dis 25:343–345
83. Gennari FJ (1994) Respiratory acidosis and alkalosis. In: Narins NG (ed) Clinical disorders of fluid and electrolyte metabolism, 5th edn. Mac Graw Hill, New-York, pp 957–989
84. Theye RA, Milde JH, Michenfelder JD (1966) Effect of hypocapnia on cardiac output during anesthesia. Anesthesiology 27:778–782

Lactate: Metabolism, Pathophysiology

8

Carole Ichai and Jean-Christophe Orban

8.1 Introduction

To understand the pathophysiology of hyperlactatemia requires to know its metabolism. Lactate metabolism is complex and depends on organs and their energetic condition. For a long time, hyperlactatemia was considered as toxic end waste, associated with lactic acidosis and tissue hypoxia-anaerobia. All these notions remain deeply anchored in our spirits but are frequently erroneous. Hyperlactatemia is really a good marker of poor outcome and a warning of energy crisis but is also a witness of a metabolic adaptative response. In many physiological and pathological conditions, lactate appears as an energetic shuttle and an efficient source of fuel.

8.2 Metabolism of Lactate

Lactate is a physiological ubiquitous and crucial metabolite which is present in humans in the levogyral form (L-lactate). This sole isomer is metabolized in humans thanks to the lactate dehydrogenase (LDH) enzyme [1–4]. The dextrogyral isomer (D-lactate) cannot be metabolized because human LDH does not recognize this form. D-lactate is specific to bacteria and can be present in case of intestinal or cerebrospinal fluid bacterial infections.

C. Ichai (✉) • J-C. Orban
Intensive Care Unit, Hôpital Pasteur 2, 30 Voie Romaine, 06001 Nice, Cédex 1, France

IRCAN (INSERM U1081, CNRS UMR 7284), University Hospital of Nice, Nice, France
e-mail: ichai@unice.fr

C. Ichai et al. (eds.), *Metabolic Disorders and Critically Ill Patients*,
http://doi.org/10.1007/978-3-319-64010-5_8

8.2.1 Metabolic Pathways of Lactate Production

Lactate is produced in cytosol from pyruvate [1–5]. The interconversion pyruvate-lactate is regulated by LDH according to the following reaction:

Pyruvate + NADH + $H^+ \rightleftarrows$ Lactate + NAD. According to the law of mass action, [Lactate] = K x [Pyruvate] x [NADH]/NAD + H^+. This reaction of oxidoreduction is close from the equilibrium, K being the constant of equilibrium. In aerobic condition, lactate/pyruvate ratio (L/P) is a good marker of the cytosolic redox potential and is <10. The increase of each three parameters favors pyruvate reduction in lactate.

– *Pyruvate* is mainly generated by glycolysis in cytosol (Fig. 8.1). Glycolytic flux is closely regulated by three enzymes: (1) hexokinase (HK) is essential for glucose to enter this pathway thanks to its initial phosphorylation in glucose 6-phosphate; (2) phosphofructokinase (PFK) allows fructose 6-phosphate conversion into fructose 1,6-biphosphate; (3) and pyruvate kinase (PK) metabolizes phosphoenolpyruvate into pyruvate. The activity of these three enzymes is

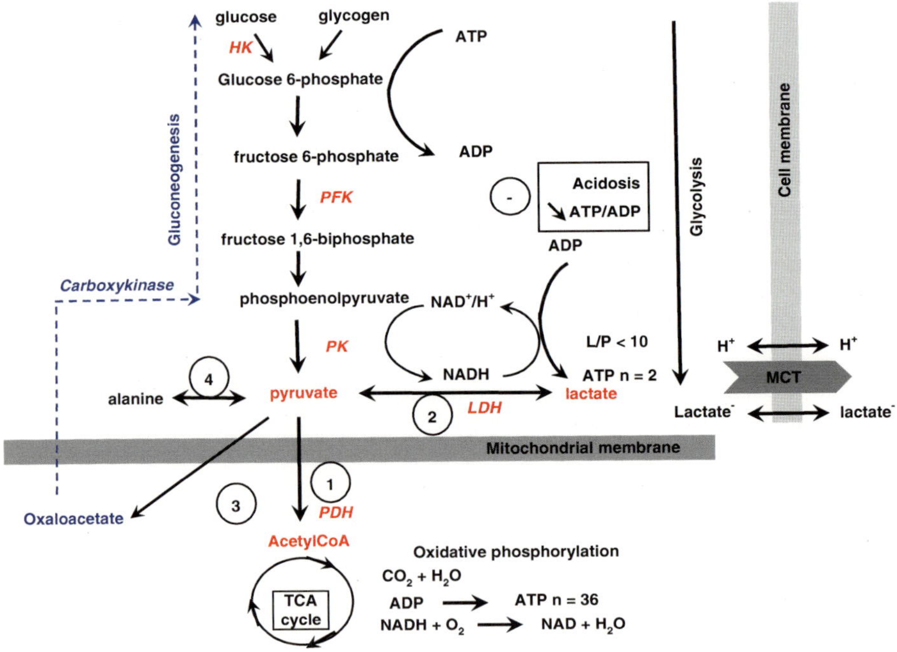

Fig. 8.1 Glycolysis and pyruvate-lactate metabolism. Cytosolic glycolysis conducts through several steps to the production of pyruvate, an essential intermediate metabolite. In the presence of oxygen, most of pyruvate enters the mitochondria to join the tricarboxylic acid (TCA or Krebs) cycle and the oxidative phosphorylation leading to release 36 molecules of ATP [1]. Cytosolic pyruvate is simultaneously reduced into lactate via the lactate dehydrogenase (LDH) enzyme [2]. Secondary pathways of pyruvate metabolism are the mitochondrial decarboxylation [3] and the cytosolic transamination [4]. *G-6P* glucose 6-phosphate, *HK* hexokinase, *PFK* phosphofructokinase, *PK* pyruvate kinase, *PDH* pyruvate dehydrogenase, *MCT* monocarboxylate transporter

controlled by an allosteric regulation leading to an inhibition of the pathway in case of accumulation of each of their respective metabolite. Acidosis and a decreased ATP/ADP ratio exert also an allosteric inhibition of PFK and PK (and conversely). In aerobic conditions, the major metabolic pathway of pyruvate is the intramitochondrial oxidative phosphorylation; pyruvate enters the mitochondrion after crossing its membrane and is oxidized into acetyl coenzyme A (acetylCoA) thanks to the pyruvate dehydrogenase (PDH) enzyme, to finally join the tricarboxylic acid (TCA or Krebs) cycle pathway. The final result is a generation of 36 ATP molecules, CO_2, and water thanks to the regeneration of NADH which allows to complete the respiratory chain pathway. Pyruvate may also join other pathways that are secondary in physiological conditions: alanine production by intracytosolic transamination (reversible) and oxaloacetate production by intramitochondrial decarboxylation. Pyruvate is also an intermediate substrate of hepatic (and in less proportion renal) gluconeogenesis.

- *NADH-H$^+$/NAD* ratio represents the intracytosolic redox potential. In the presence of oxygen (O_2), NADH issued from glycolysis is consumed in mitochondria during oxidative phosphorylation. This metabolic pathway enables to simultaneously generate ATP and resynthesize NAD which is required to maintain glycolysis. In the absence of O_2, reduction of pyruvate into lactate is the unique reaction which allows the essential reoxidation of NADH in NAD required to perpetuate glycolysis. Therefore, even not really cost-effective for energy generation (only two molecules of ATP are produced), the reduction of pyruvate into lactate is the sole able to produce energy in this situation.
- *[H$^+$]* concentration plays a complex role because it favors lactate production from pyruvate, but it slows down simultaneously pyruvate production by inhibiting PFK.

8.2.2 Turnover of Lactate

8.2.2.1 Lactate Production

In adults, basal serum lactate concentration (lactatemia) remains stable, approximately equal to 0.5–1.5 mmol/L, with a half-life of 10 min [2]. This concentration is finally the resultant of the instantaneous steady state between production and elimination from the organism at a given time. It is essential to distinguish lactate turnover from lactatemia. Indeed, normal lactatemia may be associated with a high turnover, while a normal turnover may be associated with a very high lactatemia caused by a disequilibrium between generation and removal of lactate [2].

In a 70 kg adult in basal condition, lactate production represents 1300–1500 mmol/day including 50% issued from glycolysis and the other 50% from amino acids and glycogen metabolism. Most lactate is usually produced by organs that work under anaerobic conditions, i.e., red blood cells, brain, intestine, and muscles which are classical "producing" organs. In normal conditions, there is an equilibrium between its release and its consumption, 80% by oxidation and 20% glucose synthesis (gluconeogenesis).

8.2.2.2 Lactate Clearance

Eighty percent of lactate is metabolized by oxidation (Krebs cycle and oxidative phosphorylation) essentially after an initial conversion into pyruvate. Contrary to old beliefs, lactate is not confined in cytosol and does not require obligatory to its conversion into pyruvate in cytosol to enter the intramitochondrial Krebs cycle to produce energy [3, 6, 7]. Indeed, lactate enables to cross the mitochondrial membrane thanks to monocarboxylate transport proteins (MCT) and undergoes its oxidation into pyruvate in the mitochondrion thanks to a mitochondrial LDH [2, 6]. In this way, lactate appears as a real fuel source for tissues [3, 7]. The liver is the main organ involved in approximately 70% lactate removal by oxidation. Only severe hepatic liver dysfunction or hepatic blood flow impairment enables to reduce lactate clearance and in turn to increase serum lactate level [8–10]. Moreover, the threshold of saturation of the hepatic enzymes responsible for lactate metabolism reaches a plateau above 5 mmol/L of lactatemia. In normal conditions, the removal of lactate by the kidney is secondary as it is usually totally reabsorbed in tubules. On the other hand, in some pathological conditions such as anhepatic situations, the kidney can remove and metabolize more than 30% of lactate production [11].

Conversion of lactate into glucose, i.e., Cori cycle, participates commonly to 20% of lactate removal [3, 7]. Lactate is the major glucogenic precursor of gluconeogenesis, followed by glycerol and amino acids. The liver and kidneys are approximately involved in 50% of gluconeogenesis each.

The distinguishing between "producer" and "consumer" organs is finally complex and artificial, because the same organ can exert simultaneously lactate release and uptake the ratio between both depending on metabolic conditions, leading to a net lactate uptake (consumption) or to a net release (production) [12]. Therefore, the kidney can participate to lactate consumption thanks to renal gluconeogenesis performed by cortical proximal cells. Moreover, renal gluconeogenesis increases when the hepatic one is strongly impaired [11]. On the other hand, renal medullar physiologically works in anaerobic and produces lactate. Skeletal muscle is usually a producer of lactate but becomes a consumer when the energetic demand increases, such as during physical exercise [13]. The brain can also become a lactate consumer [12, 14].

In summary: acetylCoA is the key substrate linked between carbohydrate and lipid oxidation (ß-oxidation) which enters the Krebs cycle and oxidative phosphorylation. Pyruvate is the obligatory unique intermediate metabolite that allows the oxidation of all carbon hydrates (glucose, lactate) in the TCA cycle. All reasons for an increased pyruvate production (rapid glycolysis, Krebs cycle breakdown) would cause in turn an increase in lactate production. Lactate appears as an end metabolic molecule, and it is consumed only through a reoxidation into pyruvate or through the gluconeogenetic pathway. When oxidative phosphorylation is blocked (hypoxia, anaerobia, tissues without mitochondrion), the only way to produce ATP and to perpetuate glycolysis is to regenerate NAD thanks to the reduction of pyruvate into lactate [1, 3]. Even not cost-effective, this metabolic pathway remains the sole possible in tissues not containing mitochondrion or for those in energetic crisis conditions. In these conditions, lactate may become a fuel source thanks to MCT which allows lactate to enter directly into the mitochondrion for metabolization and energy production. The simultaneous production and reuptake of lactate by tissues or organs can be explained by the metabolic compartmentation of cells and by the energetic shuttling capacity of lactate (cf infra).

8.2.3 Lactate Measurement

Various devices can perform blood lactate level measurements (central laboratory, point of care with blood gas analyzers) with an acceptable limit of agreement. Not only devices but various sampling sites (arterial, venous, capillary) are proposed. Arterial sample remains the gold standard site for lactate level determination. It has been suggested that venous or capillary measurements could be less expansive, time-consuming, and easily available [15, 16]. Therefore, such a technique could be interesting to triage patients in emergency departments. Despite acceptable relationship, venous and capillary lactatemia always overestimates values as compared with arterial measurements [17, 18]. Two recent studies do not really support the use of venous measurements due to inacceptable bias, a high number of misinterpretation, and a low agreement [19, 20]. The capillary measurement of lactate by finger blood sticks in patients with shock has been reported to be closely correlated to the arterial one in a sole monocentric small observational study [21].

The interchangeability of sampling site cannot be recommended for short interval measurements requiring very accurate value determinations. Therefore, the substitution of arterial by venous or capillary samples requires further investigations to be suggested in routine practice. Such a procedure is all the most justified since unstable patients need an arterial catheter for arterial pressure and repetitive biological monitoring [20].

8.3 Hyperlactatemia: A Marker of Both Poor Prognosis and Appropriate Metabolic Response

There are numerous clinical trials confirming that hyperlactatemia (>4 mmol/L) is a good marker of poor prognosis [21–25]. Elevated serum lactate levels on admission are associated to an increased morbi-mortality in all types of critically ill patients, including patients in severe sepsis or septic shock and surgical or trauma patients [17, 21–25, 26, 27]. In a large retrospective study including 13,932 critically ill patients, 40% of them presented hyperlactatemia during their hospitalization [25]. The median peak value was 1.8 mmol/L [1.2–2.9]. Hyperlactatemia was more frequent in trauma patients (45%), followed by medical and surgical patients.

In a cohort of 7155 patients, Nichol et al. [22] reported that hyperlactatemia, even moderate (> 0.75 mmol/L), was associated to a high mortality rate. In septic patients, lactate levels >4 mmol/L on admission are associated with a six higher risk of death, while a lower level has no impact. More than the initial serum lactate, the length of hyperlactatemia and its delay for normalization seem to be more accurate risk factors [22, 28, 29]. Therefore, several studies evaluated the predictive value of lactatemia decrease over time in patients with shock. In all of these studies, the decrease of lactate within time is inappropriately called "lactate clearance," but this parameter is not really measured. Most data are in agreement, reporting that the absence of sufficient decrease or normalization of lactatemia over time is an independent risk factor of high mortality [4, 30–33]. A recent observational trial has shown that severe hyperlactatemia (>10 mmol/L) was associated with a high mortality (78.2%). Moreover, a 33% decrease of lactatemia over 12 h was associated with a lower ICU mortality [30]. Such results have been confirmed in a recent systematic review [31]. Based on these data, the implementation of such a monitoring in an "early goal-directed therapy" has been evaluated in various studies [22, 32, 33]. In a multicenter, controlled study, 300 patients were randomized to compare whether a "lactate clearance" ≥10% as a goal of resuscitation could be superior to the central venous oxygen saturation ($SvcO_2$) one [33]. The authors failed to demonstrate any difference between the two groups in terms of in-hospital mortality or treatments administered. In septic patients treated in an emergency department, Arnold et al. [29] reported that the evolution of lactate clearance and $SvcO_2$ was not parallel: 79% of patients presenting a lactatemia decrease <10% had a concomitant $SvcO_2$ > 70%. These results underline that there is no obligatory relationship between oxygen delivery and oxygen tissue consumption. Such results were further confirmed in a multicenter open-label controlled trial, aiming to treat septic patients based on $SvcO_2$ versus $SvcO_2$ + lactate-guided therapy over 8 h [32]. In the lactate group, the additional goal was to reach at least a 20% decrease in lactatemia per 2 h using vasodilators when $SvcO_2$ was >70% and lactate clearance insufficient. Results showed a trend toward a higher survival rate in the lactate group. Lactate-guided therapy was significantly associated with an ICU and hospital lower mortality rate (HR = 0.66 and 0.61, respectively). Patients of the lactate group received more fluids and more vasodilators within the first 8 h of resuscitation. But, despite this beneficial effect, the course of lactatemia was similar in both groups, leading to question about the causal relationship between these effects. Few recent studies seem to disagree with these data [34, 35]. Some patients can present septic shock without normal lactatemia, while macrohemodynamics were similar with those presenting hyperlactatemia. Indeed, patients without elevated lactatemia exhibit less impairment of their microcirculation and less organ failure [35]. Another randomized trial failed to demonstrate an advantage of lactate monitoring-guided therapy over care based on clinical judgment [34]. Moreover, most of the positive studies have methodological bias: heterogenous magnitude of lactate decrease, no consensus on the appropriate interval for lactate measurement, no difference between groups in terms of therapeutic protocols and treatments.

In summary: the decrease in serum lactate level monitoring is helpful for evaluating the prognosis and the efficiency of therapeutic management of patients with shock, regardless of the cause of the shock. There is no doubt that this parameter is useful to guide the treatment [4, 5, 17, 31, 36]. However, lactatemia and changes in lactate clearance do not reflect only tissue hypoperfusion or anaerobic metabolism. Therefore, lactate-guided therapy must be one of the multimodal guided therapies, including usual biological parameters, $SvcO_2$, and clinical signs. Measuring serum lactate level every 2 h within the first 8 h of treatment seems to be appropriate [5].

Even if hyperlactatemia is an accurate warning indicator of severity, lactate is not responsible of high mortality. Indeed, lactate is a physiological substrate without any toxicity, and an increased production appears as an appropriate response during acute conditions with energetic crisis such as in shock. Several studies support the fact that hyperlactatemia or more precisely an increased turnover of lactate represents a metabolic adaptation [28, 29, 37, 38]. In critically ill septic patients, Levraut et al. [28, 39] evaluated lactate metabolism using a "hyperlactatemia test" induced by an exogenous infusion of lactate. Their result shows that for an equivalent hyperlactatemia, survivals were those with a high lactate turnover, consisting in an increase of both release and consumption of lactate compared with non-survivals. Another retrospective trial including 100 patients in shock has shown that patients which enabled to increase lactatemia during epinephrine infusion presented a higher survival rate compared with those who maintained a stable lactatemia [37]. These results support that hyperlactatemia is a metabolic adaptative response in case of energetic impairment. Lactate is an efficient alternative substrate and allows to spare glucose which becomes available for cell or organs in anaerobic metabolism (cf infra). The absence of enough lactate production aiming to cover needs is the marker of the severity of the situation.

8.4 Lactate and Tissue Hypoxia

Lactate production issued from glycolysis is purely anaerobic in the cytosolic cell compartment. This is the sole pathway possible to work in the absence of O_2. The systematic relationship between hyperlactatemia and hypoxia (or energy deficit) is based on these biochemical data [1, 40]. This relationship is so deeply anchored in our minds that hyperlactatemia associated with acidosis is classified into two groups according to the deficit or not in O_2 (Table 8.1) [41]. But lactatemia not only depends on macrocirculation and macrohemodynamics. The best example is sepsis which is characterized by alterations in microcirculatory perfusion which can induce a reduction in tissue oxygen delivery and cause hyperlactatemia despite normal parameters of systemic hemodynamic [42]. However, this relationship is not really always true, because independently of O_2 changes, any excessive production of pyruvate (caused

Table 8.1 Common classification and causes of hyperlactatemias

Type A: hyperlactatemias related to tissue hypoxia
– *Decrease in oxygen delivery*
• Reduction of cardiac output : cardiogenic shock, septic shock, hypovolemic shock
• Reduction of arterial content in oxygen: severe anemia, hemoglobin abnormalities, severe hypoxemia, asphyxia
– *Impaired oxygen extraction or utilization*: severe sepsis, multiple organ failure, cyanide poisoning
Type B1: hyperlactatemias and systemic diseases
– Liver failure, diabetes, cancers, alkalosis, sepsis
Type B2: hyperlactatemias and poisoning
• Biguanides, fructose
• Ethanol, methanol, ethylene glycol
• Salicylates, cyanure, paracetamol
Type B3: hyperlactatemias and increase in oxygen demand
• Status epilepticus
• Sustained muscular exercise

by an increased glycolysis) induces a simultaneous proportional increased production of lactate according to the constant of equilibrium. Therefore, a stimulated aerobic glycolysis can be responsible of an excessive lactate (and pyruvate) production, in the absence of tissue hypoxia. In these situations, the L/P ratio, a marker of the cytosolic redox potential (NADH/NAD), remains ≤ 10. A high value of L/P ratio is the sole accurate parameter of the presence of an anaerobic condition or an energetic deficit [13]. The absence of linear relationship between lactatemia and L/P ratio is well illustrated in a study that has compared these parameters during various type of shock [43]. Results showed that refractory septic shock presented a severe hyperlactatemia with a moderately elevated L/P ratio, whereas cardiogenic shock was characterized by a moderate hyperlactatemia associated with a very high L/P ratio. Several studies support against this link between hyperlactatemia and tissue hypoxia [3, 38, 44, 45]. The muscular tissue PO_2 is more elevated in septic patients than in cardiogenic shock or in controlled patients [46]. In rabbits, the decrease in cardiac output induces various metabolic modifications according to the cause of low output. For a similar increase in O_2 delivery (DO_2), consumption (VO_2), and tissue PO_2, lactatemia was higher in septic animals than in those with a low cardiac output induced by an intraventricular balloon inflation. Moreover, treatments that increase DO_2 have no effect on lactatemia, and conversely, treatments enabled to decrease lactatemia such as dichloroacetate have no effect on oxygenation [31]. Finally, hyperlactatemia without hypoxia is real and is called “stress hyperlactatemia” [7, 13, 47].

8.5 Stress Hyperlactatemia

Stress hyperlactatemia results from multiple mechanisms that induce lactate hyperproduction or lactate clearance impairment [13]. This condition is well illustrated during sepsis [7].

8.5.1 Hyperlactatemia and Overproduction of Lactate

Sepsis is characterized by an increased glucose consumption associated with a reduction in stock of glycogen and an increase in reuptake of glucose by the muscle. These modifications associate with a higher glycolytic flux which can result from changes in enzymatic activities involved in glycolysis pathway or in cytokine mediation. In this situation, the accelerating glycolysis is totally independent of O_2 supply and conducts to an overproduction of pyruvate and in turn of lactate [7]. The accumulation of pyruvate can also be caused by a decrease in pyruvate dehydrogenase (PDH) activity, PDH being the enzyme that catalyzes the conversion of pyruvate into acetylCoA and allows its entry in the Krebs cycle. In septic rats, the inactive form of PDH increases leading to an accumulation of pyruvate and in turn of lactate [48]. Moreover, during sepsis, some organs that usually consume lactate can release it and participate to the high concentration of lactate [12, 49].

8.5.2 Hyperlactatemia and Decrease of Lactate Clearance

Globally, total body enables to clear large lactate loads (1500 moles/day) (leverve curren opin, et cardiac surg). Only severe hepatic dysfunctions can induce severe hyperlactatemia related to a reduction in hepatic clearance. However, for a similar hepatic dysfunction, hyperlactatemia is higher during sepsis. In hemodynamically stable septic patients, hyperlactatemia seems to be essentially caused by an impairment in clearance rather than by an excessive production [28]. This disturbance could be the consequence of a decreased hepatic blood flow or an impairment in hepatic metabolic functions [8, 10].

8.5.3 Hyperlactatemia and Energy Cell Compartmentalization

The cell is not a uniform structure in which energy and substrate exchanges are similar everywhere in the cell. A real intracellular compartmentalization has been described [50]. It is classical to describe a glycolytic and an oxidative cell compartment. The oxidative compartment is close from the mitochondria, and the low concentration of pyruvate in this part of the cell favors lactate oxidation via the mass action of the equilibrium enzyme LDH [2, 7]. Some experimental studies have shown that a channeling glycolysis pathway is identified inside the cell [51, 52]. This glycolysis is functionally and structurally isolated from other structures of the cells, as pyruvate issued from this pathway does not disseminate equally in cytosol but it produces lactate. This specific lactate produced by an "aerobic glycolysis" in the oxidative compartment is exported outside the cell or inside the mitochondria by specific MCT transporters (Fig. 8.2).

Lactate production issued from the aerobic glycolysis is needed to resynthesize NAD^+ which is essential to maintain glycolysis. It is also essential and closely linked with the membrane Na-K-ATPase activity. Indeed, only ATP issued from this

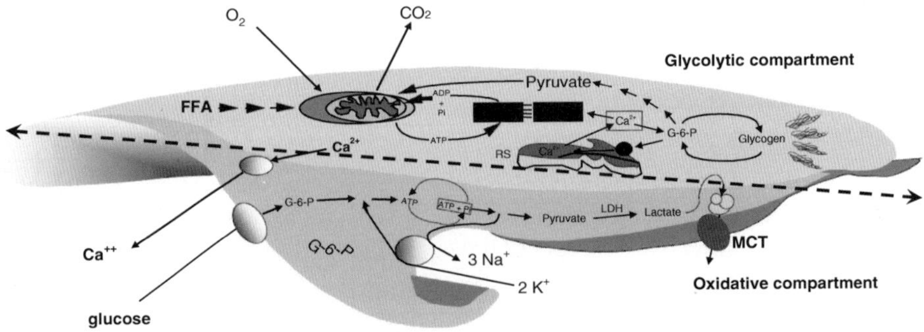

Fig. 8.2 Cellular energetic compartmentalization. Glycolysis which is performed in membranes remains a channeling pathway in which pyruvate and lactate production do not enter cytosol compartment. ATP issued from this membrane glycolysis is dedicated specifically to allow the work of the membrane Na-K-ATPase pump. *FFA* free fatty acids, *SR* sarcoplasmic reticulum

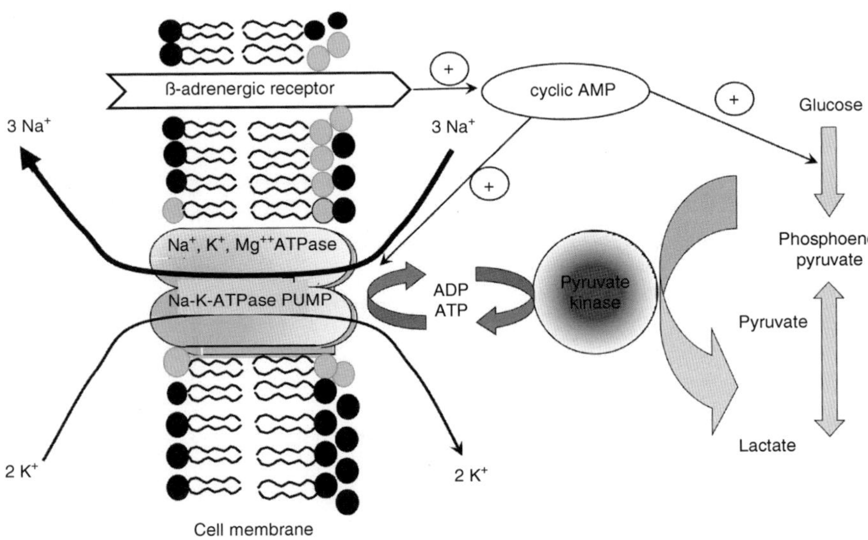

Fig. 8.3 The coupling glycolytic lactate/ATP and membrane Na-K-ATPase pump. Only ATP issued from glycolysis with lactate production allows the Na-K-ATPase pump to work. Catecholamines, by stimulating ß-adrenergic receptors, trigger the production of cyclic AMP and simultaneously accelerate glycolysis and the Na-K-ATPase pump activity. This is the mechanism by which catecholamines cause an elevation in lactatemia

channeling aerobic glycolysis allows the pump to work (Fig. 8.3). Finally, aerobic lactate production is strongly linked with Na-K-ATPase activity but totally independent of oxygen [3, 52]. Such a relation is clearly demonstrated in clinical situations, such as during sepsis [37, 53]. In a study including 14 patients in septic shock, Lévy et al. [53] reported that muscle lactate concentrations decreased significantly when the muscle was in the presence of ouabain which is an inhibitor of Na-K-ATPase pump. The absence of any role for oxygen in this trial was supported by a concomitant absence of any change in intramuscular PO_2 muscular and in muscular and plasma L/P ratio.

Such an independent evolution between hyperlactatemia and hypoxia is also described as the "Warburg" effect. This is due to an interaction between cytosolic glycolysis and hexokinase, and it can be observed during muscle exercise or some cancers. The first step of glycolysis consists in a phosphorylation of glucose into glucose 6-P which is closely regulated thanks to the hexokinase enzyme: in normal conditions, any excessive glucose 6-P production inhibits the hexokinase activity allowing to prevent an excessive glycolysis and ATP consumption and exhaustion. In some cancers, hexokinase which is usually located in the cytosol binds to the external mitochondrial membrane on a channel called "a porine" [54, 55]. This abnormal bound modifies the hexokinase structure which becomes in turn insensitive to glucose 6-P and causes the absence regulation of this step. The resulting effect of such an absence of autoregulation leads to an excessive production of both pyruvate and lactate, independently from oxygen delivery.

In summary: hyperlactatemia during sepsis results commonly from an overproduction (stress hyperlactatemia) and a reduction in its clearance [2, 7]. The excessive production is increased by the administration of catecholamines which stimulates the Na-K-ATPase pump [45, 56] (Fig. 8.3). On the other hand, at the initial phase of sepsis in unstable patients or if hyperlactatemia is severe or persists with hemodynamic instability (hypovolemia, hypokinesia), the contribution of tissue hypoxia or anaerobic condition remains possible. In this context, a persisting severe hyperlactatemia and an impaired clearance keep its poor prognosis value. However, hyperlactatemia should not be confused with lactate turnover: a transitory increased production of lactate in these conditions appears as an adaptative response, and patients unable to increase their lactate production are those with a poor prognosis [37].

8.6 Lactate and Acidosis

The association between hyperlactatemia and acidosis is deeply accepted as most physicians think that lactic acid is in our body. Lactic acid is a strong acid as its pK is very low (3.9) indicating that in large values of plasma pH, blood cannot contain the undissociated form of lactic acid but only the dissociated strong anion lactate. The increase in lactate can decrease the pH by decreasing the strong ion difference (SID): lactate accumulation causes a decrease in HCO_3, the major plasma buffer, to maintain electroneutrality [57–59]. In this way, lactate can be responsible for a metabolic acidosis. But, some data demonstrate that the relationship between hyperlactatemia and pH is often weak [4]. Indeed, proton production is not due to lactate but is secondary to ATP hydrolysis coupled with glycolysis and conversion of pyruvate into lactate on contrary consumes H^+. The net flux of glycolysis is a

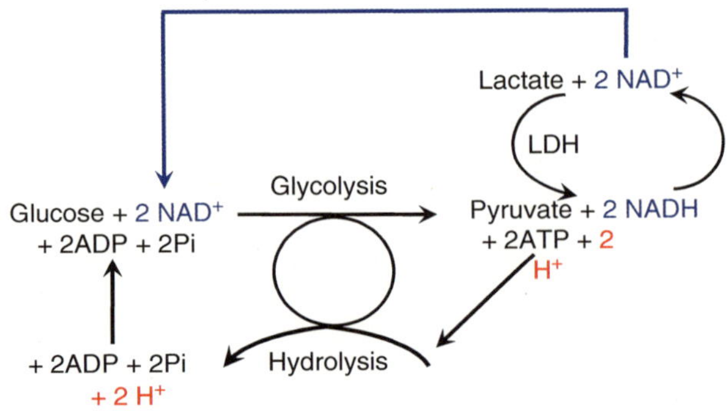

Fig. 8.4 Lactate production and acid-base equilibrium. Production of pyruvate from glucose is associated with the metabolism of ADP in ATP + 2 protons. In the same time, NAD^+ is reduced in NADH. The reduction of pyruvate into lactate does not produce any protons but is required to regenerate NAD^+ for maintaining glycolysis. Finally, ATP hydrolysis into ADP produces two protons H^+ and explains the development of acidosis

production of 1 pyruvate +2 NADH +2 H^+ and 2 ATP from 2 glucose +2 NAD^+ and 2 ADP. In the presence of oxygen, the final result is the production of 2ATP, 2 H_2O, and CO_2. In the same time, reduction of pyruvate into lactate resynthesizes NAD^+ allowing glycolysis to continue. Finally ATP will be hydrolyzed into ADP which is also needed for glycolysis, leading to a production of 2 H^+ (Fig. 8.4). Moreover, as lactate is a metabolizable anion, it leaves plasma and enters in the cell for metabolization. The resulting effect is a re-increase of plasma SID to maintain electroneutrality thanks to an increased bicarbonate level and an increase in plasma pH with a possible metabolic alkalosis. Therefore, it is more realistic to abandon the term lactic acidosis and use the term of hyperlactatemia associated with or without metabolic acidosis. Exogenous administration of lactate salts such as sodium lactate has been largely reported to cause metabolic alkalosis. In these situations, lactate and sodium are dissociated in strong anion and cation, while $lactate^-$ is metabolized in the cell, Na^+ remains in plasma leading to increase SID and create a metabolic alkalosis [60, 61].

8.7 Lactate: An Energetic Fuel

The role of lactate in the energetic metabolism is complex, because it is conditioned by the needs of each organ (or cell) in various situations. Thanks to its recycling, lactate exerts its role of shuttle allowing intra- and interorgan energy exchanges. The famous cycles lactate-glucose of Cori and lactate-alanine of Felig are essential, as they allow to some organs to cover the metabolic demand of those unable to do it. Therefore, even if some organs or cells work in anaerobic conditions, the body metabolism can only be globally aerobic. In this way, lactate cannot be considered as a toxic end waste product but on contrary as an essential substrate [2, 13, 44].

8.7.1 Lactate: An Energy Source in Physiological Situations

Considering its capacity of carbon shuttle, lactate is a real essential or preferential energetic substrate [13, 44]. The Cori lactate-glucose cycle is the most physiological proof of the involvement of lactate as a fuel source [13]: indeed this cycle is the sole pathway to produce ATP by organs without mitochondrion. Red blood cells represent the best illustration of an exclusive anaerobic cytosolic glycolysis, leading to a production of lactate, the final metabolite. The liver which is an exclusive aerobic organ resynthesizes glucose from lactate which is released by red blood cells, thanks to ATP issued from ß-oxidation of lipids (Fig. 8.5). The energetic yield is of course not poor (production of two ATP in red blood cells versus consumption of six ATP in the liver) but is the sole available.

Lactate is a source of carbohydrate useful during muscle exercise [12, 13, 38]. In this situation, changes in muscle metabolism have been summarized to a high rate of glycolysis and glycogenolysis leading to an excessive release of pyruvate and lactate. However, modifications in muscle metabolism are more complex, as a bidirectional lactate metabolism is present: indeed there is a simultaneous lactate uptake and release by the muscle [12]. The net result is a decrease in lactate release caused by a decreased in lactate production, while lactate consumption remains stable. Briefly, during exercise, lactate production is related to the metabolic rate of muscle, while lactate uptake is related to arterial lactate concentration. It is suggested that such a simultaneous production and uptake of lactate are possible thanks to the compartmentalization of cell metabolism: lactate production is performed in the glycolytic compartment close from myofibrils, while lactate consumption is performed in the oxidative compartment. This example of intra-organ cooperation is completed by an

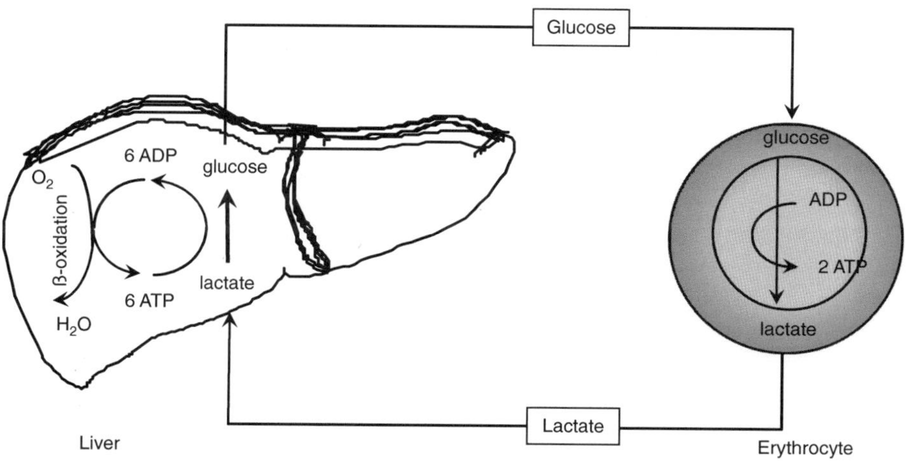

Fig. 8.5 The glucose lactate Cori cycle. ATP produced by the red blood cells is obligatory issued from the glycolytic production of lactate. This lactate is reuptake by liver and further metabolized into glucose (gluconeogenesis) with oxygen. The energetic efficiency is low but essential, and ATP produced in the liver comes from the aerobic ß-oxidation of free fatty acids: "the liver breaths for the red blood cells"

interorgan cooperation too as lactate produced by the muscle in local anaerobic condition can be aerobically metabolized into glucose (Cori cycle) in the liver or muscles at rest [2, 13]. Therefore, depending on its activity, the muscle enables to switch rapidly from a consumer to a producer organ. It can also uptake and consume exogenous lactate when lactatemia increases, leading to decrease glucose consumption. Considering these data, it appears that lactate is an intermediary metabolite that can be rapidly exchanged between various organs to supply energy.

8.7.2 Lactate: An Energy Source in Pathological Situations

The role of lactate as a source of energy in pathological conditions is largely described, especially during energetic crisis such as in sepsis or ischemia-reperfusion (shock) and for various organs such as the heart and the brain. Theoretical biochemical data strongly support that lactate is a preferential source of energy in these situations. During ischemia (or hypoxia), glycolysis favors lactate production at the expense of the Krebs cycle which is blocked [44]. In the same time, the ATP/ADP ratio collapses. Reperfusion occurs in an ATP-deficient cells, and the immediate recovery of glycolysis with an oxidative phosphorylation is not possible (Fig. 8.6).

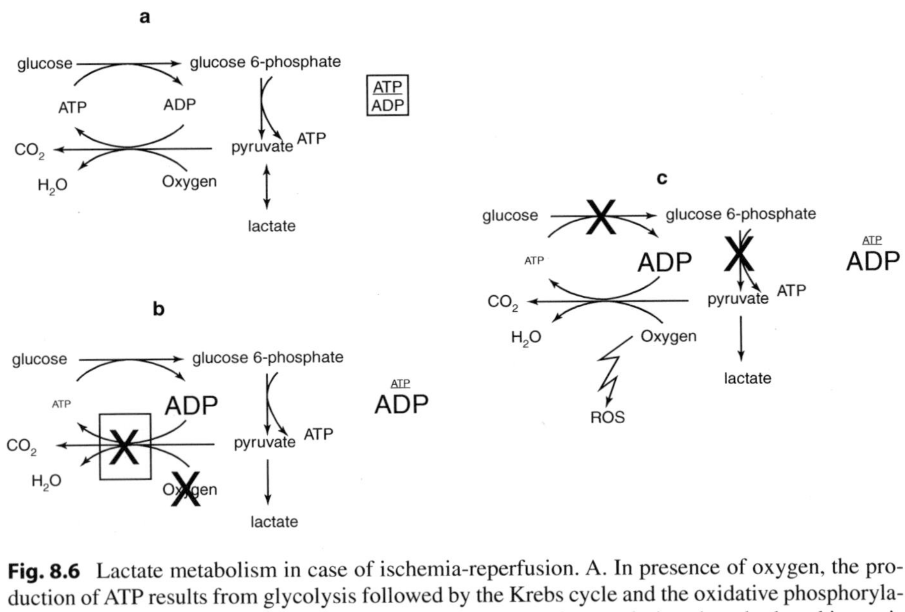

Fig. 8.6 Lactate metabolism in case of ischemia-reperfusion. A. In presence of oxygen, the production of ATP results from glycolysis followed by the Krebs cycle and the oxidative phosphorylation. This pathway, especially glucose phosphorylation in glucose 6-phosphate by hexokinase, is not limited as the cell contains large amount of ATP. B. In case of ischemia or hypoxia, pyruvate cannot be produced because the first step of glucose phosphorylation is not possible due to the low concentration in ATP. The sole metabolic issue is the oxidation of lactate into pyruvate which is associated to a low ATP/ADP ratio. C. During reperfusion, the first step of glucose phosphorylation cannot begin initially because ATP supply is not sufficient for hexokinase. On the other hand, lactate can be immediately reoxidized in pyruvate and enters in the Krebs cycle, allowing therefore the consumption of oxygen and preventing the production of oxygen reactive species (ROS)

Indeed, the first step of glucose phosphorylation into glucose 6-P is essential for glucose to enter in glycolysis and cannot begin without ATP. The oxygen which cannot be consumed in the Krebs cycle induces an oxidative stress with a production of oxygen reactive species. Only lactate, carbohydrate accumulated during ischemia, can rapidly be reoxidized without ATP to produce pyruvate, promote oxidative phosphorylation, and reload cell with ATP. This intermediate step allows to reach ATP production through the Krebs cycle in presence of oxygen while having the possibility to re-initiate glycolysis.

8.7.2.1 Lactate: A Myocardial Source of Energy

At rest, the heart presents an oxidative metabolism. Most of the substrates (60–90%) comes from the ß-oxidation of fatty acids, but lactate is also uptaken and oxidizes [62, 63]. When myocardial consumption (VO_2) increases (exercise, tachycardia, sepsis, adrenergic stimulation) or when myocardial oxygen delivery (DO_2) decreases (anemia, shock), the myocardial metabolism shifts from fatty acids toward carbohydrates oxidation, allowing to provide a higher energy production. Indeed, lactate becomes a preferential fuel which can account for up to 60% and exceeds the glucose one for pyruvate production [2, 63].

In an experimental model of rat's endotoxin shock, Levy et al. [64] have demonstrated that systemic lactate deprivation was associated with an impaired myocardial hemodynamics and energetics and a higher mortality. These data were confirmed in patients with septic and cardiogenic shock [65]. In patients undergoing cardiac surgery for coronary artery bypass grafting, a postoperative administration of exogenous sodium lactate was associated with an elevation in cardiac index (CI) and DO_2, while cardiotropic drugs and fluid balance concomitantly decreased compared with ringer lactate [66]. Compared with hypertonic sodium chloride, sodium lactate was responsible for a similar increase in CI but a lower oxygen extraction [60]. In a recent randomized controlled trial, sodium lactate was compared to ringer lactate infusion in patients presenting acute heart failure [67]. The authors reported that CI and right ventricular systolic function improved significantly within 2 days following sodium lactate administration but did not change with ringer lactate. Moreover, sodium lactate reduced significantly fluid balance.

8.7.2.2 Lactate: A Cerebral Source of Energy

For a long time, it was considered that glucose was the sole energetic substrate available for the brain. There are now growing experimental and clinical data against this theory, which demonstrate clearly that lactate is a part of energy source in human non-damaged brain and also a preferential if not obligatory source of fuel during cerebral energetic crisis [68].

In a postabsorptive period, the brain releases a net amount of 50 μmol/min, while after exercise, the brain shows a net uptake of lactate of 150 μmol/min [12]. In non-injured human brain, lactate was found to contribute to cover 7–10% of energy requirements and can reach up to 25% during exercise [12, 69, 70]. In healthy volunteers, Bouzmebeur et al. [70], using nuclear magnetic resonance spectroscopy, demonstrated that lactate is metabolized for 80% in neurons. Moreover, net cerebral lactate oxidation is linearly related with arterial lactate concentration; in case of hyperlactatemia, lactate transporters activity elevates, and lactate contribution to brain metabolism can reach up to 60% of the global brain metabolism [12, 69, 70]. Lactate cerebral metabolism has been assessed in vivo in noninjured stimulated brain of rats (sensory stimulation) [71]. The authors demonstrated that (1) stimulated brain enables to provide a sustained neuronal activity for several hours in the absence of glucose if lactate was present; (2) the brain oxidizes lactate in an activity-dependent manner; and (3) lactate was preferred over glucose in non-stimulated and stimulated brain as glucose consumption decreased was lactatemia dependent.

Schurr et al. were the first, more than 30 years ago, to demonstrate that cerebral tissue enables to consume only lactate aerobically to maintain normal neuron function. Since this time, many studies have supported the essential role of lactate in cerebral energy metabolism, especially in injured brain [14, 72–74]. These authors assessed the role of lactate on brain metabolism, using rat hippocampal slices under various conditions of ischemia-reperfusion and neuronal activation. Slices were placed in artificial cerebrospinal fluid (aCSF) containing various concentrations of glucose and lactate and inhibitors of their metabolism. We can summarize most of their result as follows [75]:

- During ischemia-reperfusion, aCSF containing lactate is associated with a better neuronal function recovery as compared with aCSF containing glucose [14].
- Glial cells play a major role in producing lactate during hypoxia as demonstrated using blockers of lactate transport. Neuronal function recovery is strongly impaired and delayed when lactate transport is blocked as compared with control conditions with lactate [74].
- The role of lactate has been assessed in hippocampal slices exposed to an excitotoxic dose of glutamate (activation of neurons) in the presence of aCSF containing glucose with or without lactate transport blockers. Regardless of the glutamate and glucose concentrations, an increased lactate concentration in aCSF develops in slices, while neuronal function dramatically impairs. As suggested by low concentration of lactate in control slices, neurons consume probably lactate rather than they decrease its production. These data indicate that the activation of neural tissue with excitatory neurotransmitter activates aerobic glycolysis and in turn increases lactate production (stress hyperlactatemia). Moreover lactate issued from this glycolytic pathway becomes the oxidative energetic substrate, allowing the neuronal function to recover.

At last, multiple data support that lactate is the essential end substrate of aerobic and anaerobic glycolysis in the brain: cytosolic glycolysis produces pyruvate which is reduced in lactate via the cytosolic LDH (cLDH); lactate enters the mitochondria thanks to its MCT and is oxidized in pyruvate via a mitochondrial LDH (mLDH), to join finally the TCA cycle [75]. Moreover, neuronal recovery function occurs only with astrocytic lactate (Fig. 8.7).

The modern concept of Schurr which consider lactate as the end product of cerebral aerobic glycolysis is in agreement with the Pellerin and Magistretti

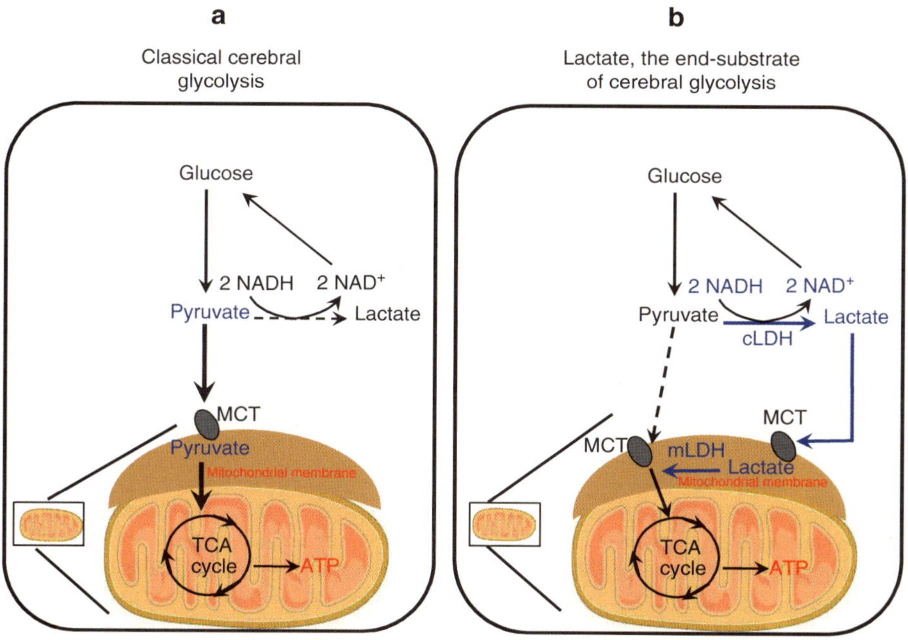

Fig. 8.7 The two concept of cerebral aerobic glycolysis. A. The classical pathway of cerebral aerobic glycolysis considers that pyruvate is the end product of the cytosolic glycolysis: pyruvate enters through the mitochondrial membrane thanks to its transporter, the monocarboxylate transporter (MCT); after penetrating the mitochondria, pyruvate joins the tricarboxylic acid cycle (TCA) and the oxidative phosphorylation to release ATP. B. The second concept considers that not pyruvate but lactate is the end substrate or cerebral aerobic glycolysis: cytosolic reduction of pyruvate into lactate is performed thanks to a cytosolic lactate dehydrogenase (cLDH); lactate (endogenous or exogenous) further enters the mitochondrial membrane thanks to its transporter MCT and is reoxidized into pyruvate via a mitochondrial LDH (mLDH), to join finally the TCA cycle and release ATP

astrocyte-neuron lactate shuttle (ANLS) model [76]. This concept highlights the coupling activity between astrocytes and neurons, especially during synaptic activity which corresponds to glutamate release [77]. Since more than 15 years, this team has provided many experimental data which support the role of lactate as a pivotal substrate for maintaining neuroenergetics [78, 79]. When released in the neuronal synaptic cleft, glutamate triggers different pathways simultaneously in both neurons and asytrocytes. Aerobic astrocytic glycolysis is activated leading to release lactate and ATP. ATP is used for glutamate reuptake by astrocytes via an activation of glutamate-sodium cotransporters followed by an extrusion of sodium by Na-K-ATPase pump. In the same time, the synaptic cleft glutamate activates postsynaptic receptors, which triggers the entry of sodium in neuronal dendrites and creates an excitatory potential. Neurons use astrocytic lactate to enter the oxidative phosphorylation leading to produce ATP. This ATP is needed to extrude excessive sodium by

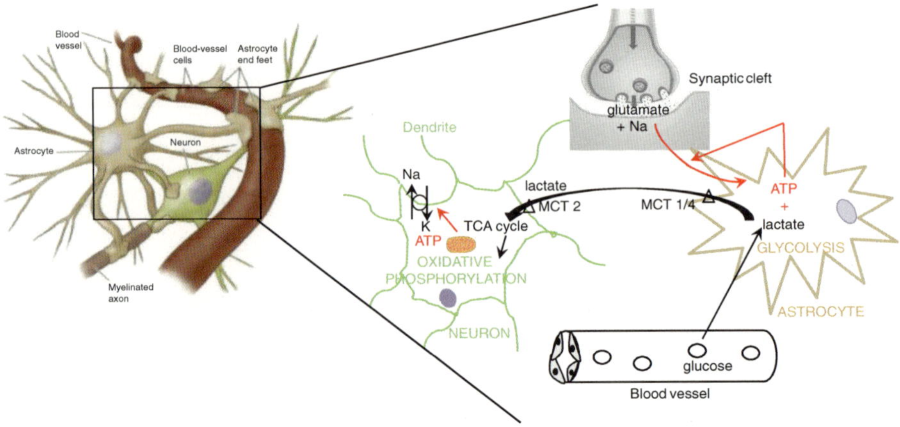

Fig. 8.8 Coupling astrocyte-neuron energetics in activated neurons [27]. Glutamate reuptake from the synaptic cleft is performed with a simultaneous reuptake of sodium through specific receptors. This phenomenon activates different but coupling metabolic pathways in astrocytes and in neurons. In the astrocyte, ATP production is issued from glycolysis, leading concomitantly to lactate production. Astrocytic ATP allows Na-K-ATPase pump to work for glutamate reuptake. Activated neurons trigger a dendritic potential via voltage-gated sodium channels and Na-K-ATPase work which requires energy. Therefore, lactate extrudes from astrocytes and enters in the neuron thanks to its monocarboxylate transporters (MCT 1/4 and 2, respectively) and joins the oxidative phosphorylation. ATP issued from the neuronal oxidative phosphorylation delivers the required energy for the activation of the dendritic potential and Na-K-ATPase pump

Na-K-ATPase pump (Fig. 8.8). Such a lactate shuttling between neurons and astrocytes is possible thanks to cell metabolism compartmentalization which contain specific substrate transporters and enzymes. The increased glutamate activates preferentially astrocytic glycolysis with lactate production: astrocytic GLUT 1 transporters favor glucose uptake which is thereafter metabolized in lactate thanks to LDH 5. The extrusion of lactate from astrocytes is performed by MCT 1–4, and its entry in neurons is activated by MCT 2, while neuronal glucose uptake is very low. Finally lactate is oxidized into pyruvate by neuronal LDH 1.

In summary: lactate is a major end product of cerebral aerobic glycolysis. Contrary to the classical concept, lactate (endogenous as well as exogenous) but not pyruvate enters the mitochondria and is further metabolized in the TCA cycle and oxidative phosphorylation. Cerebral lactate consumption is linearly correlated with arterial lactatemia. During cerebral energetic crisis (ischemia-reperfusion, neuronal activation), lactate acts as an energetic shuttle required for coupling astrocyte and neuron energetic metabolism as follows: astrocytic cytosolic glycolysis produces lactate and ATP which are consumed for neuronal mitochondrial oxidative phosphorylation and glutamate reuptake from the synaptic cleft, respectively [76, 80].

Brain lactate metabolism has been assessed in humans with cerebral injury using functional cerebral imaging techniques and microdialysis [81–84]. All data support that brain lactate increased is mostly caused by aerobic glycolysis rather than by hypoxia. This seems to be an appropriate response aiming to spare glucose in case of impaired cerebral oxidative metabolism. Moreover, hypertonic lactate therapy enables to conduct a preferential utilization of lactate as suggested by the reduction of both brain glutamate and intracranial pressure (ICP), coupled with an increased extracellular pyruvate and glucose in patients with traumatic brain injury (TBI) [81, 83, 85]. The beneficial role of exogenous lactate infusion has been reported in various experimental and clinical trials. In rat model of TBI, the administration of sodium lactate (SL) is associated with an improved cognitive function at 15 days posttrauma as compared with sodium chloride [86, 87]. In patients with severe TBI, the administration of boluses of hypertonic SL is associated with a higher reduction in raised ICP and a better neurological outcome after 1 year as compared with equiosmotic boluses of mannitol [61]. The same authors further showed that the infusion of hypertonic SL within the first 48 h of severe TBI prevented intracranial hypertensive episodes (with a reduction of 50% of episodes) [88]. Other studies have found a significant improvement of neurological dysfunction during severe hypoglycemia treated with exogenous lactate infusion [89, 90]. Considering these data strongly support that brain is capable to metabolize lactate and consider it as a major source of energy.

8.7.2.3 Sodium Lactate: A Possible Fluid Resuscitation

Not only the brain (or heart) but many organs can use lactate as an energy substrate [91, 92]. SL presents additional theoretical advantages: poor chloride concentration, hypertonic solution, alkalinizing effect, and vasodilation related to lactate. Therefore, it has been hypothesized that hypertonic SL could be an interesting fluid for vascular load in shock. In a model of porcine hypodynamic endotoxin shock, Duburcq et al. [93] have compared the effects on hemodynamics of equiosmotic SL and sodium bicarbonate versus 0.9% sodium chloride. They found that SL improved macrohemodynamic and oxygenation, microvascular reactivity while reducing significantly fluid balance. But recent data report different results in a model of sheep with hyperdynamic septic shock [94]. Animals were randomized to receive a bolus followed by a continuous infusion during 10 h of hypertonic SL, hypertonic saline, normal saline, or ringer lactate. Fluid balance was lower in the hypertonic groups (lactate and saline) within the first 8 h; macrohemodynamics (cardiac index and mean arterial pressure) were comparable during this period but worsened after in the SL group as compared with hypertonic saline one. Moreover, impaired tissue perfusion and death occurred earlier in the SL group. At last, early resuscitation of dengue shock syndrome by hypertonic SL allowed to reach a comparable hemodynamic recovery within 48 h. Moreover, children receiving SL presented a one third lower fluid balance and an improved endothelia dysfunction as compared with those receiving ringer lactate [95].

In summary: numerous data highlight beneficial effects provided by the exogenous administration of sodium lactate in various critically ill conditions such as shock, brain injury, and heart failure. The mechanism by which the solution exerts its potential beneficial effects is probably complex, not only as a source of fuel but also by vasodilating circulation, controlling fluid balance, decreasing systemic inflammation, and reducing cell edema.

Conclusion

Recent biochemical knowledges clearly demonstrate that lactate is not only a harmful end waste product of an anaerobic glycolysis. Lactatemia represents serum concentration at an instantaneous time. It must be distinguished from the body lactate turnover which results from its production and consumption. The simple view that hyperlactatemia indicates always tissue hypoxia and causes metabolic acidosis is wrong. Lactate is a physiological nontoxic metabolite. It represents a carbohydrate source of energy that allows to spare other energy resources. Hyperlactatemia and hyperproduction of lactate must not be interpreted as the cause of a high mortality but rather as an adaptative response. Hyperlactatemia must be viewed as a total body metabolic response leading to order metabolic redistribution and priorities between organs.

Numerous data demonstrate that lactate is a preferential source of energy for various organs, especially for the heart and brain. The beneficial effects of the exogenous administration of sodium lactate in patients with acute heart failure, severe traumatic brain injury, and septic shock are encouraging and seem to be promising.

Acknowledgments No conflict of interest.

References

1. De Backer D (2003) Lactic acidosis. Intensive Care Med 29:699–702
2. Gladden LB (2004) Lactate metabolism: a new paradigm for the third millennium. J Physiol 558:5–30
3. Leverve X (1999) Lactic acidosis a new insight. Minerva Anesthesiol 65:205–209
4. Bakker J, Mijsten MWN, Jansen TC (2013) Clinical use of lactate monitoring in critically ill patients. Ann Intensive Care 3:12
5. Reddy AJ, Lam SW, Bauer SR, Guzman JA (2015) Lactic acidosis: clinical implications and management strategies. Cleveland Clin J Med 82:615–624
6. Halestrap A, Price NT (1999) The proton-linked monocarboxylate transporter (MCT) family: structure, function and regulation. Biochem J 343:281–299
7. Garcia-Alvarez M, Marik P, Bellomo R (2014) Sepsis-associated hyperlactatemia. Crit Care 18:503
8. Chioléro R, Tappy L, Gillet M et al (1999) Effect of a major hepatectomy on glucose and lactate metabolism. Ann Surg 4:505–513
9. Carvalho RA, Jones JG, McGuirk C, Sherry AD, Malloy CR (2002) Hepatic gluconeogenesis and Krebs cycle fluxes in CCl_4 model of acute liver failure. NMR Biomed 15:45–51

10. Tapia P, Soto D, Bruhn A et al (2015) Impairment of exogenous lactate clearance in experimental hyperdynamic septic shock is not related to total liver hypoperfusion. Ann Intensive Care 19:188
11. Joseph SE, Heaton N, Potter D, Pernet A, Umpleby MA, Amiel SA (2000) Renal glucose production compensates for the liver during the anhepatic phase of liver transplantation. Diabetes 49:450–456
12. Van Hall G (2010) Lactate kinetics in human tissues at rest and during exercise. Acta Physiol 199:499–508
13. Leverve XM (1999) From tissue perfusion to metabolic marker: assessing organ competition and co-operation in critically ill patients. Intensive Care Med 25:890–892
14. Schurr A, Payne RS, Miller JJ, Rigor BM (1997) Brain lactate is an obligatory aerobic energy substrate for functional recovery after hypoxia: further in vitro validation. J Neurochem 69:423–426
15. Lavery RF, Livingston DH, Tortella BJ, Sambol JT, Slomovitz BM, Siegel JH (2000) The utility of venous lactate to triage injured patients in the trauma center. J Am Coll Surg 190:656–664
16. Boldt J, Kumle B, Suttner S, Haisch G (2001) Point-of-care (POC) testing of lactate in the intensive care patient. Accuracy, relability, and coasts of different measurement systems. Acta Anaesth Scand 45:194–199
17. Kruse O, Grunnet N, Barfod C (2011) Blood lactate as a predictor for in-hospital mortality in patients admitted acutely in hospital: a systematic review. Scand J Trauma Resuscitation Emerg Med 19:74
18. Andersen LW, Mackenhauer J, Roberts JC, Berg KM, Cocchi MN, Donnino MW (2013) Etiology and therapeutic approach to elevated lactate. Mayo Clin Proc 88:1127–1140
19. Theerawit P, Na Petvicharn C, Tangsujaritvijit V, Sutherasan Y (2016) The correlation between arterial and venous lactate in patients with sepsis and septic shock. J Intensive Care Med 18(Suppl 1):P177
20. Paquet AL, Valli V, Philippon AL, et al (2016) Agreement between arterial and venous lactate in emergency department patients: a prospective study of 157 consecutive patients. Eur J Emerg Med
21. Sabat J, Gould S, Gillego E et al (2016) The use of finger-stick blood to assess lactate in critically ill surgical patients. Ann Med Surg 10:41–48
22. Nichol AD, Egi M, Pettila V et al (2010) Relative hyperlactatemia and hospital mortality in critically ill patients: a retrospective multi-centre study. Crit Care 14:R25
23. Jansen TC, Van Bommel J, Woodward R, Mulder PG, Bakker J (2009) Association between blood lactate levels, sequential organ failure assessment subscores, and 28-day mortality during early and late intensive care unit stay: a retrospective observational study. Crit Care Med 37:2369–2374
24. Khosravani H, Shahpori R, Stelfox T, Kirkpatrick AW, Laupland KB (2009) Occurrence and adverse effect on outcome of hyperlactatemia in the critically ill. Crit Care 13:R90
25. Nguyen HB, Rivers EP, Knoblich BP et al (2004) Early lactate clearance is associated with improved outcome in severe sepsis and septic shock. Crit Care Med 31:1637–1642
26. Mikelsen ME, Miltiades AN, Gaieski DF et al (2009) Serum lactate is associated with mortality in severe sepsis independent of organ failure and shock. Crit Care Med 37:1670–1677
27. Donnino MW, Andersen LW, Giberson T et al (2014) Initial lactate and lactate change in post-cardiac arrest: a multicenter validation study. Crit Care Med 42:1804–1811
28. Levraut J, Ichai C, Petit I, Ciebiera JP, Perus O, Grimaud D (2003) Low exogenous lactate clearance as an early predictor of mortality in normolactatemic critically ill patients. Crit Care Med 31:705–710
29. Arnold RC, Shapiro NI, Jones AE et al (2009) Multicenter study of early lactate clearance as a determinant of survival in patients with presumed sepsis. Shock 32:35–39
30. Haas SA, Lange T, Saugel B et al (2016) Severe hyperlactatemia, lactate clearance and mortality in unselected critically ill patients. Intensive Care Med 42:202–210
31. Vincent JL, Quintairos e Silva A, Couto L, Taccone FS (2016) The value of blood lactate kinetics in critically ill patients: a systematic review. Crit Care 20:257
32. Jansen TC, van Bommel SFJ et al (2010) Early lactate-guided therapy in intensive care unit patients: a multicenter, open-label, randomized controlled study. Am J Resp Crit Care Med 182:752–761

33. Jones AE, Shapiro NJ, Trzeciak S et al (2010) Lactate clearance vs central venous oxygen saturation as goals of early sepsis therapy: a randomized clinical trial. JAMA 303:739–746
34. Investigators PCESS, Yealy DM, Kellum JA, Huang DT et al (2014) A randomized trial of protocol-based care for early septic shock. N Engl J Med 370:1683–1693
35. Hernandez G, Bruhn A, Castro R et al (2012) Persistent sepsis-induced hypotension without hyperlactatemia: a distinct clinical and physiological profile within the spectrum of septic shock. Crit Care Res Pract 2012:536852
36. Rhodes A, Evans LE, Alhazzani W et al (2017) Surviving sepsis campaign: international guidelines for management of sepsis and septic shock: 2016. Intensive Care Med 43(3):304–377
37. Wutrich Y, Barraud D, Conrad M et al (2009) Early increase in arterial lactate concentration under epinephrine infusion is associated with a better prognosis during shock. Shock 34:4–9
38. Brooks GA (2002) Lactate shuttles in nature. Biochem Soc Trans 30:258–264
39. Levraut J, Ciebiera JP, Chave S et al (1998) Mild hyperlactatemia in stable septic patients is due to impaired lactate clearance rather than overproduction. Am J Resp Crit Care Med 157:1021–1026
40. Fuller BM, Dellonger RP (2012) Lactate as hemodynamic marker in critically ill. Curr Opin Crit Care 18:267–272
41. Cohen RD, Woods HF (1976) Clinical and biochemical aspects of lactic acidosis. Blackwell, London
42. De Backer D, Creteur J, Dubois MJ et al (2006) The effects of dobutamine on microcirculatory alterations in patients with septic shock are independent of its systemic effects. Crit Care Med 34:403–408
43. Levy B, Sadoune LO, Gelot AM, Bollaert PE, Nabet P, Larcan A (2000) Evolution of lactate/pyruvate and arterial ketone body ratios in the early course of catecholamine-treated septic shock. Crit Care Med 28:114–119
44. Leverve XM (1999) Energy metabolism in critically ill patients: lactate is a major oxidizable substrate. Curr Opin Clin Nutr Metab Care 2:165–169
45. James JH, Luchette FA, Mc Carter FD, Fischer JE (1999) Lactate is an unreliable indicator of tissue hypoxia in injury or sepsis. Lancet 354:505–508
46. Boekstegers P, Weidenhöfer S, Kaspner D, Werdan K (1994) Skeletal muscle partial pressure of oxygen in patients with sepsis. Crit Care Med 22:640–650
47. Stacpoole PW, Lorenz AC, Thomas RG, Harman EM (1998) Dichloroacetate in the treatment of lactic acidosis. Ann Intern Med 108:58–63
48. Vary TC (1996) Sepsis-induced alterations in pyruvate dehydrogenase complex activity in rat skeletal muscle: effects on plasma lactate. Shock 6:89–94
49. Routsi C, Bardouniotou H, Delivoria-Ioannidou V, Kazi D, Roussos C, Zakynthinos S (1999) Pulmonary lactate release in patients with acute lung injury is not attributable to lung tissue hypoxia. Crit Care Med 27:2469–2467
50. Saks V, Dos Santos P, Gellerich FN, Diolez P (1998) Quantitative studies of enzyme-substrate compartmentation, functional coupling and metabolic channeling in muscle cells. Mol Cell Biochem 184:291–307
51. Luchette FA, Friend LA, Brown CC, Upputori RK, James JH (1998) Increased skeletal muscle Na^+, K^+-ATPase activity as a cause of increased lactate production after hemorrhagic shock. J Trauma 44:796–803
52. James JH, Fang CH, Schranz SJ, Hausselgren PO, Paul RJ, Fischer JE (1996) Linkage of aerobic glycolysis to sodium-potassium transport in rat skeletal muscle. Implications for increased muscle lactate production in sepsis. J Clin Invest 98:2288–2297
53. Levy B, Gibot S, Franck P, Cravoisy A, Bollaert PE (2005) Relation between muscle Na^+-K^+-ATPase activity and raised lactate concentrations in septic shock: a prospective study. Lancet 365:871–875
54. Oudard S, Boitier E, Miccoli M, Rousset S, Dutrillaux B, Poupon MF (1997) Gliomas are driven by glycolysis putative roles of hexokinase, oxidative phosphorylation and mitochondrial ultrastructure. Anticancer Res 17:1903–1911

55. Mathupala SP, Ko YH, Pedersen PL (2009) Hexokinase-2 bound mitochondria: cancer's stygian link to the "Warburg effect" and a pivotal target foe effective therapy. Semin Cancer Biol 19:17–24
56. Michaeli B, Martinez A, Revelly JP et al (2012) Effects of endotoxin on lactate metabolism in humans. Crit Care R16:139
57. Stewart PA (1978) Independent and dependent variables of acid-base control. Resp Physiol 33:9–26
58. Quintard H, Hubert S, Ichai C (2007) Qu'apporte le modèle de Stewart à l'interprétation des troubles acidobasiques? Ann Fr Anesth Réanim 26:423–433
59. Ichai C, Massa H, Hubert S (2006) Troubles de l'équilibre acidobasique chez l'adulte. Encycl Med Chir (Paris-France) 36-860-A-50:17
60. Mustafa I, Leverve XM (2002) Metabolic and hemodynamic effects of hypertonic solutions: sodium-lactate versus sodium chloride infusion in postoperative patients. Shock 18:306–310
61. Ichai C, Armando G, Orban JC et al (2009) Sodium-lactate vs mannitol in the treatment of intracranial hypertensive episodes in severe traumatic brain-injured patients. Intensive Care Med 35:471–479
62. Beadle RM, Frenneaux M (2010) Modification of myocardial substrate utilisation: a new therapeutic paradigm in cardiovascular disease. Heart 96:824–830
63. Ichai C, Leverve X, Orban JC (2008) Lactate and acute heart failure syndrome. In: Mebazaa A, Gheorghiade M, Zannad FM, Parrillo JE (eds) Acute heart failure. Spinger, London, pp 768–780
64. Levy B, Mansart A, Montenmont C, Gibot S, Mallie JP, Lacolley P (2007) Myocardial lactate deprivation is associated with decreased cardiovascular performance, decreased myocardial energetics and early death in endotoxin shock. Intensive Care Med 33:495–505
65. Revelly JP, Tappy L, Martinez A et al (2005) Lactate and glucose metabolism in severe sepsis and cardiogenic shock. Crit Care Med 33:2235–2240
66. Leverve XM, Boon C, Hakim T, Anwar M, Siregar E, Mustafa I (2008) Half-molar sodium-lactate solution has a beneficial effect in patients after coronary artery bypass grafting. Intensive Care Med 34:1796–1803
67. Nalos M, Leverve XM, Huang SJ et al (2014) Half-molar sodium lactate infusion improves cardiac performance in acute heart failure: a pilot randomised controlled clinical trial. Crit Care 18:R48
68. Dienel GA (2012) Brain lactate metabolism: the discoveries and the controversies. J Cereb Blood Flow Metab 32:1107–1138
69. van Hall G, Stromstad M, Rasmussen P et al (2009) Blood lactate is an important energy source for the human brain. J Cereb Blood Flow Metab 29:1121–1129
70. Boumezbeur F, Petersen KF, Cline GW et al (2010) The contribution of blood lactate to brain energy metabolism in humans measured by dynamic ^{13}C nuclear magnetic resonance spectroscopy. J Neurosci 30:13983–13990
71. Wyss MT, Jolivet R, Buck A, Magistretti PJ, Weber B (2011) *In vivo* evidence for lactate as a neuronal energy source. J Neurosci 31:7477–7484
72. Schurr A, Payne RS, Miller JJ, Rigor BM (1999) An increase in lactate output by brain tissue serves to meet the energy needs of glutamate-activated neurons. J Neurosci 19:34–39
73. Schurr A, Rigor BM (1998) Brain anaerobic lactate production: a suicide note or a survival kit? Dev Neurosci 20:348–357
74. Schurr A, Payne RS, Miller JJ, Tseng MT, Rigor BM (2001) Blockade of lactate transport exacerbates delated neuronal damage in a rat model of cerebral ischemia. Brain Res 895:268–272
75. Schurr A (2014) Cerebral glycolysis: a century of persistent misunderstanding and misconception. Front Neurosci 8:1–18
76. Pellerin L, Magistretti PJ (2012) Sweet sixteen for ANLS. J Cereb Blood Flow Metab 32:1152–1166
77. Pellerin L, Pellegri G, Bittar PG et al (1998) Evidence supporting the existence of an activity-dependent astrocyte-neuron lactate shuttle. Dev Neurosci 120:291–299

78. Pellerin L, Pellegri G, Martin JL, Magistretti PJ (1998) Expression of monocarboxylate transporter mRNA in mouse brain: support for a distinct role of lactate as an energy substrate for the neonatal vs adult brain. Proc Natl Acad Sci U S A 95:3990–3995
79. Amaral AI, Meisingset TW, Kotter MR, Sonnewald U (2013) Metabolic aspects of neuron-oligodendrocyte- astrocyte interactions. Front Endocrinol 4:1–5
80. Figley CR (2011) Lactate transport and metabolism in the human brain: implications for the astrocyte-neuron shuttle hypothesis. J Neurosci 31:4768–4770
81. Bouzat P, Sala N, Suys T et al (2014) Cerebral metabolic effects of exogenous lactate supplementation in the injured human brain. Intensive Care Med 40:412–421
82. Oddo M, Levine JM, Frangos S et al (2012) Brain lactate metabolism in humans with subarachnoid hemorrhage. Stroke 43:1418–1421
83. Quintard H, Patet C, Zerlauth JB et al (2016) Improvement of Neuroenergetics by hypertonic lactate therapy in patients with traumatic brain injury is dependent on baseline cerebral lactate/pyruvate ratio. J Neurotrauma 33:681–687
84. Patet C, Quintard H, Suys T et al (2015) Neuroenergetic response to prolonged cerebral glucose depletion after severe brain injury and the role of lactate. J Neurotrauma 32:1560–1566
85. Sala N, Suys T, Zerlauth JB et al (2013) Cerebral extracellular lactate increase is predominantly non ischemic in patients with severe traumatic brain injury. J Cereb Blood Flow Metab 33:1815–1822
86. Rice AC, Zsoldos R, Chen T et al (2002) Lactate administration attenuates cognitive deficits following traumatic brain injury. Brain Res 928:156–159
87. Holloway R, Zhou Z, Harvey HB et al (2007) Effect of lactate therapy upon cognitive deficits after traumatic brain injury in the rat. Acta Neurochir 149:919–927
88. Ichai C, Payen JF, Orban JC et al (2013) Half-molar sodium lactate infusion to prevent intracranial hypertensive episodes in severe traumatic brain injured patients: a randomized controlled trial. Intensive Care Med 39:1413–1422
89. Maran A, Cranston I, Lomas J, Macdonald I, Amiel SA (1994) Protection by lactate of cerebral function during hypoglycaemia. Lancet 343:16–20
90. King P, Kong MF, Parkin H, MacDonald IA, Barber C, Tattersall RB (1998) Intravenous lactate prevents cerebral dysfunction during hypoglycaemia in insulin-dependent diabetes mellitus. Clin Sci (Lond) 94:157–163
91. Ichai C, Orban JC, Fontaine E (2014) Sodium lactate for fluid resuscitation: the preferred solution for the coming decades? Crit Care 18:163
92. Fontaine E, Orban JC, Ichai C (2014) Hyperosmolar sodium-lactate in the ICU: vascular filling and cellular feeding. Crit Care 18:599
93. Duburcq T, Favory R, Mathieu D et al (2014) Hypertonic sodium lactate improves fluid balance and hemodynamics in porcine endotoxin shock. Crit Care 18:467
94. Su F, Xie K, He X et al (2016) The harmful effects of hypertonic sodium lactate administration in hyperdynamic septic shock. Shock 46:663–671
95. Somasetia DH, Setiati TE, Sjahrodji AM et al (2014) Early resuscitation of dengue shock syndrome in children with hyperosmolar sodium-lactate: a randomized single blind clinical trial of efficacy and safety. Crit Care 18:466

Part III

Kidney and Metabolic Disorders

Metabolism and Renal Functions

9

Aurélien Bataille and Laurent Jacob

9.1 Introduction

The kidney is the principal organ that ensures homeostatic control of fluid and electrolytes in the human body, contributing to regulation of blood volume and pressure. To perform these critical functions, the kidney possesses a remarkable anatomical organization. Renal vascularization is very specific and is restricted based on metabolic needs. In fact, there exists heterogeneity in the renal tissue with regard to perfusion and energy demand. In order to understand the coupling between these distinct requirements, the specific role of each part of the nephron, as well as its functional and regulatory mechanisms, must be considered. Notably, properties of renal circulation have been highlighted by several studies investigating pathological situations as well as therapeutic interventions.

Overall, renal blood perfusion exceeds global oxygen demand, leading to low oxygen extraction by the kidney. However, reabsorption of filtered primitive urine imparts a high metabolic burden. Thus, glomerular filtration rate (GFR) is a major determinant of renal oxygen consumption, explaining the importance of the coupling that exists between blood flow, GFR, and oxygen consumption. This coupling system includes an arteriovenous shunt for oxygen in the medulla. This anatomical area is associated with a high risk of hypoxia/ischemia when GFR increases or medullary perfusion decreases. In the following chapter, we review the physiological principles that contribute to metabolic challenges of the kidney.

A. Bataille • L. Jacob (✉)
Département d'Anesthésie-Réanimation, Hôpital Saint-Louis, Paris, France
e-mail: laurent.jacob@aphp.fr

C. Ichai et al. (eds.), *Metabolic Disorders and Critically Ill Patients*,
http://doi.org/10.1007/978-3-319-64010-5_9

9.2 Determinants of Renal Metabolism

9.2.1 General Characteristics of Renal Blood Flow (RBF)

The kidney is an organ characterized by high blood flow (i.e., approximately 1200 mL/min/1.73 m^2), accounting for 20–25% of total cardiac output. With regard to metabolic supply, it represents a macroscopically privileged organ, receiving the highest infusion rate of all perfused organs (i.e., 4 mL/min/g of tissue). This is 5–50 times more than other organs relative to weight (Table 9.1). Furthermore, this flow is much larger than the actual energy requirements of the kidney, which is reflected by the fact that the overall extraction rate for oxygen is 8% [1].

Overall oxygen consumption in the kidney is low relative to input, as confirmed by low arteriovenous differences in oxygen blood content. However, renal hyperperfusion is required to perform the primary function of the kidney, which is plasma filtration. Indeed, it requires high rates of perfusion, filtration, and tubular reabsorption.

Renal vascularization is terminal and sequential, connected directly to the aortocaval system. The number of renal arteries for each kidney is variable (i.e., one to four) and divided successively into segmental, interlobar, arcuate, and interlobular arteries. Flow then continues via a portal system (the renal portal system), comprised of a series of double capillary networks. Therefore, this anatomy represents a succession of two resistive systems, the afferent and efferent arterioles of the glomerulus. Notably, a high and stable capillary pressure (glomerular filtration pressure) exists between these systems, with a low capillary pressure downstream (tubular reabsorption pressure).

Although all nephrons have the same basic structure, they show some differences based on their positions within the renal cortex. Schematically, juxtacortical nephrons are small and numerous (constituting 85%) and display a short loop of Henle. Blood flow in glomerular capillaries is significant, fast, and under high pressure. In addition, efferent arterioles from these superficial nephrons give rise to all of the peritubular capillary networks.

Within these nephrons, the essential process of tubular reabsorption of electrolytes into the peritubular capillaries occurs, which correlates with GFR (i.e.,

Table 9.1 Rat kidney oxygen consumption compared to other organs according to Brezis [1]

	Blood flow in mL/min/100 g	O_2 delivery (DO_2) in mL/min/100 g	O_2 uptake (VO_2) in mL/min/100 g	O_2 extraction VO_2/DO_2 in %
Heart	87	16.8	11	65
Liver	58	11.6	2.2	18
Brain	54	10.8	3.7	34
Skin	13	2.6	0.4	15
Skeletal muscle	2.7	0.5	0.2	34
Kidney	420	84	6.8	8
Medulla	190	7.6	6.9	79

glomerular tubular coupling). In contrast, the juxtamedullary nephrons are larger and fewer (representing 15%) and display a long loop of Henle that dives into the medulla. There is less blood flow within these nephrons, which is slower and under low pressure. The efferent arterioles of these nephrons supply the vasa recta, diving parallel to the loops of Henle within different medullary layers. These juxtamedullary nephrons play a vital role in creating and maintaining an osmotic gradient that allows for the cortico-papillary process of urine concentration and dilution.

Blood flow distribution, and thus oxygen transport, is heterogeneous in the renal parenchyma, with 90% distributed to the cortex and 10% to the medulla.

In the past, methods involving diffusible radioactive indicators, such as krypton-85 or xenon-133, were used to study the intrarenal blood distribution. For this, a radioactive gas was fixed within the renal parenchyma by single-pass diffusion, and a decreasing curve of the gas level was measured in the blood by externally recording the radioactivity. Analysis of the kinetic curve allowed the identification of three main compartments: cortical flow (5 mL/min/g), outer medullary flow (1.5 mL/min/g), and internal medullary flow (0.2 mL/min/g). Collectively, downstream from the glomeruli, 80–85% of the perfusion is distributed to the cortical peritubular capillaries, with only 15–20% reaching the medullary [1]. Thus, more than one renal circulation system exists, with cortical and medullar circulation, initially, and glomerular and peritubular circulation, secondarily. Moreover, these microcirculation systems are regulated differentially at each level of the nephron and adapted to renal function.

The cortico-medullary osmotic gradient is created by a countercurrent concentration phenomenon, which involves active reabsorption against an electrolyte concentration gradient in the thick ascending limb of Henle's loop. The vasa recta recirculate a portion of solutes reabsorbed at the medullary level to maintain a constant cortico-medullary osmotic gradient. Insufficient flow within the vasa recta causes medullary ischemia and loss of the osmotic gradient. If flow within the vasa recta becomes too much, it leads to washing out of medullary osmotic content. Both these cases lead to loss in the ability to concentrate urine. Gradient magnitude not only depends on medullary blood flow but also on loop length and the action of the antidiuretic hormone.

9.2.2 Intra-glomerular Hemodynamics

Ultrafiltration of plasma within the glomerulus constitutes the initial step of primitive urine formation. In this regard, it is important to note that GFR is high, on the order of 120 mL/min/1.73 m^2 (i.e., 180 liters per day). Determinants of GFR include the following:

- Glomerular blood flow
- Net ultrafiltration pressure (i.e., the difference between hydrostatic pressure and oncotic pressure)
- Physical characteristics of the glomerular filtration membrane (Kf: exchange surface and permeability)

Hence, glomerular filtration is a convective phenomenon, and its determinants obey the law of Starling. Glomerular filtration can be summarized using the following formula:

$DFG = Kf \times Puf$

Puf is the net ultrafiltration pressure (driving force for filtration):

$DFG = Kf \times (\Delta P - \Delta \pi)$

P is the hydrostatic pressure and π the oncotic pressure.

Kf is the filtration glomerular coefficient:

$Kf = K \times S$

K is the hydraulic permeability.

S is the filtration modular surface (vasodilatation, vasoconstriction).

In summary, 600 mL/min of plasma enters into the kidneys. A total of 20% will be filtered in primitive urine (filtration fraction = 20%). A total of 99% of this filtered load is reabsorbed in the tubules, with 599 mL/min of plasma ultimately flowing back into renal venous circulation.

The net ultrafiltration pressure and glomerular blood flow are under the influence of both afferent and efferent arteriolar resistance. However, it is mainly at the afferent arterioles (at the level of the cortical nephrons) where modulation is possible due to self-regulation, which persists following denervation of the kidney or isolated kidney perfusion [2]. Within certain limits of perfusion pressure (i.e., 80–200 mmHg), the blood flow is not concomitantly altered along with the perfusion pressure, but instead remains constant. Increased blood pressure can cause vasoconstriction of the afferent arteriole, whereas hypoperfusion induces vasodilatation of the renal afferent arteriolar (i.e., pre-glomerular control).

Prostaglandins are mediators of reduced afferent arteriole resistance in the case of low-pressure perfusion. Nonsteroidal anti-inflammatory drugs inhibit cyclooxygenase and decrease prostaglandin synthesis, thus reducing GFR when it is dependent on vasodilatation of the afferent arteriole. Changes in vascular tone of the afferent arteriole allow maintenance of stable glomerular perfusion, ultrafiltration pressure, and GFR.

Autoregulation of RBF is related to two main mechanisms acting in synergy, a local myogenic reflex and tubulo-glomerular feedback.

9.2.3 Myogenic Reflex

The local myogenic reflex involves the smooth muscle cells in the afferent arteriole walls and is activated via stretch-sensitive calcium channels. In response to an increase in intraluminal blood pressure, calcium-induced vasoconstriction of the afferent arterioles occurs in order to avoid downstream increases in pressure [3, 4].

This local myogenic reflex accounts for 30% of the self-regulation of the RBF. In addition, its response time is short (approximately 2 s), and cortical nephrons are involved [5]. Thus, it is linked to mechanical stress and is more related to peak systolic pressure than mean arterial pressure [6]. This reflex, known as the Bayliss effect, is also present in other arteries of the body.

9.2.4 Tubulo-glomerular Feedback

Tubulo-glomerular feedback shows a slower response time (10–15 s), as its involvement is determined by metabolic stress. It is closely related to the anatomical disposition of the vessels and glomerular renal tubules. Indeed, the distal portion of the thick ascending limb of Henle's loop is in contact with afferent and efferent arterioles of the glomerulus (i.e., the juxtaglomerular apparatus) and contains specialized cells, which are called the macula densa. This area responds to variations in flow rate and concentration of urinary sodium and chloride. In fact, an increase in the flow or ion concentration causes opposite tubular glomerular filtration in a sigmoidal relationship via vasoconstriction of the afferent arteriole as well as decrease of the permeability variation coefficient through mesangial cell contraction [7]. Reabsorption of sodium in the macula densa is linked to an apical tubular transporter of $Na^+/K^+/2Cl^-$ that consumes oxygen and ATP. Therefore, ATP (or its metabolite, adenosine) mediates contraction of the afferent arteriole, and probably of the mesangium, through binding to the purinergic receptors [8]. These two responses subsequently lead to decreased blood flow and glomerular filtration in an attempt to retain sodium and water. Between the renal perfusion pressure of 70/80 mmHg and 160 mmHg, GFR and RBF are conserved (Fig. 9.1).

9.2.5 Microcirculation

Micropuncture studies performed in animals have led to a better understanding of intrarenal hemodynamics and revealed that renal microcirculation is complex. In particular, Wistar–Munich rats have been used for such studies due to the fact that their glomeruli are located immediately under the renal capsule and therefore more easily accessible. However, anesthesia used during micropuncture alters vascular tone and

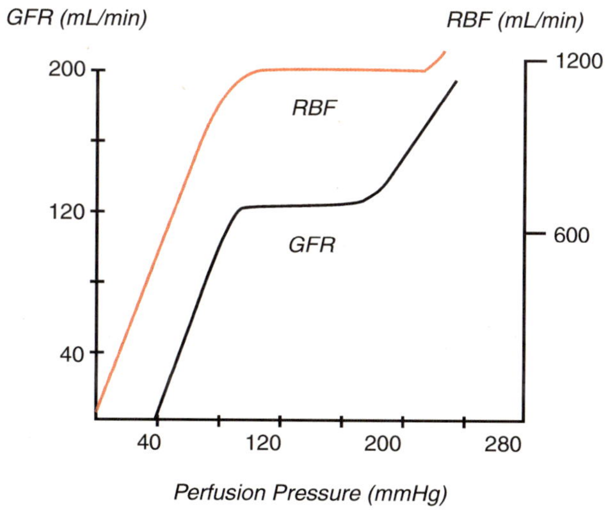

Fig. 9.1 Autoregulation of renal blood flow (RBF) and glomerular filtration rate (GFR)

reactivity. Thus, exploration is restricted to subcapsular nephrons, and the interpretation and extrapolation of data obtained by this procedure to man are limited.

For example, in a situation involving anesthesia-induced relative hypovolemia, pressure ultrafiltration is null before the end of the glomerular capillary due to a decrease in hydrostatic pressure and a rapid increase in oncotic pressure. Therefore, GFR becomes dependent on RBF and is highly influenced by its variations. However, unlike in rats, the ultrafiltration pressure in dogs is not canceled until the end of the capillary (conservation of a positive filtration gradient), such that the GFR to RBF dependence is less marked. Indeed, the same is likely true for humans.

Techniques using microspheres can only be used in experimental models, which tend to overestimate flows of external cortical areas in the axis of the vessels due to connections between interlobular and efferent arteries.

9.2.6 Oxygen

The kidneys represent less than 1% of the total human body weight but receive 25% of the cardiac output. In terms of energy balance, RBF at baseline is approximately five times that of coronary flow, while the oxygen consumption by the heart at baseline is about twice that of the kidney. Indeed, tubular reabsorption of sodium is the main determinant of oxygen consumption (VO_2) in the kidney. Thus, VO_2 varies with glomerular filtration, reflecting an intrinsic mechanistic coupling between input and oxygen requirements.

If any mechanism limits oxygen supply to the renal tissue, the oxygen partial pressure in the cortex should be high. This implies that oxygen reactive species would be produced because cellular oxidative stress in the kidney is highly dependent on oxygen availability. In fact, the mammalian kidney is not hyper-oxygenated. Cortical PO_2 is 50 mmHg, and medullary PO_2 may even be lower (25 mmHg) [9]. In mammalian kidneys, the arteriovenous shunt of oxygen by diffusion appears to represent a structural antioxidant mechanism. However, this is not the case in birds, where an alternative mechanism was developed to address this issue: the majority of RBF is due to venous blood.

These arteriovenous diffusion shunts are possible in tissues where arteries and veins are closely parallel to each other in opposite directions: muscles and kidneys. Evidence of the existence of these shunts is based on direct visualization and mathematical models of venous PO_2, which is greater than capillary PO_2. These shunts seem possible in both the cortex and the medulla. Moreover, this mechanism adapts itself to changes in blood flow under physiological conditions and accounts for susceptibility to hypoxia [9].

9.3 Pathophysiological Consideration

9.3.1 Sensitivity Zone (S3 Segment)

In the medulla, the vasa recta are arranged parallel to the tubules, and due to the diffusion of oxygen from the descending branch to the ascending branch, there is a further depletion of the oxygen content when these vessels plunge into the medulla. This results in a very low O_2 partial pressure in the deepest parts of the medulla (10–20 mmHg PO_2 vs. 50 mmHg at the cortical level) [10, 11]. Also, the relative ischemia of this nephron segment is offset by a high oxygen extraction rate (i.e., 79%) [12]. Although the medulla is highly vulnerable to renal hypoperfusion, there is a redistribution of cortical blood flow to the spinal cord layers in cases involving hypotension. In contrast, an increase in load sodium promotes cortical redistribution.

This zone is also a place of high-energy constraints related to sodium reabsorption in the terminal portion (S3 segment) of the proximal convoluted tube as well as the thick ascending limb of Henle's loop. In fact, the tubular metabolic stress imposed by active reabsorption mechanisms is the principal factor influencing medullary ischemia, which is due to both low oxygen delivery and high oxygen demand.

In models of postischemic or toxic renal failure, experimental studies have identified that the earliest cellular lesions are localized in the right portion (S3 segment) of the proximal convoluted tubule and the ascending limb off the loop of Henle. Notably, this location displays strain energy at its maximum. Although cells of the convoluted cortical S1 and S2 segments seem less affected, they also lose their brush border. Nevertheless, necrotic lesions are less extensive in these locations. The degree of influence on the other tube segments is more controversial, particularly with regard to the medullary portion of the ascending branch of the fine loop of Henle.

9.3.2 Protective Role of the L-Arginine/Nitric Oxide (NO) System

Endothelial cells synthesize NO from L-arginine through the activity of NO synthase (NOS). NO is involved in adaptation of glomerular flow, particularly the autoregulation of RBF and GFR [13]. Both constitutive isoforms of NO synthase are distributed throughout the kidney but particularly in the glomerulus [14]. In humans, NOS III is activated by stretching forces and calcium agonists and is expressed in the endothelium of cortical and medullary vessels. In rats, NO is involved in the regulation of glomerular filtration via two mechanisms: it modifies the vascular resistance of afferent and efferent arterioles and regulates the ultrafiltration coefficient, Kf [13]. Inhibition of NO synthesis leads to a 50% decrease in Kf and increased vascular resistance in the afferent arteriole. Indeed, NO is considered to be a vasodilator messenger, which is opposed to tubulo-glomerular feedback. It also has the potential to influence the myogenic component of RBF autoregulation, promoting vasodilatation in the case of low perfusion pressure. In fact, a study in humans has shown that in the presence of an NO antagonist (L-NMMA), there was a 79% decrease in RBF without modification of GFR [15]. Therefore, NO is not the main vasodilator of glomerular vessels, and other mechanisms are involved, including the cyclooxygenase pathway, which may explain GFR maintenance in situations where the NO pathway is inhibited [16]. It should be noted that NOS I (neuronal) is expressed in granular juxtaglomerular cells that are in contact with afferent arterioles [17]. Furthermore, the NO produced by the macula densa inhibits $Na^+/K^+/2Cl^-$ cotransport in the distal tubule and therefore tubulo-glomerular feedback [18]. It could also be involved in the release of renin, integrating the long-term control of sodium metabolism and regulation of blood pressure [19].

NO is also an important physiological factor in renal medullary microcirculation, which may even constitute its primary function. Indeed, its vasodilator properties are linked to cGMP (a myosin kinase-inactivating phosphorylation) and activation of calcium-dependent potassium channels of smooth muscle cells, which oppose vasoconstrictors (e.g., angiotensin II, endothelin, and norepinephrine) [20–22]. NO maintains medullary blood flow and represents an important factor preserving medullary oxygenation to compensate for the relative ischemia of this area in both physiological and pathological conditions. During sepsis, NO production is high due to the activation of NOS II (inducible NOS), but its rapid interaction with superoxide anion can result in reduced availability of NO when antioxidant mechanisms are exceeded [23]. This deficit is enhanced by the action of TNF and endotoxin, which accelerate the degradation of messenger RNA of endothelial NOS. This phenomenon could partly explain the intrarenal vasoconstriction observed during sepsis, especially in the medulla. On the other hand, the production of peroxynitrite anion (i.e., a reactive form of nitrogen) is cytotoxic and may exacerbate the ischemic cell damage occurring during acute septic renal failure [24].

Notably, inhibition of the L-arginine/NO system during experimental models of septic renal failure led to a dramatic increase in ischemic medullary tubular structures [25].

9.3.3 Glucose Production

Gluconeogenesis is the production of glucose from noncarbohydrate molecules, including amino acids and glycerol (from fat metabolism). This process is stimulated by decreased intracellular and blood glucose, as well as cortisol and catecholamines. The liver is the primary site for this glucose production. In patients in the anhepatic phase of liver transplantation, a de novo production of glucose by the kidney was observed from amino acid precursors. This extrahepatic production was quantitatively comparable to that of healthy subjects in the fasting phase, and the kidney was producing up to 70% of the total glucose synthesized, making it the main source of extrahepatic glucose production. This renal involvement shows close reciprocity with other organs, especially the liver.

9.4 Main Data on Therapeutic Interventions

9.4.1 Diuretics

Under normal conditions, when medullary PO_2 is lower than cortical PO_2, it was shown that furosemide inhibits sodium reabsorption in the renal medulla, increasing the medullary PO_2 without altering cortex PO_2. This increase is a direct consequence of lost oxygen consumption resulting from inhibition of tubular transporters [26]. Therefore, the use of diuretics in situations of renal aggression is based on these findings. However, several meta-analyses have demonstrated no beneficial effect in humans. Instead, diuretics may even be harmful in this context, especially under unstable volemic conditions.

9.4.2 Dopamine

Dopamine, which is released by postganglionic fibers of the sympathetic nervous system or synthesized locally, plays a principal role in the regulation of sodium metabolism. Under physiological conditions, dopamine increases RBF and GFR, not only by increasing cardiac output but also by decreasing renal vascular resistance. It also has a direct natriuretic activity via inhibition of the Na^+/K^+ ATPase in the proximal tubule. Peripheral dopamine receptors (D) belong to two major families: type 1 and type2. Type 1 receptors are located in the cytoplasm of the postsynaptic compartment and are recruited to the membrane by either dopamine or atrial natriuretic peptide (ANP) through activation of adenylate cyclase. Type 2 receptors are expressed by the presynaptic cell. Stimulation of type 1 dopamine receptors (D1 and D5) causes direct vasodilation, whereas activation of type 2 dopamine receptors (D2, D3, and D4) induces vasodilation by indirect inhibition of norepinephrine release. In humans, expression of these five receptors is distributed heterogeneously in the kidney, both in vascular and tubular structures. Notably, defects in the dopamine receptor system can be associated with some forms of hypertension [27–29].

Dopamine has been proposed as a treatment for acute ischemic renal failure due to its ability to reduce ATP use and oxygen requirements in the medulla. After the work of D'Orio [30], dopamine at "renal dose" (i.e., a dose lower than 5 μg/kg/min to induce renal vasodilatation and increased diuresis without increasing blood pressure) was widely used in ICU patients [30]. However, recent studies in both healthy adults and ICU patients have highlighted the lack of correlation between the rate of dopamine infusion and plasma concentrations. In fact, several meta-analyses have now demonstrated the ineffectiveness of this therapy for preventing or curing acute renal failure [31, 32]. Dopamine may even be deleterious, as electrolyte reabsorption in the medulla compensates for the inhibition of the proximal tubular dopamine reabsorption. This increases the oxygen demand for an area that is already experiencing relative ischemia. Similarly, in the mesenteric territory of septic patients, dopamine, which is a splanchnic vasodilator, can promote digestive mucosa ischemia by redistribution of blood flow [33, 34]. Fenoldopam is a selective D1 receptor agonist used as a vasodilator during hypertensive emergency. Due to its renal effects, it tends to show efficacy in animals for the prevention of acute renal failure induced by toxins (cyclosporine, contrast agents); however, this has not yet been demonstrated in humans [35, 36].

9.4.3 Noradrenaline

The kidney receives a rich vegetative innervation. However, under physiological conditions, the sympathetic nervous system has little influence on intrarenal hemodynamics. This is likely due to the dominant action of local mediators. However, under stress, activation of the sympathetic system enhances renal vascular resistance via increased intracellular calcium, decreasing RBF [37–39]. Regardless of its vasoactive activity, the sympathetic system promotes renin secretion and sodium reabsorption in different segments of the tubule, especially the ascending limb of the loop of Henle [40]. At this level, noradrenaline binds to alpha-1 receptors and increases the activity of the Na^+/K^+ ATPase. This anti-natriuretic effect participates in the formation of edema and congestive heart failure [41]. Therefore, the autonomic nervous system plays a more important role in the control of blood pressure (i.e., by modulating tubular functions and sodium metabolism), than in the regulation of RBF.

9.4.4 Atrial Natriuretic Factor (ANF)

ANF is a potent endogenous diuretic and natriuretic [42], which can improve the renal function/perfusion in both animal models and cases involving ischemic renal failure in humans. It belongs to a family of peptides synthesized by atrial myocytes.

Human-specific studies of ANF have revealed increases in GFR, renal filtration fraction (GFR/renal plasma flow), fractional sodium excretion, and urine output. However, this was also accompanied by enhanced tubular reabsorption and therefore O_2 consumption [43]. Its use during acute renal failure is based on the induction of vasodilation of the pre-glomerular artery through antagonism of the renin–angiotensin axis. Also, it leads to prostaglandin release in the initiation phase of renal aggression and during acute renal failure. These prostaglandins have a natriuretic effect that prevents tubular obstruction. Notably, ANF also likely reduces renal inflammation [44]. Furthermore, ANF treatment was analyzed in a meta-analysis [45] of the Cochrane Database, which included 1861 patients in 19 studies (11 preventative, 8 therapeutic). Overall, it was found that ANF did not reduce mortality.

Low doses (<100 ng/kg/min) showed efficacy in preventing the onset of acute renal failure (RR 0.32, 95% CI 0.14–0.71). Also, in the treatment of established acute renal failure, low doses of ANF were associated with a reduction in the use of renal replacement techniques (RR 0.54, 95% CI 0.30–0.98). However, contrast nephropathy and oliguric acute renal failure escaped this effectiveness. It should be noted that arrhythmias and hypotension were observed during treatment with ANF.

9.4.5 Glycemic Control and Insulin Therapy

The benefit of glycemic control by insulin therapy on renal function has been demonstrated. In fact, insulin therapy led to a lower need for dialysis [46] and reduction in peak plasma creatinine [47]. Nevertheless, these benefits have not been found in larger-scale studies [48]. Although injury mechanisms and pro-apoptotic effects have been highlighted as possible explanations for positive findings associated with insulin [49], future investigation will be needed to confirm the efficacy of this therapeutic strategy.

Conclusion

Understanding the mechanisms involved in the metabolic balance of the kidney has been gradual. Many different models have been used, resulting in the lack of a paradigm to integrate the data obtained from basic research. Also, these findings need to be tested for consequences in terms of clinical intervention for patients. Recently, meta-analyses have refocused clinical practice.

We hope that clinical advances yield a better understanding of renal physiology. In this regard, some important areas of recent development include improved monitoring of renal aggression and the emergence of new markers of renal cell injury.

References

1. Brenner BM, Coe FL, Rector FC (1987) Renal physiology in health and disease. Saunders, Philadelphia
2. Navar LG (1978) Renal autoregulation: perspectives from whole kidney and single nephron studies. Am J Phys 234(5):F357–F370
3. Takenaka T, Harrison-Bernard LM, Inscho EW, Carmines PK, Navar LG (1994) Autoregulation of afferent arteriolar blood flow in juxtamedullary nephrons. Am J Phys 267(5 Pt 2):F879–F887
4. Carmines PK, Inscho EW, Gensure RC (1990) Arterial pressure effects on preglomerular microvasculature of juxtamedullary nephrons. Am J Phys 258(1 Pt 2):F94–102
5. Flemming B, Seeliger E, Wronski T, Steer K, Arenz N, Persson PB (2000) Oxygen and renal hemodynamics in the conscious rat. J Am Soc Nephrol 11(1):18–24
6. Loutzenhiser R, Bidani A, Chilton L (2002) Renal myogenic response: kinetic attributes and physiological role. Circ Res 90(12):1316–1324
7. Ren Y, Garvin JL, Carretero OA (2001) Efferent arteriole tubuloglomerular feedback in the renal nephron. Kidney Int 59(1):222–229
8. Zou AP, Nithipatikom K, Li PL, Cowley AW Jr (1999) Role of renal medullary adenosine in the control of blood flow and sodium excretion. Am J Phys 276(3 Pt 2):R790–R798
9. Evans RG, Gardiner BS, Smith DW, O'Connor PM (2008) Intrarenal oxygenation: unique challenges and the biophysical basis of homeostasis. Am J Physiol Renal Physiol 295(5):F1259–F1270
10. Lote CJ, Harper L, Savage CO (1996) Mechanisms of acute renal failure. Br J Anaesth 77(1):82–89
11. Zhang W, Edwards A (2002) Oxygen transport across vasa recta in the renal medulla. Am J Physiol Heart Circ Physiol 283(3):H1042–H1055
12. Brezis M, Rosen S (1995) Hypoxia of the renal medulla—its implications for disease. N Engl J Med 332(10):647–655
13. Raij L, Baylis C (1995) Glomerular actions of nitric oxide. Kidney Int 48(1):20–32
14. Bachmann S, Bosse HM, Mundel P (1995) Topography of nitric oxide synthesis by localizing constitutive NO synthases in mammalian kidney. Am J Phys 268(5 Pt 2):F885–F898
15. Wolzt M, Schmetterer L, Ferber W et al (1997) Effect of nitric oxide synthase inhibition on renal hemodynamics in humans: reversal by L-arginine. Am J Phys 272(2 Pt 2):F178–F182
16. Beierwaltes WH (2002) Cyclooxygenase-2 products compensate for inhibition of nitric oxide regulation of renal perfusion. Am J Physiol Renal Physiol 283(1):F68–F72
17. Bachmann S, Theilig F (2000) Juxtaglomerular apparatus, nitric oxide, and macula densa signaling. Adv Nephrol Necker Hosp 30:95–107
18. Kovacs G, Komlosi P, Fuson A, Peti-Peterdi J, Rosivall L, Bell PD (2003) Neuronal nitric oxide synthase: its role and regulation in macula densa cells. J Am Soc Nephrol 14(10):2475–2483
19. Braam B, Turkstra E, Koomans HA (2000) Concerted actions of renal endothelial and macula densa NO systems in the maintenance of extracellular fluid volume. Acta Physiol Scand 168(1):125–132

20. Dickhout JG, Mori T, Cowley AW Jr (2002) Tubulovascular nitric oxide crosstalk: buffering of angiotensin II-induced medullary vasoconstriction. Circ Res 91(6):487–493
21. Cowley AW Jr, Mori T, Mattson D, Zou AP (2003) Role of renal NO production in the regulation of medullary blood flow. Am J Physiol Regul Integr Comp Physiol 284(6):R1355–R1369
22. Zou AP, Cowley AW Jr (2000) Alpha(2)-adrenergic receptor-mediated increase in NO production buffers renal medullary vasoconstriction. Am J Physiol Regul Integr Comp Physiol 279(3):R769–R777
23. Wang W, Jittikanont S, Falk SA et al (2003) Interaction among nitric oxide, reactive oxygen species, and antioxidants during endotoxemia-related acute renal failure. Am J Physiol Renal Physiol 284(3):F532–F537
24. Cohen RI, Hassell AM, Marzouk K, Marini C, Liu SF, Scharf SM (2001) Renal effects of nitric oxide in endotoxemia. Am J Respir Crit Care Med 164(10 Pt 1):1890–1895
25. Brezis M, Heyman SN, Dinour D, Epstein FH, Rosen S (1991) Role of nitric oxide in renal medullary oxygenation. Studies in isolated and intact rat kidneys. J Clin Invest 88(2):390–395
26. Brezis M, Agmon Y, Epstein FH (1994) Determinants of intrarenal oxygenation. I. Effects of diuretics. Am J Phys 267(6 Pt 2):F1059–F1062
27. Amenta F, Ricci A, Tayebati SK, Zaccheo D (2002) The peripheral dopaminergic system: morphological analysis, functional and clinical applications. Ital J Anat Embryol 107(3):145–167
28. Brismar H, Holtback U, Aperia A (2000) Mechanisms by which intrarenal dopamine and ANP interact to regulate sodium metabolism. Clin Exp Hypertens 22(3):303–307
29. Hussain T, Lokhandwala MF (2003) Renal dopamine receptors and hypertension. Exp Biol Med (Maywood) 228(2):134–142
30. D'Orio V, el Allaf D, Juchmes J, Marcelle R (1984) The use of low doses of dopamine in intensive care medicine. Arch Int Physiol Biochim 92(4):S11–S20
31. Bellomo R, Chapman M, Finfer S, Hickling K, Myburgh J (2000) Low-dose dopamine in patients with early renal dysfunction: a placebo-controlled randomised trial. Australian and new Zealand Intensive Care Society (ANZICS) clinical trials group. Lancet 356(9248):2139–2143
32. Kellum JA (2001) J MD. Use of dopamine in acute renal failure: a meta-analysis. Crit Care Med 29(8):1526–1531
33. Marik PE, Mohedin M (1994) The contrasting effects of dopamine and norepinephrine on systemic and splanchnic oxygen utilization in hyperdynamic sepsis. JAMA 272(17):1354–1357
34. Neviere R, Mathieu D, Chagnon JL, Lebleu N, Wattel F (1996) The contrasting effects of dobutamine and dopamine on gastric mucosal perfusion in septic patients. Am J Respir Crit Care Med 154(6 Pt 1):1684–1688
35. Brooks DP, Drutz DJ, Ruffolo RR Jr (1990) Prevention and complete reversal of cyclosporine A-induced renal vasoconstriction and nephrotoxicity in the rat by fenoldopam. J Pharmacol Exp Ther 254(2):375–379
36. Bakris GL, Lass NA, Glock D (1999) Renal hemodynamics in radiocontrast medium-induced renal dysfunction: a role for dopamine-1 receptors. Kidney Int 56(1):206–210
37. DiBona GF, Kopp UC (1997) Neural control of renal function. Physiol Rev 77(1):75–197
38. Barrett CJ, Navakatikyan MA, Malpas SC (2001) Long-term control of renal blood flow: what is the role of the renal nerves? Am J Physiol Regul Integr Comp Physiol 280(5):R1534–R1545
39. Salomonsson M, Arendshorst WJ (1999) Calcium recruitment in renal vasculature: NE effects on blood flow and cytosolic calcium concentration. Am J Phys 276(5 Pt 2):F700–F710
40. Lebedev AA, Kantariia VA, Kuz'min OB (1976) Effect of catecholamines on sodium resorption and oxygen tension in rat kidneys. Fiziol Zh SSSR Im I M Sechenova 62(8):1229–1233
41. DiBona GF, Sawin LL (1991) Role of renal nerves in sodium retention of cirrhosis and congestive heart failure. Am J Phys 260(2 Pt 2):R298–R305
42. Goetz KL (1988) Physiology and pathophysiology of atrial peptides. Am J Phys 254(1 Pt 1):E1–15
43. Sward K, Valsson F, Sellgren J, Ricksten SE (2005) Differential effects of human atrial natriuretic peptide and furosemide on glomerular filtration rate and renal oxygen consumption in humans. Intensive Care Med 31(1):79–85

44. Roson MI, Toblli JE, Della Penna SL et al (2006) Renal protective role of atrial natriuretic peptide in acute sodium overload-induced inflammatory response. Am J Nephrol 26(6):590–601
45. Nigwekar SU, Navaneethan SD, Parikh CR, Hix JK (2009) Atrial natriuretic peptide for preventing and treating acute kidney injury. Cochrane Database Syst Rev 4:CD006028
46. Van den Berghe G, Wouters P, Weekers F et al (2001) Intensive insulin therapy in the critically ill patients. N Engl J Med 345(19):1359–1367
47. Van den Berghe G, Wilmer A, Hermans G et al (2006) Intensive insulin therapy in the medical ICU. N Engl J Med 354(5):449–461
48. Finfer S, Chittock DR, Su SY et al (2009) Intensive versus conventional glucose control in critically ill patients. N Engl J Med 360(13):1283–1297
49. Ortiz A, Ziyadeh FN, Neilson EG (1997) Expression of apoptosis-regulatory genes in renal proximal tubular epithelial cells exposed to high ambient glucose and in diabetic kidneys. J Investig Med 45(2):50–56

Extrarenal Removal Therapies in Acute Kidney Injury

10

Olivier Joannes-Boyau and Laurent Muller

10.1 Theory and Principles

Renal replacement therapy (RRT) was the first technique that replaced an organ, more precisely the exocrine function of kidney. John Jacob Abel first demonstrated the feasibility of the concept of the "artificial kidney" in dogs in 1913 [1, 2]. During the World War 2, Kohler developed the human application of artificial kidney that was subsequently widely used in the USA in the early 1950s [1, 3]. In 1960, Scribner and Quinton invented and developed the arteriovenous shunt that allowed repeated connections of patients to machines, rapidly replaced by subcutaneous fistula [4, 5]. The combination of fistula and artificial kidney was the start signal for intermittent hemodialysis (IHD) as the first-line treatment of end-stage kidney disease (ESKD). From 1980 to the early 1990s, both continuous hemofiltration and continuous hemodialysis were advocated in intensive care units (ICUs), during acute kidney injury (AKI) because of a better hemodynamic stability and simplicity [6–8]. Renal replacement therapy is based on the concept that water and solute can cross a semi-permeable membrane from blood to extracorporeal compartment, allowing elimination of undue fluid and electrolyte accumulation induced by AKI. It is usual to oppose conventional hemodialysis, mainly based on diffusion principle, and hemofiltration, mainly based on convection principle. In fact, numerous RRT techniques have been developed, using both diffusive and convective techniques at different degrees. This can be confusing for ICU physicians and nurses. In this chapter, we will summarize general principles and main RRT techniques that can be used in

O. Joannes-Boyau, M.D. (✉)
Magellan Hospital, Haut Leveque University Hospital of Bordeaux, 33600 Pessac, France
e-mail: olivier.joannes-boyau@chu-bordeaux.fr

L. Muller, M.D., Ph.D.
Intensive Care, anesthesia and emergency medicine department, Nîmes - Caremeau Regional University Hospital, Place du Pr Debré, 30029 Nîmes, France

C. Ichai et al. (eds.), *Metabolic Disorders and Critically Ill Patients*,
http://doi.org/10.1007/978-3-319-64010-5_10

ICU to treat AKI, the timing to start RRT, the dose that should be used, and the short review on anticoagulation strategies. Before starting a RRT session, all reversible causes of AKI must have been eliminated. First, physical examination, focused ultrasound, and/or CT scan must systematically eliminate acute bladder retention and/or hydronephrosis. Second, hemodynamic analysis and monitoring must guarantee an adequate level of mean arterial pressure (ranging from 65 to 85 mmHg) and normalization of blood volume ("volume-unresponsive AKI") [9, 10].

10.2 Diffusion and Convection Principles (Fig. 10.1)

10.2.1 Diffusion Principle (Fig. 10.1a)

Diffusion is the main principle used during conventional intermittent or continuous hemodialysis. Diffusion occurs when a semipermeable membrane separates two aqueous solutions. In this case, small molecules cross the membrane from higher to lower concentration compartment. In case of RRT, a dialysis membrane separates blood and dialysate, allowing creatinine, urea, potassium, and phosphorus excess elimination from blood to dialysate compartment. In the same time, bicarbonates move from dialysate to blood compartment, which allows correction of AKI-induced acidosis. When diffusive principle is uniquely applied, water elimination is negligible. Diffusion efficacy can be summarized by the diffusion flux of a given solute across the membrane (Qx), which depends on the following equation:

$$\mathrm{Qx} = \mathrm{Ko} \times \mathrm{A} \times \left(\mathrm{Gx} / \mathrm{t}\right)$$

With Ko = Kb × T / 6π × μ × R (*t = dialysate temperature, Ko = diffusion (mass transfer) coefficient, A = membrane area, Gx = concentration gradient between blood and dialysate compartments, t = membrane thickness*). Ko depends on the effective radius of the considered molecule (R), the temperature of medium (T) the viscosity of the medium (μ) and the Boltzmann constant (Kb), which represent the entropic kinetic energy of the considered molecule [11].

Other factors may influence solute transport, such as protein binding and electrical charges of each solute.

10.2.2 Convection Principle (Fig. 10.1b)

Convection is the principle used during hemofiltration. Convection is the movement of a given fluid (mainly plasma water during RRT) across the membrane, driven by a gradient of hydrostatic pressure and the transmembrane pressure (TMP). More precisely, the TMP is the difference between blood compartment hydrostatic pressure (Pb) and ultrafiltrate compartment hydrostatic pressure (Puf), minus the plasma oncotic pressure (π):

$$\mathrm{TMP} = \left(\mathrm{Pb} - \mathrm{Puf}\right) - \pi$$

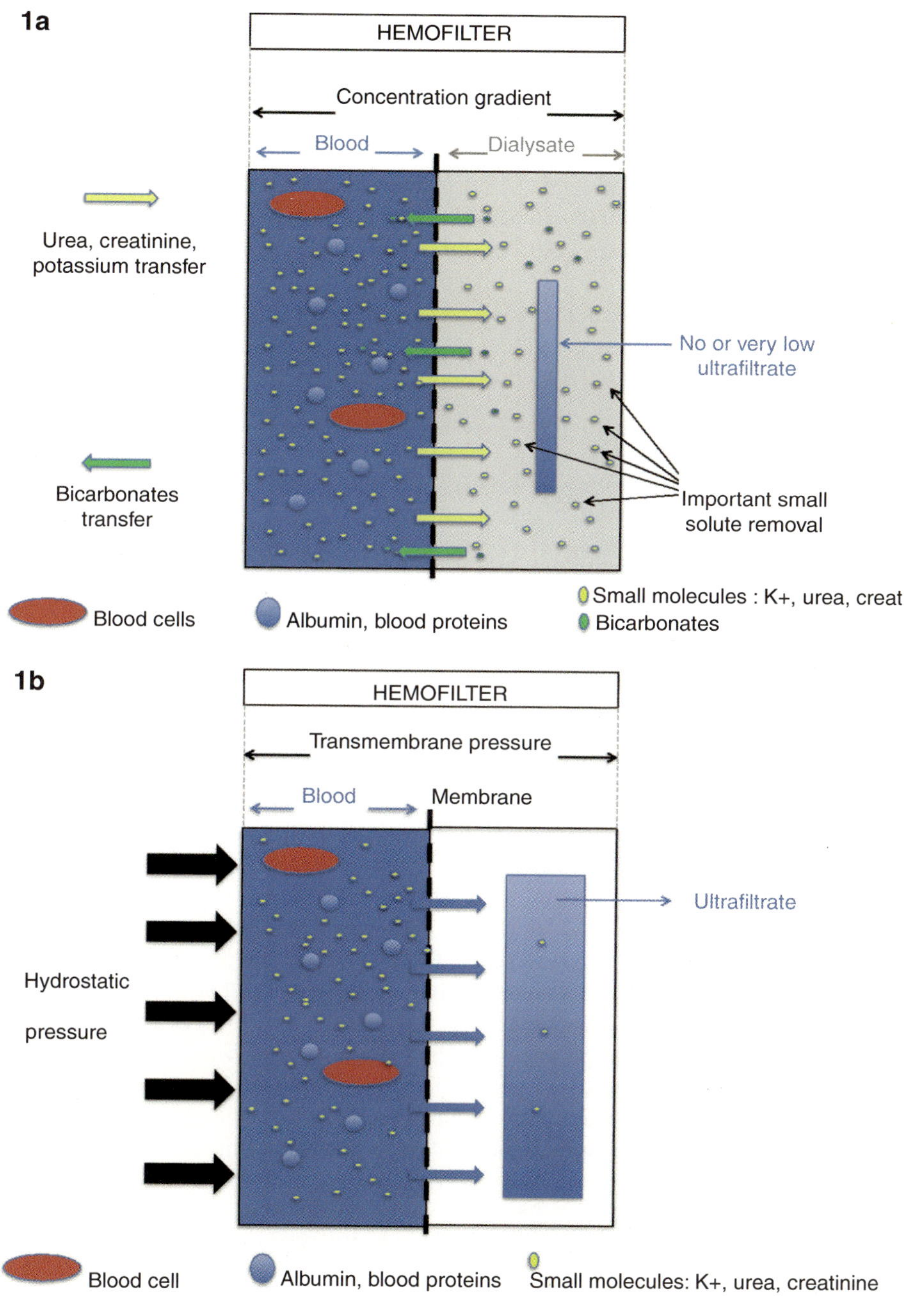

Fig. 10.1 Schematic representation of diffusion (**1a**) and convection (**1b**) principles

The fluid transport across the membrane is called ultrafiltration. The convective flux (ultrafiltration rate, *Quf*) across the membrane depends on the following equation:

$$\text{Quf} = \text{TMP} \times \text{Kuf} \times \text{A}$$

In this equation, Kuf represents the intrinsic water permeability of the hemofilter membrane and A the membrane area.

During convective therapy, besides fluid removal, a small amount of solutes moves to ultrafiltrate (Fig. 10.1b). This solute removal during convective therapy depends on the sieving coefficient (SC) of membrane that will be discussed in the following chapter. Therefore, the global efficiency (on water and solutes) of convective therapy can be summarized by the following equation:

$$\text{Convection efficiency} = \text{SC} \times \text{TMP} \times \text{Kuf} \times \text{A}$$

All the previous equations highlight the importance of the characteristics of membrane for RRT efficiency.

10.3 Postdilution, Predilution, and Net Patient Fluid Loss

As mentioned in the previous chapter, continuous convective therapy is based on large plasma water removal, generally 25–30 ml/Kg/h (see chapter "RRT Dose"). This exposes to critical hypovolemia that must be compensated by reinjection of partial to total (zero-balanced hemofiltration) of the removed volume. This substitution can be done before filter (predilution) or after filter (postdilution). Predilution offers the theoretical advantage of reducing blood viscosity along filter that could reduce the risk of filter obstruction and consequently increase the filter half-time. In contrast, predilution reduces global clearance of the technique. Postdilution leads to maximal hemoconcentration in filter that could lead to early filter clogging but preserves a maximal clearance. Therefore, both techniques have theoretical advantages and disadvantages. No clinical study has addressed in which situations pre- or postdilution should be used [12]. Net patient fluid loss is a key issue as fluid overload is strongly associated with excess mortality during AKI, especially when weight gain is >10% of body weight [13–17]. Control of fluid balance can only be achieved when hemodynamic stability is obtained. The maximal fluid loss per hour depends on patient's conditions, and closed hemodynamic monitoring must be done when fluid removal is decided. In a controlled study that compared alternate-day dialysis to daily hemodialysis, episodes of per-dialysis hypotension were 25% when hour depletion was 1000 ml/h, whereas hypotension incidence was 5% for a fluid loss of 400 ml/h [18].

10.4 Filtration Fraction (FF)

This parameter is of paramount importance during continuous convection therapy (hemofiltration, hemodiafiltration), while it is negligible during hemodialysis. It represents the concentration ratio of blood along filter. The FF is the ratio between ultrafiltrate flow rate and blood flow rate. During convection technique, because of a high plasma water removal (generally 25–30 ml/Kg/h—see part about “RRT Dose”), significant blood concentration occurs along filter. This hemoconcentration increases blood viscosity that promotes filter obstruction and early filter loss. All modern devices display FF value on machine screen. Medical and nurses staff must be conscious of the importance of monitoring FF value that must be kept below 25%. Filtration fraction is summarized by the following equation:

$$FF = \left(Q_{pre} + Q_{post} + Q_{net}\right) / \left(Qs + Q_{pre}\right)$$

In this equation, Q_{pre} = predilution flow rate, Q_{post} = postdilution flow rate, Q_{net} = net patient fluid loss, and Qs = blood flow rate.

Increasing blood flow is the first mean to reduce filtration fraction. This can be limited by the capacity of catheter to deliver adequate flow. If very low pressure (<100 mmHg) is measured on the “arterial” lumen of the catheter, the catheter flow will probably be less than what is prescribed on machine. In this case, the second mean to decrease FF is to limit ultrafiltration rate. This option is preferable in case of negative “arterial” pressure.

10.5 Characteristics of Filters

The vast majority of modern RRT filters are cylinders in which blood circulates in multiple hollow fibers [19]. The fiber wall is the filter membrane.

10.5.1 Membrane Permeability

Filter membrane permeability (Kuf) is characterized by length, mean inner radius, wall thickness (t), mean inner radius of pore (Rp), and the number of pores (Np). The membrane area (A) depends on the sum of fibers. According to the Quf formula, the Kuf unit is ml/h/mmHg/m^2. It is generally admitted that membranes can be classified in low-flux membranes (Kuf < 10 ml/h/mmHg/m^2), middle-flux membranes (10 < Kuf < 25 ml/h/mmHg/m^2), and high-flux membranes (Kuf > 25 ml/h/mmHg/m^2). This mainly describes the hydraulic permeability of membrane but does not describe the solute permeability of membrane, which depends on density, size, and distribution of pores. A membrane with high solute permeability is a highly permeable membrane. The terms high-flux and highly permeable membrane are not interchangeable. High-flux dialysis membranes are now widely used, especially polysulfone membranes, both in nephrology and ICU [20].

10.5.2 Mass Transfer Coefficient

This coefficient (Ko) represents the ability of a membrane to provide diffusive transport over the entire filter. As mentioned previously, it is one of the key issues of diffusive principle. It can be altered over time because of a progressive loss of membrane permeability during treatment.

10.5.3 Sieving Coefficient

The SC represents the ability of a convective therapy to remove solutes, regardless of diffusive transport (Fig. 10.1b). During convective therapy, SC can be compared to mass transfer coefficient during diffusive therapy. The SC is the ratio of concentrations of a given solute between ultrafiltrate (CUF) and plasma compartments of filter. As concentrations at the inlet (Cpi) and outlet (Cpo) plasma compartment of filter are different, it is admitted that the mean concentration (Cpi + Cpe/2) better represents blood solute concentration over filter.

10.5.4 Membrane Cutoff

The cutoff is a specific characteristic of a given membrane. It represents the maximal molecular weight blocked by the membrane. Above the cutoff value, the larger molecules cannot cross the membrane. Because membrane pore size is not totally homogeneous, cutoff value is statistically defined as the molecular weight of a solute with a SC of 0.1 (less than 10% of such molecules are eliminated in ultrafiltrate). In clinical practice, a high cutoff membrane usually describes a membrane with a cutoff value closed to the molecular weight of albumin (60–70 kd).

$$\mathrm{SC} = \mathrm{CUF} / \left(\mathrm{Cpi} + \mathrm{Cpo}\right) / 2$$

Therefore, the efficacy of a convective technique must be defined by its ability both to remove water and to remove solutes.

10.5.5 Membrane Adsorption

Adsorption is the adhesion of macromolecules to the membrane surface without penetration, and it primarily depends upon the internal pore structure and the hydrophobicity of the membrane [21]. It is a property of new synthetic membranes. Adsorption decreases complement activation and therefore limits the inflammatory reaction due to contact between blood and membranes, enhancing the biocompatibility of membranes [22]. If adsorption could have potential interest for cytokine blood removal during sepsis or light-chain elimination during myeloma, the clinical usefulness such membrane characteristic remains unclear [23]. Because adsorption membranes are generally high cutoff membranes, they may also have significant side effects as hormones, coagulation factors, growth factors, or albumin undue loss. Moreover, a highly adsorptive membrane may reduce the diffusive and convective capacities over time. A moderate level of protein adsorption combined with the ability to bind protein-bound uremic toxins is sometimes recommended [24].

Coupled plasma filtration and adsorption (CPFA) aims at separating plasma from cells. Plasma passes through a synthetic resin-sorbent cartridge and then returns to the blood, and a second filter allows conventional RRT. No study has demonstrated a clinical interest of this technique [12].

10.5.6 Molecular Composition of Membranes and Biocompatibility

Filter membranes are composed of semipermeable compounds that allow the separation of solutes between blood and dialysate or ultrafiltrate compartments. Historically, the membranes were cellulose based or cellulose derived. The non-modified cellulosic (natural) such as cuprophane membranes were predominantly low-flux membranes, with a very low cutoff, below 5 kd. Their performances were therefore limited [19, 22]. Moreover, their biocompatibility was poor. Biocompatibility can be defined as an inflammatory response syndrome due to complement activation mediated by the contact between blood and cellulosic membrane. This phenomenon has been well described during dialysis session with cellulose membrane, by measuring complement activation and increased levels of interleukine-1, interleukine-6, tumor necrosis factor, and C-reactive protein [25]. This syndrome was initially related to dialysis hypotension episodes. Modified cellulosic membranes as cellulose triacetate (CTA) improved the membrane biocompatibility. New synthetic membranes were developed during the past decades, with improved permeability, improved elimination of medium molecular weight molecule such as beta-2 microglobulin. Removal of beta-2 microglobulin is of paramount importance during chronic dialysis in order to limit dialysis-related amyloidosis. In contrast, the concept of cytokine removal by RRT during sepsis was not reported as effective [26, 27]. No guidelines support the routine use of RRT during sepsis in the absence of AKI [12, 28]. The most popular synthetic membranes are polysulfone, polyethersulfone, and polyacrylonitrile (AN-69). During ESKD, even if the use of synthetic membranes is not clearly associated with less hypotension, it is widely admitted that such membranes limit the inflammatory reaction to dialysis session, limit the risk of amyloidosis, and could improve long-term survival [25]. These results are generally extended to critically ill patients. In ICU, the most popular membranes are polysulfone, polyethersulfone, and AN-69. The biocompatibility of synthetic membranes is not perfect. The AN-69 membrane is a negatively charged membrane that induces coagulation factor XII activation and subsequently produces bradykinin [29]. Because bradykinin is broken down by angiotensin-converting enzyme (ACE), negatively charged membranes may cause anaphylactic-like shock in patients taking ACE inhibitors, due to the accumulation of bradykinin [30]. Therefore, dialysis treatment with AN-69 membranes is contraindicated for patients using ACE inhibitors. This side effect was corrected by treating AN-69 membrane by polyethylenimine, a positively charged molecule that neutralizes the internal surface of hollow filter membrane. This membrane (AN-69 ST) is widely used for continuous RRT in ICU [22].

10.5.7 Polymyxin B Membrane Hemoperfusion

During hemoperfusion, there is no renal replacement therapy. The blood only crosses a polymyxin B-coated filter that decreases macrophage and monocyte activity. Despite promising results of the first randomized small study [31] and prospective cohort studies [32], recent randomized controlled multicenter study did not find any survival benefit in septic shock secondary to peritonitis [33], and these results seem to be confirmed by the last trial (EUPHRATES study preliminary presentation during ESICM congress 2016).

10.6 Main RRT Techniques Used in ICU (Table 10.1)

Continuous renal replacement techniques (CRRT) represent more than two-thirds of RRT in ICU patients [34, 35]. The rationales for using continuous technique are better hemodynamic stability and better fluid balance control in ICU patients as compared to IHD [9, 12, 17, 28]. Continuous techniques are defined by duration over 24 h, whereas IHD is generally performed over a 3–4-h period. Continuous techniques also limit the risk of dialysis disequilibrium syndrome that consists in acute cerebral edema due to acute blood osmolarity decrease induced by IHD. With continuous techniques, this risk is below 0.5% [36]. The superiority of continuous technique over IHD has not been demonstrated in terms of mortality [11, 21, 22, 37]. Nevertheless, two recent meta-analyses suggest a possible favorable impact of continuous techniques in terms of renal function recovery [38, 39]. The more frequently used techniques for CRRT are continuous venovenous hemofiltration (CVVH), hemodiafiltration (CVVHDF), and hemodialysis (CVVHD) [35]. Extended daily dialysis (EDD) and sustained low-efficiency dialysis (SLED) are hybrid techniques, between intermittent and continuous methods. Schematically, these techniques consist in prolonged sessions of IHD and seem to have a comparable interest than CVVH or CVVHDF [40, 41]. As they have been less studied than continuous technique and because they are only used in a small number of centers, hybrid techniques cannot be recommended in routine, especially in nonspecialized centers [12]. Table 10.1 summarizes the characteristics of all RRT techniques that can be used in ICU.

10.7 Dialysate Bath: Solutions for Continuous RRT

During conventional IHD, dialysate bath generators are necessary due to very high volume of dialysate per time unit: 30–40 l/h. The ideal composition of dialysate bath is summarized in Table 10.2 [42]. Dialysate temperature must be kept below 1–2 °C of the patient temperature in order to limit hypotension.

Continuous RRT in ICU may have considerable effects on potassium, phosphate, and magnesium over time. Up to 25% of continuous RRT sessions are associated with severe hypokalemia. Severe hypophosphatemia occurs in more than 55% of

Table 10.1 Overview of technical and clinical characteristics of RRT techniques that can be used in ICU

	Intermittent	Continuous			Hybrid
	IHD	CVVH	CVVHDF	CVVHD	SLED, EDD
Duration (h)	4–6	>24	>24	>24	6–16
Blood flow (mL/min)	200–350	100–250	100–250	100–250	100–300
Diffusion	++++	–	++ (50%)	++++	+++
Convection	+	++++	++ (50%)	+	+
Effluent flow (mL/min)	18–50 l/h	30 ml/kg/h	30 ml/kg/h* *15 ml/kg/h diffusion, 15 ml/kg/h convection	30 ml/kg/h	12–18 ml/h
Urea clearance (ml/min)	150–200	20–45	20–45	20–45	90–140
Urea start (mg/dL)	110	110	110	110	110
Urea end (mg/dL)	30	90	90	90	–
Filtration fraction (%)	<5	20–25	15–20	<5	<5
Fluctuations of ICP	++++	–	–	–	++
Hemodynamic stability	–	++++	++++	++++	+
Fluid balance control over time	++	++++	++++	++	++
pH stability over time	+=	++++	++++	++++	+
Needs for anticoagulation	+	+++	++	++	+
Membrane	Synthetic or modified cellulosic	Synthetic	Synthetic	Synthetic	Synthetic

ICP intracranial pressure, *IHD* intermittent hemodialysis, *CVVH* continuous venovenous hemofiltration, *CVVHDF* continuous venovenous hemodiafiltration, *CVVHD* continuous venovenous hemodialysis, *SLED* sustained low-efficiency dialysis, *EDD* extended daily dialysis. Effluent flow represents the global volume of treatment

Table 10.2 Ideal composition of dialysate bath for IHD and solutions dedicated to CRRT in ICU [48–50]

Dialysate bath composition for IHD		Composition of solutions for CRRT solutions	
Sodium	150 mmol/l	Sodium	140 mmol/l
Bicarbonate	31 mmol/l	Bicarbonate	30 mmol/l
Potassium	3–4 mmol/l	Potassium	3–4 mmol/l
Calcium	1.75 mmol/l	Calcium	1.25 mmol/l
Glucose	5.5 mmol/l	Phosphate	1
Temperature	35 °C	Glucose	0 mmol/l
		Magnesium	0.6 mmol/l
		Chloride	115 mmol/l

IHD intermittent hemodialysis, *CRRT* continuous renal replacement therapy, *ICU* intensive care unit cases [36]. Significant hypomagnesemia can also be observed [43]. During continuous techniques, special solutions are used to compensate plasma water removal during CVVH or for dialysate during CVVHDF or CVVHD. Because volumes per time unit are much lower than that for IHD (20–30 ml/Kg/h (see chapter "RRT Dose")), sterile 5 l bags of solutions closed to plasma concentration are used. The use of solutions that contain predefined concentrations of potassium and phosphate significantly decreases the risk of hypokalemia, hypophosphatemia, and hypomagnesemia [43–46]. The use of such solutions is associated with mild hyperphosphatemia, relative hypocalcemia, and metabolic acidosis with no clinical impact [45]. Despite the absence of glucose, these solutions are not associated with hypoglycemia. Such solutions cannot be used in case of severe hyperkalemia. The ideal composition of such solution is summarized in Table 10.2.

10.8 Timing

The decision to initiate RRT is often multifactorial; however, the ideal timing in the absence of any urgent clinical or metabolic complications is still debated. Some experts promote early initiation to assure immediate adequate control of metabolic, fluid, and pro-inflammatory parameters. Adepts of a delayed initiation strategy adhere to more in-depth diagnostic and therapeutic "fine-tuning" which could even obviate the need for RRT. Thus, there is an agreement to start RRT as soon as possible in the presence of life-threatening fluid overload, hyperkalemia, uremia, or metabolic acidosis [47], but the triggers to start in other situations remain unknown. The first problem is that there is a lack of consensus about the definition of "early" and "late" initiation. In the past, due to the absence of clear definition or staging of AKI, and even now, despite new definitions used worldwide as Risk, Injury, Failure, Loss, and End-stage (RIFLE) or Kidney Disease Improving Global Outcomes (KDIGO) score, some experts consider early an initiation at the injury level or stage 2, while others consider that early is as soon as you reach the failure level or stage 3 (that could be "late" for the advocates of early initiation).

The supporters of early initiation push the potential beneficial effects of RRT as better electrolyte, acid-base, and uremic homeostasis and better control of extracellular volume accumulation and potentially modulate systemic inflammation and may prevent the development of life-threatening complications (hyperkalemia or pulmonary edema). However, those benefits are mainly supported by data from observational studies [48, 49], globally weak, and not by strong randomized controlled trials (RCTs). The perceived benefits of RRT have to naturally be balanced with the potential harm attributable to RRT, argue the defenders of late initiation, including risks associated with iatrogenic episodes of hemodynamic instability, insertion of a dialysis catheter in central vein, coagulation and inflammatory activation by the extracorporeal circuit, the need for anticoagulation, unpredictable drug removal, and unwanted depletion of micronutrients (trace elements and amino acids). More, a waiting strategy may avoid RRT to patients that will recover renal function spontaneously that decrease the exposure to an unnecessary treatment, nurses' workload, and incremental costs [50].

As discussed previously, very few randomized clinical trials and numerous observational studies with methodological issues have explored the best timing for RRT initiation in critically ill patients with AKI [49, 51]. More importantly, most of these studies have their own criteria for defining "early" and "late" RRT as many of them were done before the wide dissemination of new definitions of AKI (RIFLE, KDIGO). Thus, some studies used "early" definition that was considered as "late" for other studies, making impossible reliable meta-analysis. We will not describe all these observational studies (most of them suggested taht "early" initiation of RRT was associated with improved outcomes) but more focused on RCTs, in particular the recent ones.

The first RCT, done by Bouman et al., randomized 106 critically ill predominantly cardiac surgical patients with oliguric AKI despite fluid resuscitation and inotropic support, to a strategy of early versus late initiation of RRT [52]. The early group started RRT when inclusion criteria were reached: oliguria (<30 ml/h for 6 h and no response to a diuretic challenge or hemodynamic optimization) or a creatinine clearance <20 ml/min. The late group started RRT if patient faced one of the following threatening situation: serum urea >40 mmol/L, potassium of >6.5 mmol/L, or evidence of pulmonary edema. In this study, there were no differences in terms of survival, renal recovery, or length of stay. However, this trial was not adequately designed to assess these outcomes, the global mortality was low due to the specific population studied (mainly post-cardiac surgery), and the trial was underpowered.

Two recently published prospective randomized trials have assessed the impact of different timings of RRT on the outcome of severely ill ICU patients with AKI but acute life-threatening complications. The Artificial Kidney Initiation in Kidney Injury (AKIKI) study [53], which randomized KDIGO stage 3 AKI patients, found no significant difference in 60-day mortality between an early (RRT initiation immediately after obtaining KDIGO stage 3 criteria) and delayed (RRT initiation after KDIGO stage 3 associated with a clinical complication such as pulmonary edema, severe hyperkalemia, severe acidosis, oliguria >72 h) RRT strategy (48.5% vs. 49.7%; $p = 0.79$). Catheter-related infection occurred less frequently in the delayed treatment arm, and more hypophosphatemia occurred in the early group, but hyperphosphatemia was not addressed (probably higher in the delayed group). Length of ICU and hospital stay was not different between groups. Interestingly, half of patients in the delayed treatment group did not need RRT at any time. The major concern is that the study did not report a protocol for hemodynamic improvement or fluid filling, implying that some patients may face transient AKI more due to hypovolemia or renal vasoconstriction than organic insult. In the other hand, the early versus late initiation of renal replacement therapy in critically ill patients with acute kidney injury (ELAIN) trial [54] reported a significantly reduced 90-day mortality in patients receiving early (within 8 h of diagnosis of KDIGO stage 2) as compared with delayed (within 12 h of stage 3 AKI or no initiation) RRT (39.3% vs. 54.7%; $p = 0.03$). Early initiation of RRT resulted in a more rapid recovery of renal function, significantly shortened duration of hospitalization, but did not affect future dialysis dependence or length of ICU stay. The major concern here is that more than half of the patients recruited were post-cardiac surgery patients with a large amount of fluid overload that is known to be successfully treated by RRT.

These studies do not contribute so much to an optimal RRT timing strategy in critically ill patients who develop AKI despite the fact that these trials were very well conducted. The AKIKI trial was a multicenter trial conducted in 31 ICUs screening 5528 predominantly medical patients for 29 months to finally randomize 620 (11%) patients. The ELAIN trial was a single-center trial conducted for 23 months screening 604 almost exclusively postsurgical and trauma patients to include 231 (38%) patients. This suggests potential patient selection, inclusion, and treatment bias. Also, the modest difference in RRT initiation time in the ELAIN trial is difficult to reconcile with the amazing positive effects on outcome. Last, RRT modalities substantially differed between both studies. All patients in the ELAIN trial underwent CVVHDF mode when only 30% of the AKIKI patients received continuous RRT. Mostly, choice of methods for RRT or parameters was let to the appreciation of physician in each center. Continuous RRT has not been shown to improve mortality but may be beneficial for patients with severe fluid overload or unstable cardiogenic/septic shock. Finally, it is just the idea that we could choose to start or not RRT based only on KDIGO stage that is unrealistic. These two studies showed that early initiation may be beneficial for some patients (cardiogenic shock, post-cardiac surgery, fluid overload) when others will never need RRT and will recover alone.

That underlines the importance of individualized strategy, based not only on the stage of AKI evidently but also on the rapidity of AKI progression, comorbidities, cause of AKI, presence of shock, and many other variables [55], and, anyway, RRT initiation should not be based only on renal score stratification as KDIGO, RIFLE, or AKIN.

10.9 RRT Dose

Twenty years ago, standard hemofiltration was often given at 1 or 2 l/h of ultrafiltration treatment and only in predilution mode. Practices began to change with the Ronco et al. study in 2001 proving the beneficial effect on outcome of increasing the ultrafiltration rate to 35 ml/kg/h in patients with acute kidney injury in ICU [56]. At that time, the old definition of high-volume hemofiltration (HVHF) became the standard of care, and volumes used to treat septic patients in ICU with AKI increased dramatically from 35 to 70 ml/kg/h or more [57–59]. But few years later, two large RCTs, the VA/NIH study and the RENAL study [36, 60], demonstrated that high intensity of hemofiltration was not beneficial comparing to 25 ml/kg/h, the dose currently recommended. Indeed, the first RCT from the USA compared high-intensity treatment represented by IHD or SLED 6 days a week or CVVHDF at 35 ml/kg/h versus low-intensity treatment as IHD or SLED thrice a week or CVVHDF at 20 ml/kg/h; no difference in terms of mortality or other important secondary endpoints was found but more hypokalemia or hypophosphatemia in the high intensive group [60]. Same results came from Australia and New Zealand with the RENAL study that compared CVVHDF at 40 ml/kg/h versus 25 ml/kg/h [36].

During this period, two different HVHF methods became common: continuous high-volume treatment providing 50–70 ml/kg/h 24 h a day and intermittent high-volume hemofiltration with brief, very high-volume treatment at 100–120 ml/kg/h for 4–8 h which used to be called "pulse" high-volume hemofiltration. Both came under the heading HVHF despite their concepts and results were somewhat different [61–66]. In the 2015 Vicenza Nomenclature Standardization Initiative (NSI) [11], they defined HVHF as a continuous convective treatment with a (prescribed) target dose greater than 35 ml/kg/h. A dose exceeding 45 ml/kg/h represents very HVHF (VHVHF). Intermittent procedures using brief VHVHF episodes (100–120 ml/kg/h for 4–8 h), followed by conventional CVVH, are identified as "pulse" HVHF.

The first positive randomized controlled study on HVHF was performed by Laurent and coll in post-cardiac arrest patients, with clear positive results in favor of the experimental arm [67], but this study has never been reproduced or confirmed and recently challenged by an animal study that did not show any beneficial impact of HVHF on post-cardiac arrest in rat population [68]. After these preliminary observational studies, the first positive RCT in septic patients was done by Boussekey, 20 patients randomized in two groups (65 vs. 35 ml/kg/h), with beneficial impact of HVHF on hemodynamic parameters [66]. The first large RCT on HVHF came from China by Zhang and coll, who randomized 280 septic patients with AKI in a single center in two groups, one treated by HVHF at 50 ml/kg/h and the other by very HVHF at 80 ml/kg/h [69]. They did not find any difference in terms of mortality or hemodynamic improvement. In 2013, a large multicenter RCT, the IVOIRE study, conducted by Joannes-Boyau and coll, included 140 patients with AKI and septic shock randomized in two groups: 35 vs. 70 ml/kg/h [26]. The authors definitely demonstrated that HVHF had no beneficial effect in terms of hemodynamic parameter improvement or mortality at 28 or 90 days. They also found that a large amount of antibiotics was removed by hemofiltration and might be an explanation of the negative results of the HVHF studies, as the benefice of high volume might be counteracted by the harm effect of drug removal. However, a recent study using a specific technique, the cascade HVHF, which allows very HVHF (120 ml/kg/h) with removal of only middle-sized molecules, contradicts this argument [27]. This technique uses a large-pore-size filter (40 kDa) upstream of a low-pore-size membrane (15 kDa) refiltrating the ultrafiltrate. The majority of the ultrafiltrate containing small-sized molecules (antibiotics, drugs, vitamins, etc.) is then re-administrated to the patient, while a little part of the ultrafiltrate containing middle-sized molecules (and cytokines) is retained in the effluent bag. In this multicenter RCT, Quenot and coll included 60 septic shock patients randomized in two groups: cascade HVHF versus standard care. The authors failed to demonstrate any beneficial effect in terms of catecholamine drug requirement, mortality, or even the cytokine removal except for IL-8. In cardiogenic and distributive shock post-cardiac surgery, Combes and coll published the HEROICS trial studying the effect on mortality of HVHF (80 ml/kg/h) in post-cardiac surgery patients. Two hundred and twenty-four patients were included and randomized in two groups: HVHF versus standard treatment [70]. Again, the authors did not find differences in terms of mortality between groups; HVHF patients only experienced faster correction of metabolic acidosis and tended to be more rapidly weaned from catecholamine despite more frequent hypophosphatemia, metabolic alkalosis, and thrombocytopenia.

Finally, regarding recommendations for clinical practice, patients with AKI should receive a renal replacement dose of 25 ml/kg/hour delivered (level I evidence and grade A recommendation) that imply to prescribe more, about 30–35 ml/kg/h, to take into account the downtime (expected and unexpected) during a treatment day [28]. A higher dose when patients suffer from sepsis and AKI is not recommended outside research programs.

10.10 Anticoagulation

Coagulation and treatment breakdown are the major concerns during continuous methods. However, two-thirds of these problems are independent of anticoagulation management. Indeed, if we summarize, 50% of hemofiltration breakdown are due to problems with vascular access, the treatment management and the use of the machine are responsible for 15%, and the anticoagulation choice and management are the points for the last one-third of the machine break. For clinical practice, the following checklist may help to avoid most current problems. After checking these criteria, ICU physician can focus on anticoagulation management.

It is crucial to have a good checklist with key point elements to "pilot" correctly continuous hemofiltration; each aspect has to be respected to obtain efficiency.

- **Excellent vascular access**: It is the most important point; efficient blood flow cannot be obtained without adapted catheter. Large catheter (13.5–15.5 French) is mandatory, with adequate location and correlated length (15–20 cm in the right jugular is the best equivalent to 24–28 cm in femoral approach, while the subclavian route should be avoided) and good structure (coaxial double kidney and shotgun termination with large arterial intake) [71–73].
- **Nursing**: Efficient position should be found for the patient to obtain the best blood flow (avoid catheter torsion or angulation), and treatment should be stopped during nursing or patient position change (just keep blood pump running).
- **Filtration fraction (FF) below 25%**: Adapted blood flow is necessary to maintain this level of filtration fraction; a level above is prone to clogging in the membrane.
- **Restitution fluid**: All in postdilution. If you have clotting problems in the filter or you use HVHF = one-third in predilution and two-thirds in postdilution. **Restitution fluid should not be given all in predilution**, which decreases treatment efficiency and does not prevent circuit clotting.

When you have checked all these items and you do not face trouble, you can concentrate on anticoagulation:

- **Heparin**: 5–10 UI/kg/h. Monitoring efficiency by ACT, heparinemy, or anti-Xa activity. Monitoring toxicity by platelet count. **Mandatory coenzyme is**

antithrombin, monitoring is recommended, and supplementation if the activity level drops below 60% is suggested (grade D, levels 3 and 4) [74, 75].

- **Benefits**: Easy to use, reversed by protamine, low cost.
- **Risks**: Heparin-induced thrombocytopenia (HIT), hemorrhage (but theoretical, very low risk in the latest study if heparin is correctly managed with an ACT target at 1.5 maximum).

– **Low molecular weight heparin (LMWH): Renal removal excludes this technique for continuous methods** (toxicity if treatment stops). This anticoagulation is interesting for dialysis in chronic renal failure patients.

– **Citrate: Probably the best anticoagulant, recommended as first choice** [28]. It is a calcium chelator. Hepatic metabolism. **Monitoring is essential**: Ionized calcium, pH and bicarbonate, magnesium, and hepatic functions.

- **Benefits: REGIONAL anticoagulation.** Cheap. Best anticoagulant effect.
- **Risks: Do not use for hepatic failure patients with PT below 26% or septic shock patients with tissue hypoxia and hyperlactatemia** [76, 77]. Use good protocol. Use only dedicated machines with dedicated pumps for citrate and calcium infusion in strict relation with blood pump. Be aware of Stewart theory to understand the possible acid-base disorders due to citrate anticoagulation: **Acidosis** caused by citrate accumulation due to lack of metabolization, where the first sign will be progressive patient hypocalcemia and increase compensation over time and a total of ionized calcium ratio above 2.5. **Alkalosis** in relation to hypernatremia occurs when concentrate citrate is used for hypochloremia with dilute citrate.

Conclusion

Renal replacement therapy is now a daily and mandatory technique in ICU, but it is also one of the procedures that has been less studied and known in the past. Effort has been done recently to enhance knowledge and recommendations in this field, but many questions remain unanswered. We will conclude by a list of some important recommendations and tips to try to increase the good RRT treatment delivery to the patients.

- Good venous access, right jugular (15–20 cm) or femoral (24–30 cm), at least 12 French.
- Use biocompatible membranes.
- Use adapted dialysis or restitution fluids with ionic composition closest to the plasma one.
- Use intermittent and continuous RRT as complementary techniques, but prefer continuous ones for hemodynamic unstable or brain injury patients.
- Recommended dose for AKI patients in ICU is 25 ml/kg/h for continuous hemofiltration that implies to prescribe 30–35 ml/kg/h.
- High-volume hemofiltration is not recommended outside research programs.
- Remain with a filtration fraction below 25% with heparin and 30% with citrate anticoagulation.
- Use citrate as first-choice anticoagulation method in the absence of contraindication, but monitor carefully the metabolic status of the patients.

References

1. Rettig RA (2011) Special treatment—the story of Medicare's ESRD entitlement. N Engl J Med 364(7):596–598
2. Eknoyan G (2009) The wonderful apparatus of John Jacob Abel called the "artificial kidney". Semin Dial juin 22(3):287–296
3. Flexner J, Chassin MR (1941) Clinical studies on pyridoxine (vitamin B(6)). J Clin Invest mai 20(3):313–316
4. Blagg CR, Hickman RO, Eschbach JW, Scribner BH (1970) Home hemodialysis: six years' experience. N Engl J Med 283(21):1126–1131
5. Scribner BH, Cole JJ, Christopher TG, Vizzo JE, Atkins RC, Blagg CR (1970) Long-term total parenteral nutrition. The concept of an artificial gut. JAMA 212(3):457–463
6. Dodd NJ, O'Donovan RM, Bennett-Jones DN, Rylance PB, Bewick M, Parsons V et al (1983) Arteriovenous haemofiltration: a recent advance in the management of renal failure. Br Med J Clin Res Ed 287(6398):1008–1010
7. Gibney RT, Stollery DE, Lefebvre RE, Sharun CJ, Chan P (1988) Continuous arteriovenous hemodialysis: an alternative therapy for acute renal failure associated with critical illness. Can Med Assoc J 139(9):861–866
8. Bellomo R, Mansfield D, Rumble S, Shapiro J, Parkin G, Boyce N (1992) Acute renal failure in critical illness. Conventional dialysis versus acute continuous hemodiafiltration. ASAIO J Am Soc Artif Intern Organs 38(3):M654–M657
9. Khwaja A (2012) KDIGO clinical practice guidelines for acute kidney injury. Nephron Clin Pract 120(4):c179–c184
10. Ad-hoc working group of ERBP, Fliser D, Laville M, Covic A, Fouque D, Vanholder R et al (2012) A European renal best practice (ERBP) position statement on the kidney disease improving global outcomes (KDIGO) clinical practice guidelines on acute kidney injury: part 1: definitions, conservative management and contrast-induced nephropathy. Nephrol Dial Transplant 27(12):4263–4272
11. Neri M, Villa G, Garzotto F, Bagshaw S, Bellomo R, Cerda J et al (2016) Nomenclature for renal replacement therapy in acute kidney injury: basic principles. Crit Care Lond Engl 20(1):318
12. Ronco C, Ricci Z, De Backer D, Kellum JA, Taccone FS, Joannidis M et al (2015) Renal replacement therapy in acute kidney injury: controversy and consensus. Crit Care Lond Engl 19:146
13. Bouchard J, Soroko SB, Chertow GM, Himmelfarb J, Ikizler TA, Paganini EP et al (2009) Fluid accumulation, survival and recovery of kidney function in critically ill patients with acute kidney injury. Kidney Int 76(4):422–427
14. Grams ME, Estrella MM, Coresh J, Brower RG, Liu KD, National Heart, Lung, and Blood Institute Acute Respiratory Distress Syndrome Network (2011) Fluid balance, diuretic use, and mortality in acute kidney injury. Clin J Am Soc Nephrol CJASN 6(5):966–973
15. Payen D, de Pont AC, Sakr Y, Spies C, Reinhart K, Vincent JL et al (2008) A positive fluid balance is associated with a worse outcome in patients with acute renal failure. Crit Care Lond Engl 12(3):R74
16. Teixeira C, Garzotto F, Piccinni P, Brienza N, Iannuzzi M, Gramaticopolo S et al (2013) Fluid balance and urine volume are independent predictors of mortality in acute kidney injury. Crit Care Lond Engl 17(1):R14
17. Bagshaw SM, Darmon M, Ostermann M, Finkelstein FO, Wald R, Tolwani AJ et al (2017) Current state of the art for renal replacement therapy in critically ill patients with acute kidney injury. Intensive Care Med 43(6):841–854
18. Schiffl H, Lang SM, Fischer R (2002) Daily hemodialysis and the outcome of acute renal failure. N Engl J Med 346(5):305–310
19. Sakai K, Matsuda M (2011) Solute removal efficiency and biocompatibility of the high-performance membrane - from engineering points of view. Contrib Nephrol 173:11–22

20. Bowry SK, Gatti E, Vienken J (2011) Contribution of polysulfone membranes to the success of convective dialysis therapies. Contrib Nephrol 173:110–118
21. Krummel T, Hannedouche T (2013) Clinical potentials of adsorptive dialysis membranes. Blood Purif 35(Suppl 2):1–4
22. Kokubo K, Kurihara Y, Kobayashi K, Tsukao H, Kobayashi H (2015) Evaluation of the biocompatibility of dialysis membranes. Blood Purif 40(4):293–297
23. Santoro A, Guadagni G (2010) Dialysis membrane: from convection to adsorption. NDT Plus mai 3(Suppl 1):i36–i39
24. Aucella F, Gesuete A, Vigilante M, Prencipe M (2013) Adsorption dialysis: from physical principles to clinical applications. Blood Purif 35(Suppl 2):42–47
25. Kerr PG, Toussaint ND, Kidney Health Australia, Caring for Australasians with Renal Impairment (2013) KHA-CARI guideline: dialysis adequacy (haemodialysis): dialysis membranes. Nephrol Carlton Vic 18(7):485–488
26. Joannes-Boyau O, Honoré PM, Perez P, Bagshaw SM, Grand H, Canivet J-L et al (2013) High-volume versus standard-volume haemofiltration for septic shock patients with acute kidney injury (IVOIRE study): a multicentre randomized controlled trial. Intensive Care Med 39(9):1535–1546
27. Quenot J-P, Binquet C, Vinsonneau C, Barbar S-D, Vinault S, Deckert V et al (2015) Very high volume hemofiltration with the Cascade system in septic shock patients. Intensive Care Med 41(12):2111–2120
28. Vinsonneau C, Allain-Launay E, Blayau C, Darmon M, Ducheyron D, Gaillot T et al (2015) Renal replacement therapy in adult and pediatric intensive care : recommendations by an expert panel from the French Intensive Care Society (SRLF) with the French Society of Anesthesia Intensive Care (SFAR) French Group for Pediatric Intensive Care Emergencies (GFRUP) the French dialysis society (SFD). Ann Intensive Care 5(1):58
29. Verresen L, Fink E, Lemke HD, Vanrenterghem Y (1994) Bradykinin is a mediator of anaphylactoid reactions during hemodialysis with AN69 membranes. Kidney Int 45(5):1497–1503
30. Tielemans C, Madhoun P, Lenaers M, Schandene L, Goldman M, Vanherweghem JL (1990) Anaphylactoid reactions during hemodialysis on AN69 membranes in patients receiving ACE inhibitors. Kidney Int 38(5):982–984
31. Cruz DN, Antonelli M, Fumagalli R, Foltran F, Brienza N, Donati A et al (2009) Early use of polymyxin B hemoperfusion in abdominal septic shock: the EUPHAS randomized controlled trial. JAMA 301(23):2445–2452
32. Chang T, Tu Y-K, Lee C-T, Chao A, Huang C-H, Wang M-J et al (2017) Effects of Polymyxin B Hemoperfusion on mortality in patients with severe sepsis and septic shock: a systemic review, meta-analysis update, and disease severity subgroup meta-analysis. Crit Care Med 45(8):e858–e864
33. Payen DM, Guilhot J, Launey Y, Lukaszewicz AC, Kaaki M, Veber B et al (2015) Early use of polymyxin B hemoperfusion in patients with septic shock due to peritonitis: a multicenter randomized control trial. Intensive Care Med 41(6):975–984
34. Uchino S, Kellum JA, Bellomo R, Doig GS, Morimatsu H, Morgera S et al (2005) Acute renal failure in critically ill patients: a multinational, multicenter study. JAMA 294(7):813–818
35. Friedrich JO, Wald R, Bagshaw SM, Burns KEA, Adhikari NKJ (2012) Hemofiltration compared to hemodialysis for acute kidney injury: systematic review and meta-analysis. Crit Care Lond Engl 16(4):R146
36. RENAL, Replacement Therapy Study Investigators, Bellomo R, Cass A, Cole L, Finfer S, Gallagher M et al (2009) Intensity of continuous renal-replacement therapy in critically ill patients. N Engl J Med 361(17):1627–1638
37. Vinsonneau C, Camus C, Combes A, Costa de Beauregard MA, Klouche K, Boulain T et al (2006) Continuous venovenous haemodiafiltration versus intermittent haemodialysis for acute renal failure in patients with multiple-organ dysfunction syndrome: a multicentre randomised trial. Lancet Lond Engl 368(9533):379–385
38. Schneider AG, Bellomo R, Bagshaw SM, Glassford NJ, Lo S, Jun M et al (2013) Choice of renal replacement therapy modality and dialysis dependence after acute kidney injury: a systematic review and meta-analysis. Intensive Care Med 39(6):987–997

39. Schoenfelder T, Chen X, Bleß H-H (2017) Effects of continuous and intermittent renal replacement therapies among adult patients with acute kidney injury. GMS Health Technol Assess 13:Doc01
40. Zhang L, Yang J, Eastwood GM, Zhu G, Tanaka A, Bellomo R (2015) Extended daily dialysis versus continuous renal replacement therapy for acute kidney injury: a meta-analysis. Am J Kidney Dis 66(2):322–330
41. Kovacs B, Sullivan KJ, Hiremath S, Patel RV (2017) Effect of sustained low efficient dialysis versus continuous renal replacement therapy on renal recovery after acute kidney injury in the intensive care unit: a systematic review and meta-analysis. Nephrol Carlton Vic 22(5):343–353
42. Schortgen F (2003) Hypotension during intermittent hemodialysis: new insights into an old problem. Intensive Care Med 29(10):1645–1649
43. Godaly G, Carlsson O, Broman M (2016) Phoxilium(®) reduces hypophosphataemia and magnesium supplementation during continuous renal replacement therapy. Clin Kidney J 9(2):205–210
44. Besnard N, Serveaux M, Machado S, Daubin D, Brunot V, Amigues L et al (2016) Electrolytes-enriched Hemodiafiltration solutions for continuous renal replacement therapy in acute kidney injury: a crossover study. Blood Purif 42(1):18–26
45. Chua H-R, Schneider AG, Baldwin I, Collins A, Ho L, Bellomo R (2013) Phoxilium vs Hemosol-B0 for continuous renal replacement therapy in acute kidney injury. J Crit Care 28(5):884.e7–884.14
46. Broman M, Carlsson O, Friberg H, Wieslander A, Godaly G (2011) Phosphate-containing dialysis solution prevents hypophosphatemia during continuous renal replacement therapy. Acta Anaesthesiol Scand 55(1):39–45
47. Ostermann M, Dickie H, Barrett NA (2012) Renal replacement therapy in critically ill patients with acute kidney injury—when to start. Nephrol Dial Transplant 27(6):2242–2248
48. Karvellas CJ, Farhat MR, Sajjad I, Mogensen SS, Leung AA, Wald R et al (2011) A comparison of early versus late initiation of renal replacement therapy in critically ill patients with acute kidney injury: a systematic review and meta-analysis. Crit Care Lond Engl 15(1):R72
49. Wierstra BT, Kadri S, Alomar S, Burbano X, Barrisford GW, Kao RLC (2016) The impact of "early" versus "late" initiation of renal replacement therapy in critical care patients with acute kidney injury: a systematic review and evidence synthesis. Crit Care Lond Engl 20(1):122
50. Shiao C-C, Ko W-J, Wu V-C, Huang T-M, Lai C-F, Lin Y-F et al (2012) U-curve association between timing of renal replacement therapy initiation and in-hospital mortality in postoperative acute kidney injury. PLoS One 7(8):e42952
51. Seabra VF, Balk EM, Liangos O, Sosa MA, Cendoroglo M, Jaber BL (2008) Timing of renal replacement therapy initiation in acute renal failure: a meta-analysis. Am J Kidney Dis 52(2):272–284
52. Bouman CSC, Oudemans-Van Straaten HM, Tijssen JGP, Zandstra DF, Kesecioglu J (2002) Effects of early high-volume continuous venovenous hemofiltration on survival and recovery of renal function in intensive care patients with acute renal failure: a prospective, randomized trial. Crit Care Med 30(10):2205–2211
53. Gaudry S, Hajage D, Schortgen F, Martin-Lefevre L, Pons B, Boulet E et al (2016) Initiation strategies for renal-replacement therapy in the intensive care unit. N Engl J Med 375(2):122–133
54. Zarbock A, Kellum JA, Schmidt C, Van Aken H, Wempe C, Pavenstädt H et al (2016) Effect of early vs delayed initiation of renal replacement therapy on mortality in critically ill patients with acute kidney injury: the ELAIN randomized clinical trial. JAMA 315(20):2190–2199
55. Bagshaw SM, Cruz DN, Gibney RN, Ronco C (2009) A proposed algorithm for initiation of renal replacement therapy in adult critically ill patients. Crit Care 13:317
56. Ronco C, Bellomo R, Homel P, Brendolan A, Dan M, Piccinni P et al (2000) Effects of different doses in continuous veno-venous haemofiltration on outcomes of acute renal failure: a prospective randomised trial. Lancet Lond Engl 356(9223):26–30
57. Honore PM, Joannes-Boyau O (2004) High volume hemofiltration (HVHF) in sepsis: a comprehensive review of rationale, clinical applicability, potential indications and recommendations for future research. Int J Artif Organs 27(12):1077–1082

58. Bellomo R, Honoré PM, Matson J, Ronco C, Winchester J (2005) Extracorporeal blood treatment (EBT) methods in SIRS/sepsis. Int J Artif Organs 28(5):450–458
59. Tetta C, Bellomo R, Kellum J, Ricci Z, Pohlmeiere R, Passlick-Deetjen J et al (2004) High volume hemofiltration in critically ill patients: why, when and how? Contrib Nephrol 144:362–375
60. VA/NIH Acute Renal Failure Trial Network, Palevsky PM, Zhang JH, O'Connor TZ, Chertow GM, Crowley ST et al (2008) Intensity of renal support in critically ill patients with acute kidney injury. N Engl J Med 359(1):7–20
61. Cole L, Bellomo R, Hart G, Journois D, Davenport P, Tipping P et al (2002) A phase II randomized, controlled trial of continuous hemofiltration in sepsis. Crit Care Med 30(1):100–106
62. Cole L, Bellomo R, Journois D, Davenport P, Baldwin I, Tipping P (2001) High-volume haemofiltration in human septic shock. Intensive Care Med 27(6):978–986
63. Honore PM, Jamez J, Wauthier M, Lee PA, Dugernier T, Pirenne B et al (2000) Prospective evaluation of short-term, high-volume isovolemic hemofiltration on the hemodynamic course and outcome in patients with intractable circulatory failure resulting from septic shock. Crit Care Med 28(11):3581–3587
64. Joannes-Boyau O, Rapaport S, Bazin R, Fleureau C, Janvier G (2004) Impact of high volume hemofiltration on hemodynamic disturbance and outcome during septic shock. ASAIO J 50(1):102–109
65. Cornejo R, Downey P, Castro R, Romero C, Regueira T, Vega J et al (2006) High-volume hemofiltration as salvage therapy in severe hyperdynamic septic shock. Intensive Care Med 32(5):713–722
66. Boussekey N, Chiche A, Faure K, Devos P, Guery B, d'Escrivan T et al (2008) A pilot randomized study comparing high and low volume hemofiltration on vasopressor use in septic shock. Intensive Care Med 34(9):1646–1653
67. Laurent I, Adrie C, Vinsonneau C, Cariou A, Chiche J-D, Ohanessian A et al (2005) High-volume hemofiltration after out-of-hospital cardiac arrest: a randomized study. J Am Coll Cardiol 46(3):432–437
68. Shinozaki K, Lampe JW, Kim J, Yin T, Da T, Oda S et al (2016) The effects of early high-volume hemofiltration on prolonged cardiac arrest in rats with reperfusion by cardiopulmonary bypass: a randomized controlled animal study. Intensive Care Med Exp 4(1):25
69. Zhang P, Yang Y, Lv R, Zhang Y, Xie W, Chen J (2012) Effect of the intensity of continuous renal replacement therapy in patients with sepsis and acute kidney injury: a single-center randomized clinical trial. Nephrol Dial Transpl 27(3):967–973
70. Combes A, Bréchot N, Amour J, Cozic N, Lebreton G, Guidon C et al (2015) Early high-volume hemofiltration versus standard Care for Post-Cardiac Surgery Shock. The HEROICS study. Am J Respir Crit Care Med 192(10):1179–1190
71. DiCarlo JV, Auerbach SR, Alexander SR (2006) Clinical review: alternative vascular access techniques for continuous hemofiltration. Crit Care Lond Engl. 10(5):230
72. Naka T, Egi M, Bellomo R, Baldwin I, Fealy N, Wan L (2008) Resistance of vascular access catheters for continuous renal replacement therapy: an ex vivo evaluation. Int J Artif Organs 31(10):905–909
73. Joannidis M, Oudemans-van Straaten HM (2007) Clinical review: patency of the circuit in continuous renal replacement therapy. Crit Care Lond Engl. 11(4):218
74. Lafargue M, Joannes-Boyau O, Honoré PM, Gauche B, Grand H, Fleureau C et al (2008) Acquired deficit of antithrombin and role of supplementation in septic patients during continuous veno-venous hemofiltration. ASAIO J Am Soc Artif Intern Organs 1992 54(1):124–128
75. du Cheyron D, Bouchet B, Bruel C, Daubin C, Ramakers M, Charbonneau P (2006) Antithrombin supplementation for anticoagulation during continuous hemofiltration in critically ill patients with septic shock: a case-control study. Crit Care Lond Engl. 10(2):R45
76. Schultheiß C, Saugel B, Phillip V, Thies P, Noe S, Mayr U et al (2012) Continuous venovenous hemodialysis with regional citrate anticoagulation in patients with liver failure: a prospective observational study. Crit Care Lond Engl 16(4):R162
77. Tan JN, Haroon SWP, Mukhopadhyay A, Lau T, Murali TM, Phua J, et al. Hyperlactatemia predicts citrate intolerance with regional citrate anticoagulation during continuous renal replacement therapy. J Intensive Care Med. 2017; 885066617701068. 10.1177/0885066617701068

Strategies for Preventing Acute Renal Failure

11

Malik Haddam, Carole Bechis, Valéry Blasco, and Marc Leone

11.1 Introduction

The acute renal failure (ARF) is due to a decline in glomerular filtration rate, leading to the inability of the kidney to eliminate the degradation products of nitrogen metabolism. This is a common situation in anesthesiology and intensive care unit. We propose to detail the different measures of prevention of ARF. Three areas are emerging in our daily activities: prevention of contrast-induced nephropathy (CIN), prevention of ARF after major surgery, and prevention of ARF in intensive care unit (ICU).

11.2 Extrarenal Strategies

11.2.1 Hemodynamic Monitoring

No strategy for hemodynamic monitoring resulted in a direct impact on renal function [1]. However, future options of monitoring probably offer opportunity to be efficient in terms of ARF prevention. Doppler ultrasonography and resistive index measurements of the renal arteries may facilitate the determination of the optimal perfusion pressure, thereby preventing ARF in high-risk patients [2, 3]. Large studies are required to confirm this hypothesis.

M. Haddam • C. Bechis • M. Leone (✉)
Service d'anesthésie et de réanimation, Hôpital Nord, AP-HM, Aix Marseille Université, 13015 Marseille, France
e-mail: marc.leone@ap-hm.fr

V. Blasco
Service d'anesthésie et de réanimation, Hôpital La Conception, AP-HM, 13005 Marseille, France

C. Ichai et al. (eds.), *Metabolic Disorders and Critically Ill Patients*,
http://doi.org/10.1007/978-3-319-64010-5_11

11.2.2 Hydration and Intravenous Fluids

11.2.2.1 Sodium Bicarbonate

With respect to the prevention of CIN in patients undergoing coronary procedure, the prehydration of sodium bicarbonate is more effective than the prehydration of sodium chloride [4, 5]. However, a randomized study of 353 patients did not confirm this result in patients with moderate-to-severe chronic renal failure (CRF) undergoing coronary angiography [6]. In patients undergoing cardiac surgery, sodium bicarbonate loading and continuous infusion were associated with a lower incidence of ARF [7]. This preliminary finding was not confirmed in a large study. In conclusion, prophylactic use of sodium bicarbonate should not be recommended in current practice [8].

11.2.2.2 Colloids

Volume resuscitation using hydroxyethyl starch (HES) has been largely assessed in recent years. In severe sepsis and septic shock, the rate of patients requiring renal replacement therapy was increased in the groups of patients receiving HES, as compared to those receiving crystalloids [9, 10]. In a randomized clinical trial, the mortality rate was increased in the patients treated with HES (day 90) [9]. This finding was not confirmed in another randomized clinical trial including a large number of patients [10]. In a study comparing colloids and crystalloids, no detrimental effect was reported in the patients treated with HES. The 90-day mortality was reduced in the colloid group [11]. In operating room, no effect was reported on the renal function [12]. In the light of those studies [13–17], the French health authorities, based on European health authorities' recommendations, restricted the use of HES by excluding:

- Patients with sepsis
- Burn patients
- Patients with renal insufficiency or renal replacement therapy continue
- Cases of intracranial or cerebral hemorrhage
- Patients in intensive care
- Patients with fluid overload, including patients with pulmonary edema
- Dehydrated patients
- Case of severe coagulopathy
- Case of severe hepatic impairment

In addition, HES should be used at the lowest effective dose, for the shortest possible time. In brief, they can be administered during the first 24 h after an acute blood loss [12]. Renal function should be monitored 90 days after their administration. Their use should be discontinued at the first sign of kidney damage. To date, in critically ill patients, HES cannot be used for preventing ARF.

11.2.3 Maintaining Perfusion Pressure by Vasopressors

Renal hypoperfusion is the leading cause of ARF. Increasing renal perfusion pressure improves creatinine clearance in patients with septic shock [18, 19]. The optimal level of mean arterial pressure in septic patients is between 65 and 85 mmHg. It seems that the goal of mean arterial pressure of patients with a prior history of arterial hypertension should be around 85 mmHg, in order to avoid the development of ARF. In contrast, in the patients without prior history of arterial hypertension, a goal around 65 mmHg is probably sufficient. In order to improve organ perfusion, the first step should always be the preload assessment. In patients without criteria for fluid loading, norepinephrine is the vasopressor of choice [20]. In septic patients its administration was associated with improved renal function [21]. In trauma patients, its use did not affect creatinine clearance [21]. Vasopressin is an alternative vasopressor with a potent vasoconstricting effect at the level of efferent glomerular artery. This property resulted in improved renal function of patients with septic shock [22]. In septic patients with moderate renal dysfunction, the administration of low-dose vasopressin was associated with improved outcomes in a post hoc analysis [23].

11.2.4 Nephrotoxic Anti-infective Agents

Anti-infective agents are largely administered to patients at high-risk of ARF. Worldwide, it is an avoidable cause of renal dysfunction in the critically ill patients. Whichever the drugs, the optimal dosage of anti-infective agents should be determined with regard to renal function. Of note, the first (loading) dosage of anti-infective agents does not depend of renal function.

11.2.4.1 Aminoglycosides

With respect to aminoglycosides, several meta-analyses show an equivalence or superiority of a once-daily schema of administration, as compared to a multiple-daily administration schema [24]. The monitoring of plasma peak and trough concentrations should be performed in cases of impaired renal function in order to determine the best timing for reinjections. This option prevents the occurrence of ARF. The combination of an aminoglycoside with beta-lactam antibiotics in the treatment of septic patients should be restricted to the treatments of shock, neutropenia, or suspected infections due to multidrug-resistant pathogens. Even in the patients at risk of renal dysfunction, aminoglycosides remain the first choice for a combined therapy.

11.2.4.2 Amphotericin

The renal toxicity of amphotericin B is due to a dual indirect effect by vasoconstriction of the afferent arteriole by glomerular and tubular direct toxicity. This affects approximately 30% of the patients. This toxicity is dose-dependent but it appears for doses <0.5 mg/kg/day and a cumulative dose <600 mg. In clinical practice, the majority of teams abandoned the use of amphotericin B in the critically ill patients. The lipid form is associated with a reduced nephrotoxicity [25, 26].

11.2.5 Iodinated Contrast Media

The CIN is the third leading cause of ARF. The contrast agents act by direct tubular toxicity. In addition, they induce intrarenal vasoconstriction. Several authors hypothesized that the reduction in osmolality of contrast would be associated with a reduced incidence in ARF. This hypothesis was tested in patients undergoing cardiac catheterization. In a first randomized clinical trial, the use of low-osmolality contrast medium reduced the rate of renal dysfunction in a subgroup of patients with pre-existing renal insufficiency and diabetes mellitus [27]. In a second randomized clinical trial, the use of low-osmolality contrast medium iopamidol was tested in patients with chronic kidney disease undergoing cardiac catheterization procedure. The incidence of CIN was similar in both groups, even among the patients with diabetes mellitus [28]. Hence, strategies aiming at reducing the osmolality of contrast did not result in positive outcomes.

11.2.6 Glycemic Control

Strict glycemic control showed a reduction in mortality in medical ICU patients with a significant decrease in the incidence of ARF [29, 30]. This is explained by a reduced activation of the vascular endothelium. Elsewhere, the results were dissimilar to those reported above. They show an increased mortality in the tight control group, due to sudden variation glucose [31, 32]. To prevent the occurrence of ARF, it is therefore necessary to control blood sugar, avoiding sudden changes in glucose.

11.2.7 Angiotensin-Converting Enzyme Inhibitors

In aortic and cardiac surgery, studies show that treatment with angiotensin-converting enzyme inhibitors was significantly associated with poorer renal function [33, 34]. However, there is a protective effect in patients with diabetes mellitus. In a meta-analysis, it was concluded that the effect of these drugs was inefficient in terms of renal prevention [35]. It is recommended to stop their administration for 48 h before surgery, except in the case of heart failure.

11.2.8 Thoracic Epidural Anesthesia

In the context of cardiac surgery, only one study assessed postoperative complications comparing thoracic epidural analgesia and intravenous morphine. ARF was less frequent in the thoracic epidural group than in the morphine group. This effect seems explained by improved cardiac recovery [36]. This effect was not found for other surgeries, including colorectal or orthopedic knee surgery (spinal anesthesia).

11.3 Renal Strategies

11.3.1 Dopamine and Its Analogues

There is no argument recommending the use of low-dose dopamine to prevent ARF [37, 38]. In a large randomized clinical trial, dopamine did not improve renal function more efficiently than norepinephrine [20]. In contrast, the rate of side effects was higher in the patients treated with dopamine, as compared with norepinephrine [20]. Fenoldopam is a selective D1 dopamine receptor agonist. In two studies, the administration of fenoldopam tended to reduce the incidence of ARF and the need for recourse to renal replacement therapy [39, 40]. However, the extensive analysis of the literature does not support the use of dopamine and its analogues for preventing renal failure [35, 41, 42].

11.3.2 Diuretics

Diuretics associated with hydration do not prevent the occurrence of CIN, as compared to a simple hydration. In contrast, there is an increase of ARF incidence [43]. In surgical patients, the use of diuretics showed no benefit for preventing ARF [44]. These drugs are associated with deleterious effects and an increased use of renal replacement therapy [45].

Meta-analysis showed disappointing results with the use of diuretics [35, 46]. Diuretics do not serve for improving recovery of renal function. There is no excess mortality associated with their use, except in one study [47]. Of note, this result was reported from a nonrandomized and retrospective study. The effects were observed in patients who were unresponsive to diuretics. However, the use of high doses increases the risk of side effects ototoxicity (tinnitus, hearing loss, deafness) [48].

11.3.3 Acetylcysteine

N-acetylcysteine (NAC) is the prodrug of L-cysteine, which acts as biologic antioxidant. Its role in the prevention of CIN has been reported in two meta-analyses [49, 50]. In contrast, it is an inefficient drug to prevent postoperative renal dysfunction [35].

Conclusion

Prevention of CIN relies on an intravenous hydration. The administration of NAC may have a positive effect. The use of low doses of moderately hyperosmolar contrast may probably be preferred, although the level of evidence is low.

In the critically ill patients, there is no specific treatment for preventing ARF. However, the rules should be to monitor adequately these patients in order to optimize the renal pressure perfusion and to avoid drugs with renal toxicity and unnecessary contrast administration. Those simple rules, used as a preventive bundle, may result in a decrease incidence of ARF in those patients.

References

1. Gan TJ, White PF, Scuderi PE et al (2002) FDA "black box" warning regarding use of droperidol for postoperative nausea and vomiting: is it justified? Anesthesiology 97:287
2. Deruddre S, Cheisson G, Mazoit JX et al (2007) Renal arterial resistance in septic shock: effects of increasing mean arterial pressure with norepinephrine on the renal resistive index assessed with Doppler ultrasonography. Intensive Care Med 33:1557–1562
3. Dewitte A, Coquin J, Meyssignac B et al (2012) Doppler resistive index to reflect regulation of renal vascular tone during sepsis and acute kidney injury. Crit Care 16:R165
4. Masuda M, Yamada T, Mine T et al (2007) Comparison of usefulness of sodium bicarbonate versus sodium chloride to prevent contrast-induced nephropathy in patients undergoing an emergent coronary procedure. Am J Cardiol 100:781–786
5. Merten GJ, Burgess WP, Gray LV et al (2004) Prevention of contrast-induced nephropathy with sodium bicarbonate: a randomized controlled trial. JAMA 291:2328–2334
6. Brar SS, Shen AY, Jorgensen MB et al (2008) Sodium bicarbonate vs sodium chloride for the prevention of contrast medium-induced nephropathy in patients undergoing coronary angiography: a randomized trial. JAMA 300:1038–1046
7. Haase M, Haase-Fielitz A, Plass M et al (2013) Prophylactic perioperative sodium bicarbonate to prevent acute kidney injury following open heart surgery: a multicenter double-blinded randomized controlled trial. PLoS Med 10:e1001426
8. Haase M, Haase-Fielitz A, Bellomo R et al (2009) Sodium bicarbonate to prevent increases in serum creatinine after cardiac surgery: a pilot double-blind, randomized controlled trial. Crit Care Med 37:39–47
9. Perner A, Haase N, Guttormsen AB et al (2012) Hydroxyethyl starch 130/0.42 versus Ringer's acetate in severe sepsis. N Engl J Med 367:124–134
10. Myburgh JA, Finfer S, Bellomo R et al (2012) Hydroxyethyl starch or saline for fluid resuscitation in intensive care. N Engl J Med 367:1901–1911
11. Annane D, Siami S, Jaber S et al (2013) Effects of fluid resuscitation with colloids vs crystalloids on mortality in critically ill patients presenting with hypovolemic shock: the CRISTAL randomized trial. JAMA 310:1809–1817
12. Martin C, Jacob M, Vicaut E et al (2013) Effect of waxy maize-derived hydroxyethyl starch 130/0.4 on renal function in surgical patients. Anesthesiology 118:387–394
13. Haase N, Perner A, Hennings LI et al (2013) Hydroxyethyl starch 130/0.38-0.45 versus crystalloid or albumin in patients with sepsis: systematic review with meta-analysis and trial sequential analysis. BMJ 346:f839
14. Perel P, Roberts I, Ker K (2013) Colloids versus crystalloids for fluid resuscitation in critically ill patients. Cochrane Database Syst Rev 2:CD000567
15. Zarychanski R, Abou-Setta AM, Turgeon AF et al (2013) Association of hydroxyethyl starch administration with mortality and acute kidney injury in critically ill patients requiring volume resuscitation: a systematic review and meta-analysis. JAMA 309:678–688
16. Schortgen F, Lacherade JC, Bruneel F et al (2001) Effects of hydroxyethyl starch and gelatin on renal function in severe sepsis: a multicentre randomised study. Lancet 357:911–916
17. Brunkhorst FM, Engel C, Bloos F et al (2008) Intensive insulin therapy and pentastarch resuscitation in severe sepsis. N Engl J Med 358:125–139

18. Martin C, Eon B, Saux P et al (1990) Renal effects of norepinephrine used to treat septic shock patients. Crit Care Med 18:282–285
19. Martin C, Papazian L, Perrin G et al (1993) Norepinephrine or dopamine for the treatment of hyperdynamic septic shock? Chest 10:1826–1831
20. De Backer D, Biston P, Devriendt J et al (2010) Comparison of dopamine and norepinephrine in the treatment of shock. N Engl J Med 362:779–789
21. Albanèse J, Leone M, Garnier F et al (2004) Renal effects of norepinephrine in septic and nonseptic patients. Chest 126:534–539
22. Patel BM, Chittock DR, Russell JA et al (2002) Beneficial effects of short-term vasopressin infusion during severe septic shock. Anesthesiology 96:576–582
23. Gordon AC, Russell JA, Walley KR et al (2010) The effects of vasopressin on acute kidney injury in septic shock. Intensive Care Med 36:83–91
24. Beauchamp D, Labrecque G (2001) Aminoglycoside nephrotoxicity: do time and frequency of administration matter? Curr Opin Crit Care 7:401–408
25. Harbarth S, Pestotnik SL, Lloyd JF et al (2001) The epidemiology of nephrotoxicity associated with conventional amphotericin B therapy. Am J Med 111:528–534
26. Walsh TJ, Finberg RW, Arndt C et al (1999) Liposomal amphotericin B for empirical therapy in patients with persistent fever and neutropenia. N Engl J Med 340:764–771
27. Rudnick MR, Goldfarb S, Wexler L et al (1995) Nephrotoxicity of ionic and nonionic contrast media in 1196 patients: a randomized trial. The Iohexol cooperative study. Kidney Int 47:254–261
28. Solomon RJ, Natarajan MK, Doucet S et al (2007) Cardiac Angiography in Renally Impaired Patients (CARE) study: a randomized double-blind trial of contrast-induced nephropathy in patients with chronic kidney disease. Circulation 115:3189–3196
29. Van den Berghe G, Wouters P, Weekers F et al (2001) Intensive insulin therapy in critically ill patients. N Engl J Med 345:1359–1367
30. Van den Berghe G, Wilmer A, Hermans G et al (2006) Intensive insulin therapy in the medical ICU. N Engl J Med 354:449–461
31. NICE-SUGAR Study Investigators (2012) Hypoglycemia and risk of death in critically ill patients. N Engl J Med 367:1108–1118
32. NICE-SUGAR Study Investigators (2009) Intensive versus conventional glucose control in critically ill patients. N Engl J Med 360:1283–1297
33. Cittanova ML, Zubicki A, Savu C et al (2001) The chronic inhibition of angiotensin-converting enzyme impairs postoperative renal function. Anesth Analg 93:1111–1115
34. Mouton R, Finch D, Davies I (2008) Effect of aprotinin on renal dysfunction in patients undergoing on-pump and off-pump cardiac surgery: a retrospective observational study. Lancet 371:475–482
35. Zacharias M, Mugawar M, Herbison GP et al (2013) Interventions for protecting renal function in the perioperative period. Cochrane Database Syst Rev 9:CD003590
36. Scott NB, Turfrey DJ, Ray DA et al (2001) A prospective randomized study of the potential benefits of thoracic epidural anesthesia and analgesia in patients undergoing coronary artery bypass grafting. Anesth Analg 93:528–535
37. Friedrich JO, Adhikari N, Herridge MS (2005) Meta-analysis: low-dose dopamine increases urine output but does not prevent renal dysfunction or death. Ann Intern Med 142:510–524
38. Rafouli-Stergiou P, Parissis JT, Anastasiou-Nana M (2012) Inotropes for the management of acute heart failure patients with renal dysfunction. Still an option? Expert Opin Pharmacother 13:2637–2647
39. Morelli A, Ricci Z, Bellomo R et al (2005) Prophylactic fenoldopam for renal protection in sepsis: a randomized, double-blind, placebo-controlled pilot trial. Crit Care Med 33:2451–2456
40. O'Hara JF Jr, Mahboobi R, Novak SM et al (2013) Fenoldopam and renal function after partial nephrectomy in a solitary kidney: a randomized, blinded trial. Urology 81:340–345
41. Landoni G, Biondi-Zoccai GG, Tumlin JA (2007) Beneficial impact of fenoldopam in critically ill patients with or at risk for acute renal failure: a meta-analysis of randomized clinical trials. Am J Kidney Dis 49:56–68

42. Landoni G, Biondi-Zoccai GG, Marino G (2008) Fenoldopam reduces the need for renal replacement therapy and in-hospital death in cardiovascular surgery: a meta-analysis. J Cardiothorac Vasc Anesth 22:27–33
43. Solomon R, Werner C, Mann D (1994) Effects of saline, mannitol, and furosemide to prevent acute decreases in renal function induced by radiocontrast agents. N Engl J Med 331:1416–1420
44. Cantarovich F, Rangoonwala B, Lorenz H et al (2004) High-dose furosemide for established ARF: a prospective, randomized, double-blind, placebo-controlled, multicenter trial. Am J Kidney Dis 44:402–409
45. Lassnigg A, Donner E, Grubhofer G et al (2000) Lack of renoprotective effects of dopamine and furosemide during cardiac surgery. J Am Soc Nephrol 11:97–104
46. Sampath S, Moran JL, Graham PL et al (2007) The efficacy of loop diuretics in acute renal failure: assessment using Bayesian evidence synthesis techniques. Crit Care Med 35:2516–2524
47. Mehta RL, Pascual MT, Soroko S et al (2002) Diuretics, mortality, and nonrecovery of renal function in acute renal failure. JAMA 288:2547–2553
48. Ho KM, Sheridan DJ (2006) Meta-analysis of frusemide to prevent or treat acute renal failure. BMJ 333:420
49. Alonso A, Lau J, Jaber BL, Weintraub A (2004) Prevention of radiocontrast nephropathy with N-acetylcysteine in patients with chronic kidney disease: a meta-analysis of randomized, controlled trials. Am J Kidney Dis 43:1–9
50. Shyu KG, Cheng JJ, Kuan P (2002) Acetylcysteine protects against acute renal damage in patients with abnormal renal function undergoing a coronary procedure. J Am Coll Cardiol 40:1383–1388

Part IV

Brain and Metabolic Disorders

Cerebral Metabolism and Function 12

Lionel Velly and Nicolas Bruder

The brain has an extremely active metabolism. The weight of the adult brain is approximately 1400 g representing 2% of body weight and at the same time accounts for 20% of oxygen (3 to 5 ml • 100 g^{-1} • min^{-1}) and 25% of glucose consumption in a subject at rest (31 μmol • 100 g^{-1} • min^{-1}). This brain metabolism requires a high cerebral blood flow (CBF) of approximately 750 mL • min^{-1} or 50 mL • 100 g^{-1} • min^{-1} equivalent to 15% of cardiac output at rest. The oxygen supply is in excess of oxygen consumption explaining a low cerebral extraction of oxygen (25–30%), but the brain has very little energy stores. This requires a very accurate and fast adaptation of CBF to cerebral metabolism. Another important anatomic characteristic of the brain is its containment in a rigid structure meaning that a change in volume gives rise to an exponential change in intracranial pressure (ICP) after volume compensation mechanisms are exceeded. Hence, the status of the cerebral circulation and its consequences on brain metabolism are very specific to this organ.

12.1 Relations of Cerebral Blood Flow and Metabolism

12.1.1 Cerebral Metabolism at the Cellular Level

Brain metabolism is mainly oxidative. Glucose is the main energy supply for the brain, but only a small amount of neuron metabolism comes directly from glucose. In 1994 Pellerin and Magistretti suggested a main role for astrocyte-neuron cooperation and a fundamental role of lactate (Fig. 12.1) [1, 2].

Glutamate, the main excitatory neurotransmitter of the brain, is released in the synaptic cleft upon depolarization and has to be rapidly removed to allow the next

L. Velly • N. Bruder (✉)
Département d'Anesthésie-Réanimation, CHU Timone, 264 rue St-Pierre,
13385 Marseille, Cedex, France
e-mail: nicolas.bruder@ap-hm.fr

C. Ichai et al. (eds.), *Metabolic Disorders and Critically Ill Patients*,
http://doi.org/10.1007/978-3-319-64010-5_12

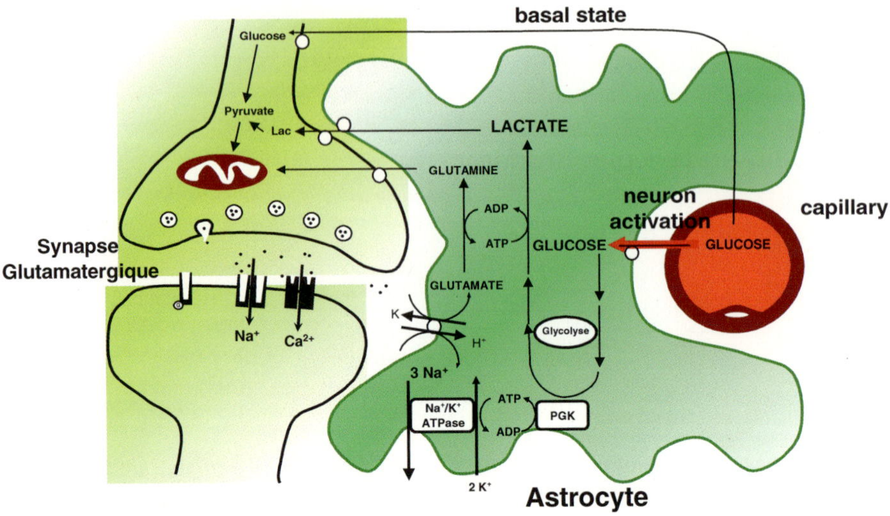

Fig. 12.1 Schematic representation of the astrocyte-neuron lactate shuttle. During neuron depolarization, glutamate is released in the synapse, activating glutamatergic receptors. Most of the glutamate released is taken up by astrocytes via specific transporters (EAAT, GLT1, GLAST), together with three Na^+. This increased intracellular Na+ is eliminated by the action of the Na^+/K^+ ATPase. This consumes ATP, produced through glycolysis. The lactate produced is shuttled to neurons through monocarboxylate transporters. In neurons, lactate is converted to pyruvate by LDH1 (Adapted from Pellerin and Magistretti [2])

transmission. This is accomplished by astrocyte uptake via specific transporters *(excitatory amino acid transporter* (EAAT)) using the electrochemical gradient of Na^+, resulting in a tight coupling between glutamate and Na^+ uptake. Glutamate is recycled in glutamine and taken up by neurons. The Na + gradient is maintained by activation of the Na^+/K^+ ATPase pump. Activation of glutamate transporters and activation of the Na^+/K^+ ATPase stimulate glucose uptake into astrocytes, undergoing glycolysis and releasing lactate. Lactate is taken up by neurons to be converted in pyruvate as the energy source of neurons. During short-lasting neuronal activity, oxidative metabolism is the default response to increased neural activity. After a longer period (> 10 s), astrocytic glycolysis is activated [3]. This astrocyte to neuron lactate shuttle allows a fast energy supply during neuron activation. At rest, the contribution of systemic lactate to cerebral energy metabolism is 8% but can increase up to 27% at high lactate blood concentrations [4]. After an acute traumatic brain injury, a study using brain microdialysis at the bedside showed that increased cerebral lactate was nonischemic but associated with increased glycolysis. This supports the idea that lactate can be used as an energy substrate by neurons [5]. In addition, lactate has been shown to be essential for long-term memory formation in rats. Thus, astrocytes are not only supporting cells but have a key role in maintaining brain homeostasis, delivering essential metabolites to neurons, and synthetizing or recycling neurotransmitters (glutamate) [6]. In fact, the confinement of glycolysis to astrocytes implies that ^{18}F-fluorodeoxyglucose PET studies measure glucose uptake into the glial instead of the neuronal compartment. The tight anatomical connections between astrocytes, capillaries, and blood vessels make astrocyte the ideal cell for the control and regulation of brain energy demand. The astrocytic end feet cover approximately 90% of the arterial surface of brain vessels making these cells ideal for the supply of nutrients to other cells.

12.1.2 Flow-Metabolism Coupling

In 1890, Roy and Sherrington hypothesized that brain blood flow should vary according to variations in functional activity and metabolism. Although there is a close coupling between regional CBF and cerebral metabolic rate of glucose (CMR_{glc}), cerebral oxygen consumption does not increase to the same extent than CMR_{glc}. This explains increased oxygen tension in response to activation. This uncoupling of flow and oxidative metabolism is the basis for the BOLD (blood-oxygenation-level dependent) effect used for functional magnetic resonance imaging. There are major variations in flow and metabolism between different areas of the brain. For example, gray matter CBF is 2–4 times white matter CBF. Nevertheless, cerebral oxygen extraction is uniform throughout the brain showing a tight coupling between metabolic supply and demand [7, 8]. During cognitive tasks, local CBF in activated tissue is limited to a 5% increase. There are several arguments for glutamate as the initial starter of neurovascular coupling. Glutamate is the main excitatory neurotransmitter in the brain, and the rate of the glutamate/glutamine cycle is 80% the rate of glucose oxidation in the cortex [9]. In addition, the increase in the glutamine/glutamate flux is tightly coupled to glucose oxidation. Astrocytes link neurons to vessels and are responsible for flow-metabolism coupling. According to the model proposed by Zonta et al., increased synaptic activity leads to glutamate release, activating metabotropic glutamate receptors. This activation triggers a calcium-dependent signal transmitted to other astrocytes and to astrocyte end feet [10]. The rise in intracellular calcium concentration activates phospholipase A2, leading to the production of prostaglandins inducing vasodilation. Thus, neurovascular coupling is a glutamate-mediated calcium-dependent mechanism [11]. Mitochondrial calcium homeostasis probably plays an important role in neurometabolic and neurovascular coupling [12].

CBF has to decrease more than 40% ($< 22\ mL \cdot 100\ g^{-1} \cdot min^{-1}$) to give rise to cerebral ischemia. This ischemic threshold has been questioned [13]. After an ischemic stroke, the ischemic threshold in the penumbra is around $8\ mL \cdot 100\ g^{-1} \cdot min^{-1}$ [14]. After a traumatic brain injury, the threshold for ischemia was $15\ mL \cdot 100\ g^{-1} \cdot min^{-1}$ for CBF, $36.7\ \mu mol \cdot 100\ g^{-1} \cdot min^{-1}$ for $CMRO_2$, and 25.9% for oxygen extraction [15, 16]. All studies showed considerable heterogeneity between and within patients and marked overlap between viable and ischemic brain tissue. The reason why no specific CBF threshold can be determined is that many metabolic pathways can lead to cell necrosis independently of tissue perfusion.

12.2 Regulation of CBF

12.2.1 Pressure Autoregulation of CBF

The stability of CBF for a large range of blood pressure values is a characteristic of the cerebral circulation. It is usually accepted that CBF is constant for mean arterial pressure (MAP) between 50 and 150 mmHg, corresponding to the plateau of autoregulation (Fig. 12.2).

In pathological states, it is important to consider cerebral perfusion pressure (CPP = MAP – ICP) instead of MAP when ICP may be high. However, the first publication by Lassen leading the way to the concept of autoregulation was a compilation of several studies in few subjects, including very few points toward the lower limit of autoregulation [17]. Further studies found various lower thresholds for autoregulation from less than 40–100 mmHg in individuals [18]. In a more recent study using transcranial Doppler to assess relative changes in CBF, the authors found a close relation between MAP and CBF, with a mean change in CBF velocity of 0.82% per millimeter of mercury change in mean blood pressure [19]. In addition, pulsatility index increased as MAP decreased indicating that diastolic velocity is affected more than systolic velocity during hypotension. Changes in cortical oxygenation index (near-infrared spectroscopy) were inversely related to

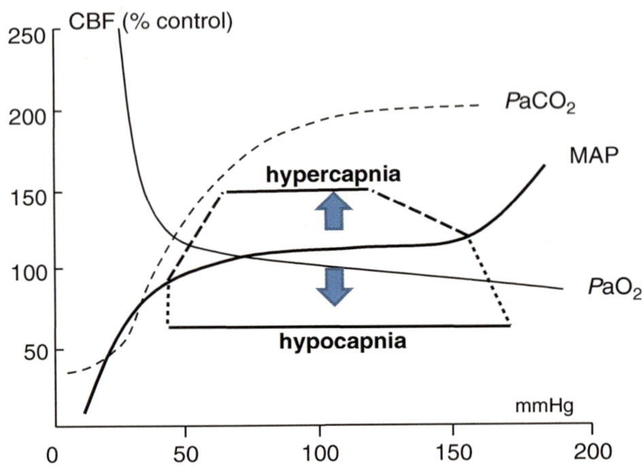

Fig. 12.2 Influence of PaO_2 and $PaCO_2$ mean arterial pressure (MAP) on cerebral blood flow (CBF). The effect of decreasing PaO_2 (hypoxia) is significant only for low values, less than 58 mmHg. A PaO_2 value at 30 mmHg nearly doubles CBF. CBF increases 2–5% for every mm change in $PaCO_2$. Below 20 mmHg or above 80 mmHg, $PaCO_2$ has little effect on CBF. CBF remains constant for MAP values between 50 and 150 mmHg, corresponding to the plateau of autoregulation. Hypercapnia increases CBF, shifts the plateau upward, and shifts the lower limit of autoregulation to the right and the upper limit to the left, reducing the plateau. Hypocapnia decreases CBF, has no effect on the lower limit of autoregulation, and shifts the upper limit to the right, increasing the length of the plateau

changes in MAP. These data show that changes in CBF in the presence of fluctuations of MAP do not imply a defective cerebral autoregulation.

12.2.2 Cardiac Output and Cerebral Blood Flow

Obviously, there should be a relation between cardiac output (CO) and CBF. However, this relation is confounded by the influence of CO on blood pressure. Grossly, there is about a 10% CBF decrease for a 30% CO reduction [20]. However, differences in methodologies used to vary CO and assess CBF make interpretation of results from different studies difficult. CBF is reduced in patients with chronic heart failure and may be related to cognitive dysfunction. However, the relationship between CO and CBF is complex and also involves changes in sympathetic tone, blood pressure, cardiac rhythm, and hormonal changes [21]. In other situations like awakening from general anesthesia [22] or after a brain injury [23], CBF is maintained despite significant changes in CO. The conceptual framework on the influence of CO on CBF is a shift of the plateau of autoregulation downward when CO is reduced and upward when CO is augmented. The autonomic nervous system plays an important role in CBF regulation during acute changes in CO [20].

12.2.3 Myogenic, Neurogenic, and Metabolic Regulation of CBF

The first suggestion of smooth muscle contraction of the vessel wall in response to an increase in intraluminal pressure has been formulated more than a century ago [24]. The demonstration of pressure-induced myogenic responses in human cerebral arteries is more recent [25]. Myogenic regulation refers to the influence of mechanical stress or strain on vascular smooth muscle tone. Transmural pressure elevation gives rise to vasoconstriction and pressure reduction to vasodilation [26]. This response has been demonstrated for arterioles of 300 μm diameter and for a pressure range between 20 and 90 mmHg. This response did not depend on an intact endothelium showing a pure myogenic mechanism. This regulation is very rapid with a time constant of a few seconds, typically less than 10 s. Increased shear stress on the vessel wall stimulates NO release by the endothelium. This produces vessel relaxation, reducing shear stress. This response has been shown at the arterial and arteriolar level. This is a slow response with a time constant around 60 s. Intracarotid infusion of a NO synthase inhibitor (N-monomethyl-L-arginine (L-NMMA)) induces a 20% decrease in CBF [27, 28]. By contrast, intracarotid infusion of a NO donor (sodium nitroprusside) does not change CBF [29].

Many metabolic pathways have been implicated in cerebral autoregulation. Carbon dioxide (CO_2) has a major influence on the cerebral circulation. It has been postulated that venous CO_2 produced by metabolism can diffuse to the arterioles causing vasodilation. The role of CO_2 on the cerebral circulation will be summarized later in this review. Many other metabolites (potassium, H^+, adenosine, NO, etc.) have been implicated as playing a role in cerebral autoregulation. As mentioned earlier, astrocytes participate in the metabolic regulation of autoregulation by releasing K^+ or downstream metabolites of arachidonic acid.

Cerebral vessels are extensively innervated by adrenergic and cholinergic fibers. A role of the autonomic nervous system in the regulation of CBF has been demonstrated although its importance remains controversial. Activation of the sympathetic nervous system decreases CBF. Surgical stellate ganglionectomy showed increased CBF, and excision of the inferior cervical ganglion was shown to reduce cerebrovascular resistances [30]. Superior cervical ganglionectomy with carotid perivascular sympathectomy has been used in patients with vasospasm after SAH to induce vasodilation. Most studies using stellate ganglion block show an increased CBF, mostly on the ipsilateral side of intervention. Both direct innervation of the cerebral arteries from cervical ganglia and stimulation of adrenergic receptors by circulating sympathomimetics prevent sudden increases of CBF associated with hypertension and hypercapnia. It may be that under normal physiological conditions, myogenic control of cerebral vasomotor tone is dominant and that neurogenic control has little influence [31]. Sympathetic activation may have deleterious consequences on the brain. During hemorrhage it may explain that hypotension is less well tolerated than pharmacological-induced hypotension at the same blood pressure level [32]. Conversely, sympathetic stimulation could protect the brain in hypertensive crisis. The rich distribution of cholinergic nerve terminals near cerebral vessels suggests a role of the parasympathetic nervous system on autoregulation. However, little is known on the role of the cholinergic control in cerebral autoregulation.

12.2.4 CO_2 Regulation of CBF

CBF is highly sensitive to changes in $PaCO_2$. There is an approximate 3–6% change in CBF per mmHg change in $PaCO_2$ in a large range of values, approximately from 20 to 70 mmHg. Hypercapnia causes vasodilation and increases CBF, and hypocapnia causes vasoconstriction and decreases CBF. There is no significant change in oxidative metabolism during $PaCO_2$ variations [33]. The effect of CO_2 is mainly on pial arteries, but some changes in large vessel diameter have also been demonstrated [30]. The mechanism of the arterial response to CO_2 is independent on the arterial pH and is probably due to the diffusion of CO_2 across the blood-brain barrier inducing a change in pH in the extracellular space of the vessel. Since cerebral autoregulation is based on changes in vasomotor tone, it is not surprising that changes in $PaCO_2$ affect the lower and upper limit of autoregulation. Hypercapnia causes cerebral vasodilation and shifts the lower limit of autoregulation to the right and the upper limit to the left, thus reducing the plateau of autoregulation. The threshold at which $PaCO_2$ significantly impaired autoregulation ranged from 50 to 66 mmHg in anesthetized patients [34]. Hypocapnia decreases CBF by cerebral vasoconstriction. Hypocapnia does not seem to shift the lower limit of autoregulation. It is possible that vasodilation caused by hypotension overrides hypocapnic vasoconstriction. It is not clear whether hypocapnia changes the upper limit of autoregulation or not [35]. The blood pressure level has an important effect on the cerebrovascular response to

CO_2. The cerebrovascular reactivity to CO_2 is attenuated or abolished at a MAP of 50 mmHg either due to hemorrhage or drug induction. In pathological conditions, modest hypocapnia may give rise to cerebral ischemia by reducing CBF without affecting cerebral metabolism [36]. Hypercapnia may worsen intracranial pressure by increasing blood brain volume in patients with intracranial hypertension and cause cerebral vasogenic edema [37]. However, hypercapnia may also afford neuroprotection in rat models of ischemia/reperfusion [38, 39]. This neuroprotection is not related to changes in CBF but to reduced apoptosis due to modulation of apoptosis-regulating proteins (Bax and Bcl-2).

12.3 Vasoactive Agents and CBF

The literature on vasoactive agents and CBF is difficult to interpret due to methodological concerns. Intravenous infusion of vasoconstrictive and vasodilating agents may change the cerebral circulation either by a direct effect on cerebral vessels or by activation of autoregulation. Noninvasive assessment of cerebral oxygenation by near-infrared spectroscopy may also be disturbed by changes in skin blood flow [40]. In the intact brain, vasoconstrictors (norepinephrine, phenylephrine) do not cross the blood-brain barrier and do not cause cerebral vasoconstriction [41]. Following norepinephrine infusion in volunteers, cerebrovascular resistance increased due to an increase in MAP (normal autoregulation) but not to an alpha-receptor-mediated cerebral vasoconstriction [42]. In anesthetized patients, the response may vary depending on the anesthetic used and its impact on autoregulation. In healthy volunteers, sympathomimetic agents (ephedrine, dobutamine, or dopexamine) did not change the strength of autoregulation or the reactivity to CO_2 [43]. Conversely, calcium blockers have a direct vasodilatory effect on the cerebral circulation. Conversely, intracarotid verapamil decreases both proximal and distal cerebrovascular resistances and gives rise to a 40% increase in CBF [44]. Beta-adrenergic blocking agents have no effect on the cerebral circulation and do not affect cerebral vasoreactivity and cerebral autoregulation [45]. This is true only in physiological conditions. In animals or humans during stress and activation of the sympathetic nervous system, beta-blockers mitigate the increase in CBF related to the stressful event. A clinical example is recovery from general anesthesia after neurosurgery where esmolol blunted early postoperative cerebral hyperemia related to recovery from anesthesia [46, 47].

12.4 Physiological Factors Affecting CBF

12.4.1 Age

In adults, CBF decreases with age. The mean CBF in subjects aged 19–29 years is 748 mL • min^{-1} and decreases to 474 mL • min^{-1} between 80 and 89 years [48]. The yearly decrease in age is 4.8 mL • min^{-1} or approximately 0.5% per year [7]. This decrease is related to neuronal loss and brain metabolism explaining that the ratio of CBF and brain weight remains constant. The decrease in CBF is variable among brain regions. CBF and CMRO2 decrease mostly in association areas (frontal and parietal cortices) but are relatively spared in the primary motor and sensory areas [49]. However, considerable variations may occur in patients with cerebrovascular disease. In children, CBF reaches a maximum value toward 10 years after birth [50]. Studies using transcranial Doppler have shown that CBF increases rapidly between birth and 3 weeks of age and then more slowly and finally decreases from adolescence to older age [51].

12.4.2 Hypoxia

Unlike the cerebrovascular response to changes in PaCO2, hypoxemia causes little change in CBF until a very low hemoglobin saturation in oxygen (80% arterial saturation of O2). In the physiological range for oxygenation, arterial oxygen content has not influenced on CBF. However, severe hypoxemia ($PaO_2 < 50$ mmHg) is a potent stimulus of arterial vasodilation [52]. During hypoxia, CBF increases in order to maintain oxygen delivery to the brain [53]. The mechanisms of vasodilation during hypoxia include activation of membrane potassium channels, interference with transmembrane calcium flux, adenosine release, and nitric oxide synthesis [30]. The effect of hypoxia on CBF is confounded by extracellular acidosis and hypocapnia due to hyperventilation.

12.4.3 Hemodilution

CBF varies inversely with hematocrit in order to maintain oxygen delivery to the brain. The increase is 2% for every decrease in hematocrit value of 1% and for hematocrit values between 40% and 30% [54]. CBF augmentation is due to both a decrease in blood viscosity and a decrease in arterial oxygen content [55]. Arterial oxygen content has the main influence on CBF during hemodilution, but CBF augmentation does not fully compensate for the decrease in oxygen content, reducing oxygen delivery [56]. For hematocrit values below 20%, compensatory mechanisms for reduced oxygen content are exhausted, and CBF depends only on changes in blood viscosity [57]. Pial arteriolar reactivity to hypocapnia but not to hypercapnia is impaired during hemodilution [58].

12.4.4 Temperature

Cerebral blood flow and metabolism are extremely sensitive to changes in temperature. The brain temperature is approximately 1 °C higher than body temperature, but a higher gradient may be found in diseases inducing brain inflammation as brain trauma, subarachnoid hemorrhage, stroke, meningitis, etc. Thus, the role of the cerebral circulation is to cool the brain. Hypothermia decreases CBF and metabolism. $CMRO_2$ and CMR_{glc} decrease by between two- and fourfold with a 10 °C reduction in temperature from 37 °C to 27 °C [59]. Within this temperature range, CBF declines in parallel with $CMRO_2$ or CMR_{glc}. This suggests that cerebral autoregulation is maintained until a temperature around 27 °C. Below 27 °C, there are controversies on the relation between brain temperature and metabolism. Some studies find a linear decrease in metabolism during hypothermia; others report a much larger decrease in metabolism below 27 °C [60]. This may be real or due to methodological or species differences. The decrease in CMR_{glc} is parallel to the $CMRO_2$ reduction. The low brain metabolism under 20 °C allows prolonged periods of circulatory arrest (> 30 min), without any ischemic brain damage, for the purpose of cardiac or aortic repair. Below 27–28 °C, the decrease in metabolic rate is larger than the decrease in CBF showing uncoupling between flow and metabolism. CBF depends on acid-base management (α-stat versus pH-stat management). Uncoupling between CBF and metabolism is much larger with pH-stat management, where $PaCO_2$ is increased. During mild hypothermia, $PaCO_2$ changes may explain most of CBF variations [61].

12.5 CBF After Acute Brain Injury

12.5.1 Cerebral Autoregulation in Disease States

A considerable literature has been published on cerebral autoregulation after brain injury (brain trauma, stroke, subarachnoid hemorrhage, encephalitis, brain edema, etc.). It is only possible here to give some clues on the impact of diseases on CBF regulation.

While non-injured brain present cerebral autoregulation which is directly, all pathological states affecting cerebral vasomotor tone disturb autoregulation. Obviously, chronic arterial hypertension or vascular disease alters autoregulation [62, 63]. Chronic hypertension shifts the lower limit of autoregulation to the right with an impaired tolerance to pressure decrease. With chronic antihypertensive treatment, CBF autoregulation may readapt toward normal. Conversely, severe hypertension with autoregulation failure may lead to severe cerebral edema and encephalopathy [62].

Cerebral autoregulation may be altered after any kind of acute brain injury. Even a mild brain trauma may result in loss of autoregulation [64]. Altered autoregulation has been demonstrated after brain trauma, stroke and subarachnoid hemorrhage (SAH), meningitis or encephalitis, and hepatic failure. Autoregulation failure has been shown to have prognostic value. After SAH, poor-grade patients exhibit autoregulatory failure, while autoregulation is preserved in good-grade patients. At the subacute phase of SAH, delayed cerebral vasospasm can cause failure of autoregulation. This explains that the brain is at high risk of delayed ischemia especially with fluctuations in blood pressure [65]. Monitoring of autoregulation at the bedside may help screening patients at high risk of delayed cerebral ischemia and put more attention on blood pressure management.

12.5.2 Assessment of CBF and Autoregulation

12.5.2.1 Arterio-jugular Difference of Oxygen Content ($AJDO_2$)

Assessment of CBF derived from AJDO2 is derived from Kety and Schmidt's original work [66]. Their technique is based on the Fick principle as for the measure of cardiac output. Kety and Schmidt used 15% N_2O as an inert tracer and draw blood samples in the jugular bulb. More recently, other methods using radioactive tracers as ^{85}Krypton or ^{133}Xenon have been developed [67]. The main limitation to these methods is the use of radioactive agents. The same principle may be adapted to thermodilution techniques. Several methods have been described but have not gained popularity due to poor accuracy or technical complexity [68, 69]. Assuming constant arterial oxygenation and hemoglobin concentration, jugular venous bulb saturation in oxygen (SjO_2) variations reflect changes in CBF. Jugular venous desaturation indicates cerebral hypoperfusion and has been associated with poor outcome after head injury [70]. Elevated SjO_2 is common and difficult to interpret as it may be related to hyperemia or low cerebral oxygen consumption. It has been also associated with poor outcome [71]. Finally, there are large differences in SjO_2 between the right and the left jugular veins, without any agreement between measurements on both sides [72], explaining that this monitoring technique is seldom used nowadays.

12.5.2.2 Positron Emission Tomography (PET)

It is the reference method for the measurement of cerebral blood flow and metabolism. It uses markers labeled with isotopes that emit radiations. For example, a popular tracer, ^{18}F-deoxyglucose (^{18}FDG), is used to measure glucose metabolism, and $H_2{}^{15}O$ may be used to measure CBF (half-life of oxygen-15 2 min). Hence, a real assessment of flow-metabolism coupling is possible with PET. The association of radiation measurement and a CT scan allows measurement of regional differences in flow and metabolism. With this technique, gray matter CBF was 60 ml • 100 g^{-1} • min^{-1} and white matter CBF 20 ml • 100 g^{-1} • min^{-1} [73]. High costs and exposure to ionizing radiations limit the use of this technique in intensive care. PET analysis in anesthetized patients revealed a decrease in $CMRO_2$ and CBF to 50–70% of the baseline with sevoflurane or propofol. However, these agents had a different effect on cerebral blood volume, which was reduced by propofol only [74]. In disorders of consciousness, 18FDG PET showed high sensitivity to detect minimally conscious state. Patients with locked-in syndrome are clearly identified as conscious by PET imaging (Fig. 12.3) [75].

12.5.2.3 Single Photon Emission Computed Tomography (SPECT)

SPECT detects emitted photon with gamma cameras of an injected radionuclide to quantify regional CBF. Technecium-99m-hexamethylpropyleneamine oxime

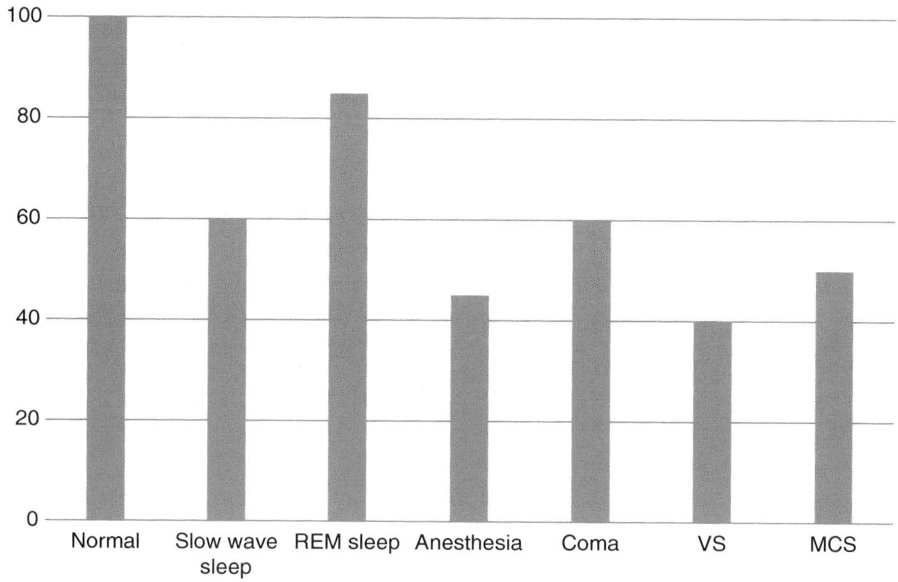

Fig. 12.3 Schematic representation of brain metabolism compared to normal awake subjects (100%) during sleep, anesthesia, coma, vegetative state (VS), and minimally conscious state (MCS)

(^{99m}Tc-HMPAO) is the most popular radionuclide to measure CBF. It has a relatively long halftime precluding repeated measurements within a short time period.

12.5.2.4 Magnetic Resonance Imaging (MRI)

Arterial spin labeling (ASL) is a promising MRI technique to measure CBF. Blood water is magnetically labeled in the carotid artery by applying radiofrequency pulses and used as a tracer to measure CBF. Because ASL is noninvasive, the measure is repeated several times in order to improve the signal to noise ratio. Studies comparing ASL to ^{15}O-water PET found good accuracy and reproducible CBF measurements [76]. This method has still to be improved and validated in patients to be used clinically. Functional MRI (fMRI) has been used to detect consciousness in unresponsive patients for the differential diagnosis of minimally conscious state and vegetative state. However, fMRI is more technically challenging than PET for this purpose and has a lower sensitivity. The appropriate cognitive task to use in patients in minimally conscious state is probably crucial to obtain results, because the patients may not understand the task or do not have the drive to participate [75].

12.5.2.5 Transcranial Doppler

Transcranial Doppler (TCD) ultrasonography was introduced in clinical practice by Aaslid in 1982. It measures the velocity of red blood cells in the cerebral arteries. Velocity depends on CBF and vessel diameter, which is unknown. Hence the correlation between CBF velocity and absolute CBF is very poor. However, providing that the vessel diameter remains constant, changes in velocities closely reflect changes in flow

(Table 12.1). Thus, TCD has been extensively used to study static and dynamic autoregulation or response to CO_2. There are several methods to assess cerebrovascular reactivity with TCD. Velocities may be used as a surrogate of flow to calculate changes in cerebrovascular resistance (MAP/CBF velocity). The percentage change in estimated cerebrovascular resistance per 1% change in MAP gives an index of autoregulation. Continuous monitoring of TCD allows calculation of correlation coefficients between flow velocity and cerebral perfusion pressure [77]. A low coefficient (no correlation) indicates maintained autoregulation, and a high coefficient indicates that flow is pressure dependent. Another simple test using TCD to assess autoregulation is the transient hyperemic response test (Fig. 12.4). This test uses carotid compression to induce downstream arteriolar vasodilation due to reduced perfusion pressure. After release of the compression, a transient hyperemia is observed related to arteriolar vasodilation. The THR ratio is normally above 1:10. TCD is noninvasive and can be repeated as often as needed at the bedside or for continuous monitoring [78]. There are studies showing that TCD upon admission of patients with mild or moderate head injury may predict neurologic outcome a few days later [79]. After a traumatic brain injury, zero-flow diastolic velocity indicates impending cerebral circulatory arrest requiring emergency treatments to improve CBF [80]. Vasospasm after SAH is characterized by high TCD velocities. There is no association between CBF or changes in CBF and blood flow velocities in this case. Decreasing velocities may indicate improvement of vasospasm or, on the opposite, very severe ischemic vasospasm with reduced CBF [81]. Finally, there are specific TCD patterns of cerebral circulatory arrest for the diagnosis of brain death.

Table 12.1 Cerebral blood flow velocities and pulsatility index: normal values

	Depth (mm)	Mean	Diastolic	Systolic	RI	PI
MCA	40–55	62 ± 12	45 ± 10	90 ± 16	0.4–0.7	0.90 ± 0.24
ACA	60–75	50 ± 13	35 ± 10	71 ± 18		0.83 ± 0.17
PCA	55–80	37 ± 10	26 ± 7	53 ± 11		0.88 ± 0.20
BA	85–100	39 ± 9	31 ± 9	52 ± 9		

MCA middle cerebral artery, *ACA* anterior cerebral artery, *PCA* posterior cerebral artery, *TB* basilar artery, *RI* resistivity index, *PI* pulsatility index

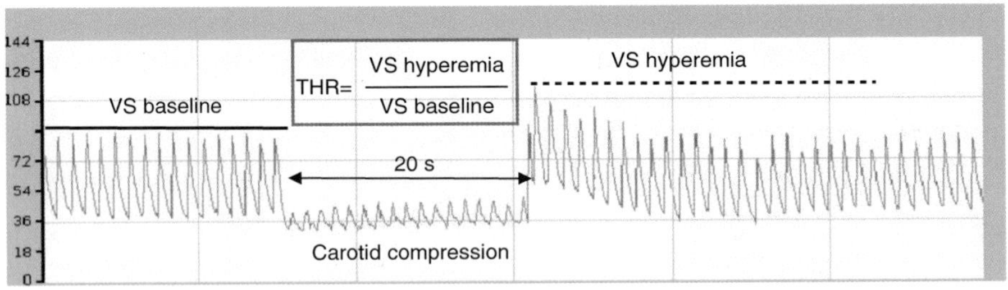

Fig. 12.4 Recording of cerebral blood flow velocity in the middle cerebral artery at the baseline, during carotid compression and after release of the compression. A ratio between the systolic velocity after and before the compression above 1:10 indicates maintained cerebral autoregulation

In conclusion, a precise and fast-acting regulation of CBF is critical to maintain cerebral metabolism and function. Several regulatory mechanisms act together to supply adequate oxygen and nutrient delivery to the brain, at rest and during activation. For clarity, these mechanisms are often reviewed independently. However, the final effect is mostly arteriolar vasodilation or vasoconstriction, which is anatomically limited. Thus, CO_2 reactivity, for example, cannot induce any change in CBF in the context of maximal vasodilation due to low blood pressure. In pathological states, assessment of cerebrovascular reactivity and autoregulation is important for prognostication and also to individualize hemodynamic and respiratory management in brain-injured patients. At present, transcranial Doppler is most used at the bedside, but there is no reliable noninvasive monitoring of brain oxygenation. Development of new monitoring of metabolism and flow is expected to improve our understanding of brain circulation changes after an acute brain injury.

References

1. Magistretti PJ (2009) Neuroscience. Low-cost travel in neurons. Science 325:1349–1351
2. Magistretti PJ, Pellerin L, Rothman DL, Shulman RG (1999) Energy on demand. Science 283:496–497
3. Kasischke KA, Vishwasrao HD, Fisher PJ et al (2004) Neural activity triggers neuronal oxidative metabolism followed by astrocytic glycolysis. Science 305:99–103
4. van Hall G, Stromstad M, Rasmussen P et al (2009) Blood lactate is an important energy source for the human brain. J Cereb Blood Flow Metab 29:1121–1129
5. Sala N, Suys T, Zerlauth JB et al (2013) Cerebral extracellular lactate increase is predominantly nonischemic in patients with severe traumatic brain injury. J Cereb Blood Flow Metab 33:1815–1822
6. Belanger M, Allaman I, Magistretti PJ (2011) Brain energy metabolism: focus on astrocyte-neuron metabolic cooperation. Cell Metab 14:724–738
7. Leenders KL, Perani D, Lammertsma AA et al (1990) Cerebral blood flow, blood volume and oxygen utilization. Normal values and effect of age. Brain 113(Pt 1):27–47
8. Fazekas F, Niederkorn K, Schmidt R et al (1988) White matter signal abnormalities in normal individuals: correlation with carotid ultrasonography, cerebral blood flow measurements, and cerebrovascular risk factors. Stroke 19:1285–1288
9. Shen J, Petersen KF, Behar KL et al (1999) Determination of the rate of the glutamate/glutamine cycle in the human brain by in vivo 13C NMR. Proc Natl Acad Sci U S A 96:8235–8240
10. Zonta M, Angulo MC, Gobbo S et al (2003) Neuron-to-astrocyte signaling is central to the dynamic control of brain microcirculation. Nat Neurosci 6:43–50
11. Attwell D, Buchan AM, Charpak S et al (2010) Glial and neuronal control of brain blood flow. Nature 468:232–243
12. Kannurpatti SS (2017) Mitochondrial calcium homeostasis: implications for neurovascular and neurometabolic coupling. J Cereb Blood Flow Metab 37:381–395
13. Botteri M, Bandera E, Minelli C, Latronico N (2008) Cerebral blood flow thresholds for cerebral ischemia in traumatic brain injury. A systematic review. Crit Care Med 36:3089–3092
14. Bandera E, Botteri M, Minelli C et al (2006) Cerebral blood flow threshold of ischemic penumbra and infarct core in acute ischemic stroke: a systematic review. Stroke 37:1334–1339
15. Coles JP, Cunningham AS, Salvador R et al (2009) Early metabolic characteristics of lesion and nonlesion tissue after head injury. J Cereb Blood Flow Metab 29:965–975
16. Cunningham AS, Salvador R, Coles JP et al (2005) Physiological thresholds for irreversible tissue damage in contusional regions following traumatic brain injury. Brain 128:1931–1942

17. Lassen NA (1959) Cerebral blood flow and oxygen consumption in man. Physiol Rev 39:183–238
18. Drummond JC (1997) The lower limit of autoregulation: time to revise our thinking? Anesthesiology 86:1431–1433
19. Lucas SJ, Tzeng YC, Galvin SD et al (2010) Influence of changes in blood pressure on cerebral perfusion and oxygenation. Hypertension 55:698–705
20. Meng L, Hou W, Chui J et al (2015) Cardiac output and cerebral blood flow: the integrated regulation of brain perfusion in adult humans. Anesthesiology 123:1198–1208
21. Gruhn N, Larsen FS, Boesgaard S et al (2001) Cerebral blood flow in patients with chronic heart failure before and after heart transplantation. Stroke 32:2530–2533
22. Grillo P, Bruder N, Auquier P et al (2003) Esmolol blunts the cerebral blood flow velocity increase during emergence from anesthesia in neurosurgical patients. Anesth Analg 96:1145–1149
23. Bouma G, Muizelaar J (1990) Relationship between cardiac output and cerebral blood flow in patients with intact and with impaired autoregulation. J Neurosurg 73:368–374
24. Bayliss W (1902) On the local reaction of the arterial wall to changes in intraluminal pressure. J Physiol 28:220–231
25. Wallis SJ, Firth J, Dunn WR (1996) Pressure-induced myogenic responses in human isolated cerebral resistance arteries. Stroke 27:2287–2290. discussion 2291
26. Spronck B, Martens EG, Gommer ED, van de Vosse FN (2012) A lumped parameter model of cerebral blood flow control combining cerebral autoregulation and neurovascular coupling. Am J Physiol Heart Circ Physiol 303:H1143–H1153
27. Joshi S, Young WL, Duong DH et al (2000) Intracarotid infusion of the nitric oxide synthase inhibitor, L-NMMA, modestly decreases cerebral blood flow in human subjects. Anesthesiology 93:699–707
28. Thompson BG, Pluta RM, Girton ME, Oldfield EH (1996) Nitric oxide mediation of chemoregulation but not autoregulation of cerebral blood flow in primates. J Neurosurg 84:71–78
29. Joshi S, Young WL, Duong H et al (2002) Intracarotid nitroprusside does not augment cerebral blood flow in human subjects. Anesthesiology 96:60–66
30. Willie CK, Tzeng YC, Fisher JA, Ainslie PN (2014) Integrative regulation of human brain blood flow. J Physiol 592:841–859
31. Umeyama T, Kugimiya T, Ogawa T et al (1995) Changes in cerebral blood flow estimated after stellate ganglion block by single photon emission computed tomography. J Auton Nerv Syst 50:339–346
32. Pearce WJ, D'Alecy LG (1980) Hemorrhage-induced cerebral vasoconstriction in dogs. Stroke 11:190–197
33. Chen JJ, Pike GB (2010) Global cerebral oxidative metabolism during hypercapnia and hypocapnia in humans: implications for BOLD fMRI. J Cereb Blood Flow Metab 30:1094–1099
34. McCulloch TJ, Visco E, Lam AM (2000) Graded hypercapnia and cerebral autoregulation during sevoflurane or propofol anesthesia. Anesthesiology 93:1205–1209
35. Meng L, Gelb AW (2015) Regulation of cerebral autoregulation by carbon dioxide. Anesthesiology 122:196–205
36. Menon DK, Coles JP, Gupta AK et al (2004) Diffusion limited oxygen delivery following head injury. Crit Care Med 32:1384–1390
37. Joyce RR, McGee WT (2011) Hypercapnic cerebral edema presenting in a woman with asthma: a case report. J Med Case Rep 5:192
38. Tao T, Liu Y, Zhang J et al (2013) Therapeutic hypercapnia improves functional recovery and attenuates injury via antiapoptotic mechanisms in a rat focal cerebral ischemia/reperfusion model. Brain Res 1533:52–62
39. Zhou Q, Cao B, Niu L et al (2010) Effects of permissive hypercapnia on transient global cerebral ischemia-reperfusion injury in rats. Anesthesiology 112:288–297
40. Sorensen H, Secher NH, Siebenmann C et al (2012) Cutaneous vasoconstriction affects near-infrared spectroscopy determined cerebral oxygen saturation during administration of norepinephrine. Anesthesiology 117:263–270

41. Strebel SP, Kindler C, Bissonnette B et al (1998) The impact of systemic vasoconstrictors on the cerebral circulation of anesthetized patients. Anesthesiology 89:67–72
42. Kimmerly DS, Tutungi E, Wilson TD et al (2003) Circulating norepinephrine and cerebrovascular control in conscious humans. Clin Physiol Funct Imaging 23:314–319
43. Moppett IK, Wild MJ, Sherman RW et al (2004) Effects of ephedrine, dobutamine and dopexamine on cerebral haemodynamics: transcranial Doppler studies in healthy volunteers. Br J Anaesth 92:39–44
44. Joshi S, Meyers PM, Pile-Spellman J et al (2004) Intracarotid verapamil decreases both proximal and distal human cerebrovascular resistance. Anesthesiology 100:774–781
45. Heinke W, Zysset S, Hund-Georgiadis M et al (2005) The effect of esmolol on cerebral blood flow, cerebral vasoreactivity, and cognitive performance: a functional magnetic resonance imaging study. Anesthesiology 102:41–50
46. Bruder N, Pellissier D, Grillot P, Gouin F (2002) Cerebral hyperemia during recovery from general anesthesia in neurosurgical patients. Anesth Analg 94:650–654
47. Bryan RMJ (1990) Cerebral blood flow and energy metabolism during stress. Am J Phys 259:H269–H280
48. Buijs PC, Krabbe-Hartkamp MJ, Bakker CJ et al (1998) Effect of age on cerebral blood flow: measurement with ungated two-dimensional phase-contrast MR angiography in 250 adults. Radiology 209:667–674
49. Aanerud J, Borghammer P, Chakravarty MM et al (2012) Brain energy metabolism and blood flow differences in healthy aging. J Cereb Blood Flow Metab 32:1177–1187
50. Kennedy C, Sokoloff L (1957) An adaptation of the nitrous oxide method to the study of the cerebral circulation in children; normal values for cerebral blood flow and cerebral metabolic rate in childhood. J Clin Invest 36:1130–1137
51. Fischer A, Truemper E (1993) Transcranial Doppler applications in the neonate and child. In: Babikian V, Wechsler L (eds) Transcranial Doppler ultrasonography. Mosby, St-Louis, pp 282–302
52. Brown MM, Wade JP, Marshall J (1985) Fundamental importance of arterial oxygen content in the regulation of cerebral blood flow in man. Brain 108(Pt 1):81–93
53. Shapiro W, Wasserman AJ, Baker JP, Patterson JL Jr (1970) Cerebrovascular response to acute hypocapnic and eucapnic hypoxia in normal man. J Clin Invest 49:2362–2368
54. Bruder N, Cohen B, Pellissier D, Francois G (1998) The effect of hemodilution on cerebral blood flow velocity in anesthetized patients. Anesth Analg 86:320–324
55. Tomiyama Y, Jansen K, Brian JE Jr, Todd MM (1999) Hemodilution, cerebral O2 delivery, and cerebral blood flow: a study using hyperbaric oxygenation. Am J Phys 276:H1190–H1196
56. Hoiland RL, Bain AR, Rieger MG et al (2016) Hypoxemia, oxygen content, and the regulation of cerebral blood flow. Am J Physiol Regul Integr Comp Physiol 310:R398–R413
57. Rebel A, Lenz C, Krieter H et al (2001) Oxygen delivery at high blood viscosity and decreased arterial oxygen content to brains of conscious rats. Am J Physiol Heart Circ Physiol 280:H2591–H2597
58. Rebel A, Ulatowski JA, Kwansa H et al (2003) Cerebrovascular response to decreased hematocrit: effect of cell-free hemoglobin, plasma viscosity, and CO2. Am J Physiol Heart Circ Physiol 285:H1600–H1608
59. Erecinska M, Thoresen M, Silver IA (2003) Effects of hypothermia on energy metabolism in mammalian central nervous system. J Cereb Blood Flow Metab 23:513–530
60. Michenfelder JD, Milde JH (1991) The relationship among canine brain temperature, metabolism, and function during hypothermia. Anesthesiology 75:130–136
61. Vigue B, Ract C, Zlotine N et al (2000) Relationship between intracranial pressure, mild hypothermia and temperature-corrected PaCO2 in patients with traumatic brain injury. Intensive Care Med 26:722–728
62. Strandgaard S (1993) The cerebral circulation in the elderly: the influence of age, vascular disease, and antihypertensive treatment. Am J Geriatr Cardiol 2:32–36
63. Paulson OB, Waldemar G, Schmidt JF, Strandgaard S (1989) Cerebral circulation under normal and pathologic conditions. Am J Cardiol 63:2C–5C

64. Strebel S, Lam AM, Matta BF, Newell DW (1997) Impaired cerebral autoregulation after mild brain injury. Surg Neurol 47:128–131
65. Budohoski KP, Czosnyka M, Kirkpatrick PJ et al (2013) Clinical relevance of cerebral autoregulation following subarachnoid haemorrhage. Nat Rev Neurol 9:152–163
66. Kety SS, Schmidt CF (1945) The determination of cerebral blood flow in man by the use of nitrous oxide in low concentrations. Am J Phys 14:353
67. Young WL, Prohovnik I, Schroeder T et al (1990) Intraoperative 133Xe cerebral blood flow measurements by intravenous versus intracarotid methods. Anesthesiology 73:637–643
68. Melot C, Berre J, Moraine JJ, Kahn RJ (1996) Estimation of cerebral blood flow at bedside by continuous jugular thermodilution. J Cereb Blood Flow Metab 16:1263–1270
69. Wietasch GJ, Mielck F, Scholz M et al (2000) Bedside assessment of cerebral blood flow by double-indicator dilution technique. Anesthesiology 92:367–375
70. Gopinath S, Robertson C, Contant C et al (1994) Jugular venous desaturation and outcome after head injury. J Neurol Neurosurg Psychiatry 57:717–723
71. Cormio M, Valadka A, Robertson C (1999) Elevated jugular venous oxygen saturation after severe head injury. J Neurosurg 90:9–15
72. Metz C, Holzschuh M, Bein T et al (1998) Monitoring of cerebral oxygen metabolism in the jugular bulb: reliability of unilateral measurements in severe head injury. J Cereb Blood Flow Metab 18:332–343
73. Huang SC, Carson RE, Hoffman EJ et al (1983) Quantitative measurement of local cerebral blood flow in humans by positron computed tomography and 15O-water. J Cereb Blood Flow Metab 3:141–153
74. Kaisti KK, Langsjo JW, Aalto S et al (2003) Effects of sevoflurane, propofol, and adjunct nitrous oxide on regional cerebral blood flow, oxygen consumption, and blood volume in humans. Anesthesiology 99:603–613
75. Stender J, Gosseries O, Bruno MA et al (2014) Diagnostic precision of PET imaging and functional MRI in disorders of consciousness: a clinical validation study. Lancet 384:514–522
76. Fan AP, Jahanian H, Holdsworth SJ, Zaharchuk G (2016) Comparison of cerebral blood flow measurement with [15O]-water positron emission tomography and arterial spin labeling magnetic resonance imaging: a systematic review. J Cereb Blood Flow Metab 36:842–861
77. Czosnyka M, Balestreri M, Steiner L et al (2005) Age, intracranial pressure, autoregulation, and outcome after brain trauma. J Neurosurg 102:450–454
78. Donnelly J, Budohoski KP, Smielewski P, Czosnyka M (2016) Regulation of the cerebral circulation: bedside assessment and clinical implications. Crit Care 20:129
79. Bouzat P, Almeras L, Manhes P et al (2016) Transcranial Doppler to predict neurologic outcome after mild to moderate traumatic brain injury. Anesthesiology 125:346–354
80. Varsos GV, Budohoski KP, Kolias AG et al (2014) Relationship of vascular wall tension and autoregulation following traumatic brain injury. Neurocrit Care 21:266–274
81. Aaslid R (2002) Transcranial Doppler assessment of cerebral vasospasm. Eur J Ultrasound 16:3–10

Cerebral Ischemia: Pathophysiology, Diagnosis, and Management

13

Lionel Velly, D. Boumaza, and Pierre Simeone

13.1 Introduction

In industrialized countries, stroke represents the third cause of death after cardiopathies and cancers, and the first cause of long-term disability in adults [1].

It is well established that stroke has to be considered as a medical emergency. Every year in France, about 130,000 patients present with a stroke. Among them, we schematically estimate that 30,000 will die during the days or months following the stroke and 60,000 will present a handicap of variable severity. Ischemic stroke or cerebral infarction represents 85% of overall stroke [2]. The management of stroke is today an absolute neurological emergency. It is important to know the main decisional steps in order to evaluate patients with ischemic stroke evolving since less than 4 h and eligible for thrombolytic treatment.

13.2 Pathophysiology of Cerebral Infarction

Healthy brain insures its needs in energy almost exclusively by oxidation of glucose [3]. An interruption in blood flow leads to a decrease in oxygen (O_2) supply and in glucose in brain and then a disruption of the energetic balance. Normal cerebral blood flow (CBF), measured with the clearance of Xenon 133 in tomoscintigraphy is 51.2 ± 8.8 mL/min/100 g of cerebral tissue [4] which represents about 15% of the cardiac output for an oxygen consumption (CMRO2) of 3.5 mL/min/100 g of cerebral tissue. But this value of CBF is a global value and it varies importantly depending on the functional areas. In the grey matter, a normal value is 75 ± 10 mL/min/100 g (thalamus: 86 ± 13 mL/min/100 g and frontolaterodorsal

L. Velly (✉) • D. Boumaza • P. Simeone
Département d'Anesthésie-Réanimation, CHU Timone,
264 rue Saint Pierre, 13385 Marseille, Cedex, France
e-mail: LionelJean.VELLY@ap-hm.fr; pierre.simeone@ap-hm.fr

C. Ichai et al. (eds.), *Metabolic Disorders and Critically Ill Patients*,
http://doi.org/10.1007/978-3-319-64010-5_13

cortex: 64 ± 4 mL/min/100 g) and in the white matter 30 ± 3 mL/min/100 g. Cerebral function and CMRO2 are preserved as long as the global CBF remains above or equal to 25-30 mL/min/100 g because the defect in tissular perfusion is then compensated by an increase in oxygen extraction. The ischemic threshold is defined by the value of the ratio CBF/CMRO2 below which aerobic metabolism cannot be maintained. For an ischemic distress related to an insufficiency in CBF to appear, CBF has to decrease more than 40%. Also, when CBF decreases below 15 mL/min/100 g for more than 1 or 2 min, the cortical electric activity slows down (disappearance of Beta-wave rhythm and occurrence of Delta-wave) and below 10 mL/min/100 g and evident failure of the cellular ionic pump occurs.

Stroke is the most studied clinical situation in clinic because the assessment of the impairment in cerebral perfusion is the basis of therapeutic decision in emergency.

During an arterial occlusion, three different areas (Fig. 13.1) are observed: the ischemic core where CBF is between 8 and 8.4 mL/100 g/min, the penumbra zone were CBF is between 14.1 and 35 mL/100 g/min and the oligemic zone with a CBF between 35 and 50 mL/100 g/min [5]. In the ischemic core, the complete lack of blood supply causes irreversible cellular damages; we observe then a massive necrotic zone. In the penumbra, blood flow is decreased but not entirely disrupted. It seems too weak though for an electric activity to be maintained, but sufficient to preserve ionic gradients. Even though neurons are functionally inactive their structure are intact and they stay temporarily viable. However, the concept of ischemic threshold is not univocal and we must distinguish the global threshold, varying from an individual to another and local ischemic threshold deeply dependent to the injured tissue and variable from a zone to another in the same patient and from pathology to another.

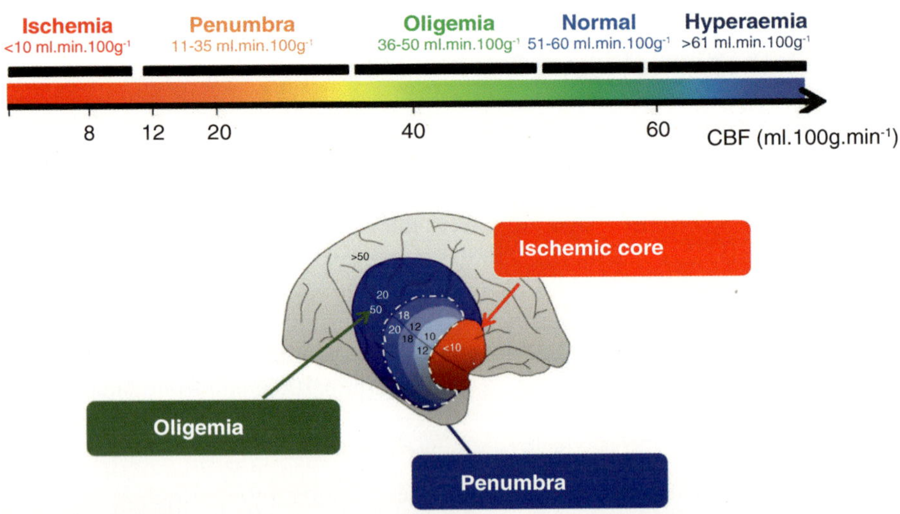

Fig. 13.1 Following an arterial occlusion, damage is composed of three regions: ischemic core, penumbra zone, and the oligemic zone

For example, in traumatic brain injury, the threshold value allowing to differentiate areas evolving toward an ischemic damage from healthy areas is 15 mL/100 g/min [6], with an important overlap in values between injured and health zones, allowing to define an abnormal pathophysiological situation rather than an absolute threshold [7]. After a subarachnoid hemorrhage due to an aneurysm rupture, a vasospasm becomes symptomatic for CBF under 25 mL/100 g/min [8, 9] with also important regional variability [10]. This explains certainly the difficulties to generalize the therapeutic concept of those patients.

13.2.1 Main Cellular Mechanisms in Cerebral Ischemia

The extension of the ischemic core is a time-dependent phenomenon. Cells die in the hours or days following a series of events named the ischemic cascade [11]. The main mechanisms of this series are excitotoxicity, peri-infarction depolarization which damages irreversibly neurons, glial and endothelial cells in the core of ischemia. In the penumbra zone, other mechanisms are involved such as oxidative stress, and then, lately on, inflammation and apoptosis [11, 12]. Each of these pathophysiological process occurs at a define time in the ischemic phenomenon, some occurring after a few minutes and others after several hours or days [12] (Fig. 13.2). The longer CBF is disrupted, the more important is the extension of ischemic core to the detriment of the penumbra zone which requires to be reperfused as quickly as possible. In ischemic core, where CBF is more severely limited, excitotoxicity and cellular death occur after a few minutes. On the periphery of ischemic core, in the penumbra zone, when parallel blood flow can limit the effects of stroke, the degree of ischemia and the delay before reperfusion determine the individual outcome of each cell. In this zone, cellular death through apoptosis or inflammation occurs less quickly [12]. Shortly after the occlusion of the middle cerebral artery (MCA), penumbra is approximately the same size than the ischemic core. After 3 h, penumbra only represents 50% of the ischemic core and 6–8 h later, almost all the penumbra zone disappears and is part of the irreversible damages in the ischemic core [13]. Although the length of ischemia is a determinant element in the intensity of

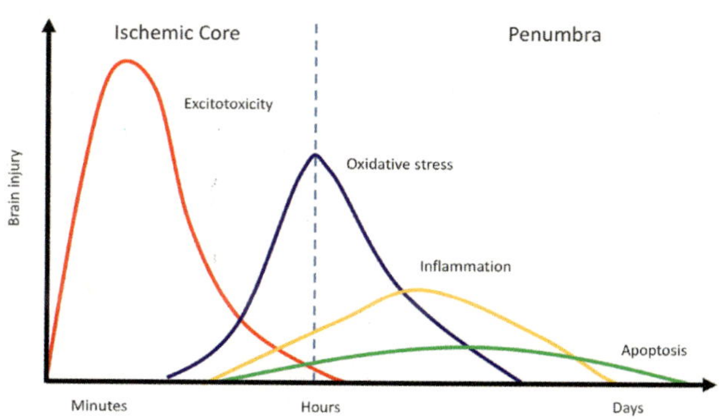

Fig. 13.2 Spatiotemporal evolution of mechanism involved in cerebral ischemia

damages, reperfusion plays also an important role in damage distribution. During reperfusion, a consequent amount of oxygen reaches the brain, which is responsible for formation of free radicals (oxygen-activated species ROS) and leads to additional oxidative stress.

13.2.1.1 Excitotoxicity and Calcium: Initials Determinants of Cellular Death

This expression was first used by Olney [14] in order to describe the potential of destruction of glutamatergic neurons. Beneviste was the first in 1984 to observe an increase in extracellular glutamate concentration, measured by microdialysis during global ischemia in rats [15]. This phenomenon has been since more precisely described and also observed in animal models of focal ischemia. This increase starts 1–2 min after the beginning of ischemia and reaches its maximum (16–30 μM) at the 15th minute [15] although extracellular glutamate amount remains below 6 μM in the periphery zone [16]. A correlation has been observed between extracellular glutamate concentration and the severity of neurological deficit in patients with cerebral ischemia [17]. The explications of this rise in extracellular glutamate are controversial. Two theories confront; the first is using the vesicular exocytosis path [18] depending on cytosolic presynaptic calcium concentration. The second implies the decrease in glutamate uptake or even the inversion of glutamate transport related to the inhibition of ATPase [19].

Cytotoxic Edema

Ischemia causes a massive entry of sodium within the cells because the decrease in ATP level induces a stopping of the ATPase Na/K and the activation by extracellular glutamate (in excess) of ionotropic glutamatergic receptors AMPA and Kaïnate (Fig. 13.3). This entry of Na fastly induces a postsynaptic membrane depolarization, followed by an entry of Chlore maintaining thus the ionic balance, and water according to an osmotic gradient. This induces a rise in cellular volume (osmotic swelling). The final consequence of this swelling is cellular lysis with release of cellular components, including glutamate, in the extracellular space, establishing then a vicious circle. However, this osmotic component of excitotoxicity is a reversible phenomenon if the depolarizing stimulus is abolished.

Calcic Influx and Its Consequences

Increased intracellular concentration in calcium (Ca) is one of the main and fastest consequences of ischemia within cerebral tissue, leading quickly to necrosis. This cellular destruction occurs through several enzymatic systems (protein kinase, protease, No synthase NOS) responsible for an inhibition of protein synthesis, free radicals formation and altered cytoskeletal proteins. Calcic invasion is triggered by cellular energetic depletion and anoxia and is responsible for an abnormal depolarization. It is sustained by massive release of excitating amino acids and in particular glutamate. Calcium is one of the main second messengers among neuronal cells. It is involved in the control of neurotransmitters release mechanisms, neuronal excitability, and in modulation of numerous metabolic processes. Calcium concentration is about 10,000 times more important in extracellular than in intracellular

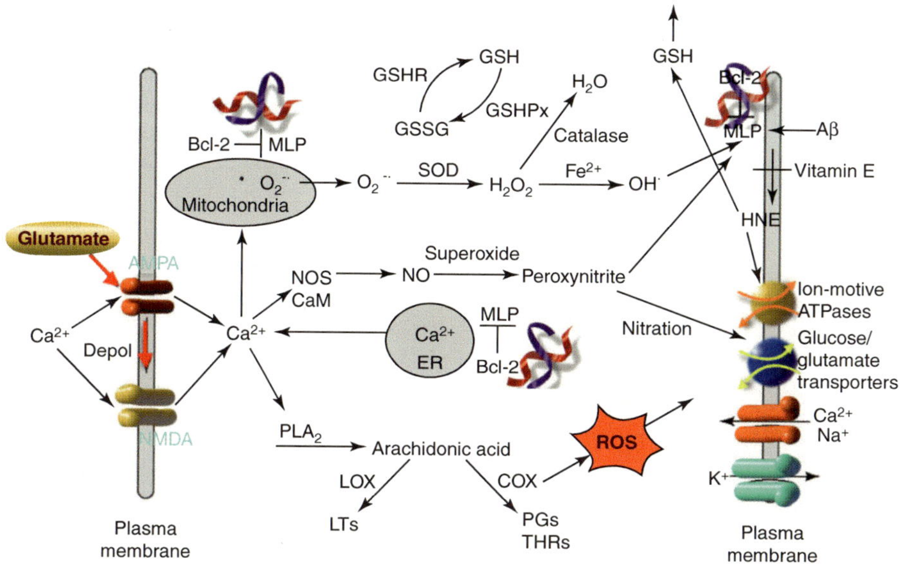

Fig. 13.3 Involvement of excitotoxicity in neuronal death. In case of cerebral ischemia, increased glutamate concentration by exocytosis and/or decrease or inversion of its transport leads to an activation by AMPA and NDMA receptors, osmotic swelling, and a massive entry of calcium ions in neurons

space. The preservation of a low cytosolic calcium concentration against extracellular concentration gradient is insured under physiological conditions by Na+/Ca^{2+} and by Ca^{2+} ATPase and Na+/K+ ATPase transporters in parallel with passive channels Na+/Ca^{2+} [20]. Involvement of these different systems has a high cost in energy. Energetic depletion caused by cerebral ischemia disrupts suddenly Ca homeostasis. Moreover, postsynaptic membrane depolarization due to the massive influx in intracellular sodium, by inhibiting ATPase, allows deactivating magnesium blockade on ionotropic glutamatergic receptors NMDA. In the presence of excess in glutamate, activated NMDA receptors also allow a calcium influx (Fig. 13.3) [20]. A brief but superior at 3 min activation of these NMDA receptors is sufficient to induce neuronal death by excitotoxicity. An extended activation of AMPA receptors (over 60 min) is in contrast necessary to induce such a neuronal death. A decrease or an absence of ATP inhibits also its sequestration in endoplasmic reticulum or its extrusion throughout the plasma membrane by calcium ATPase. Calbindin, calmodullin, and phospholipids tampon activities are decreased during ischemia, due to the diminished pH following lactic acid formation. H+ ion competes with Ca to bind these different molecules [21]. In these conditions, massive rise in intracellular calcium concentration initiates a cascade of molecular deleterious events (Fig. 13.4) for cerebral tissue among them a mitochondrial dysfunction (energetic deficit and toxic free radicals synthesis), involvement of enzymatic systems able to damage different structures of the cells (lipase, endonuclease, and protease), or activation of cytotoxic nitric oxide (NO) synthesis by the neuronal isoform of type 1 NO synthase (NOS) [22]. Calpaïne is the main protease activated by excess in Ca. It is responsible for the cleavage of numerous proteins essential in cellular function such as Ca^{2+} ATPase, PKC, and NF-KB. Proteolytic activity of calpaïne is deeply overwhelmed during ischemia, leading to a loss of synaptic density and cytoskeletal destruction by cleavage of its constituting proteins [23]. Activated PLA2 by excess in CA during ischemic process leads to a disrupted phospholipidic metabolism with degraded glycerophospholipids and massive formation of free fatty acids. This rise in free fatty acids during global ischemia occurs in the first 5 min and reaches a plateau within 15 min with 8–10 times the normal level [24]. Arachidonic acid is the principal free fatty acid produced during ischemia. It is then metabolized by cyclooxygenase (COX) in prostaglandin (PG) by the lipooxygenase in leukotriene (both of them are pro-inflammatory lipidic mediators) but also in lysophospholipids (precursor of the platelet activating factor) and in superoxide anions responsible for free radical formation [25].

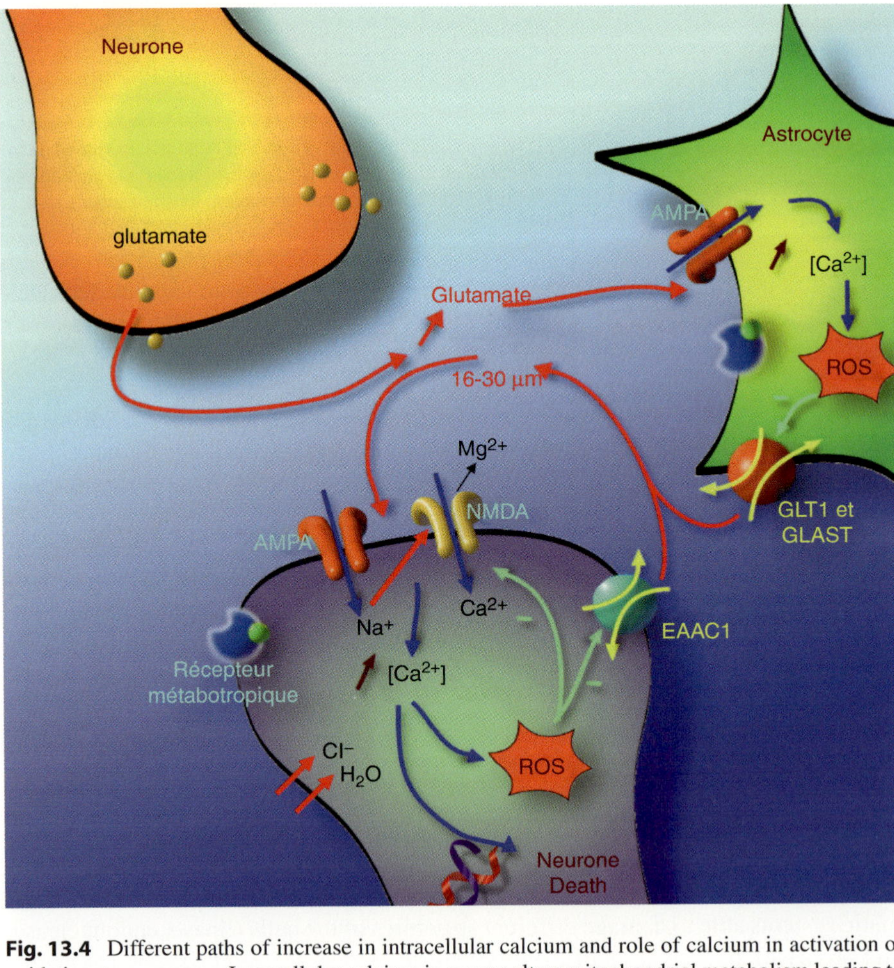

Fig. 13.4 Different paths of increase in intracellular calcium and role of calcium in activation of oxidative stress process. Intracellular calcium in excess alters mitochondrial metabolism leading to the production of free radicals, activated nitric oxide synthase (NOS) leading to formation of peroxynitrites and PLA-2 with production of prostaglandins and ROS

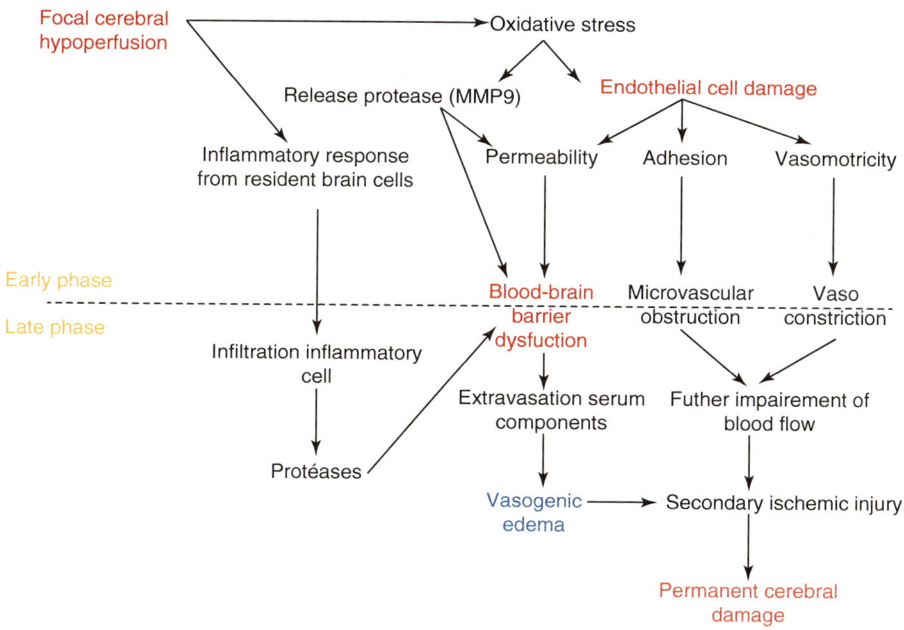

Fig. 13.5 Alteration of the blood–brain barrier during cerebral ischemia

13.2.1.2 Oxidative Stress and Nitric Oxide

Oxidative stress is represented by the whole reactions using ROS, which are characterized by the presence of a very reactive unpaired electron (free radical). Oxidative stress results of an imbalance between free radicals formation and cells anti-oxidative capacity. Cerebral ischemia and reperfusion in particular are responsible for oxidative stress leading to free radicals production and to deleterious effects during pathogenesis. Brain is extremely sensible to damages caused by free radicals due to its high content in lipids. This phenomenon prevails in the penumbra [26] and results in serious and immediate damages in cellular proteins, DNA, and lipids. In post-ischemic reperfusion, free radicals formation is enhanced by a great amount of oxygen supply [27]. Free radicals produced during reperfusion are principally activated species of oxygen. Main generated ROS are: superoxide anion $O_2^{-\bullet}$, hydroxyle radical ($OH^{\bullet}$ the most reactive oxygen-free radicals), hydrogen peroxide (H_2O_2), nitric oxide, and peroxynitrite ($ONOO^{\bullet}$). During ischemia, ionic homeostasis disruption, excitotoxicity, local anoxia, and inflammation facilitate oxygen-derivated free radicals production by several complex mechanisms. Altered mitochondria constitute an important source of free radicals [28]. Mitochondria produce ATP by using 90% of oxygen gathered by neurons. During the electrons transfer in mitochondrial chain, electrons spontaneously flee in order to react with oxygen and produce free radical. These reactive species are normally controlled by protective reduction enzymes such as superoxide dismutase (SOD) or glutathiase peroxidase (GPx). However, in case of ischemia and reperfusion, excess in cytosolic Ca^{2+} and in mitochondria leads to an accumulation of free radicals. Storaged free radicals in mitochondria will be able to react with oxygen when reperfusion occurs in order to produce superoxide ions ($O_2^{-\bullet}$). Free radicals thus produced inhibit electron transport in mitochondria and intensify the free radicals formation by mitochondria. Production of hydrogen peroxide (H_2O_2) involves the presence of nitric oxide (NO) which is produced by NOS through an oxygen-dependent reaction and activated by Ca^{2+}/calmodulin binding. It has been shown that neuronal and inductible NOS (nNOS and iNOS) are over-expressed during cerebral ischemia [29]. NO thus produced diffuses freely across membranes and can react with superoxide ion ($O_2^{-\bullet}$) to produce peroxynitrite ($ONOO^-$). $ONOO^-$ is able to induce cellular damage by nitration of DNA and proteins but also by lipids, DNA, and proteins oxidation; NO may also act as an electron acceptor inhibiting the ATP production by mitochondria.

Metallic ions are also an important factor of free radicals formation. Fe^{2+} released during ischemia by transport proteins can convert hydrogen peroxide (H_2O_2) in hydroxyl radical ($OH^\bullet$). They can also induce a lipid peroxidation during reperfusion. Also, Zn^{2+} stored in presynaptic vesicles of glutamatergic neurons and released in glutamate exocytosis induces a cellular death during ischemic phenomenon by producing free radicals via the activation of COX and PKC [30].

Finally, during oxidative stress, this fast overproduction of free radicals overwhelmed protective mechanisms of detoxification and the inhibition capacity of anti-oxidative enzymes such as catalase (CAT), SOD, GPx, and nonenzymatic anti-oxidative agents such as vitamin E, C, and glutathione (GSH).

13.2.1.3 Post-Ischemic Inflammation

High intracellular calcium concentration, NO and free radicals production, and hypoxia induce the activation of numerous nuclear transcription factors and particularly NF-KB factor [31]. Activation of this factor leads to many deleterious effects: an increase in NO synthesis via Type II NOS; re-enforcing the side effects of these, COX 2 expression; this enzyme involved in toxic and oxidative prostanoïdes synthesis; expression of numerous cytokines such as tumor necrosis factor alpha (TNFα) and Interleukine 1S (IL-1S), cytokines that are involved in glial cells and macrophages activation (Type II NOS and COX 2 synthesis) and also in process favoring polynuclears and monocytes adhesion to vascular endothelia (activation of adhesion proteins ICAM-1, selectine P and E) and their migration through cerebral tissue inducing in this manner the increase in ischemic damages [32].

13.2.1.4 Activation of Apoptotic Phenomenon

Apart from the mechanism of cellular necrosis which occurs early, in particular in the ischemic core, the increase in intracellular calcium, NO, free radicals, and inflammation mediators production are likely to induce the process of programmed cellular death called apoptosis [33]. This process is by definition delayed, prevails in the penumbra, and implies complex biological mechanisms. This type of cellular death is different from necrosis in its functional aspects, which are organized and anatomical. Apoptosis is defined morphologically by cytoplasm condensation (membrane changes and cytoskeletal re organization), by condensation and aggregation of chromatin in the periphery of nucleus under the nuclear membrane and occurrence of membrane gemmules containing nuclear fragments. They are precursors to apoptotic bodies aimed to be phagocytosed by macrophages or other adjacent cells. On a nuclear level, DNA is fragmented in multiple fractions by specific cleavage between nucleosomes. Abundance and relative activity of pro- and anti-apoptotic proteins determine at a given time the outcome (death or survival) of the cell. We can distinguish proteins that expression facilitates apoptosis (pro-apoptotic proteins: Bax, Bid) and proteins that on the contrary limit this type of cell death (anti-apoptotic proteins: Bcl-2, Bcl-XL). In pathological conditions such as cerebral ischemia, the balance between these proteins represents the ability of decision of the cell and can lead to cellular death. We described the different trigger signal transduction pathways in apoptosis: the extrinsic pathway (receptors mediated), the intrinsic pathway (mitochondrial), and the caspase-independent pathway (cysteine aspartate-specific protease). Caspase-3 is the terminal determinant in the caspase cascade and favors numerous DNA catalysis pathways [33].

13.2.1.5 Cerebral Edema

Cerebral ischemia leads to a membrane ionic pump dysfunction which triggers complex mechanisms leading to cell swelling and cellular-related cerebral edema: cytotoxic edema. Ionic disruption triggers a passive osmotic flow of water toward the cells. The rise in water into cerebral tissue affects both grey and white matter which leads macroscopically to an increase in volume. There exists also specific system of water transport playing a role in the occurrence of cerebral edema, aquaporines (AQP), and particularly AQP4 mostly found in central nervous system. The density of these channels is particularly high at the interface between brain and liquid spaces (blood, subarachnoid space, ventricles). AQP4 is expressed in astrocytes, endothelial cells, and ependymal cells. Neurons are free from AQP4. The role of cerebral AQP in pathology is yet not fully understood but these channels ease water flow. In rodents, AQP4 expression varies following a cerebral ischemic damage or traumatic injury [34, 35]; the level of AQP4 expression decreases the first moments after an ischemic or traumatic damage and increases then [36]. These results suggest that AQP4 contributes to edematous process but the positive or negative role of AQP4 in edema formation is not completely elucidated. In parallel, ischemia-reperfusion alters vessels and the blood–brain barrier which leads to the formation of an edema which origin is a capillary leak: the vasogenic edema [37]. When blood–brain barrier is disrupted, liquid, plasmatic proteins, and inflammatory cells enter in brain tissue. Most of the biological pathways leading to edema are observed during ischemia: excessive release in glutamate, oxidative stress, and inflammatory cascade. Moreover, an increase in cerebral volume generates an increased intracranial pressure and a decreased cerebral perfusion pressure which enhance the ischemic phenomenon. Edema grows to its maximal development the fourth day and declines during the second week. The "mass effect" is proportional to the volume of the infarction. Finally, cytotoxic edema, as vasogenic edema can be worsened by reperfusion due to the intensification of oxidative stress and inflammatory response but also due to the brain–blood barrier disruption. Some other works has reported the interest of bumetanide in order to regulate the expression of couple of kinase proteic channel NKCC1 and KCC2 and the chloric homeostasis control [38].

13.3 Diagnosis of Ischemic Stroke

At first, the semiology analysis stays the essential tool of the physicians and the accuracy of the diagnosis stays related to a good anatomical, clinical, and pathophysiological knowledge.

Diagnosis of stroke has to be evoked in case of sudden neurological deficit. In 15–20% of cases, we observe diagnostic errors, and this false diagnosis also need a specific assessment and management (seizure, nonvascular sudden neurological deficits, tumoral or infectious). In practice, in case of a patient suspected to have a stroke, the first step is, after interviewing the patient or its relatives and clinical examination, to determine if the neurological deficit is compatible with a stroke; that is to say: the sudden onset or rapidly progressive (over a few hours) of the following symptoms: hemiparesia or hemiplegia, unilateral sensitive disorders, language disorder, balance disorders, dizziness, total loss of vision, or bilateral partial or monocular loss of vision. It is also really important to keep in mind that brainstem stroke could occur with a clinical loss of vigilance and consciousness. It is then necessary to insure by asking to the patient or a witness the exact time of symptoms onset. If the patient woke up with the deficit, the hour of onset is the last hour where he has been seen without deficit. Patients must be then transferred as quickly as possible toward a reference hospital, where cerebral imaging will allow immediately to differentiate an ischemic from an hemorrhagic stroke.

The second step concerns the strategy of neuro-imaging explorations that could vary depending on the level of equipment more or less sophisticated of the different hospitals, but that should always be guided by the clinical expertise in order to ask precise questions according to the temporal data of symptoms onset. We have to determine most precisely and quickly the nature of stroke (ischemic or hemorrhagic), the anatomical and vascular territory, the possible mechanism responsible (thromboembolic or hemodynamic), and the pathophysiological stage (reversible damage or irreversible) which determine the prognosis and the therapeutic options. At present, magnetic resonance imaging (MRI) is the gold-standard diagnostic test in emergency concerning stroke according to the official guidelines. Cerebral tomodensitometry (CT scan) is only used by lack of access to MRI (except from contraindications).

13.3.1 Diffusion and Perfusion-Weighted MRI

Only the MRI weighted with diffusion and perfusion sequences allows to diagnose ischemic stroke and to evaluate the penumbra zone. Indeed, during the first 6 h, CT imaging and conventional MRI imaging are at this stage normal or show only discrete abnormalities of cerebral tissue while the ischemic zone is clearly identified by diffusion-MRI from the first minutes after clinical onset and hypoperfused zone is immediately detectable in perfusion-MRI.

13.3.1.1 Diffusion-Weighted MRI

Diffusion-MRI estimates the mobility of water molecules and allows detecting early the cellular dysfunction secondary to ischemia. At the acute phase of cerebral ischemia, the disruption in CBF leads very quickly to a failure in energetic metabolism. It results a massive water influx from the extracellular space toward the intracellular space, resulting in the cytotoxic edema. Thus, the mobility of free water from interstitial space toward the cells is reduced, and this phenomenon can be seen from the first minutes by diffusion-MRI in the form of a hyper signal (white). This technique presents an excellent sensibility (over 90%) for the detection of acute ischemic damages.

13.3.1.2 Perfusion-Weighted MRI

Perfusion-MRI provides information on regional cerebral hemodynamic on a microvascular scale and gives an estimation of CBF. This method studies the kinetic of a nondiffusible contrast agent (chelate of gadolinium) in the brain and allows visualizing the cerebral hypo perfusion zones [39]. Many measures have been suggested and studied: the time at peak (Tmax), medium time to transit (MTT), cerebral blood volume (CBV), and cerebral blood flow (CBF) (Fig. 13.6).

To simplify, Tmax corresponds to the delay to reach the peak concentration of gadolinium in each regions compared to the arrival of gadolinium in cerebral arteries. At present, it seems to be the measure offering the strongest results in published therapeutical trials [40].

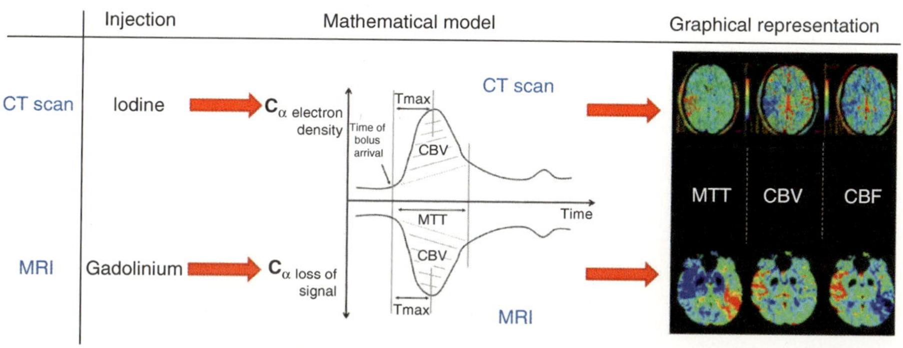

Fig. 13.6 Methods of perfusion-weighted MRI and CT scan: middle time to transit (MTT): middle time of crossing capillaries (unit: sec); cerebral blood volume (CBV): area under the curve and measure of autoregulation (unit: mL/100 g of cerebral tissue/min): cerebral blood flow (CBF) is equal to the ratio CBV/MTT (unit: mL/100 g of tissue/min). During an ischemia, we observe in the involved territory a longer MTT and of Tmax and a decrease in CBV and CBF

13.3.1.3 The Concept of "Mismatch"

The coupled analysis of perfusion and diffusion-weighted MRI allows to identify the penumbra zone risking to evolve toward infarction. The tally zone with a decrease in cerebral perfusion without signs of necrosis in diffusion-MRI is called the "mismatch." It is considered as a substitute to the ischemic penumbra [41]. The concept of mismatch based on the subtraction of diffusion and perfusion volumes appeared as a simple way to identify in emergency the zone at risk (Fig. 13.7) [42]. Schematically, the necrotic zone is assimilated to the damage volume observed in diffusion-imaging. In the absence of rapid reperfusion, sequential studies have showed an extension of the initial damage at the expense of the hypo perfused zone. This evaluation, coupled with the analysis of intracranial angio-MRI (in order to search a vascular occlusion) allows selecting patients likely to benefit from a fibrinolysis. However, unlike PET-imaging, perfusion-MRI does not allow a quantitative evaluation: the main parameters used (Tmax, MTT, CBV, CBF) only give a qualitative hemodynamic information. Moreover, the different attempts in order to establish the tissular viability threshold using MRI parameters failed to determine a precise approach of the at-risk zone. No consensus has been established on the choice of hemodynamic parameters, neither on the relevance of the criteria defining the zone of mismatch. To answer these questions, numerous

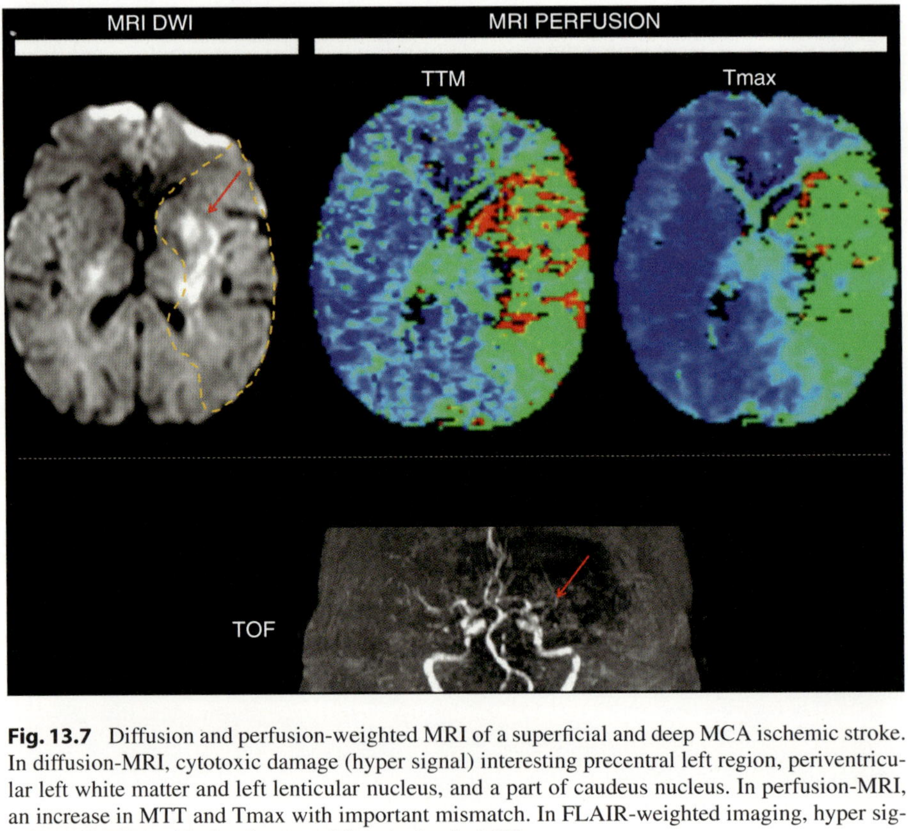

Fig. 13.7 Diffusion and perfusion-weighted MRI of a superficial and deep MCA ischemic stroke. In diffusion-MRI, cytotoxic damage (hyper signal) interesting precentral left region, periventricular left white matter and left lenticular nucleus, and a part of caudeus nucleus. In perfusion-MRI, an increase in MTT and Tmax with important mismatch. In FLAIR-weighted imaging, hyper signal in left MCA with the absence of flow in Angio-MRI

modelization programs using multiple parameters to study tissular suffering are currently in the course of elaboration. Addition of imaging exploring metabolism such as spectroscopy, determination of the regional oxygen consumption (CMRO2) by Bold effect could allow to complete relevantly the evaluation of the at-risk tissue, under the condition that it does not lengthen the test duration.

13.3.2 Tomodensitometry Imaging

Recognizing early scanographic signs of ischemic stroke is often difficult, explaining the great variability of the detection rate observed in literature (56–94%). Two types of early signs can be found: intravascular irregularities (intra-arterial hyper density) and parenchymatous abnormalities (softened contrast and mass effect).

13.3.2.1 Intravascular Abnormalities

Intra-arterial thrombus is responsible for an increased density of the artery corresponding to the spontaneous arterial hyper density and in theory visible on every of the artery constituting Willis polygon and this from the early stage of stroke. This intravascular hyper density traduces the presence of a thrombotic clot, or more often an embolic clot. Occlusion of the middle cerebral artery (MCA) is the most frequent.

13.3.2.2 Parenchyma Abnormalities

These parenchymatous signs include: softened contrast and cerebral edema. The decrease in contrast is by definition due to a loss of contrast spontaneously visible between densities in the white and the grey matter. In physiological condition, white matter appears spontaneously more hypo dense than the grey matter constituent the cortical zone and the basal ganglia. According to the localization of the softening in contrast, several signs have been described. The disappearance of the lentiform nucleus corresponds to a softening of the precise outline of this nucleus and is correlated to the development of an infarction in the deep territory of MCA. Disappearance of the insular band corresponds to a loss of definition between the grey and the white matter in the insula and is associated to infarction in the superficial territory of MCA. This sign is frequently associated with the others due to the strategic location of insular region which match with the distal territory of the superficial MCA territory. Erasure of cortical sulcus results in a modification in the contrast of cortex. It is correlated to the development of a cortical infarction of MCA. Association between these softening of contrast predicts the development of an extended infarction. The global subjective assessment of a threshold volume of more or less 33% of suffering territory has been studied, particularly in order to be used as an inclusion or exclusion criteria in therapeutical trials of anti-thrombotic agents. This approach stays however speculative because of the great variability in the definition of the middle cerebral artery territory. Mass effect is revealed by the compression exerted on the reference structures (ventricular system or cortical sulcus). A discrete ventricular compression can affect the frontal pole, and the mass effect results in a disappearance of the middle cerebral artery valley or of cortical sulcus. These localized mass effects are more easily detected when we observe a clear hypo density.

13.3.2.3 Perfusion CT Scan

Recently, in order to obtain a better sensitivity of the technique, the principle of CT perfusion has been suggested as an alternative for measuring the ischemic penumbra or in detection of a vasospasm after subarachnoid hemorrhage [43].

It is based on the measure of cerebral perfusion according to the same principle than perfusion-MRI with an iode-contrast product (Fig. 13.6). Thus, ischemic cerebral zones have a decreased regional CBF and CBV and longer MTT. In stroke, the criteria have been defined depending on their ability to predict the size of the final infarction. The mismatch between regions with a CBV below 2 mL/100 g/min (ischemic core) and those with an MTT one and a half times greater than the one measured in the contralateral hemisphere (hypo perfusion) would represent a substitute of ischemic penumbra [44]. The main advantage of CT perfusion is its easy use with integrated software in most of equipment, able to create in real time, 24 h/7 in most of centers, a "perfusion map." Yet, except from last-generation CT scans, Perfusion CT only allows to cover 2 cm thick in four slices when perfusion-MRI covers 8–12. The second major limit of its use in everyday practice in stroke is the absence of validation of these criteria by prospective trials such as in cerebral MRI. However, comparing the values of each region at interest previously defined and establishing a ratio between ischemic region and equivalent contralateral regions seems to present a great interest.

13.4 Therapeutic Management of Ischemic Stroke

Regardless of the severity of the stroke, patients need to be admitted into hospital as soon as possible (from the first hours) in a specialized ward because this management constitutes at present the most efficient therapeutic measure in order to improve outcome of patients with stroke. Indeed, neurovascular wards dedicated and specifically organized for stroke management allow alone to reduce 25% of inpatients ischemic stroke mortality and 17% of one-year mortality of hemorrhagic stroke. This benefit applies for every stroke, regardless of their type (ischemic or hemorrhagic) or their severity, or the patient's age. Almost the entire benefit is obtained during the first 30 days [45]. For more critical patients, needing ICU, admission in a neuro-ICU, used to stroke management is associated with a decrease in mortality for a 3:4 ratio [46]. It seems then evident that an early and oriented management has a major impact on stroke patient's outcome.

At present, two ministerial memorandums (3rd November 2003 and 22nd March 2007) have precised the path of management of stroke and particularly in special neurovascular units (21 in 2005, 77 in 2009). But we estimated that only a few proportion of patients have access to those units at the present time. According to a survey of the French Neurovascular Society, 1080 patients have been treated in 2005 in France so less than 1% of the overall strokes. Expected progresses are related to acceleration in the outpatients care, an increase in the number of candidate and use of new treatments. Mobile units of emergency are largely aware of neurovascular emergency. Yet, the delay in outpatients care is often very important and results usually from a late alert. The involvement from the prehospital phase and the formation of health care professionals, emergency physicians, emergency medical service, and emergency fire assistance in particular are of capital interest in order to allow the fast selection of patients who have to be admitted in neurovascular units.

13.4.1 Thrombolytic and Anticoagulant Treatments

The main mechanism of stroke being an arterial thromboembolic occlusion, the key point of every therapeutic strategy in emergency is to suppress as soon as possible the arterial occlusion in order to reperfuse the arterial ischemic territory still viable (ischemic penumbra) before definitive neuronal death occurs. The European authorization for intravenous thrombolysis by tissular activator of recombinant plasminogen (rt-PA) in the first 3 h of cerebral infarction represented in 2002 an absolute revolution: for the first time in this pathology, an efficient emergency treatment (less than 20% of patients disabled) was available. According to the marketing authorization, only a trained neurologist is authorized to prescribe rt.-PA. The recommended dose is 0.9 mL/kg with a maximal dose of 90 mg (10% in a bolus in 1 min and 90% in a 1-h perfusion). The combined analysis of randomized trials (ATLANTIS, ECASS, NINDS) including over 5000 patients showed that the benefit of thrombolysis is all the more important since the treatment is early administrated, with a maximal benefit when fibrinolytic agent is administrated in the first 90 min [47]. However, the benefit is obtained at a high price, which is a significant increase in symptomatic cerebral hemorrhage. Thrombolysis is a potentially dangerous treatment: the risk of hemorrhagic transformation varies from 6 to 11% regarding the administrated protocols for intravenous thrombolysis (vs. 0.6–3% in placebo groups) [48]. Hemorrhagic transformations related to thrombolysis are more voluminous, severe, and fatal or responsible for a major handicap in 50–75% of cases. Secondary analysis of rt.-PA trials allowed identifying risk factors of severe hemorrhagic transformation under rt.-PA. These factors are: age, previous treatment with aspirin, extended hypo density on initial CT scan, high blood pressure, and uncontrolled hyperglycemia [49]. In order to limit this risk, it is fundamental to respect scrupulously all the contraindications (Table 13.1). During European Marketing Authorization, it was intended to evaluate by a European register all symptomatic intracranial hemorrhage risk in everyday practice and to compare it to the particular situation of randomized trials. The results of this register, named "Safe Implementation of Thrombolysis monitoring study" (SITS-MOST) including 6483 patients founds an efficiency (preserved independent living skills in 55% of patients) and a safety to use (risk of cerebral hemorrhage 7.3%) of thrombolysis with rt.-PA, congruent with the results of randomized trials [50]. Since then, several therapeutic trials showed that there exists a therapeutic window for rt.-PA after the third hour (until about four and a half hour), even if the benefit decreases quickly with time [51]. We know today that the risk of hemorrhage does not increase between the third and the sixth hour [52]. These results encourage the implementation of a European study (ECASS III) including 821 patients in order to compare thrombolysis with rt.-PA to a placebo administrated in the third to the fourth and a half hours following the onset of stroke symptoms [53]. In these conditions, a treatment with rt.-PA increases compared to the placebo at 28% the chances to recover a complete independence with 14 patients to treat to obtain a favorable neurological outcome. The risk of hemorrhagic transformation was 7.9% in the rt.-PA group (vs. 6.4% in the NINDS study) but only 2.4% of hemorrhagic transformations were considered responsible for a neurologic deterioration. Since a large observational study (SITS-ISTR) including 650 patients confirmed the

Table 13.1 Indications and contraindications of use of Alteplase (rt-PA) in ischemic stroke at acute phase

Indications:
– Diagnosis of ischemic stroke responsible for neurological deficit
– Onset of symptoms less than 4.5 h before the instauration of the treatment
Contraindications:
Clinical:
• High blood pressure with systolic pressure over >185 mmHg or diastolic >110 mmHg
• Symptoms suggesting a subarachnoidal hemorrhage even in the absence of evidence at CT scan
• History of intracranial hemorrhage
• History of myocardial infarction in the last 3 months
• History of brain injury or stroke in the last 3 months
• Majors surgery in the last 14 days
• Digestive hemorrhage or urinary tract hemorrhage in the last 21 days
• Arterial punction in uncompressible site in the last 7 days
• Seizures at the onset of stroke
• Angiography or arterial pressure monitoring authorized if needed
• Minor neurological deficit or symptoms improving quickly before treatment
Radiological
• Signs of intracranial hemorrhage at imaging
• Hypo density superior at 33% of a cerebral hemisphere
Biological
• Oral anticoagulation with INR over 1.7
• Heparin intake in the last 48 h with prolonged TCA
• Platelets <100,000
• Glycemia <2.7 mmol/l or >22 mmol/l
Supplementary contraindications for thrombolysis between the 3rd and the 4.5th hour
• Age > 80 years
• Severe neurological deficit (NIHSS > 25)
• Diabetic patients with history of stroke

Likewise other thrombolytic agents, rt.-PA should not be used in case with a high risk of hemorrhage

safety of use of rt.-PA between the third and the fourth and a half hour [54]. We should however notice that additional exclusion criteria must be used in this time between the third and the fourth and a half hour (Table 13.1). Currently, a large literature still tries to enlarge the potential candidates to thrombolysis. In these different situations, out of marketing authorization, cerebral MRI could be a precious tool through information on cerebral tissue, by selecting patients according to the size of penumbra zone. The prospective observational study DEFUSE, including 74 patients thrombolysed between the third and the sixth hour with rt.-PA, all of them having a diffusion and perfusion-weighted MRI (with no influence on the decision of thrombolysis) showed a benefit to thrombolysis in patients with a large hypo perfusion and a restricted region of limited diffusion (mismatch). On the contrary, an unacceptable hemorrhagic risk was found in patients with a large region of limited diffusion [55]. Several new thrombolytic agents including desmoteplase are also currently tested and could allow to reduce the hemorrhagic risk [56]. Thus, a pilot study shows a benefit to use desmoteplase between the third and the ninth hour after symptoms onset in selected patients based on the penumbra zone on MRI [57]. However, these results were not confirmed by a recent prospective study in phase III DIAS-2 [58]. Other approaches seem to emerge such as the association of a low dose of intravenous rt.-PA with an intra-arterial thrombolytic bolus, on contact with the clot [59]. Even if the first studies were negative, since 2013, five studies proved the interest of mechanical thrombectomy (Mr CLEAN, ESCAPE, EXTEND-IA, SWIFT-PRIME and REVASCAT) with better outcome at 90 days regarding mortality and functional mRS score, even for the elderly patients. New guidelines encourage the realization of mechanical thrombectomy in the first 4h30 hours for the anterior circulation [60].

Aspirin is the only antiplatelet drug which proved its efficiency in randomized trials to prevent early ischemic recurrence and improve outcome in ischemic stroke at the acute phase [61]. In fact, aspirin reduces mortality by 4 for 1000 patients treated and death or major disability by 12 for 1000 patients at a price of 2 for 1000 severe hemorrhagic complications [62]. A treatment with aspirin (160 and 300 mg) is then instituted as soon as possible after a cerebral infarction following the contraindications (gastro duodenal ulcer, allergy, and unexplained microcytic anemia). In order to reduce the risk of intracerebral hemorrhagic complications, prescription of aspirin is delayed of 24 h if a thrombolytic agent has been administrated to the patient. Systematic use of heparin (unfractionned heparin, low molecular-weight heparin or heparinoïd) at curative doses is not recommenced at the acute phase of ischemic stroke, including in non-valvular atrial fibrillation. Curative dose heparin can be used in selected indications, presumed at high risk of recurrence or extension such as high embolic risk cardiopathy, several arterial stenosis, intra-luminal thrombus, or extra-cranial arterial dissection.

In conclusion, thrombolysis largely contributes to change the "wait and see" behavior in stroke treatment ate the acute phase. Its place is considerable, even if too few patients can nowadays benefit from it. Its development in the future years is inseparable of development of neurovascular units.

13.4.2 General Measures

Ischemic stroke treatment aims at first at avoiding that the penumbra zone evolve toward neuronal death, which allows to limit the final size of infarction and thus neurological sequels. Main aggravating factors needing a close surveillance and correction have been identified. These factors are arterial hypertension, hypo, and more importantly hyperglycemia, hyperthermia, and hypoxia. General measures aim also at preventing and treating neurological or general complications. Evaluation of swallowing disorders and early mobilization allow preventing from aspiration pneumonia and decubitus complications.

First, if a perfusion is needed, isotonic fluid will be favored (isotonic salted solution) in order to avoid the occurrence or aggravation of a cerebral edema. Furthermore, it is recommenced at the acute phase of cerebral infarction to treat hyperglycemia which is associated with a poor neurological outcome, whenever it occurs in diabetic or nondiabetic patients. However, a recent study (GIST-UK) did not show a benefit effect on insulin treatment on reduction of mortality [63].

Hyperthermia is treated if temperature exceeds 37.5 °C. The cause of the fever has to be explored. Another alternative could be mild hypothermia (33–34 °C) using external or invasive cooling devices. Feasibility studies have been realized such as COOLAID (Colling for Acute Ischemic Brain Damage) but at present this device has not proved its efficiency during cerebral ischemia [64, 65]. Arterial hypertension is frequent at initial phase of ischemic stroke and should be respected. If blood pressure is at several successive measures above 220 mmHg for systolic pressure and above 120 mmHg for diastolic pressure, it is recommenced to treat using intravenous medication, in order to reach a progressive decrease in blood pressure. It is important to keep in mind that the tensional objectives are different regarding the fact that the mechanical thrombectomy is done if indicated. Before thrombectomy, the tensional aim is 200 mmHg for systolic pressure and 100-120 for mean pressure. After the mechanical thrombectomy, it is better to lower the pressure around 150 mmHg for systolic pressure to avoid rebleeding or vasogenic oedema. A brutal decrease is likely to aggravate ischemic stroke. In case of hypoxia, the European Stroke Initiative and the American Stroke Association recommend introduction of oxygen [66, 67]. Anticonvulsant treatment is not recommended in prevention of seizure. In case of seizure at the acute phase, an anticonvulsant treatment is recommended in order to prevent recurrence of seizures. The different medications have not been studied specifically in the context of stroke, including in status epilepticus. Optimal treatment duration has not been evaluated. There is no evidence for a long-term treatment. Systematical use of anti-edematous agents (mannitol, glycerol, diuretics, or corticosteroids) is not justified because none has made the proof of its efficiency in cerebral ischemia and all present potential side effects (hydro electrolytes disorders, pulmonary edema, acute renal failure, allergy, hemolysis, infection, and hyperglycemia). Mannitol can however be used in patients with an acute degradation of neurological state and before a decompressive surgical treatment.

13.4.3 Neuroprotective Treatment Prospects

During the past 6 years, 1000 experimental studies and 400 clinical studies have been published about this subject [68]. There is an important amount of neuroprotective agents studied at different phases of clinical trials, based on experimental models reproducing cerebral vascular pathology and on pathophysiological mechanisms during ischemia (antiglutamatergic agents, anti-oxidative agents, etc.). Even if the explored leads by these trials were very promising, most of these molecules have not shown a significant efficiency or a limited efficiency. Some of them even appeared to be deleterious [69]. The fail of these molecules contributes to take an interest in other neuroprotective molecules already used in human clinic in other indications (minocycline derivated, magnesium, immunosuppressive agents, etc). Human recombinant erythropoietin (rhEPO) seemed to be the most promising lead. A randomized monocentric study (phase III) including 40 patients presenting a right middle cerebral artery ischemic stroke from less than 8 h found in patients treated with high dose of rhEPO (33,000 UI/day during 3 days) a significant improvement of their motor deficit and functional recovery [70]. However, a second multicentric, prospective randomized trial (phase III) from the same group (German Multicenter EPO Stroke Trial) including 522 patients, did not proved an improvement in neurological outcome on Barthel and Rankin scale, nor on NIHSS score [71]. It has been shown also that in the group receiving concomitantly rt.-PA and rhEPO an increased mortality (rt-PA placebo 16.4% vs. rt.-PA-EPO 9% $p = 0.01$). EPO therapy has also been responsible for an increased occurrence of side effects (cerebral hemorrhage, cerebral edema, thromboembolic events). Only the analysis in subgroups founds in non-thrombolysed patients that EPO improves, compared to the placebo, variation of the NIHSS score between Day 1 and Day 90. This study questions seriously the safety of use of hematopoietic EPO in ischemic stroke. A current multicentric study (phase II) on the use during ischemic stroke of non-hematopoietic EPO (carbamyled EPO) (clinicaltrials.gov NCT00870844) could bring other encouraging results. No neuroprotective treatment can be recommended yet.

13.4.4 Specific Management of Malignant Middle Cerebral Artery Infarction

A cerebral life-threatening edema complicates 1–10% of supratentorials infarction. It is the first cause of early death after cerebral infarction [72, 73]. Cytotoxic edema occurs in the first hour after infarction and is followed by vasogenic edema which reaches its maximum between the second and the fifth day [74]. Voluminous hemispheric infarction secondary to complete occlusion of middle cerebral artery (MCA) or of internal carotid artery just as cerebellum infarction have an edematous and rapidly compressive evolution, exposing the patient to a risk of temporal engagement or an acute hydrocephalus (Fig. 13.8a,b). The term of malignant infarction defines those infarction compromising the immediate vital prognosis of the patient with a mortality rate between 50 and 78% the first week [74]. An MCA infarction has to be suspected and requires an ICU management in case of a sudden complete hemiplegia, associated to a forced deviation of head and eyes toward the opposite side, somnolence, and depending on the affected side, global aphasia or hemineglect. The clinical situation evolves in the following hours toward a fast worsening of vigilance and occurrence of signs of temporal engagement (unilateral then bilateral mydriasis, Cheyne Stokes dyspnea, alveolar hypoventilation, tachycardia, agitation, and then decerebration signs). This worsening is related to the increase in ischemic edema. Radiological predictive signs of malignant MCA infarction are the presence on the CT scan in the initial 6 h of early signs of ischemia in more than 50% of the MCA territory or presence on CT scan during the first 48 h of a softened density of the entire MCA territory or an horizontal displacement of the pineal gland of more than 4 mm [75]. Nevertheless, the best

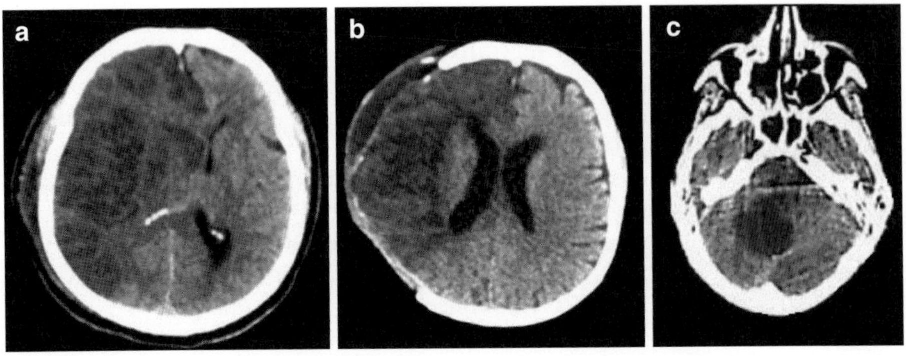

Fig. 13.8 Malignant infarction in MCA territory before (**a**) and after decompressive hemi-craniectomy (**b**) and cerebellum infarction (**c**)

predictive factor of a malignant edema is the volume of infarction measured in diffusion-weighted MRI. A volume over 145cm^3 before the 14th hour is a predictive indicator of evolution toward malignant edema with a 100% sensitivity and a 94% specificity [76]. Three randomized trials in Europe (HAMLET, DESTINY, and DECIMAL) and one meta-analysis studied decompressive hemi-craniectomy in MCA malignant infarction [77]. Hemi-craniectomy realized in 93 patients from 18 to 65 years in the first 48 h allows a significant increase in survival (78% vs. 29% in the group treated medically) with a survival probability with a score of Rankin under or equal to 3 (that is to say with mild handicap, allowing to walk without assistance) doubled. The decision of craniectomy has to be discussed on individual cases with family and relatives, explaining the reduction of mortality but the major risk of dependence. These data only concerns patients under the age of 65 years.

13.4.5 Specific Management of Edematous Infarction of Cerebellum

Cerebellum infarction represents 4.2–15% of overall cerebral infarction. Benign forms are the most frequent. However, a particularly severe complication to fear at the acute phase (between the second and the fifth day but sometimes delayed to the 8th–10th day after infarction) is compressive ischemic edema, responsible for a compression of brainstem and an acute hydrocephalus leading to death (Fig. 13.8c). Surgical treatment consists in a suboccipital craniectomy associated or not with an excision of the ischemic lesion and an external ventricular drainage and can prevent mortality. Published series show a survival rate of 100% with a variable functional result, often very good but sometimes with a mild to severe handicap [78]. Factors associated with a poor result of surgery are the coexistence of a brainstem ischemia, age over 60, and importance of the brainstem compression (motor dysfunction, eyes deviation, vigilance disorders) at the time of the surgery and delayed surgery but not the cerebellar territory of infarction [79]. However, a prolonged brainstem compression should not exclude surgical treatment because observation of comatous patients with signs of cerebral engagement having recovered after surgery has been reported [80]. The delay and surgical strategy are still debated. For some teams, external ventricular derivation is the first intention method, followed by suboccipital craniectomy in case of neurological worsening. In all cases, those patients need a close surveillance in ICU according to the probability of very fast neurological worsening on a few hours.

Conclusion

Passivity and fatalism have no more places in stroke management. Acute management of severe stroke stays difficult, due to the prognosis uncertainty and the perspective of severe sequels. It requires knowledge on therapeutics in the acute phase, individual reflection for a multidisciplinary decision. The improvement in individual outcome assessment stays a major stake in this management. It would allow to precise the place of resuscitation or considerable therapeutics (decompresisve hemi-craniectomy, ventricular derivation).

References

1. Feigin VL, Lawes CM, Bennett DA, Anderson CS (2003) Stroke epidemiology: a review of population-based studies of incidence, prevalence, and case-fatality in the late 20th century. Lancet Neurol 2:43–53
2. Qureshi AI, Tuhrim S, Broderick JP, Batjer HH, Hondo H, Hanley DF (2001) Spontaneous intracerebral hemorrhage. N Engl J Med 344:1450–1460
3. Hossman KA (2006) Pathophysiology and therapy of experimental stroke. Cell Mol Neurobiol 26:1057–1083
4. Vernooij MW, van der Lugt A, Ikram MA, Wielopolski PA, Vrooman HA et al (2008) Total cerebral blood flow and total brain perfusion in the general population: the Rotterdam Scan Study. J Cereb Blood Flow Metab 28:412–419
5. Bandera E, Botteri M, Minelli C, Sutton A, Abrams KR, Latronico N (2006) Cerebral blood flow threshold of ischemic penumbra and infarct core in acute ischemic stroke: a systematic review. Stroke 37:1334–1339
6. Cunningham AS, Salvador R, Coles JP et al (2005) Physiological thresholds for irreversible tissue damage in contusional regions following traumatic brain injury. Brain 128:1931–1942
7. Coles JP, Cunningham AS, Salvador R, Chatfield DA, Carpenter A, Pickard JD, Menon DK (2009) Early metabolic characteristics of lesion and nonlesion tissue after head injury. J Cereb Blood Flow Metab 29:965–975
8. Leclerc X, Fichten A, Gauvrit JY, Riegel B, Steinling M, Lejeune JP et al (2002) Symptomatic vasospasm after subarachnoid haemorrhage: assessment of brain damage by diffusion and perfusion-weighted MRI and single-photon emission computed tomography. Neuroradiology 44:610–616
9. Jabre A, Babikian V, Powsner RA, Spatz EL (2002) Role of single photon emission computed tomography and transcranial Doppler ultrasonography in clinical vasospasm. J Clin Neurosci 9:400–403
10. Vajkoczy P, Horn P, Thome C, Munch E, Schmiedek P (2003) Regional cerebral blood flow monitoring in the diagnosis of delayed ischemia following aneurysmal subarachnoid hemorrhage. J Neurosurg 98:1227–1234

11. Dirnagl U, Iadecola C, Moskowitz MA (1999) Pathobiology of ischaemic stroke: an integrated view. Trends Neurosci 22:391–397
12. Doyle KP, Simon RP, Stenzel-Poore MP (2008) Mechanisms of ischemic brain damage. Neuropharmacology 55:310–318
13. Hata R, Maeda K, Hermann D, Mies G, Hossmann KA (2000) Evolution of brain infarction after transient focal cerebral ischemia in mice. J Cereb Blood Flow Metab 20:937–946
14. Olney JW (1986) Inciting excitotoxic cytocide among central neurons. Adv Exp Med Biol 203:631–645
15. Benveniste H, Drejer J, Schousboe A, Diemer NH (1984) Elevation of the extracellular concentrations of glutamate and aspartate in rat hippocampus during transient cerebral ischemia monitored by intracerebral microdialysis. J Neurochem 43:1369–1374
16. Graham SH, Shirashi K, Panter SS, Simon RP, Faden AI (1990) Changes in extracellular amino acid neurotransmitters produced by focal cerebral ischemia. Neurosci Lett 110:124–130
17. Castillo J, Davalos A, Naveiro J, Noya M (1996) Neuroexcitatory amino acids and their relation to infarct size and neurological deficit in ischemic stroke. Stroke 27:1060–1065
18. Jehle T, Lagrèze WA, Blauth E, Knörle R, Schnierle P, Lücking CH, Feuerstein TJ (2000) Gabapentin-lactam (8-aza-spiro[5,4]decan-9-on; GBP-L) inhibits oxygen glucose deprivation-induced [3H]glutamate release and is a neuroprotective agent in a model of acute retinal ischemia. Naunyn Schmiedebergs Arch Pharmacol 362:74–81
19. Jabaudon D, Scanziani M, Gähwiler BH, Gerber U (2000) Acute decrease in net glutamate uptake during energy deprivation. Proc Natl Acad Sci U S A 97:5610–5615
20. Neumar RW (2000) Molecular mechanisms of ischemic neuronal injury. Ann Emerg Med 36:483–506
21. Siesjo BK (1994) Calcium-mediated processes in neuronal degeneration. Ann N Y Acad Sci 747:140–161
22. Bonde C, Noraberg J, Noer H, Zimmer J (2005) Ionotropic glutamate receptors andglutamate transporters are involved in necrotic neuronal cell death induced by oxygen–glucose deprivation of hippocampal slice cultures. Neurosciences 136:779–794
23. Pettigrew L, Holtz S, Craddocak S, Minger N, Geddes J (1996) Microtubular proteolysis in focal cerebral ischemia. J Cereb Blood Flow Metab 16:1189–1202
24. Zhang Y, Sun G (1995) Free fatty acids, neutral glycerides and phosphoglycerides in transient focal ischemia. J Neurochem 64:1688–1695
25. Sapirstein A, Bonventre JV (2000) Phospholipases A2 in ischemic and toxic brain injury. Neurochem Res 25:745–753
26. Solenski NJ, Kwan AL, Yanamoto H, Bennett JP, Kassell NF, Lee KS (1997) Differential hydroxylation of salicylate in core and penumbra regions during focal reversible cerebral ischemia. Stroke 28:2545–2552
27. Hallenbeck JM, Dutka AJ (1990) Background review and current concepts of reperfusion injury. Arch Neurol 47:1245–1254
28. Andreyev AY, Kushnareva YE, Starkov AA (2005) Mitochondrial metabolism of reactive oxygen species. Biochemistry 70:200–214
29. Iadecola C (1997) Bright and dark sides of nitric oxide in ischemic brain injury. Trends Neurosci 20:132–139
30. Suh SW, Chen JW, Motamedi M, Bell B, Listiak K, Pons NF, Danscher G, Frederickson CJ (2000) Evidence that synoptically-released zinc contributes to neuronal injury after traumatic brain injury. Brain Res 852:268–273
31. O'Neill LA, Kaltschmidt C (1997) NF-kappa B: a crucial transcription factor for glial and neuronal cell function. Trends Neurosci 20:252–258
32. Frijns CJM, Kappelle LJ (2002) Inflammatory cell adhesion molecules in ischemic cerebrovascular disease. Stroke 33:2115–2122
33. Nakka VP, Gusain A, Mehta SL, Raghubir R (2008) Molecular mechanisms of apoptosis in cerebral ischemia: multiple neuroprotective opportunities. Mol Neurobiol 37:7–38
34. Badaut J, Lasbennes F, Magistretti PJ, Regli L (2002) Aquaporins in brain: distribution, physiology, and pathophysiology. J Cereb Blood Flow Metab 22:367–378

35. Badaut J, Brunet JF, Grollimund L et al (2003) Aquaporin 1 and 4 expression after human acute subarachnoid hemorrhage. Acta Neurochir 86:495–498
36. Unterberg AW, Stover J, Kress B, Kiening KL (2004) Edema and brain trauma. Neuroscience 129:1019–1027
37. Payen JF, Fauvage B, Falcon D, Lavagne P (2003) Brain oedema following blood-brain barrier disruption: mechanisms and diagnosis. Ann Fr Anesth Reanim 22:220–225
38. Wang G, Huang H, He Y, Ruan L, Huang J (2014) Bumetanide protects focal cerebral ischemia-reperfusion injury in rat. Int J Clin Exp Pathol 7(4):1487–1494
39. Dousset V, Ménégon P, Rouanet F, Dumont E, Moonen CT, Caillé JM, Orgogozo JM (1999) Ischemic vascular accidents in the acute phase. J Neuroradiol 26:200–208
40. Davis SM, Donnan GA, Parsons MW et al (2008) Effects of alteplase beyond 3 h after stroke in the echoplanar imaging thrombolytic evaluation trial (epithet): a placebo-controlled randomised trial. Lancet Neurol 7:299–309
41. Donnan GA, Baron JC, Ma H, Davis SM (2009) Penumbral selection of patients for trials of acute stroke therapy. Lancet Neurol 8:261–269
42. Schlaug G, Benfield A, Baird AE et al (1999) The ischemic penumbra: operationally defined by diffusion and perfusion MRI. Neurology 53:1528–1537
43. Nabavi DG, Leblanc LM, Baxter B, Lee DH, Fox AJ, Lownie SP et al (2001) Monitoring cerebral perfusion after subarachnoid hemorrhage using CT. Neuroradiology 43:7–16
44. Wintermark M, Meuli R, Browaeys P et al (2007) Comparison of CT perfusion and angiography and MRI in selecting stroke patients for acute treatment. Neurology 68: 694–697
45. Ronning OM, Guldvog B, Stavem K (2001) The benefit of an acute stroke unit in patients with intracranial haemorrhage: a controlled trial. J Neurol Neurosurg Psychiatry 70:631–634
46. Diringer MN, Edwards DF (2001) Admission to a neurologic–neurosurgical intensive care unit is associated with reduced mortality rate after intracerebral hemorrhage. Crit Care Med 29:635–640
47. The ATLANTIS, ECASS, NINDS rt-PA Study Group Investigators (2004) Association of outcome with early stroke treatment: pooled analysis of ATLANTIS, ECASS, and NINDS rt-PA stroke trials. Lancet 363:768–774
48. Schellinger P, Fiebach J, Mohr A, Ringleb P, Jansen O, Hacke W (2001) Thrombolytic therapy for ischemic stroke—a review. Part I-Intravenous thrombolysis. Crit Care Med 29:1812–1818
49. Larrue V, von Kummer RR, Muller A, Bluhmki E (2001) Risk factors for severe hemorrhagic transformation in ischemic stroke patients treated with recombinant tissue plasminogen activator: a secondary analysis of the European-Australasian Acute Stroke Study (ECASS II). Stroke 32:438–441
50. Wahlgren N, Ahmed N, Davalos A, Ford GA, Grond M, Hacke W et al (2007) Thrombolysis with alteplase for acute ischaemic stroke in the safe implementation of thrombolysis in stroke-monitoring study (SITS-MOST): an observational study. Lancet 369:275–282
51. Kohrmann M, Juttler E, Fiebach JB, Huttner HB, Siebert S, Schwark C et al (2006) MRI versus CT-based thrombolysis treatment within and beyond the 3 h time window after stroke onset: a cohort study. Lancet Neurol 5:661–667
52. Thomalla G, Schwark C, Sobesky J, Bluhmki E, Fiebach JB, Fiehler J et al (2006) Outcome and symptomatic bleeding complications of intravenous thrombolysis within 6 h in MRI-selected stroke patients: comparison of a German multicenter study with the pooled data of ATLANTIS, ECASS and NINDS tPA trials. Stroke 37:852–858
53. Hacke W, Kaste M, Bluhmki E, Brozman M, Dávalos A, Guidetti D, Larrue V, Lees KR, Medeghri Z, Machnig T, Schneider D, von Kummer R, Wahlgren N (2008) Toni D; ECASS Investigators. Thrombolysis with alteplase 3 to 4.5 hours after acute ischemic stroke. N Engl J Med 359:1317–1329
54. Wahlgren N, Ahmed N, Dávalos A, Hacke W, Millán M, Muir K, Roine RO, Toni D (2008) Lees KR; SITS investigators. Thrombolysis with alteplase 3-4.5 h after acute ischaemic stroke (SITS-ISTR): an observational study. Lancet 372:1303–1309

55. Albers GW, Thijs VN, Wechsler L, Kemp S, Schlaug G et al (2006) Magnetic resonance imaging profiles predict clinical response to early reperfusion: the diffusion and perfusion imaging evaluation for understanding stroke evolution (DEFUSE) study. Ann Neurol 60:508–517
56. Furlan AJ, Eyding D, Albers GW, Al-Rawi Y, Lees KR, Rowley HA, Sachara C, Soehngen M, Warach S, Hacke W, Investigators DEDAS (2006) Dose Escalation of Desmoteplase for Acute Ischemic Stroke (DEDAS): evidence of safety and efficacy 3 to 9 hours after stroke onset. Stroke 37:1227–1231
57. Hacke W, Albers G, Al-Rawi Y, Bogousslavsky J, Davalos A et al (2005) The Desmoteplase in Acute Ischemic Stroke Trial (DIAS): a phase II MRI-based 9-hour window acute stroke thrombolysis trial with intravenous desmoteplase. Stroke 36:66–73
58. Hacke W, Furlan AJ, Al-Rawi Y, Davalos A, Fiebach JB et al (2009) Intravenous desmoteplase in patients with acute ischaemic stroke selected by MRI perfusion-diffusion weighted imaging or perfusion CT (DIAS-2): a prospective, randomised, double-blind, placebo-controlled study. Lancet Neurol 8:141–150
59. Khaja AM, Grotta JC (2007) Established treatments for acute ischaemic stroke. Lancet 369:319–330
60. Badhiwala JH, Nassiri F, Alhazzani W, Selim MH, Farrokhyar F, Spears J, Kulkarni AV, Singh S et al (2015) Endovascular Thrombectomy for Acute Ischemic Stroke: A Meta-analysis. JAMA 314(17):1832–1843. doi: 10.1001/jama.2015.13767
61. Derex L, Adeleine P, Nighoghossian N, Honnorat J, Trouillas P (2002) Factors influencing early admission in a French stroke unit. Stroke 33:153–159
62. Sandercock P, Gubitz G, Foley P, Counsell C (2003) Antiplatelet therapy for acute ischaemic stroke. Cochrane Database Syst Rev 2:CD000029
63. Gray CS, Hildreth AJ, Sandercock PA, O'Connell JE, Johnston DE, Cartlidge NE et al (2007) Glucose-potassium-insulin infusions in the management of post-stroke hyperglycaemia: the UK glucose insulin in stroke trial (GIST-UK). Lancet Neurol 6:397–406
64. Krieger DW, De Georgia MA, Abou-Chebl A, Andrefsky JC, Sila CA, Katzan IL, Mayberg MR, Furlan AJ (2001) Cooling for acute ischemic brain damage (cool aid): an open pilot study of induced hypothermia in acute ischemic stroke. Stroke 32:1847–1854
65. De Georgia MA, Krieger DW, Abou-Chebl A, Devlin TG, Jauss M, Davis SM, Koroshetz WJ, Rordorf G, Warach S (2004) Cooling for Acute Ischemic Brain Damage (COOL AID): a feasibility trial of endovascular cooling. Neurology 63:312–317
66. Adams HP Jr, del Zoppo G, Alberts MJ, Bhatt DL, Brass L, Furlan A et al (2007) Guidelines for the early management of adults with ischemic stroke. Stroke 38:1655–1711
67. Hacke W, Kaste M, Bogousslavsky J, Brainin M, Chamorro A, Lees K et al (2003) European stroke initiative recommendations for stroke management-update 2003. Cerebrovasc Dis 16:311–337
68. Ginsberg MD (2009) Current status of neuroprotection for cerebral ischemia: synoptic overview. Stroke 40:S111–S114
69. Zaleska MM, Mercado ML, Chavez J, Feuerstein GZ, Pangalos MN, Wood A (2009) The development of stroke therapeutics: promising mechanisms and translational challenges. Neuropharmacology 56:329–341
70. Ehrenreich H, Hasselblatt M, Dembowski C, Cepek L, Lewczuk P et al (2002) Erythropoietin therapy for acute stroke is both safe and beneficial. Mol Med 8:495–505
71. Ehrenreich H, Weissenborn K, Prange H, Schneider D, Weimar C, Wartenberg K et al (2009) Recombinant human erythropoietin in the treatment of acute ischemic stroke. Stroke 40:e647–e656
72. Yoshimoto T, Ogawa A, Seki H, Kogure T, Suzuki J (1986) Clinical course of acute middle cerebral artery occlusion. J Neurosurg 65:326–330
73. Ringelstein EB, Biniek R, Weiller C, Ammeling B, Nolte PN, Thron A (1992) Type and extent of hemispheric brain infarctions and clinical outcome in early and delayed middle cerebral artery recanalization. Neurology 42:289–298
74. Hacke W, Schwab S, Horn M, Spranger M, De Georgia M, Von Kummer R (1996) "Malignant" middle cerebral artery territory infarction: clinical course and prognostic signs. Arch Neurol 53:309–315

75. Von Kummer R, Meyding-Lamadé U, Forsting M, Rosin L, Rieke K, Hacke W (1994) Sensitivity and prognostic value of early CT in occlusion of the middle cerebral artery trunk. AJNR Am J Neuroradiol 15:9–15
76. Oppenheim C, Samson Y, Manaï R, Lalam T, Vandamme X, Crozier S et al (2000) Prediction of malignant middle cerebral artery infarction by diffusion-weighted imaging. Stroke 31:2175–2181
77. Vahedi K, Hofmeijer J, Juettler E, Vicaut E, George B, Algra A et al (2007) Early decompressive surgery in malignant infarction of the middle cerebral artery: a pooled analysis of three randomised controlled trials. Lancet Neurol 6:215–222
78. Hornig CR, Rust DS, Busse O, Jauss M, Laun A (1994) Space-occupying cerebellar infarction. Clinical course and prognosis. Stroke 25:372–374
79. Cioffi FA, Bernini FP, Punzo A, D'Avanzo R (1985) Surgical management of acute cerebellar infarction. Acta Neurochir 74:105–112
80. Laun A, Busse O, Calatayud V, Klug N (1984) Cerebellar infarcts in the area of the supply of the PICA and their surgical treatment. Acta Neurochir 71:295–306

Evaluation of Cerebral Blood Flow and Brain Metabolism in the Intensive Care Unit

14

Pierre Bouzat, Emmanuel L. Barbier, Gilles Francony, and Jean-François Payen

14.1 Introduction

The imbalance between oxygen supply to the brain tissue and its utilization, that is, brain tissue hypoxia, is considered the major cause for the development of secondary brain damage and hence poor neurological outcome [1, 2]. This phenomenon develops hours after the initial insult, e.g., trauma, stroke, intracerebral hematoma, and subarachnoid hemorrhage (SAH). Therefore, improving brain oxygenation after severe brain injury is the focus of modern management in the intensive care unit (ICU). It relies upon a multimodal approach of monitoring that includes assessments of brain perfusion and metabolism at the bedside and during imaging modalities.

14.2 Bedside Monitoring

Bedside monitoring of brain tissue oxygenation after the initial insult may help clinicians to initiate adequate actions when episodes of brain ischemia/hypoxia are identified. This monitoring relies upon several parameters to temptingly reflect the

P. Bouzat • G. Francony • J-F.Payen (✉)
Pôle Anesthesie-Reanimation, CHU Grenoble Alpes, F-38000, Grenoble, France

Inserm U1216, F-38000, Grenoble, France

Univ. Grenoble Alpes, Grenoble Institute ofneurosciences (GIN),
F-38000, Grenoble, France
e-mail: pbouzat@chu-grenoble.fr; gfrancony@chu-grenoble.fr; jfpayen@chu-grenoble.fr

E.L. Barbier
Inserm U1216, F-38000, Grenoble, France

Univ. Grenoble Alpes, Grenoble Institute ofneurosciences (GIN),
F-38000, Grenoble, France
e-mail: barbier@chu-grenoble.fr

C. Ichai et al. (eds.), *Metabolic Disorders and Critically Ill Patients*,
http://doi.org/10.1007/978-3-319-64010-5_14

complex heterogeneity of brain ischemia/hypoxia by providing global and/or local information of the injured brain tissue.

14.2.1 Clinical Examination

In conscious patients, a normal clinical examination is the best evidence of an adequate balance between cerebral blood flow (CBF) and metabolism at the bedside. In brain-injured patients, clinical examination should be considered first. For example, the development of a vasospasm post-SAH, which impacts on the brain perfusion, can be clinically suspected when a recent neurological deterioration is observed. Wherever possible after neurosurgical procedure, clinical examination can detect any ischemia-related postoperative complications.

14.2.2 Intracranial Pressure and Cerebral Perfusion Pressure

International guidelines emphasize the use of intracranial pressure (ICP) monitors following severe brain injury and the continuous calculation of cerebral perfusion pressure (CPP, with CPP = mean arterial pressure – ICP). To prevent brain ischemia due to elevated ICP, it is recommended to maintain CPP at 60–70 mmHg and ICP below 20 mmHg [3]. Intracranial hypertension, as defined by ICP values over 20 mmHg in adults, is indeed considered as an independent risk factor of mortality and neurological disabilities. Prolonged periods of CPP levels below 50 mmHg are usually associated with unfavorable outcome after severe TBI. However, clinical studies have demonstrated that episodes of brain ischemia/hypoxia are common despite optimization of CPP and are independently associated with poorer patient outcome [4]. In a recent trial, maintaining ICP below 20 mmHg was not superior to care based on imaging and clinical examination [5]. Although CPP and CBF can be positively correlated in normal subjects, this statement is not always verified in patients with brain disorders. The effect of hyperventilation, i.e., hypocapnia, is indeed illustrative: despite the normalization of CPP and ICP levels during hyperventilation in TBI patients, CBF was markedly reduced to ischemic levels [6]. Collectively, these data suggest that ICP and CPP monitoring is needed to avoid conditions of low brain perfusion in severely brain-injured patients, but it may be insufficient to detect brain hypoxia.

14.2.3 Transcranial Doppler

Transcranial Doppler (TCD) was introduced in 1982 [7]. The method is easy to use, is noninvasive, and measures real-time CBF velocities from basal cerebral arteries. Initially used to diagnose vasospasm after SAH, TCD is now used in other brain injuries such as TBI and stroke [8]. Most commonly insonated in clinical practice is the middle cerebral artery (MCA) that is easily accessible through the temporal window above the zygomatic arch. The MCA carries 60–70% of the ipsilateral carotid artery blood flow, so its TCD measurement can be taken to represent blood flow to that hemisphere.

Blood flow in the basal cerebral arteries has a prominent diastolic component. Diastolic blood flow velocity (FVd) reflects the degree of downstream vascular resistance, whereas systolic blood flow velocity (FVs) depends on upstream determinants, that is, cardiac output, ipsilateral carotid blood flow, and arterial blood pressure. Mean blood flow velocity (FVm) is the weighted flow velocity that takes into account the different velocities of the formed elements in the blood vessel insonated and decreases with low CBF (Table 14.1, Fig.14.1). In TBI patients, a low FVd, a peaked waveform, and higher pulsatility index [PI, with PI = (FVs-FVd)/

Table 14.1 Comparison of several perfusion imaging methods

	Iodine CT	Xenon CT	Water MRI	Gd chelate MRI	PET	SPECT	Ultrasound
Measured parameters	CBF, CBV, MTT	CBF	CBF	CBF, CBV, MTT	CBF, CBV	CBF	
Measurement type	Dynamic monitoring		Measurements before/after	Dynamic follow-up		One measurement	Dynamic follow-up
Quantification	++	+++	+++	+	+++	+	–
Spatial resolution (mm)	2	2	2	2	4–6	4–6	
Acquisition duration (min)	2	10	3	2	10	15	1
Spatial coverage	Depends on the number of detectors	Depends on the number of detectors	Whole brain	Whole brain	Whole brain	Whole brain	Under development

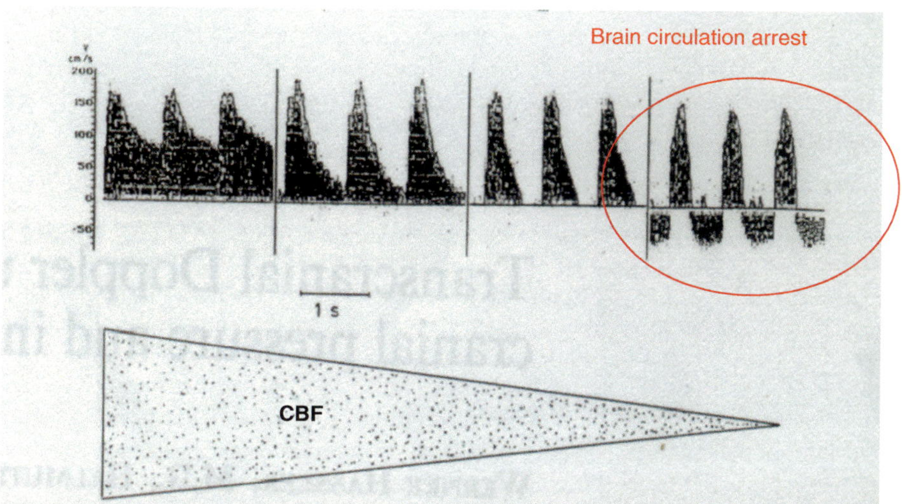

Fig. 14.1 Transcranial Doppler. *CBF* cerebral blood flow

FVm] values can be observed during high vascular bed resistance induced by elevated ICP or hypocapnia. In patients with severe TBI, TCD can detect inadequate CBF, assess cerebral autoregulation, and help indicate the need for invasive brain monitoring and of required therapies in a multimodal neuromonitoring approach [9]. In patients with mild-to-moderate TBI, TCD can be used in the emergency room, in conjunction with CT scan, to identify patients at risk for secondary neurological deterioration [10].

14.2.4 Brain Oxygenation

Measurements of brain oxygenation have been increasingly developed to measure the adequacy between oxygen supply and oxygen consumption that is not provided by ICP/CPP or TCD monitoring.

14.2.4.1 Jugular Venous Oxygen Saturation

This technique relies upon the insertion of a catheter in the internal jugular vein to measure the jugular venous oxygen saturation ($SvjO_2$) from the ipsilateral hemisphere. Arteriovenous difference of oxygen ($AVDO_2$) is then calculated from hemoglobin concentration, arterial oxygen saturation of oxygen (SaO_2), and $SvjO_2$. Cerebral metabolic rate of oxygen ($CMRO_2$) is obtained by the formula:

$$CMRO_2 = CBF \times AVDO_2$$

$SvjO_2$ measurement can be a good estimator of CBF assuming unchanged levels of hemoglobin, SaO_2, and $CMRO_2$. Furthermore, $SvjO_2$ may reflect the adequacy between CBF and metabolic requirements because any decrease in oxygen supply will raise tissue oxygen extraction fraction (OEF) and lower $SvjO_2$. $SvjO_2$ values less than 50–60% were found associated with unfavorable neurological outcome after severe TBI [11]. However, there are technical limitations that hinder its routine use: extracranial blood contamination, discontinuous measurement, global assessment of brain oxygenation, and the risk of catheter-related jugular vein thrombosis.

14.2.4.2 Brain Tissue Oxygenation

Measuring cerebral tissue oxygen tension can be safely and reliably achieved at the bedside using brain tissue PO_2 ($PbtO_2$) probes surgically inserted into the parenchyma [12, 13]. $PbtO_2$ was proved more suitable for long-term continuous monitoring than measurements of $SjvO_2$. $PbtO_2$ values lower than 15 mmHg for more than 30 minutes were shown to be an independent predictor of unfavorable outcome and death [14]. Aggressive treatment of low $PbtO_2$ was associated with improved outcome compared to standard ICP-/CPP-directed therapy in cohort studies of severely head-injured patients [15]. The use of devices to monitor brain tissue oxygenation has been suggested in the Brain Trauma Foundation's guidelines for the management of severe TBI [16]. There are several factors that may impact on the $PbtO_2$ measurements: CBF, PaO_2 levels, gradients for oxygen diffusion across tissues, and hemoglobin content [17, 18, 13]. Overall, $PbtO_2$ would reflect the diffusion of dissolved plasma oxygen across the blood-brain barrier (BBB) [19].

Monitoring the $PbtO_2$ requires a surgical procedure, and this procedure yields a local estimate of brain tissue oxygenation. The $PbtO_2$ device most widely used is the Licox® probe (Integra Neurosciences, Plainsboro, NJ), which is a safe and reliable Clark-based electrode. However, the reading surface area of the Licox catheter tip is approximately 18 mm^2. In addition, the placement site of the catheter is an issue for data interpretation. After TBI, distinct pathophysiological differences are apparent between injured, normal, and at-risk brain tissue, so PbtO2 values can vary according to whether the catheter tip is placed in contused brain tissue or normal tissue [20]. In practice, the $PbtO_2$ response can be used to guide the management of CPP at the bedside. Manipulating CPP to maintain $PbtO_2$ above 15–20 mmHg ($PbtO_2$-directed strategy) might optimize CBF and avoid secondary brain ischemia/hypoxia [16, 21].

14.2.4.3 Near-Infrared Spectroscopy

Near-infrared spectroscopy (NIRS) technique uses principles of optical spectrophotometry related to the fact that biological material is relatively transparent in the NIR range [22]. Because of the poor signal-to-noise ratio, commercially available devices use reflectance-mode NIRS in which receiving optodes are placed ipsilateral to the transmitter. Measurement of tissue oxygen saturation is determined by the difference in oxy- and deoxyhemoglobin intensities between a transmitted and received light delivered according to the Beer-Lambert law. This allows a continuous real-time monitoring of brain tissue oxygenation (StO_2) in the frontal cortex. Since the blood venous compartment reaches 70–80% of total blood volume, NIRS is believed to provide a noninvasive estimation of $SvjO_2$ in normal subjects. However, StO_2 was not correlated to $SvjO_2$ in patients with severe TBI and showed large interindividual variability [23]. There are several technical limitations with NIRS, e.g., the light scattering by tissue, the extracranial contamination of NIRS signal, and the predefined cerebral arterial/venous partitioning [22, 24]. Nevertheless, NIRS can be useful to detect cerebral ischemic conditions during specific procedures such as carotid endarterectomy or shoulder arthroscopy. In these conditions, StO_2 values <55% at baseline and/or a 20% relative decrease in StO_2 are considered as thresholds for brain ischemia [25].

14.2.4.4 Cerebral Microdialysis

Cerebral microdialysis (CMD) has largely contributed to a better understanding of the pathophysiology of acute brain dysfunction and was recently introduced as an additional bedside neuromonitoring tool in this context. CMD consists in the placement of an intraparenchymal probe with a semipermeable dialysis membrane. A cerebrospinal fluidlike solution, infused through this catheter, allows hourly sampling of patients' brain extracellular fluid for bedside analysis [26]. CMD provides monitoring of dynamic changes of main brain energy substrate (glucose) and metabolites (lactate and pyruvate). High lactate/pyruvate ratio (LPR) values would reflect either a mitochondrial dysfunction or an imbalance between oxygen supply and its tissue utilization. A LPR >40 and an extracellular glucose <0.7–1 mmol/L are usually considered as thresholds for abnormality in the clinical setting [27]. For example, these CMD abnormalities were found in patients with delayed cerebral ischemia after SAH [28]. In TBI, the LPR threshold value is considered abnormal if >25. Additionally, CMD contributed to manage blood glucose control after severe TBI [29].

14.3 Imaging Techniques

14.3.1 Perfusion Imaging

The development of brain perfusion imaging over the last 20 years is spectacular [30]. This progress is due to the development of hardware allowing larger spatial coverage, shorter acquisition times, and a better understanding of the relationship between imaging signals and the pathophysiology. It is thus possible to obtain quantitative maps of the cerebral blood flow (CBF, in mL/100 g/min) and of the cerebral blood volume (mL/100 g) [31].

14.3.1.1 Perfusion CT Scan

Cerebral perfusion CT scan has been increasingly used since the introduction of rapid, large-coverage multidetector-row CT scanners. Perfusion CT imaging is based on the signal changes induced by an intravenous bolus of iodine contrast agent [32, 33]. The temporal evolution of the signal reflects the change in iodine concentration within each voxel. If the contrast agent remains intravascular, the signal-time curve yields a quantitative estimation of CBV, CBF, and the mean transit time (MTT) of the contrast agent. Quantitative information about the BBB status can be obtained with acquisition duration lasting up to 4 min after the bolus [34].

The analysis of the bolus passage requires technical cautions: automated administration of the bolus, correct selection of arterial and venous input vessels, correct selection of brain regions of interest, and maintenance of patient's conditions during the CT acquisition, i.e., hemodynamics and ventilation. Software for post-processing perfusion CT data is now available on each CT scanner. Perfusion CT scan has limitations, in particular the necessity to have an intact blood-brain barrier to obtain MTT and CBV measurements and the calculation derived from one arterial input function. In addition to regional CBF variations, diffuse cerebral lesions may alter the correct calculation of the arterial input function. Major clinical applications of the perfusion CT scan are the diagnosis of cerebral ischemia and infarction and evaluation of vasospasm after SAH [32].

14.3.1.2 Xenon-Enhanced CT Scan

Mapping CBF can be obtained using inhaled 28% xenon [35, 36]. Because lipophilic xenon gas diffuses across the BBB, changes in the xenon concentration in brain tissue and in arterial blood allow the determination of the CBF. In patients with normal pulmonary function, the xenon arterial input function can be estimated from expired xenon fraction measurements [37].

14.3.1.3 Arterial Spin-Labeled MRI

Arterial spin labeling (ASL) is a MRI approach that has been developed and validated to quantify brain perfusion [38, 39]. In ASL techniques, arterial blood water is magnetically labeled to be an endogenous tracer. Magnetization of arterial blood water is obtained from carotid arteries or from Willis circle arteries. Arterial blood water with inverted magnetization (T1 relaxation) flows to the brain. During ASL image acquisition, repeated label and control images are interleaved. Perfusion contrast is then obtained by subtraction of the label and control acquisitions to provide quantitative measurements of CBF. Because only small amounts of arterial spin-labeled water accumulate in the brain, ~40 pairs of control/label images are required to estimate CBF with accuracy. The ASL approach is highly analogous to positron emission tomography (PET), which uses ^{15}O-labeled water as the flow tracer. Over two decades, technical developments and validation have led to the emergence of robust ASL implementations in clinical imagers, with a tenfold increase in the quality of CBF map [40]. Cerebral perfusion using ASL can be obtained in 3 min now.

14.3.1.4 Dynamic Susceptibility Contrast MRI

The principles of the dynamic susceptibility contrast MRI (DSC-MRI) are similar to those of perfusion CT scan [30, 38]. Relative cerebral blood flow (rCBF) is calculated by a model-independent deconvolution approach from the tracer concentration curves following a bolus injection of gadolinium chelate (diethylenetriaminepentaacetate) or Gd-DTPA.

The difference between DSC-MRI and perfusion CT relies on the relation between the signal and the contrast agent concentration in the voxel. While linear with CT, this relation is more complex with MRI. Indeed, Gd-DTPA shortens the relaxation times T1 and T2 of the blood as well as the T2* relaxation time of the voxel. This does not allow obtaining absolute CBF measurements. Relative CBF values are however robust [41]. Information about the BBB status can be obtained using a follow-up of T1 changes following Gd-DTP administration (dynamic contrast-enhanced MRI). Finally, DCS-MRI can estimate microvessel diameter within the voxel and/or microvessel density. This allows the characterization of tumor angiogenesis [42, 43].

14.3.1.5 Positron Emission Tomography

Brain perfusion imaging with PET requires the administration of oxygen-15-labeled water [44]. A cyclotron nearby is mandatory due to the short radioactive period of $^{15}O_2$ (2 min). $H_2{}^{15}O_2$ is injected intravenously, while $C^{15}O_2$ is inhaled for a few minutes to be converted to $H_2{}^{15}O_2$ in the blood by anhydrase carbonic. Quantifying CBF needs a correct estimation of the arterial input function. Although limited in its accessibility, PET imaging remains the reference method to map CBF, CBV, and brain metabolism in humans and may provide clues to novel pathophysiology after TBI [45].

14.3.1.6 Single Photon Emission Computed Tomography (SPECT)

Historically, CBF measurements were obtained using external scintillation cameras after ^{133}Xe inhalation, in a similar approach to xenon-enhanced CT scan [46]. The low energy of gamma photons emitted by ^{133}Xe has limited the development of the method. The use of ^{123}I-IMP (inosine-5′-monophosphate) combined with a gamma emitter, either 99^{mTc}-HMPAO (hexamethylpropyleneamine oxime) or 99^{mTc}-ECD (ethyl cysteinate dimer), has been proposed [47]. However, amounts of tracer trapped into the brain are not strictly proportional to CBF. CBF maps using SPECT are therefore not quantitative.

14.3.1.7 Dynamic Contrast-Enhanced Ultrasound

Brain perfusion can be explored with ultrasound contrast agents. Microbubbles (1–10 μm in diameter) are intravenously injected to yield brain perfusion at the capillary level [48]. This approach differs from transcranial Doppler that is limited to larger vessels with fast flow rates. Dynamic contrast-enhanced ultrasound can assess both the macro- and microcirculation. It analyzes the time-intensity curves in a region of interest, e.g., tumor, myocardium, and the brain.

14.3.2 Metabolic Imaging

Metabolic information can be obtained in humans using PET and MR spectroscopy. Research is active to develop metabolic contrast agents and optical imaging.

14.3.2.1 Positron Emission Tomography

$^{15}O_2$-PET imaging can assess $CMRO_2$ as well as CBF and CBV [45]. Fluorine-18 is an alternative tracer to map cerebral glucose consumption (fluorine-18 fluorodeoxyglucose, ^{18}F-FDG) or brain hypoxia (fluorine-18 fluoromisonidazole, ^{18}F-MISO). Because fluorine-18 has a 2-h radioactive period, it is more convenient than $^{15}O_2$. ^{18}F-FDG enters brain cells and remains trapped and non-metabolized. ^{18}F-FDG-PET tissue accumulation matches cerebral glucose consumption. ^{18}F-FMISO distributes over the entire brain and remains trapped in cells with a tissue pressure of oxygen below 10 mmHg. The tissue accumulation of ^{18}F-FMISO reflects thus hypoxic regions [49].

14.3.2.2 Magnetic Resonance Spectroscopy

Proton (^{1}H) or phosphorus (^{31}P) magnetic resonance spectroscopy (MRS) can determine the concentration ($\geq$1 mM) of brain tissue metabolites. ^{1}H-MRS can identify markers of the neuronal viability (N-acetyl-aspartate, NAA), cell membrane turnover (choline), and cell energy metabolism (creatine, Cr; lactate). Peaks most readily identified using ^{31}P-MRS are involved in the high-energy cellular metabolism (ATP; phosphocreatine, PCr; inorganic phosphate, Pi), and intracellular pH can be assessed using this technique [50]. In practice, ^{1}H or ^{31}P spectrum is obtained from single-voxel acquisition, and results are expressed as ratios, e.g., NAA/Cr and Pi/PCr. In TBI patients, NAA/Cr value in the posterior pons was found associated with neurological outcome [51].

Quantification of the blood oxygenation level-dependent (BOLD) contrast is possible now. This approach is based on an MR signal model that incorporates prior knowledge about brain tissue composition and considers signals from gray and white mattes, cerebrospinal fluid, and blood. Cerebral maps of OEF and $CMRO_2$ have been obtained in humans and after diffuse TBI in rats [52, 53].

Conclusion

To preserve injured brain from ischemia/hypoxia and its negative impact on neurological outcome, several techniques are in use to assess CBF, brain oxygenation, and metabolism. Because one technique cannot provide a comprehensive and quantitative description of brain ischemia-hypoxia, there is a need for a combination of monitoring tools and imaging modalities.

References

1. Bramlett HM, Dietrich WD (2007) Progressive damage after brain and spinal cord injury: pathomechanisms and treatment strategies. Prog Brain Res 161:125–141
2. Graham DI, Adams JH (1971) Ischaemic brain damage in fatal head injuries. Lancet 1:265–266
3. Bratton SL, Chestnut RM, Ghajar J, McConnell Hammond FF, Harris OA, Hartl R, Manley GT, Nemecek A, Newell DW, Rosenthal G, Schouten J, Shutter L, Timmons SD, Ullman JS, Videtta W, Wilberger JE, Wright DW (2007) Guidelines for the management of severe traumatic brain injury. IX. Cerebral perfusion thresholds. J Neurotrauma 24(Suppl 1):S59–S64
4. Eriksson EA, Barletta JF, Figueroa BE, Bonnell BW, Vanderkolk WE, McAllen KJ, Ott MM (2012) Cerebral perfusion pressure and intracranial pressure are not surrogates for brain tissue oxygenation in traumatic brain injury. Clin Neurophysiol 123:1255–1260
5. Chesnut RM, Temkin N, Carney N, Dikmen S, Rondina C, Videtta W, Petroni G, Lujan S, Pridgeon J, Barber J, Machamer J, Chaddock K, Celix JM, Cherner M, Hendrix T (2012) A trial of intracranial-pressure monitoring in traumatic brain injury. N Engl J Med 367:2471–2481
6. Coles JP, Minhas PS, Fryer TD, Smielewski P, Aigbirihio F, Donovan T, Downey SP, Williams G, Chatfield D, Matthews JC, Gupta AK, Carpenter TA, Clark JC, Pickard JD, Menon DK (2002) Effect of hyperventilation on cerebral blood flow in traumatic head injury: clinical relevance and monitoring correlates. Crit Care Med 30:1950–1959
7. Aaslid R, Markwalder TM, Nornes H (1982) Noninvasive transcranial Doppler ultrasound recording of flow velocity in basal cerebral arteries. J Neurosurg 57:769–774
8. Czosnyka M, Kirkpatrick PJ, Pickard JD (1996) Multimodal monitoring and assessment of cerebral haemodynamic reserve after severe head injury. Cerebrovasc Brain Metab Rev 8:273–295
9. Saqqur M, Zygun D, Demchuk A (2007) Role of transcranial Doppler in neurocritical care. Crit Care Med 35:S216–S223
10. Bouzat P, Francony G, Declety P, Genty C, Kaddour A, Bessou P, Brun J, Jacquot C, Chabardes S, Bosson JL, Payen JF (2011) Transcranial Doppler to screen on admission patients with mild to moderate traumatic brain injury. Neurosurgery 68:1603–1609
11. Gopinath SP, Robertson CS, Contant CF, Hayes C, Feldman Z, Narayan RK, Grossman RG (1994) Jugular venous desaturation and outcome after head injury. J Neurol Neurosurg Psychiatry 57:717–723
12. Beynon C, Kiening KL, Orakcioglu B, Unterberg AW, Sakowitz OW (2012) Brain tissue oxygen monitoring and hyperoxic treatment in patients with traumatic brain injury. J Neurotrauma 29:2109–2123
13. Oddo M, Villa F, Citerio G (2012) Brain multimodality monitoring: an update. Curr Opin Crit Care 18:111–118

14. Chang JJ, Youn TS, Benson D, Mattick H, Andrade N, Harper CR, Moore CB, Madden CJ, Diaz-Arrastia RR (2009) Physiologic and functional outcome correlates of brain tissue hypoxia in traumatic brain injury. Crit Care Med 37:283–290
15. Narotam PK, Morrison JF, Nathoo N (2009) Brain tissue oxygen monitoring in traumatic brain injury and major trauma: outcome analysis of a brain tissue oxygen-directed therapy. J Neurosurg 111:672–682
16. Bratton SL, Chestnut RM, Ghajar J, McConnell Hammond FF, Harris OA, Hartl R, Manley GT, Nemecek A, Newell DW, Rosenthal G, Schouten J, Shutter L, Timmons SD, Ullman JS, Videtta W, Wilberger JE, Wright DW (2007) Guidelines for the management of severe traumatic brain injury. X. Brain oxygen monitoring and thresholds. J Neurotrauma 24(Suppl 1):S65–S70
17. Nortje J, Coles JP, Timofeev I, Fryer TD, Aigbirhio FI, Smielewski P, Outtrim JG, Chatfield DA, Pickard JD, Hutchinson PJ, Gupta AK, Menon DK (2008) Effect of hyperoxia on regional oxygenation and metabolism after severe traumatic brain injury: preliminary findings. Crit Care Med 36:273–281
18. Menon DK, Coles JP, Gupta AK, Fryer TD, Smielewski P, Chatfield DA, Aigbirhio F, Skepper JN, Minhas PS, Hutchinson PJ, Carpenter TA, Clark JC, Pickard JD (2004) Diffusion limited oxygen delivery following head injury. Crit Care Med 32:1384–1390
19. Rosenthal G, Hemphill JC 3rd, Sorani M, Martin C, Morabito D, Obrist WD, Manley GT (2008) Brain tissue oxygen tension is more indicative of oxygen diffusion than oxygen delivery and metabolism in patients with traumatic brain injury. Crit Care Med 36:1917–1924
20. Ponce LL, Pillai S, Cruz J, Li X, Julia H, Gopinath S, Robertson CS (2012) Position of probe determines prognostic information of brain tissue PO2 in severe traumatic brain injury. Neurosurgery 70:1492–1502
21. Maloney-Wilensky E, Gracias V, Itkin A, Hoffman K, Bloom S, Yang W, Christian S, LeRoux PD (2009) Brain tissue oxygen and outcome after severe traumatic brain injury: a systematic review. Crit Care Med 37:2057–2063
22. Murkin JM, Arango M (2009) Near-infrared spectroscopy as an index of brain and tissue oxygenation. Br J Anaesth 103(Suppl 1):i3–13
23. Lewis SB, Myburgh JA, Thornton EL, Reilly PL (1996) Cerebral oxygenation monitoring by near-infrared spectroscopy is not clinically useful in patients with severe closed-head injury: a comparison with jugular venous bulb oximetry. Crit Care Med 24:1334–1338
24. Davie SN, Grocott HP (2012) Impact of extracranial contamination on regional cerebral oxygen saturation: a comparison of three cerebral oximetry technologies. Anesthesiology 116:834–840
25. Murphy GS, Szokol JW, Marymont JH, Greenberg SB, Avram MJ, Vender JS, Vaughn J, Nisman M (2010) Cerebral oxygen desaturation events assessed by near-infrared spectroscopy during shoulder arthroscopy in the beach chair and lateral decubitus positions. Anesth Analg 111:496–505
26. Hillered L, Vespa PM, Hovda DA (2005) Translational neurochemical research in acute human brain injury: the current status and potential future for cerebral microdialysis. J Neurotrauma 22:3–41
27. Timofeev I, Carpenter KL, Nortje J, Al-Rawi PG, O'Connell MT, Czosnyka M, Smielewski P, Pickard JD, Menon DK, Kirkpatrick PJ, Gupta AK, Hutchinson PJ (2011) Cerebral extracellular chemistry and outcome following traumatic brain injury: a microdialysis study of 223 patients. Brain 134:484–494
28. Sarrafzadeh A, Haux D, Plotkin M, Ludemann L, Amthauer H, Unterberg A (2005) Bedside microdialysis reflects dysfunction of cerebral energy metabolism in patients with aneurysmal subarachnoid hemorrhage as confirmed by 15 O-H2 O-PET and 18 F-FDG-PET. J Neuroradiol 32:348–351
29. Oddo M, Schmidt JM, Carrera E, Badjatia N, Connolly ES, Presciutti M, Ostapkovich ND, Levine JM, Le Roux P, Mayer SA (2008) Impact of tight glycemic control on cerebral glucose metabolism after severe brain injury: a microdialysis study. Crit Care Med 36:3233–3238

30. Wintermark M, Sesay M, Barbier E, Borbely K, Dillon WP, Eastwood JD, Glenn TC, Grandin CB, Pedraza S, Soustiel JF, Nariai T, Zaharchuk G, Caille JM, Dousset V, Yonas H (2005) Comparative overview of brain perfusion imaging techniques. Stroke 36:e83–e99
31. Payen JF, Lefournier V, Barbier E, Darderian F, Fauvage B, Le Bas JF (2006) Imagerie de la perfusion et du metabolisme cerebral. Ann Fr Anesth Reanim 25:722–728
32. Wintermark M, Sincic R, Sridhar D, Chien JD (2008) Cerebral perfusion CT: technique and clinical applications. J Neuroradiol 35:253–260
33. Metting Z, Cerliani L, Rodiger LA, van der Naalt J (2013) Pathophysiological concepts in mild traumatic brain injury: diffusion tensor imaging related to acute perfusion CT imaging. PLoS One 8:e64461
34. Hom J, Dankbaar JW, Schneider T, Cheng SC, Bredno J, Wintermark M (2009) Optimal duration of acquisition for dynamic perfusion CT assessment of blood-brain barrier permeability using the Patlak model. AJNR Am J Neuroradiol 30:1366–1370
35. Pindzola RR, Yonas H (1998) The xenon-enhanced computed tomography cerebral blood flow method. Neurosurgery 43:1488–1492
36. Carlson AP, Brown AM, Zager E, Uchino K, Marks MP, Robertson C, Sinson GP, Marmarou A, Yonas H (2011) Xenon-enhanced cerebral blood flow at 28% xenon provides uniquely safe access to quantitative, clinically useful cerebral blood flow information: a multicenter study. AJNR Am J Neuroradiol 32:1315–1320
37. Honda M, Sase S, Yokota K, Ichibayashi R, Yoshihara K, Masuda H, Uekusa H, Nomoto J, Sugo N, Kishi T, Seiki Y (2013) Early cerebral circulation disturbance in patients suffering from different types of severe traumatic brain injury: a xenon CT and perfusion CT study. Acta Neurochir Suppl 118:259–263
38. Barbier EL, Lamalle L, Decorps M (2001) Methodology of brain perfusion imaging. J Magn Reson Imaging 13:496–520
39. Detre JA, Rao H, Wang DJ, Chen YF, Wang Z (2012) Applications of arterial spin labeled MRI in the brain. J Magn Reson Imaging 35:1026–1037
40. Dai W, Garcia D, de Bazelaire C, Alsop DC (2008) Continuous flow-driven inversion for arterial spin labeling using pulsed radio frequency and gradient fields. Magn Reson Med 60:1488–1497
41. Liu W, Wang B, Wolfowitz R, Yeh PH, Nathan DE, Graner J, Tang H, Pan H, Harper J, Pham D, Oakes TR, French LM, Riedy G (2013) Perfusion deficits in patients with mild traumatic brain injury characterized by dynamic susceptibility contrast MRI. NMR Biomed 26:651–663
42. Beaumont M, Lemasson B, Farion R, Segebarth C, Remy C, Barbier EL (2009) Characterization of tumor angiogenesis in rat brain using iron-based vessel size index MRI in combination with gadolinium-based dynamic contrast-enhanced MRI. J Cereb Blood Flow Metab 29:1714–1726
43. Emblem KE, Mouridsen K, Bjornerud A, Farrar CT, Jennings D, Borra RJ, Wen PY, Ivy P, Batchelor TT, Rosen BR, Jain RK, Sorensen AG (2013) Vessel architectural imaging identifies cancer patient responders to anti-angiogenic therapy. Nat Med 19:1178–1183
44. Raichle ME, Martin WR, Herscovitch P, Mintun MA, Markham J (1983) Brain blood flow measured with intravenous H2(15)O. II. Implementation and validation. J Nucl Med 24:790–798
45. Menon DK (2006) Brain ischaemia after traumatic brain injury: lessons from $^{15}O_2$ positron emission tomography. Curr Opin Crit Care 12:85–89
46. Lassen NA, Henriksen L, Paulson O (1981) Regional cerebral blood flow in stroke by 133Xenon inhalation and emission tomography. Stroke 12:284–288
47. Lassen NA, Andersen AR, Friberg L, Paulson OB (1988) The retention of [99mTc]-d,l-HM-PAO in the human brain after intracarotid bolus injection: a kinetic analysis. J Cereb Blood Flow Metab 8:S13–S22
48. Cosgrove D, Lassau N (2010) Imaging of perfusion using ultrasound. Eur J Nucl Med Mol Imaging 37(Suppl 1):S65–S85
49. Padhani AR, Krohn KA, Lewis JS, Alber M (2007) Imaging oxygenation of human tumours. Eur Radiol 17:861–872
50. Payen JF, Francony G, Fauvage B, Le Bas JF (2005) Apport de la spectroscopie RMN à l'évaluation du traumatisme crânien. Ann Fr Anesth Reanim 24:522–527

51. Tollard E, Galanaud D, Perlbarg V, Sanchez-Pena P, Le Fur Y, Abdennour L, Cozzone P, Lehericy S, Chiras J, Puybasset L (2009) Experience of diffusion tensor imaging and 1H spectroscopy for outcome prediction in severe traumatic brain injury: preliminary results. Crit Care Med 37:1448–1455
52. He X, Yablonskiy DA (2007) Quantitative BOLD: mapping of human cerebral deoxygenated blood volume and oxygen extraction fraction: default state. Magn Reson Med 57:115–126
53. Bouzat P, Millet A, Boue Y, Pernet-Gallay K, Trouve-Buisson T, Gaide-Chevronnay L, Barbier EL, Payen JF (2013) Changes in brain tissue oxygenation after treatment of diffuse traumatic brain injury by erythropoietin. Crit Care Med 41:1316–1324

Part V

Endocrine Disorders in Intensive Care Unit

Acute Complications of Diabetes

15

Jean-Christophe Orban, Emmanuel Van Obberghen,
and Carole Ichai

15.1 Introduction

Incidence of diabetes grows continuously in developed and developing countries, so it is considered as an epidemic disease [1]. There are nowadays several possible criteria for diagnosing diabetes [2]: (1) clinical signs evoking diabetes associated with blood glucose level (BGL) ≥ 200 mg/dL (11.1 mmol/L) at any time of day, (2) a fasting BGL ≥ 126 mg/dL (7.0 mmol/L), (3) a 2-h postload BGL ≥ 200 mg/dL during an oral glycemia tolerance test, and (4) a plasma glycated hemoglobin (HbA1c) ≥ 6.5%. Type 1 diabetes is characterized by insulinopenia caused by an autoimmune and irreversible destruction of pancreatic ß-cells. Relative insulin deficiency and insulin resistance are the hallmarks of type 2 diabetes which is the most frequent in the world [3, 4].

Acute complications of diabetes are represented by hyperglycemic and hypoglycemic acute disorders. Beside these complications, metformin-associated lactic acidosis represents a complex metabolic complication. All of them are life-threatening complications which require an emergency management. The severity of these complications makes the knowledge of their pathophysiology essential for treating these patients.

J-C. Orban (✉) • C. Ichai
Intensive Care Unit, Hôpital Pasteur 2, 30 Voie Romaine, 06001 Nice, Cédex 1, France

IRCAN (INSERM U1081, CNRS UMR 7284), University Hospital of Nice, Nice, France
e-mail: orban.jc@chu-nice.fr

E. Van Obberghen
IRCAN (INSERM U1081, CNRS UMR 7284), University Hospital of Nice, Nice, France

C. Ichai et al. (eds.), *Metabolic Disorders and Critically Ill Patients*,
http://doi.org/10.1007/978-3-319-64010-5_15

15.2 Hyperglycemic Crises [3, 4]

Diabetic ketoacidosis (DKA) and hyperosmolar hyperglycemic nonketotic (HHNK) states, both acute hyperglycemic complications, are classically differentiated, the first being usually observed in type 1 diabetes while the second one occurs rather in type 2 diabetes. Despite some differences in terms of pathophysiology, conditions of patients, the principle of treatment is very close.

15.2.1 Epidemiology

The incidence of acute hyperglycemic crisis is estimated between 4.6 and 8 episodes per 1000 diabetic patients and occurs in 3.5–9% of diabetic patients [5, 6]. These complications represent approximately 4–9% of hospital admissions and more than 94% of acute complications of diabetic patients. Acute hyperglycemic crisis are distributed for 2/3 in DKA and 1/3 in HHNK [7]. The temporal trend of these complications varies among countries: a 50% decrease incidence is reported in Italy, i.e., a 5.7% decrease per year [5], while a 30–35% re-increase is observed in the USA and Wales, especially in patients between 10 and 29 years [3, 8] after a previous period showing a lower incidence [9]. Mortality varies between 3 and 15% depending on the countries, the nature of the complication (DKA vs HHNK), the comorbidities and age of patients, the experience of the clinical centers, and the implementation of protocols or guidelines for the management of such patients [3, 5, 7, 10–12]. Mortality rate is clearly higher in HHNK than in DKA patients: less than 2% in academic medical centers for DKA but up to 15–40% in HHNK [7, 13]. Severity of hyperosmolarity does not represent a poor prognosis factor unlike age and hemodynamic failure [14].

15.2.2 Pathophysiology

15.2.2.1 Diabetic Ketoacidosis

– Hyperglycemia: It results from the absolute insulin deficiency which is associated with an increased concentrations of counterregulatory hormones (glucagon, catecholamines, cortisol, and growth hormone) (Fig. 15.1) [3, 4, 15]. Such an imbalance causes an elevation of both gluconeogenesis and glycogenolysis and simultaneously an impaired glucose utilization by peripheral tissues (insulin resistance). Insulin deficiency stimulates lipolysis and free fatty acids release leading to elevate gluconeogenic substrates (glycerol) and in turn hyperglycemia and ketosis. Counterregulatory hormones stimulate proteolysis and inhibit protein synthesis, leading to release also gluconeogenic precursors (amino acids). Hyperglycemia causes glycosuria and osmotic diuresis, extracellular dehydration (hypovolemia), and decreased renal perfusion. Impaired renal function decreases renal glucose excretion, which is a major mechanism of defense

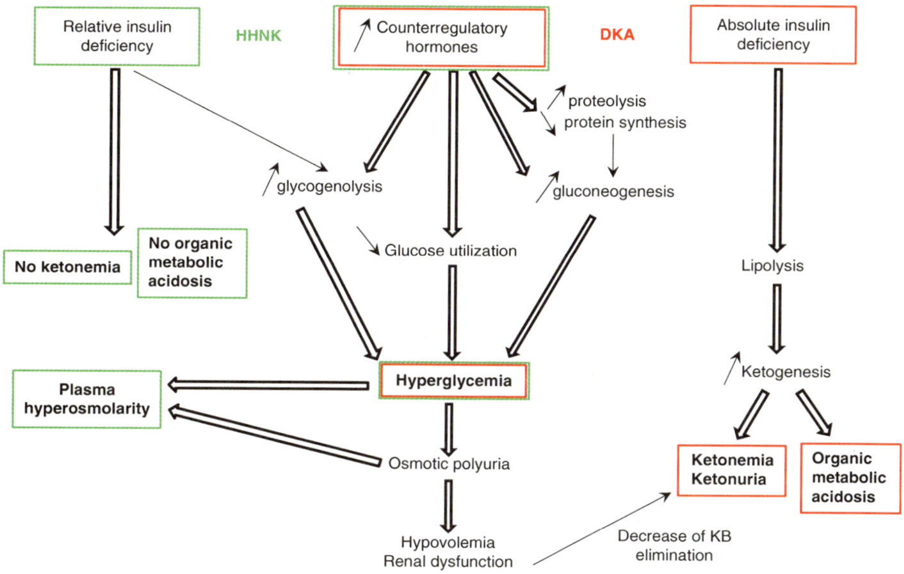

Fig. 15.1 Pathogenesis of diabetic ketoacidosis (DKA) and hyperosmolar hyperglycemic nonketotic syndrome (HHNK). DKA is caused by the association of an absolute deficit in insulin and an elevation of counterregulatory hormones. Such modifications cause (1) hyperglycemia (decrease of glucose utilization and increase of gluconeogenesis) which is responsible for hypovolemia and renal dysfunction, (2) ketonemia (increase lipolysis and decrease of ketone bodies [KB] renal elimination), and (3) organic metabolic acidosis (due to KB). HHNK is caused by the association of a relative deficit in insulin and an elevation of counterregulatory hormones. Such modifications cause (1) a severe hyperglycemia (decrease of glucose utilization and increase of glycogenolysis), (2) a severe plasma hyperosmolarity, and (3) no reason for ketonemia and metabolic acidosis

against hyperglycemia. The magnitude of hyperglycemia is enhanced by extracellular dehydration ("glucoconcentration").

– Ketonemia and metabolic organic acidosis: The imbalance between insulin deficiency and high concentrations of counterregulatory hormones activates hormone-sensitive lipase which increases lipolysis with production of high amounts of free fatty acids and glycerol (Fig. 15.1) [3, 4, 15]. Such an excessive production accelerates the ß-oxidation of fatty acids in hepatic mitochondria for producing at last ketone bodies (KB) (acetoacetate and β-hydroxybutyrate). Moreover, elevated blood KB concentration is exacerbated by a simultaneous decreased utilization and renal elimination. Metabolic organic acidosis is usually attributed to the accumulation of blood KB. Interestingly, KB might be responsible of sedative effects, which could explain partly altered consciousness and abdominal pain observed in some patients [16].
– Electrolytes and acid-base disorders: Major water losses result from several processes including osmotic diuresis due to glycosuria and ketonuria, emesis, fever, and hyperventilation. Patients usually exhibit extracellular dehydration. Such hypovolemia can be accompanied by an intracellular dehydration if hyperglycemia

is severe or if hypernatremia is associated, creating plasma hypertonicity [17]. Classically, total water body deficit reaches approximately 6 l. However, such an association is not classical during DKA. Body electrolyte deficits are common and result from various mechanisms. Sodium losses are due to osmotic diuresis, insulin deficiency, and increased glucagon levels. Osmotic diuresis, vomiting, and hyperaldosteronism secondary to hypovolemia generate potassium and phosphate (and magnesium) deficits.

15.2.2.2 Hyperosmolar Hyperglycemic Nonketotic Syndrome

As in DKA, HHNK is characterized by hyperglycemia. However, its pathogenesis differs and is less clear because of the presence of frequent severe underlying diseases and comorbidities [3]. In HHNK, pancreatic cell function is not totally absent allowing a persistent residual endogenous insulin production. As a consequence, insulin deficiency is relative, leading to reduce glucose utilization by insulin-mediated tissues or hyperglycemia, and lipolysis remains adequate allowing to prevent excessive KB production (Fig. 15.1) [3, 4]. HHNK is classically characterized by severe hyperglycemia with severe osmotic polyuria and global dehydration in the absence of ketonemia and metabolic acidosis. However such a distinction is rather theoretical, and DKA can present with severe dehydration and HHNK with metabolic acidosis related to other reasons such as hyperlactatemia.

15.2.3 Diagnosis

15.2.3.1 Context and Precipitating Factors

Near 80% of patients presenting DKA are between the ages of 18 and 45 years and 2/3 of them suffer of type 1 diabetes [3]. The most common precipitating factors of DKA are infections, discontinuation (non-adherence) or inadequate insulin therapy, and new-onset diabetes [3, 4, 18]. All drugs or stress situations that favor hyperglycemia expose to DKA decompensation (diuretics, steroids, vascular thrombosis). The relative contribution of these factors may vary depending on the type of population. Discontinuation of treatment is the most frequent cause in young adults and socially fragile people [19]. However, in 5–10% of cases, no real precipitating factor is found.

HHNK is commonly observed in type 2 diabetes and in elderly patients. Frequently, HHNK develops in patients with new-onset diabetes, and hyperglycemia is provoked by an underlying illness which induces a restriction in water intake. The most frequent precipitating factor is also infection followed by myocardial infection, surgery, cerebrovascular accident, etc. [3, 4].

15.2.3.2 Clinical Presentation

The diagnosis of both DKA and HHNK requires informations concerning the treatments, and the history must be carefully obtained from the patient or the family. A physical examination is also needed.

Clinical Signs

DKA develops rapidly over few hours. The classical clinical presentation consists in a history of polyuria-polydipsia, nausea-vomiting, abdominal pain, altered mental status, weakness, and polypnea. All of these signs are not specific and can reflect other associated disease (sepsis, stroke, etc.). Therefore, the presence of such signs must conduct to eliminate another cause before attributing them to DKA alone. Clinical signs are essentially related to hypovolemia and dehydration: skin turgor, oliguria following polyuria in case of severe and sustained hypovolemia, hypotension, and tachycardia. Altered consciousness is not constant, and its severity depends on the magnitude of hypotension and biological abnormalities (especially hypertonicity): confusion, seizures, and coma [3, 4, 14]. The classical Küssmaul polypnea only reflects the secondary respiratory response to metabolic acidosis [12, 20]. Ketotic breath is rather specific and useful to orientate the diagnosis. Nausea-vomitings, anorexia, and abdominal pain are commonly attributed to ketonemia and present in approximately 50% of patients. However, their presence can be caused by other disease (surgical abdominal complication) and should lead to perform additional complementary exams (abdominal CT scan) if they do not resolve with the normalization of metabolic disorders. Hypothermia indicates more severe DKA.

HHNK evolves over several days to weeks with a persistent polyuria, but the classical polydipsia can be absent due to an impaired perception of thirst. The underlying illness can also limit the access of oral water intake. Central nervous system alterations are more frequent than in DKA and related to the deeper hypertonicity and global dehydration. Coma and focal neurological signs are common [3, 4]. Usually, nausea-vomitings are not present as well as the Küssmaul tachypnea due to the absence of hyperketotic acidosis. However, tachypnea can be caused by many disorders such as fever, encephalopathy due to cerebral hemorrhage or stroke, pain, abdomen complication, pulmonary infection, myocardial infarction with shock, etc. Limb ischemia seems more frequent probably due to the increased blood viscosity [21].

Biological Signs

The diagnosis of DKA and HHNK is confirmed on biological abnormalities. The association of three biological disorders is classically required to diagnose DKA: hyperglycemia (> 250 mg/dL), metabolic organic acidosis, and ketonemia. On the other hand, HHNK is characterized by a severe hyperglycemia (> 600 mg/dL) associated with plasma hypertonicity (> 320 mOsm/kg) with a normal or slightly reduced pH and the absence of very low ketonemia [3] (Table 15.1).

Acid-Base Disorders

DKA is classically described as a pure metabolic organic acidosis caused by the increased blood KB concentration. Considering the Henderson-Hasselbalch approach, KB consume bicarbonates leading to the decrease in plasma pH. The presence of excessive blood KB is detected by calculating plasma anion gap (AG) which is high ($Na^+ - [Cl^- + HCO_3^-] > 12$ mEq/L). Such a high AG metabolic acidosis is associated with a secondary predictable respiratory response that leads to

Table 15.1 Diagnosis and severity parameters of diabetic ketoacidosis (DKA) and hyperosmolar hyperglycemic nonketotic syndrome (HHNK)

	DKA			
	Mild	*Moderate*	*Severe*	HHNK
Glycemia (mmol/L)	>14	>14	>14	>14
Plasma pH	7.25–7.35	7.0–7.24	<7.0	>7.3
Anion gap (mEq/L)	>12			≤12
Strong ion gap (mEq/L)	≥5			≤12
Bicarbonatemia (mmol/L)	15–18	10–14	<10	>15
Ketonemia	+	++	+++	±
Ketonuria	+++	++	+	±
Plasma tonicity (mOsm/kg)	Variable			>320

The presence of mental status alteration is a clinical sign of severity

hypocapnia (expected decrease of $PaCO_2$ = 1.3 decrease of bicarbonate) [12, 20]. To confirm that metabolic acidosis is solely due to the increased blood level of KB, it has been proposed to correlate the relationship between the variation (Δ) in plasma bicarbonate and in AG [12, 20]. Metabolic acidosis is pure if the decrease in HCO_3^- explains the increase in AG ($\Delta\ HCO_3^- = \Delta AG$) and if the actual measured $PaCO_2$ is comparable to the predictable one. However, such an approach has major pitfalls, especially because it does not consider the role of weak acids in acid-base equilibrium [22–25]. Indeed, hypoalbuminemia is the major source of misinterpretation of AG as it causes an underestimation of high values. Therefore, some authors recommend to calculate the corrected AG (cAG) which takes into account blood albumin concentration using the following formula: cAG (mEq/L) = AG + 0.25 (40—actual Alb) [22, 23]. Despite such a correction, this approach only considers the role of bicarbonate in the development of acid-base disorders and ignores totally the role of weak acids and nonvolatile buffers. It is preferred to interpret this metabolic disorder with the Stewart concept which stipulates that metabolic acid-base disorders are caused by variations of independent variables which are the strong ion difference (SID) and the weak acid content [25]. In this approach, metabolic acidosis in DKA is caused by the excessive blood KB concentration which is responsible for a decrease in SID and in turn in pH. The presence of the strong anions KB can be detected by calculating the strong ion gap (see chapter "Interpretation of Acid-Base Disorders") which is elevated. Hyperlactatemia is also another classical reason for organic metabolic acidosis during DKA which results in a high SIG as well as hyperketonemia. In a retrospective study, hyperlactatemia >2 mmol/L and >4 mmol/L has been reported to be present in 68% and 40% of DKA, respectively [26]. The presence of hyperlactatemia was not associated with a higher mortality or length of stay as compared with patients presenting hyperlactatemia in other conditions than DKA. The mechanism of this trouble is not totally understood but might be attributed to the acceleration of glycolysis induced by metabolic alkalosis or to the administration of catecholamines. In all cases whether considering the AG, cAG, or the SIG, the determination of strong anions involved in metabolic acidosis requires a specific measurement. Usually, hyperglycemic-related osmotic polyuria induces an acute renal impairment with a reduction in glomerular filtration rate (GFR) which is responsible of an accumulation of weak acids (sulfate, phosphate) that worsens metabolic acidosis. Hypoalbuminemia does not impact on the SID and the SIG but can add metabolic alkalosis leading to underestimate the severity of acidosis.

Another important point is that acid-base disorder in DKA is not rarely a pure isolated organic metabolic acidosis but frequently mixed and modifies with resolution and treatment [27]. In the early period, the reduced GFR induces a decrease in renal excretion of ketone bodies which is associated with a concomitant increase in urinary chloride excretion in order to maintain urine electroneutrality. This phenomenon is responsible of a slight hypochloremic metabolic alkalosis. Such a disorder is frequently aggravated by vomitings [12, 20]. The restoration of volemia using normal saline is responsible of a persistent metabolic acidosis which progressively moves from organic to hyperchloremic caused by two mechanisms: (1) the infusion of large volumes of normal saline which contains high chloride concentration, i.e., unbalanced solution [28, 29], and (2) the simultaneous improvement in GFR allows the urinary excretion of ketone bodies in return to chloride reuptake [30, 31]. At last, associated respiratory acidosis or alkalosis can be present. Respiratory acidosis is present if the actual $PaCO_2$ is higher than the predictable one and respiratory alkalosis if $PaCO_2$ is lower than the predictable one. Respiratory alkalosis is frequently associated caused by encephalopathy, infection, or hypoxia [24]. Respiratory acidosis may develop in case of severe hypophosphatemia and hypokalemia [32].

Patients with HHNK present classically without or a slight metabolic acidosis ($pH > 7.30$ and $HCO_3^- > 18$ mmol/L). However, the underlying illness which has precipitated the patients to HHNK is frequently responsible for a metabolic acidosis, especially lactic metabolic acidosis in patients with hypotension, hypoxia, and shock [3, 4]. In this situation, AG is also elevated, SID reduced and SIG increased. The only way to determine the nature of the strong anion which is responsible for the trouble is a specific determination.

Ketonemia and Ketonuria

Ketonemia is the key biological disorder but as explained not the sole in DKA. However, its evaluation is a cornerstone for evaluating the severity of DKA and the efficiency of the treatment. The gold standard determination of serum ketone bodies (ketonemia) in the laboratory is long, expansive, and time-consuming. Therefore, in clinical practice, it is commonly replaced by a semiquantitative and indirect but rapid detection in urines (ketonuria). The efficacy of treatment is based on the decreased rate of hyperglycemia and on the decrease of KB concentration which is frequently monitored by ketonuria [33]. But such a method shows pitfalls as ketone bodies determination by urine dipsticks uses a nitroprusside reagents which react only with acetoacetate (and acetone) [34, 35]. When ketonemia is very high, the thermodynamic reaction favors the production of ß-hydroxybutyrate from acetoacetate and conversely. This explains the discordant results between ketonuria and ketonemia (and the evaluation of DKA severity) and why it is not uncommon to observe low ketonuria in most severe patients. Also, when the patient's condition improves and ketonemia decreases, the common trap is to observe a paradoxical re-increase of ketonuria which does not indicate a worsening but simply the inverse preferential thermodynamic metabolism of ß-hydroxybutyrate into acetoacetate. Capillary measurement of ketonemia has been advocated, using point-of-care devices, which presents the advantage to be rapid, in real time, and available at bedside. However, values from these devices, even with the most recent generation, remain insufficiently precise, accurate, and dependent on the staff training [35, 36]. Finally, recommendations on the method for measuring ketone bodies production (in plasma, capillary, or urine) for the diagnosis of DKA and its severity remain debated [33]. The use of point-of-care analyzers for blood KB determination at bedside are not really recommended to guide therapy because of a lack of precision and accuracy with common available devices [4].

No or slight ketonemia and ketonuria are common in HHNK.

Electrolyte Disorders

In DKA natremia is classically normal or slightly/moderately low. Indeed, hyperglycemia can be responsible of plasma hypertonicity, leading to an osmotic extrusion of water from cell to the extracellular compartment and to a sodium dilution in plasma [3, 17]. Hyperglycemia induces a hypertonic hyponatremia and must really be distinguished from hypotonic hyponatremia by calculating plasma tonicity and the corrected natremia (cNa) [17, 37, 38]. cNa represents the predictable natremia with a normal glycemia. The formula includes a correction factor between 0.4 and 0.65: cNa (mmol/L) = actual Na + [0.4/0.65 × glycemia] mmol/L). A normal cNa (and isotonicity) indicates a normal intracellular hydration. However, even not classical, DKA can be associated with plasma hypertonicity and normo- and hypernatremia, reflecting the presence of intracellular dehydration. In more than 25% of patients, the initial serum potassium level is normal or high due to acidemia, renal dysfunction, and above all to insulinopenia [3]. However, total body potassium is in fact strongly depleted due to several disorders including digestive losses (vomitings) and renal losses (osmotic polyuria, hyperaldosteronism). The administration of insulin rapidly induces hypokalemia which reveals body potassium depletion. Phosphatemia follows the same evolution than kalemia.

In HHNK, severe hyperglycemia can be associated with hypertonic hyponatremia but is often associated with hypernatremia which reflects the severity of global dehydration. Plasma tonicity is strongly elevated.

Various nonspecific biological abnormalities can be observed in DKA and HHNK. Prerenal acute renal dysfunction is common due to hypovolemia and characterized by an increased blood urea nitrogen and creatinine concentrations. The incidence and characteristics of renal dysfunction during DKA have been assessed in a recent retrospective study including 94 patients [39]. Half of patients presented acute kidney injury on the RIFLE criteria, 50% of them being in the "risk" stage. The incidence decreased to 25% within the first 24 h. Advanced age, hyperglycemia, and hypoprotidemia were found as independent risk factor of renal dysfunction. On admission leukocytosis can be moderately elevated (10000–15,000/mm^3) without any underlying infectious problem, probably due to adrenergic stress. In all cases, infection must be investigated systematically at least by blood and urine cultures and orientated samples if required. Hyperamylasemia and hyperlipasemia have been reported to be present frequently without any real pancreatitis. However, in case of persistent elevated concentrations or suggestive clinical signs, an abdominal scan must be performed to eliminate pancreatitis which can be the precipitating factor of DKA. Troponin I can be elevated in the absence of acute coronary syndrome. This elevation seems to be correlated with an increased mortality at 2 years [40]. Due to the severe dehydration, acute kidney injury is more frequent and severe in HHNK than in DKA.

In summary: Criteria for diagnosing DKA and HHNK are theoretically different. DKA is diagnosed on the presence of hyperglycemia, metabolic acidosis caused by hyperketonemia (elevated AG or SIG), variable plasma tonicity, and possible alterations in consciousness. According to the severity of these biological disorders and mental status alterations, DKA is classified into three levels of severity, mild, moderate, and severe (Table 15.1). HHNK is characterized by severe hyperglycemia associated with severe plasma hypertonicity, no or slight ketonemia and metabolic acidosis, and mental status alterations (Table 15.1). However, in practical, frontiers in these disorders are not so clear-cut, and classical disorders of DKA can be observed in HHNK and vice versa.

15.2.4 Treatment

Treatment of DKA and HHNK is based on four principles (Table 15.2): (1) fluid replacement, (2) normalization of blood glucose level using continuous intravenous insulin infusion, (3) correction of potassium and other electrolytes imbalances, and (4) alkalinization by sodium bicarbonate [3, 11, 41]. Simultaneously, the specific treatment of underlying disease and precipitating factors and organ failure support are essential. The consideration of these principles is consensual leading to recommendations which can slightly differ in details [3, 11].

15.2.4.1 Fluid Replacement

Volume resuscitation is essential and should begin firstly to correct circulatory volume and in the same time intracellular dehydration. This intervention alone reduces hyperglycemia and ketonemia by diluting blood glucose, by decreasing the secretion of counterregulatory hormones and possible insulin resistance, and by restoring renal function. The initial route for rehydration is often parenteral, but oral intake can be added in case of the absence of any contraindication (consciousness alteration) and must be resumed as soon as possible. In DKA, mean fluid deficit represents 6–7 l in adults so that required fluid volume is approximately 15–20 mL/kg/h (1–1.5 l) within the first or 2 h [3, 4, 11]. Fluid replacement is performed using crystalloids, and 0.9% NaCl remains the reference. Recent studies underline the beneficial effects of balanced crystalloid infusion to avoid the development or worsening of hyperchloremic metabolic acidosis during treatment [29, 42, 43]. But all of them failed to report any difference in terms of DKA resolution. The subsequent

Table 15.2 General principles of diabetic ketoacidosis treatment [3, 4]

Clinical assessment of the patient
Fluid replacement
– Initial vascular load by 1000 mL of crystalloid (0.9%NaCl or balanced crystalloid) followed by a continuous infusion at a rate of 1000 mL/h; check arterial pressure and urine output; close more invasive hemodynamic monitoring if necessary
– Hemodynamic restoration → continue fluid infusion by hypo- or isotonic crystalloid according to plasma tonicity and corrected natremia at a rate of approximately 10 mL/kg/h
– Hypovolemic shock or hemodynamic worsening → increase volume of crystalloid or use macromolecules
– Cardiogenic shock → close hemodynamic monitoring
– Glycemia <11 mmol/L → add 5% dextrose in association with crystalloid
Potassium normalization
– Kalemia < 3.3 mmol/L: hold insulin infusion, potassium supplementation of 20–30 mEq/h until reaching a value >3.3 mmol/L
– Kalemia between 3.3 and 5 mmol/L: potassium supplementation of 20–30 mEq/h
– Kalemia >5 mmol/L: check kalemia every hour until reaching a value <5 mmol/L
Insulin infusion
– Always after the initial fluid replacement; use ultrarapid insulin
– Initial intravenous bolus of 0.1 U/kg without exceeding 10 U
– Followed by a continuous infusion at a rate of 0.1 U/kg/h
– Adjust the rate of infusion to reach an initial decrease of glycemia by 10% within the first hour, then approximately 3–5 mmol/L per hour
– Decrease the rate of infusion finally to 0.03–0.05 U when glycemia is <11 mmol/L
Bicarbonates
– pH > 7 → no indication
– pH < 7 → discuss the need for 250–500 mL de bicarbonate 1.4% within 1–2 h
Check
– On admission: clinical examination, EKG, blood gas analysis and electrolytes, blood urea nitrogen, creatininemia, blood cultures, leukocytes, amylasemia and lipasemia, and ketonuria (ketonemia)
– Check glycemia and ketonuria every hour until ketonuria disappears; check every 2–4 h plasma electrolytes, especially potassium and phosphate, and mental status

choice for crystalloids depends on the evolution of clinical signs and biological parameters, especially plasma tonicity and corrected serum sodium: iso- or hypotonicity/cNa must favor isotonic 0.9% NaCl or balanced solution, while hypertonicity and high cNa must favor hypotonic solutions (0.45%), all of them given at a rate of 500–1000 mL/h. In HHNK, the volume of fluid replacement is usually greater, and hypotonic crystalloid can be required to correct severe plasma hypertonicity. Indeed, volume expansion and the choice of fluid require a close clinical hemodynamic and biological monitoring. When blood glucose reaches 11 mmol/L (200 mg/dL) for DKA and 16.5 (300 mg/dL) mmol/L for HHS, 5% dextrose is needed to avoid hypoglycemia. This allows to continue insulin infusion until the disappearance of ketonemia and to maintain the appropriate speed correction of hyperglycemia. Correction of hyperosmolarity should not exceed 3–5 mOsm/L/h.

15.2.4.2 Insulin Therapy

Insulin therapy is the second principle of treatment using ultrarapid continuous intravenous infusion. This therapy must not be initiated before having restoring vascular volume and supplemented hypokalemia if present [3, 4]. Indeed, insulin is well known to cause an intracellular transfer of potassium by stimulating the Na-K-ATPase pump [44, 45]. It is also responsible for a decrease in plasma tonicity which induces an osmotic shift from the extracellular to the intracellular compartment and in turn may worsen or reveal hypovolemic shock. Numerous algorithms recommend to begin with an initial intravenous bolus of 0.1 U/kg of insulin followed by a continuous infusion of 0.1 U/kg/h [3, 4, 11]. Glucose should decrease of 10% in the first hour and after at a rate of 3–5 mmol/L/h down to 11 mmol/L. During the first hour, the administration of an additional bolus of 0.1–0.14 U is possible if the reduction in glycemia is insufficient. Once reduction of BGL is achieved (< 200 mg/dL for DKA and <300 mg/dL for HHNK), insulin infusion must not be totally stopped but reduced at a rate of 0.02–0.05 U/kg/h while introducing sugar intake or infusion to maintain blood glucose levels between 8 and 12 mmol/L (150–200 mg/dL). Uncomplicated and slight DKA can be treated with subcutaneous insulin analogs [46].

15.2.4.3 Electrolytes Normalization

Potassium

Initial blood potassium level may be normal, high, or low, despite a constant total body potassium depletion: hyperkalemia is present in 80% of patients at admission, while hypokalemia develops in 60% of cases during treatment [30]. Therefore, it is essential to delay insulin infusion until potassium measurements are obtained. In case of initial hypokalemia (< 3.3 mmol/L), intravenous potassium supplementation is needed as soon as possible at a rate of 20–30 mEq/h (1.5–2 g/h). When kalemia is between 3.3 and 5.2 mmol/L, a dose of 20–30 mEq/L of fluid is suggested. For levels >5.2 mmol/L, potassium administration should be held and checked within the following 1–2 h [3, 4]. After the initial correction of hyper- or hypokalemia, a practical method to avoid dyskalemia with continuous insulin infusion is to maintain a comparable cumulative quantity of exogenous potassium (QK in mEq/L) and of insulin infusion (QI in units): QK/QI ratio must be equal to 1. The goal is to maintain kalemia in a normal value (4–5 mmol/L).

Phosphate

Blood phosphate levels move along with potassium. Despite a constant total body phosphate depletion, there is no data supporting a systematical phosphate supplementation as it may cause hypocalcemia [47]. However, it should be provided in case of profound hypophosphatemia (<0.30 mmol/L) or in case of moderate hypophosphatemia associated with signs of poor tolerance (hypoxia, anemia, or cardiopulmonary failure) at a rate of 20–30 mEq/L [32]. In all cases, phosphate monitoring is usually required.

15.2.5 Bicarbonate Therapy

The use of bicarbonate for DKA has been strongly controversial for a long time based on potential deleterious effect of acidosis, especially cardiovascular dysfunction and worsening insulin resistance. However, some experimental studies support the absence of such deleterious effects [48]. Several studies showed that administration of bicarbonate has no beneficial effect in this indication, even in severe acidosis [49, 50]. American last guidelines from 2009 recommended the administration of sodium bicarbonate only when arterial pH was <6.9. Indeed, an adequate management with fluid replacement and insulin stops ketone bodies production and favors their metabolization causing an "endogenous alkalinization" which allows to restore a normal pH without any exogenous administration of sodium bicarbonate. A recent systematic review of 44 studies (three randomized controlled) has evaluated the impact of sodium bicarbonate in the treatment of DKA [51]. The authors conclude that sodium bicarbonate shows a trend for a higher risk of hypokalemia, a longer delay for blood lactate, and KB normalization. No beneficial effect on mortality, pH and glycemia normalization, and insulin requirements was found, but these parameters were very difficult to interpret due to a great heterogeneity in studies. At last sodium bicarbonate administration was associated with a higher risk of cerebral edema in children. Therefore, the indication of sodium bicarbonate must be considered in the context and according to the evolution of the patient with the treatment.

15.2.6 Structure of Admission, Monitoring, and Complications

Repeated clinical examination is needed especially in case of mental status alteration. Hemodynamic monitoring (at least arterial pressure, urine output) is required every hour at the beginning or until the patient becomes stable. EKG is needed to verify the absence or not of electric signs of potassium disorder. Glycemia and ketonemia/ketonuria should be assessed every hour until glycemia reaches 200 mg/dL for DKA and 300 mg/dL for HHNK and until ketonuria disappears. Arterial blood gas analysis and electrolytes concentrations (especially potassium), blood urea nitrogen, creatininemia, and plasma tonicity should be checked every 2 h until electrolytes and KB normalize. The goal is to reach resolution of DKA and HHNK within 6–12 h, the first normalization being for pH.

Such a resolution must not be too rapid, especially the decrease in glycemia which exposes to life-threatening complications. The most frequent complications of DKA and HHNK are hypoglycemia and hypokalemia (and hypophosphatemia) which are caused by high insulin dose and sodium bicarbonate infusion. A close biological monitoring associated with appropriate potassium supplementation and moderate dose of insulin allows to prevent such complications [3, 30]. The replacement of metabolic organic acidosis by a metabolic hyperchloremic acidosis is usually with no relevant clinical effect. Hyperchloremic acidosis is the most common complications of the treatment of DKA and HHS. If hyperchloremic acidosis persists, it is possible to infuse sodium bicarbonate or give water enterally. The infusion of hypotonic crystalloid in elderly or pediatric patients must be careful because of an increased risk of cerebral edema if plasma tonicity reduces too rapidly [3, 4]. Such a complication during treatment in children with DKA is responsible for an increased mortality and is related to high insulin infusion and volume fluid replacement over the first 4–6 h, severe acidemia. The mechanism by which cerebral edema develops is not really clear and might be due to various parameters: a rapid decrease in plasma tonicity caused by the intracellular ß-hydroxybutyrate with monocarboxylate transporters or by the rapid decrease in glycemia or by the infusion of electrolyte-free infusion [22]. Excessive fluid replacement must be avoided in elderly patients with cardiac or renal dysfunction as it exposes to cause acute respiratory failure [52]. This complication occurs during the treatment rather than initially. Major risk factors are (1) intracellular ions depletion including potassium, phosphate, and magnesium; (2) pulmonary edema (cardiogenic or not); and (3) respiratory infection.

Considering all of these possible complications and the need for close monitoring, there is no doubt that the management of DKA and HHNK should be performed in a high dependency unit or equivalent. Recent studies report that the primary admission of patients with DKA varies strongly according to hospitals, from 2 to 87% without difference in hospital length of stay and mortality [10, 53]. Hospital with a high rate of ICU utilization had a high volume of DKA admission, but the exact reasons for that are unknown. It is reasonable to suggest that the most appropriate unit for managing these patients depends on the severity of the patient and above all on the capacity of the unit to allow a close monitoring. Rules should be that in the unit that the staff is (1) trained to measure accurately and frequently blood glucose level and ketonuria and (2) to monitor clinical and biological parameters every 2–6 h. ICU is needed in case of severe acidosis (pH < 7.1, HCO_3^- < 5 mmol/L), severe ketonemia (> 6 mmol/L), initial hypokalemia, mental status alteration, or any organ failure [11].

15.3 Metformin-Associated Lactic Acidosis (MALA)

Lactic acidosis (LA) is an organic metabolic acidosis due to an increased blood lactate level caused by an elevation of its production and/or a reduction of its utilization. This disorder is commonly defined by the association of an organic metabolic acidosis associated to a lactate concentration > 5 mmol/L [20, 28].

15.3.1 Epidemiology of MALA

15.3.1.1 Context and Precipitating Factors

Metformin is the drug of choice in type 2 diabetes allowing to control efficiently glycemia while better preventing macrovascular complications than other oral antidiabetic drugs or insulin [55]. Its major mechanism of action is a reduction of insulin resistance. It is the first-line therapy in obese diabetic patients owing to its beneficial effects on weight. This drug seems to be also more protective than the other oral antidiabetic agents in heart failure patients or after cardiac surgery [56]. Because of a fear to precipitate lactic acidosis, physicians remain reluctant for its wide indication, and metformin is prescribed in only 65% of good candidates [57]. However, large and recent study aiming to assess MALA reports that this complication is rare [28, 58–61]. The usual incidence varies commonly between 2 and 9/100,000 patients/year of exposure. A recent systematic review confirms that this event remains rare but seems to increase (47/100,000 persons per year) [58]. In a 10-year retrospective analysis, MALA was reported to be the reason for ICU admission in 0.12% of all patients: 30% of them were voluntary intoxication and the remaining 70% were incidental intoxication [62]. The precise incidence of MALA is rather difficult to estimate and unknown because of multiple confounding factors. The real implication of metformin in the development of MALA remains a matter of debate. Indeed, more recent data failed to demonstrate any difference in MALA between diabetic patients treated with metformin and those treated with other oral antidiabetic drugs (sulfonylurea) [60, 63–65]. Confusion and complexity due to a large association of underlying conditions and drugs that predispose to lactic acidosis explain the difficulties to confirm the diagnosis. This problem is highlighted in a 15-year evaluation issued from a large pharmacological database reporting [66]. The authors report that 41.3% of patients were declared to have MALA but only 10.4% have a correct diagnosis confirmed by the presence of plasma metformin.

Mortality rate of MALA varies strongly from 5 to 61% but seems to be of 50% in most studies [58, 67, 68]. Large studies report a decrease over time with a reduction of the mean value reaching 25% in the most recent years [58, 68]. Mortality rate is markedly lower in case of intentional overdose as compared with incidental accumulation [69]: 0% without lactic acidosis and reach 10% in case of moderate lactic acidosis [62, 70], up to 80% in case of severe lactic acidosis (pH < 6.9, lactatemia >5 mmol/L) and high plasma metformin concentration (>5 mg/L) [71]. Severity of metabolic acidosis is a good predictor of fatal outcome [58, 59, 62], but mortality is lower for a comparable lactatemia and magnitude of acidosis not related to metformin overdose [64]. The prognostic value of high plasma metformin concentration remains controversial [59, 62, 72]. A recent French analysis from pharmacovigilance database reported that plasma metformin concentration was higher in non-survival patients. On the other hand, plasma metformin level was higher in patients presenting voluntary MALA as compared with those with incidental MALA, but mortality rate was higher in incidental MALA [62]. All data strongly suggest that the underlying disease, comorbidities, and organ dysfunction, especially renal and liver impairment, strongly increase the incidence of MALA and influence the outcome of these patients [58, 59, 73].

15.3.2 Pharmacokinetic and Pathophysiology of MALA

Metformin is absorbed for 40% in the upper small intestine (duodenum and proximal jejunum), while only 10% is absorbed in the ileum and colon [59]. Its bioavailability is of 50–60%, with no protein bound in plasma. Metformin is not metabolized and eliminated unchanged for 90% by kidneys (10% in feces). Metformin can accumulate in some tissues such as the kidneys, liver, and intestine. Therapeutic plasma concentration is classically <1.34 mg/L, and intra-erythrocyte concentration is <1.65 mg/L. Excessive erythrocyte concentration reflects a chronic accumulation, while plasma elevated concentration reflects rather an acute accumulation. The elevation of both signs an acute or chronic accumulation.

The mechanism by which metformin can cause MALA is multifactorial [74]. The most important is the inhibition of mitochondrial respiration which is suggested in intoxicated patients by the initial decreased VO_2 and increased oxygen venous saturation [75]. More precisely, metformin inhibits complex I of the mitochondrial respiratory chain in a concentration-dependent manner [76]. Such phenomenons associated with a suppression of glycerophosphate dehydrogenase cause a reduction in hepatic gluconeogenesis leading to increase lactate accumulation [77]. An elevation of lactate production is also possible due to (1) an acceleration of glycolysis caused by an increased NAD/NADH ratio and in turn an increased activity of pyruvate kinase [78], an increased production of lactate from the intestinal glycolysis [78, 79]. Considering these mechanisms, it seems that oxygen deficit is not involved in this disorder explaining why MALA is commonly classified as a type B lactic acidosis. However, such a classification is artificial as MALA is frequently observed in unstable and hypoxic conditions [54]. Therefore, lactic acidosis observed in metformin intoxication is frequently of a mixed origin, type A and B (with hypoxia).

15.3.3 Diagnosis of MALA

15.3.3.1 Clinical Presentation

The context frequently facilitates the diagnosis considering the history of the patient, its treatments, and comorbidities. Acute events such as sepsis, shock, cardiac heart failure, gastrointestinal disorders, or drugs which predispose for MALA must be searched. All of the predisposing factors are characterized by the presence of hypovolemia and dehydration. In more than 60% of cases, MALA occurs in patients with a worsening renal dysfunction [60, 62, 74]. The diagnosis of MALA is accepted after eliminating other diagnosis which can possibly induce lactic acidosis. However, lactic acidosis can be caused by multiple disease, and it can be difficult to know the chronology of the events ("what is the egg? what is the chicken"?). Clinical history and examination are essential to detect an underlying disease that is responsible for the development of MALA.

Clinical signs of MALA are often nonspecific signs. Frequently patients present weakness, gastrointestinal disorders (in 10–30 % of patients) such as nausea-vomitings, abdominal pain, anorexia, myalgia, altered mental status, shortness of breath, hypothermia, hemodynamic instability due to vasoplegia, or cardiac dysrhythmia [59, 80]. The diagnosis of certitude is based on the presence of a metabolic lactic acidosis (pH < 7.35 associated with hyperlactatemia >5 mmol/L) and the presence of plasma metformin. In a retrospective study including 49 MALA, good and poor outcome patients exhibited similar lactate levels [81], while in another study, lactate levels were in higher in poor outcome patients [62]. Acute kidney injury with hyperkalemia is also frequent [82]. A retrospective study found that a prothrombin activity <50% on admission was associated with a poor prognosis [62]. An supratherapeutic plasma metformin level (> 5 mg/L) allows to confirm the diagnosis. The intra-erythrocyte metformin level is interesting because it reflects the chronic accumulation of metformin and can be into account to stop renal replacement therapy [72]. But such measurements are not widely available in emergency and the treatment must not be delayed in case of suspicion of MALA.

From a practical point of view, MALA occurs in three conditions. In the first case, an underlying cause explains lactic acidosis (shock, liver failure, hypoxia), and the presence of metformin is only anecdotal. In this situation, the prognosis is poor. In the second case, metformin represents the main cause of lactic acidosis, and the prognosis is often favorable. Intentional poisoning is the main origin of this late figure [62]. In the third condition which is the most common, an underlying cause of lactic acidosis is aggravated by metformin accumulation [83].

15.3.4 Treatments of MALA

15.3.4.1 Curative Treatment

Life-threatening supportive nonspecific treatment of organ failure is needed. Renal replacement therapy (RRT) with bicarbonate buffer is the first-line treatment of MALA [62, 80, 84]. Such a management allows to support renal dysfunction which is frequent and to accelerate metformin elimination. In a population of MALA patients, the RRT group and the non-RRT group had comparable outcome despite the greater severity in the RRT group [85]. The indication of renal replacement therapy is based only on clinical cases and pharmacokinetic data showing clearly a rapid reduction in plasma metformin levels under RRT, but until now there is no real clinical comparative study showing that RRT improves morbi-mortality. However, indications for RRT include a lactate concentration greater than 20 mmol/L, pH less than or equal to 7.0, shock, failure of standard supportive measures and decreased level of consciousness [80, 85]. Extracorporeal treatment should be continued until the lactate concentration is less than 3 mmol/L and pH greater than 7.35. At each time close monitoring is warranted to determine the need for additional courses of extracorporeal treatment.

The technique of RRT is controversial [62, 80, 85]. On a theoretical point of view, because metformin is a small molecule, intermittent hemodialysis is commonly preferred and recommended initially. However, due to its large volume of distribution, there is often a rebound re-increase in plasma metformin level which requires to perform an additional session of intermittent RRT. Seidowsky et al. [62] reported that normalization of elevated plasma metformin levels needs a prolonged session of RRT of at least 15 h to avoid any rebound. Continuous renal replacement therapies may be considered if hemodialysis is unavailable and is the technique of choice in patients with hemodynamic instability. Moreover, continuous RRT offers the advantage to eliminate continuously tissue metformin accumulation as shown by the decrease of intra-erythrocyte metformin concentration. Alkalinization by sodium bicarbonate has no interest in this indication and could even worsen intracellular acidosis.

15.3.4.2 Preventive Treatment

Prevention of metformin-associated lactic acidosis is essential and is based primarily on compliance with contraindications (Table 15.3). However, several studies have shown that contraindications are not respected in 24–73% of cases [65, 86]. Judicious prescription of this treatment by doctors is not optimal [57]. Caution must be the rule in case of an association with favoring drugs (nonsteroidal anti-inflammatory molecules, phosphodiesterase inhibitors, diuretics, angiotensin-converting enzyme inhibitors, angiotensin II receptors blockers, etc.) or in case of situations at risk such as renal function impairment, conditions with a high risk of hemodynamic instability, and contrast medium products injection. Education of patients is insufficient as they do not know that they must stop temporarily metformin during these acute events [82]. The most important point is to check renal

Table 15.3 Contraindications and caution for metformin prescription

Definitive and temporarily contraindications to metformin
– Hypersensibility to metformin chlorhydrate
– Diabetic ketoacidosis, hyperosmolar hyperglycemic nonketotic syndrome
– Renal insufficiency or renal function impairment (creatinine clearance < 60 mL/min): stop temporarily metformin in case of acute renal failure until restoration of renal function
– Acute diseases predisposing to induce renal dysfunction: hypovolemia, dehydration, severe sepsis, shock, contrast iodinated medium product (stop temporarily for 24 hours, then check renal function, and decide according to renal function restoration)
– Chronic or acute disease susceptible to induce tissue hypoxia: cardiac or respiratory insufficiency, myocardial infarction, and shock
– Liver failure, acute alcohol intoxication
– Pregnancy, lactation
Caution prescription
– Age ≥ 80 years (until confirming a normal renal function)
– Liver disease
– Concomitant administration of cationic drug
– Stop temporarily metformin prescription in case of:
• Creatininemia >150 μmol/L
• All hypoxic conditions (respiratory insufficiency, sepsis, myocardial infarction, dehydration)
• During 24–48 h after an infusion of iodinated medium contrast product and checking renal function
• No stop before elective minor; stop 12–24 h before moderate surgery and after surgery until beginning oral intake and after checking renal function; stop metformin 24 h before major surgery with high risk of hemorrhage or hemodynamic instability

function after introduction of potentially nephrotoxic drugs and to stop temporarily metformin until renal function recovers.

15.4 Hypoglycemia

Hypoglycemia is an inextricable complication of diabetes treatment. Diagnosis is based on Whipple's triad involving symptoms consistent with hypoglycemia, blood glucose less than 0.5 g/L, and a rapid resolution of symptoms with normalization of glycemia. Moderate hypoglycemia is treated by the patient himself, whereas severe hypoglycemia requires external help.

15.4.1 Epidemiology

Hypoglycemia is the most common metabolic complications of diabetes. It affects both type 1 diabetes and type 2 treated with insulin or oral antidiabetic agents [87]. The incidence of hypoglycemia represents 5.6% of acute diabetic complications and decreases since 10 years [5]. This incidence is different depending on the type of diabetes, type of treatment, and glycemic targets. Risk factors for hypoglycemia are strict metabolic control assessed by a low HbA1c [88], the occurrence of episodes of severe hypoglycemia, an impaired awareness of hypoglycemia, and the absence of C-peptide and sleep.

15.4.2 Consequences of Hypoglycemia

Unlike healthy subjects, all the adaptive mechanisms to fight against hypoglycemia in type 1 diabetes are altered over time. Insulin levels resulting only from the exogenous input are no longer adjustable according to glucose levels. Moreover, hypoglycemia is no more an effective stimulus of glucagon synthesis. Then, physiological adaptation to hypoglycemia involves only the adrenergic response, which deteriorates over time, especially during episodes of hypoglycemia. In a long history of diabetes, counterregulatory mechanisms can become ineffective, and patients present a hypoglycemia without any consciousness or perception, which reflects diabetic dysautonomia [89].

Clinical symptoms of hypoglycemia depend on the activation of the autonomic nervous system and brain glucose deprivation. The autonomic nervous response to hypoglycemia leads to anxiety, palpitations, sweating, and feeling hungry. Neurological symptoms related to glycopenia are many and varied: malaise, mood and behavior troubles, cognitive dysfunction (difficulty of concentration or speech, inability to make decisions), seizures, or coma. The hypoglycemic encephalopathy is the most severe form which can be responsible directly or not of 2–4% of diabetes deaths [90].

15.4.3 Prevention of Hypoglycemia

Prevention of hypoglycemia is based on two principles. Patient education should enable the acquisition of knowledge about the disease, its treatment, and the adaptation thereof in case of hypoglycemia. Some techniques resensitize the hypoglycemia unawareness patient to hypoglycemic episodes. These are the strict avoidance of hypoglycemia for at least 3 weeks or a psychoeducational program improving the accuracy of patients to detect symptoms associated with hyper- and hypoglycemia [91].

15.4.4 Curative Treatment

Ingestion of carbohydrates by the patient is enough to correct nonsevere episodes of hypoglycemia (fruit juice, sugar, biscuit, food, etc.). This treatment has a transient effect and must be followed by a meal or a snack. Parenteral route is needed to give a glucose solution in severe hypoglycemia. Continuous glucose administration should also follow to avoid hypoglycemia recurrence. Glucagon is sometimes used in type 1 diabetic patients but has no indication in type 2 diabetic patients since it also stimulates insulin secretion.

Conclusions

Acute complications of diabetes remain relatively frequent despite improvements in their prevention. Pathophysiology of hyperglycemic crises is very close, and the fundamentals of their treatment are similar. Metformin-associated lactic acidosis remains an uncommon condition during appropriate use of this drug. In case of non-compliance to contraindications, the patient is exposed to a greater risk of developing this poor outcome complication whose treatment is based on renal replacement therapy. Finally, hypoglycemia is the most common acute complication of diabetes but also the least serious in terms of mortality.

Acknowledgments No conflict of interest.

References

1. Ricordeau P, Weill A, Vallier N et al (2003) The prevalence and cost of diabetes in metropolitan France: what trends between 1998 and 2000? Diabetes Metab 29:497–504
2. American Diabetes Association (2017) Classification and diagnosis of diabetes. Diabetes Care 40(Suppl 1):S11–S24
3. Kitabchi AE, Umpierrez GE, Miles JM, Fisher JN (2009) Hyperglycemic crises in adult patients with diabetes. Diabetes Care 32:1335–1348
4. Van Ness-Otunnu R, Hack F (2013) Hyperglycemic crisis. J Emerg Med 45:795–805
5. Lombardo F, Maggini M, Gruden G, Bruno G (2016) Temporal trend in hospitalizations for acute diabetic complications: a nationwide study, Italy, 2001-2010. PLoS One 8:e63675

6. Holman RR, Paul SK, Bethel MA, Matthews DR, Neils HA (2008) 10-year follow-up of intensive glucose control in type 2 diabetes. N Engl J Med 359:1577–1589
7. Ezeani IU, Eregie A, Ogebengbe OS (2013) Treatment outcome and prognostic indices in patients with hyperglycemic emergencies. Diabetes Metab Syndrome Obes 6:303–307
8. Abdulrahman GO, Amphlett B, Okosiemme OE (2013) Trends in hospital admissions with diabetic ketoacidosis in Wales, 1999-2010. Diabetes Res Clin Pract 100:e7–10
9. Wang J, Williams DE, Narayan KM et al (2006) Declining death rates from hyperglycemic crisis among adults with diabetes, U.S., 1985-2002. Diabetes Care 29:2018–2022
10. Barski L, Nevzorov R, Rabaev E et al (2012) Diabetic ketoacidosis: clinical characteristics, precipitating factors and outcomes of care. Isr Med Assoc 14:299–303
11. Savage MW, Dhatariya KK, Kilvert A et al (2011) Diabetes UK position statements and care recommendations. Joint british diabetes societies guideline for the management of diabetic ketoacidosis. Diabet Med 28:508–515
12. Kraut JA, Kurtz I (2005) Metabolic acidosis of CKD: diagnosis, clinical characteristics, and treatment. Am J Kidney Dis 45:978–993
13. Wachtel TJ, Tetu-Mouradjian LM, Goldman DL et al (1991) Hyperosmolarity and acidosis in diabetes mellitus: a three-year experience in Rhode Island. J Gen Intern Med 6:495–502
14. Piniés JA, Cairo G, Gaztambide S et al (1994) Course and prognosis of 132 patients with diabetic non ketotic hyperosmolar state. Diabete Metab 20:43–48
15. English P, Williams G (2004) Hyperglycaemic crises and lactic acidosis in diabetes mellitus. Postgrad Med J 80:253–261
16. Yang L, Zhao J, Milutinovic PS et al (2007) Anesthetic properties of the ketone bodies beta-hydroxybutyric acid and acetone. Anesth Analg 105:673–679
17. Spasovski G, Vanholder R, Allolio R et al (2014) Hyponatraemia guideline development group. Clinical practice guideline on diagnosis and treatment of hyponatraemia. Intensive Care Med 40:320–331
18. Weinert LS, Scheffel RS, Severo MD et al (2012) Precipitating factors of diabetic ketoacidosis at a public hospital in a middle-income country. Diabetes Res Clin Pract 96:29–34
19. Musey VC, Lee JK, Crawford R et al (1995) Diabetes in urban African-Americans. I. Cessation of insulin therapy is the major precipitating cause of diabetic ketoacidosis. Diabetes Care 18:483–489
20. Narins RG, Kupin W, Faber MD, Goodkin DA, Dunfee DP (1995) Pathophysiology, classification, and therapy of acid-base disturbances. In: Arieff AI, DeFronzo RA (eds) Fluid, electrolyte and acid-base disorders. Churchill Livingstone, New York, pp 105–198
21. Megarbane B, Marsanne C, Meas T et al (2007) Acute lower limb ischemia is a frequent complication of severe diabetic hyperosmolarity. Diabetes Metab 33:148–152
22. Kamel KS, Halperin ML (2015) Acid-base problems in diabetic ketoacidosis. N Engl J Med 372:546–554
23. Figge J, Jabor A, Kazda A, Fencl V (1998) Anion gap and hypoalbuminemia. Crit Care Med 26:1807–1810
24. Emmett M (2006) Anion-gap interpretation: the old and the new. Nat Clin Pract 2:4–8
25. Stewart PA (1978) Independent and dependent variables of acid-base control. Resp Physiol 33:9–26
26. Cox K, Cocchi MN, Salciccioli JD, Carney E, Howell M, Donnino MX (2012) Prevalence and significance of lactic acidosis in diabetic ketoacidosis. J Crit Care 27:132–137
27. Adrogue HJ, Madias NE (1995) Mixed acid-base disorders. In: Jacobson HR, Striker GE, Klarh S (eds) The principles and practice of nephrology, 2nd edn. Mosby-Year Book, St Louis, pp 953–962
28. Orban JC, Giunti C, Levraut J et al (2003) Metformin-associated lactic acidosis remains a serious complication of metformin therapy. Ann Fr Anesth Reanim 22:461–465
29. Mahler SA, Conrad SA, Wang H, Arnold TC (2011) Resuscitation with balanced electrolyte solution prevents hyperchloremic metabolic acidosis in patients with diabetic ketoacidosis. Am J Emerg Med 29:670–674

30. Nyenwe EA, Kitabchi AE (2016) The evolution of diabetic ketoacidosis: an update of its etiology, pathogenesis and management. Metabolism 65:507–521
31. Taylor D, Durward A, Tibby SM et al (2006) The influence of hyperchloraemia on acid base interpretation in diabetic ketoacidosis. Intensive Care Med 32:295–301
32. Liu P, Jeng C (2004) Case report - severe hypophosphatemia in a patient with diabetic ketoacidosis and acute respiratory failure. J Chin Med Assoc 76:355–359
33. Misra S, Oliver NS (2015) Utility of ketone measurement in the prevention, diagnosis and management of diabetic ketoacidosis. Diabet Med 32:14–23
34. Schwab TM, Hendey GW, Soliz TC (1999) Screening for ketonemia in patients with diabetes. Ann Emerg Med 34:342–346
35. Arora S, Probst MA, Agy C, Menchine M (2011) Point-of-care beta-hydroxybutyrate testing for assessing diabetic ketoacidosis severity prior to treatment in the emergency department. Diabetes Res Clin Pract 94:e86–e88
36. Sheikh-Ali M, Karon BS, Basu A, Kudva YC, Muller LA, Xu J, Schwenk WF, Miles JM (2008) Can serum betahydroxybutyrate be used to diagnose diabetic ketoacidosis? Diabetes Care 4:643–647
37. Hillier TA, Abbott RD, Barrett EJ (1999) Hyponatremia evaluating the correction factor for hyperglycemia. Am J Med 106:399–404
38. Katz MA (1973) Hyperglycemia-induced hyponatremia—calculation of expected serum sodium depression. N Engl J Med 289:843–844
39. Orban JC, Maizière EM, Ghaddab A, Van Obberghen E, Ichai C (2014) Incidence and characteristics of acute kidney injury in severe diabetic ketoacidosis. PLoS One 9:e110925
40. Al-Mallah M, Zuberi O, Arida M et al (2008) Positive troponin in diabetic ketoacidosis without evident acute coronary syndrome predicts adverse cardiac events. Clin Cardiol 31:67–71
41. Kitabchi AE, Umpierrez GE, Murphy MB et al (2006) Hyperglycemic crises in adult patients with diabetes: a consensus statement from the American Diabetes Association. Diabetes Care 29:2739–2748
42. Van Zyl DG, Rheeder P, Delport E (2012) Fluid management in diabetic-acidosis - Ringer's lactate versus normal saline: a randomized controlled trial. Q J Med 105:337–343
43. Chua HR, Venkatesh B, Stachowski E et al (2012) Plasma-Lyte 148 vs 0.9% saline for fluid resuscitation in diabetic ketoacidosis. J Crit Care 27:138–145
44. Brown RS (1986) Extrarenal potassium homeostasis. Kidney Int 30:116–127
45. Clausen T (2010) Hormonal and pharmacological modification of plasma potassium homeostasis. Fundam Clin Pharmacol 24:595–605
46. Mazer M, Chen E (2009) Is subcutaneous administration of rapid-acting insulin as effective as intravenous insulin for treating diabetic ketoacidosis? Ann Emerg Med 53:259–263
47. Fisher JN, Kitabchi AE (1983) A randomized study of phosphate therapy in the treatment of diabetic ketoacidosis. J Clin Endocrinol Metab 57:177–180
48. Maury E, Vassal T, Offenstadt G (1999) Cardiac contractility during severe ketoacidosis. N Engl J Med 341:1938
49. Viallon A, Zeni F, Lafond P et al (1999) Does bicarbonate therapy improve the management of severe diabetic ketoacidosis? Crit Care Med 27:2690–2693
50. Morris LR, Murphy MB, Kitabchi AE (1986) Bicarbonate therapy in severe diabetic ketoacidosis. Ann Intern Med 105:836–840
51. Chua HR, Schneider A, Bellomo R (2011) Bicarbonate in diabetic ketoacidosis - a systematic review. Crit Care 1:23
52. Konstantinov NK, Rohrscheib M, Agaba EI, Dorin RI, Murata GH, Tzamaloukas AH (2015) Respiratory failure in diabetic ketoacidosis. World J Diabetes 6:1009–1023
53. Gershengom HB, Iwashyna TJ, Cooke CR et al (2012) Variation in use of intensive care for adults with diabetic ketoacidosis. Crit Care Med 40:2009–2015
54. Cohen RD, Woods HF (1983) Lactic acidosis revisited. Diabetes 32:181–191

55. UK Prospective Diabetes Study Group (1998) Effect of intensive blood-glucose control with metformin on complications in overweight patients with type 2 diabetes (UKPDS 34). Lancet 352:854–865
56. Duncan AI, Koch CG, Xu M et al (2007) Recent metformin ingestion does not increase in-hospital morbidity or mortality after cardiac surgery. Anesth Analg 104:42–50
57. Trinkley KE, Malone DC, Nelson JA, Saseen JJ (2016) Prescribing attitudes, behaviors nd opinions regarding metformin for patients with diabetes: a focus group study. Ther Adv Chronic Dis 7:220–228
58. Renda F, Mura P, Finco G, Ferrazin F, Pani L, Landoni G (2013) Metformin-associated lactic acidosis requiring hospitalization. A national 10 year survey and a systematic literature review. Eur Rev Med Pharmacol Sci 17(suppl):45–49
59. DeFronzo R, Fleming GA, Chen K, Bisack A (2016) Metformin-associated lactic acidosis: current perspective on causes and risk. Metab Clin Exp 65:20–29
60. Bodmer M, Meier C, Krahenbuhl S, Jick SS, Meier CR (2008) Metformin, sulfonylurea, or other antidiabetic drugs and the risk of lactic acidosis or hypoglycemia: a nested case-control analysis. Diabetes Care 31:2086–2091
61. Misbin RJ, Lahn RG, Stadel BV et al (1998) Lactic acidosis in patients with diabetes treated with metformin. N Engl J Med 338:265–266
62. Seidowsky A, Nseir S, Houdret N et al (2009) Metformin-associated lactic acidosis: a prognostic and therapeutic study. Crit Care Med 37:2191–2196
63. Salpeter SR, Greyber E, Pasternak GA, Salpeter EE (2010) Risk of fatal and non fatal lactic acidosis with metformin use in type 2 diabetes mellitus. Cochrane Database Syst Rev 20:CD002967
64. Friesecke S, Abel P, Roser M, Felix SB, Runge S (2010) Outcome of severe lactic acidosis associated with metformin accumulation. Crit Care 14:R226
65. Kamber N, Davis WA, Bruce DG et al (2008) Metformin and lactic acidosis in an Australian community setting: the Fremantle diabetes study. Med J Aust 188:446–449
66. Kajbaf F, Lalau JD (2013) The criteria for metformin-associated lactic acidosis: the quality of reporting in a large pharmacovigilance database. Diabetes Metab 30:345–348
67. Kajbaf F, Lalau JD (2013) The prognostic value of blood pH and lactate and metformin concentrations in severe metformin-associated lactic acidosis. BMC Pharmacol Toxicol 14:22
68. Kajbaf F, Lalau JD (2014) Mortality rate in so-called "metformin-associated lactic acidosis": a review of the data since the 1960s. Pharmacoepidemiol Drug Safe 23:1123–1127
69. Chang CT, Chen YC, Fang JT, Huang CC (2002) Metformin-associated lactic acidosis: case reports and literature review. J Nephrol 15:398–402
70. Wills BK, Bryant SM, Buckley P, Seo B (2010) Can acute overdose of metformin lead to lactic acidosis? Am J Emerg Med 28:857–861
71. Dell'Aglio DM, Perino LJ, Kazzi Z, Abramson J, Schwartz MD, Morgan BW (2009) Acute metformin overdose: examining serum pH, lactate level, and metformin concentrations in survivors versus nonsurvivors: a systematic review of the literature. Ann Emerg Med 54:818–823
72. Boucaud-Maitre D, Ropers J, Porokhov B et al (2016) Lactic acidosis: relationship between metformin levels, lactate concentration and mortality. Diabet Med 33:1536–1154
73. Li L, Gopalakrishnan C, Heide-Jørgensen U et al (2017) Metformin use and risk of lactic acidosis in people with diabetes with and without renal impairment: a cohort study in Denmark and the UK. Diabet Med 34:485–489
74. Orban JC, Fontaine E, Ichai C (2012) Metformin overdose: time to move on. Crit Care 16:164
75. Protti A, Russo R, Tagliabue P et al (2010) Oxygen consumption is depressed in patients with lactic acidosis due to biguanide intoxication. Crit Care 14:R22
76. El-Mir MY, Nogueira V, Fontaine E et al (2000) Dimethylbiguanide inhibits cell respiration via an indirect effect targeted on the respiratory chain complex I. J Biol Chem 275:223–228
77. Madiraju AK, Erion DM, Rahimi Y et al (2014) Metformin suppresses gluconeogenesis by inhibiting mitochondrial glycerophosphate dehydrogenase. Nature 510:542–546
78. Argaud D, Roth H, Wiernsperger N et al (1993) Metformin decreases gluconeogenesis by enhancing the pyruvate kinase flux in isolated rat hepatocytes. Eur J Biochem 213:1341–1348

79. McCreight LJ, Bailey CJ, Pearson ER (2016) Metformin and the gastrointestinal tract. Diabetologia 59:426–435
80. Mirrakhimov AE, Barbaryan A, Gray A, Ayach T (2016) The role of renal replacement therapy in the management of pharmacologic poisoning. Int J Nephrol 2016:12
81. Lalau JD, Race JM (1999) Lactic acidosis in metformin therapy. Drugs 58:55–60
82. Arroyo D, Melero R, Panizo N et al (2011) Metformin associated acute kidney injury and lactic acidosis. Int J Nephrol 2011:749653
83. Stades AM, Heikens JT, Erkelens DW et al (2004) Metformin and lactic acidosis: cause or coincidence? A review of case reports. J Intern Med 255:179–187
84. Callelo DP, Liu KD, Wiegand TJ et al (2015) Extracorporeal treatment for metformin poisoning: systematic review and recommendations from the extracorporeal treatments in poisoning workgroup. Crit Care Med 43:1716–1730
85. Peters N, Jay N, Barraud D et al (2008) Metformin-associated lactic acidosis in an intensive care unit. Crit Care 12:R149
86. Emslie-Smith AM, Boyle DI, Evans JM et al (2001) Contra-indications to metformin therapy in patients with type 2 diabetes: a population-based study of adherence to prescribing guidelines. Diabet Med 18:483–488
87. UK Prospective Diabetes Study Group (1998) Intensive blood-glucose control with sulphonylureas or insulin compared with conventional treatment and risk of complications in patients with type 2 diabetes (UKPDS 33). Lancet 352:837–853
88. Murata GH, Duckworth WC, Shah JH et al (2004) Factors affecting hypoglycemia awareness in insulin-treated type 2 diabetes: the diabetes outcomes in veterans study (DOVES). Diabetes Res Clin Pract 65:61–67
89. Vinik AI, Maser RE, Mitchell BD et al (2003) Diabetic autonomic neuropathy. Diabetes Care 26:1553–1579
90. Laing SP, Swerdlow AJ, Slater SD et al (1999) The British diabetic association cohort study, I: all-cause mortality in patients with insulin-treated diabetes mellitus. Diabet Med 16:459–465
91. Cranston I, Lomas J, Maran A et al (1994) Restoration of hypoglycaemia awareness in patients with long-duration insulin-dependent diabetes. Lancet 344:283–287

Neuroendocrine Dysfunction in the Critically Ill Patients 16

Antoine Roquilly and Karim Asehnoune

16.1 Introduction

Thanks to the medical progress over the past decades, patients nowadays survive previously lethal sepsis, trauma, or acute illnesses [1]. About 25% of ICU patients, however, enter a chronic phase of critical illness, during which organ support is often required for weeks.

Patients with acute life-threatening conditions such as septic shock or sever trauma frequently develop organ failure even if these organs have not been directly injured by the initial stress. These organ failures are traditionally attributed to the effects of pro-inflammatory mediators that induce macro- and microcirculatory changes resulting in tissue hypoxia and cellular damages. However, if things were so simple, organ failures should be irreversible, especially for organs with low regenerative capacity such as kidneys. Although renal insufficiency frequently evolves toward an almost "*ad integrum*" restitution of renal function in survivors. It is also remarkable that the functionally injured organs remain almost normal histologically, in particular in terms of architecture and tissue structure with very few apoptotic phenomena or cell necrosis. These findings suggest that systemic inflammation induces functional alterations rather than structural impairment of organs. Cells enter a state of hibernation which allows the organ to be preserved by decreasing its function [2]. This state of "metabolic sleep" is directly attributed to the inflammatory response as well as to the neuroendocrine response, both of which are strongly entangled. This response should be beneficial, by limiting the insults of the organs during the inflammatory storm.

The endocrine system, especially the hypothalamic–pituitary axis, plays an essential role in the metabolic adaptation to aggression [3]. Even partial

A. Roquilly • K. Asehnoune (✉)
CHU de Nantes, service d'anesthésie reanimation, Hôpital Hôtel-dieu,
1 place Alexis Ricordeau, 44093 Nantes, Cedex 1, France
e-mail: karim.asehnoune@chu-nantes.fr

C. Ichai et al. (eds.), *Metabolic Disorders and Critically Ill Patients*,
http://doi.org/10.1007/978-3-319-64010-5_16

dysregulation of the endocrine response increases the morbidity and mortality associated with severe stress, resulting in increased weight loss and ICU-acquired weakness, prolonged weaning of mechanical ventilation, and susceptibility to secondary infections. Two phases of endocrine dysregulation can be defined in critically ill patients: an early phase characterized by a peripheral resistance to hypothalamic-pituitary hormones and a later one corresponding rather to a central deficit of hypothalamic hormones.

16.2 Physiological Response to Severe Stress (Table 16.1)

16.2.1 Time Course of the Response of the Hypothalamic–Anterior Pituitary Axes to Acute Stress

Early phase. The first phase of the endocrine response lasts for 7–10 days. In the early hours of a stress, inflammatory mediators (such as TNF-α, Interleukins 1 and 6) are released by innate immune cells, mainly dendritic cells and monocytes, and epithelial cells. These cytokines powerfully activate the hypothalamic–pituitary axis and trigger a complex endocrine response that must allow the organism to survive the aggression. This early endocrine response initiates the consummation of the body's protein mass of up to 10% of total muscle mass in 1 week [4]. The objective of this hormone-induced catabolism is to provide injured tissues and organs with poor stock of energy (brain, heart) with endogenous energetic substrates allowing rapid healing despite the decrease in exogenous caloric intake. The releases of amino acids, fatty acids, and glucose consecutive to proteolysis, lipolysis, and gluconeogenesis is therefore a phenomenon of adaptation to acute stress [5].

Late phase. This second period, which begins after the seventh day, lasts for several months. It is characterized by an endocrine status very different from the

Table 16.1 Neuroendocrine dysfunction in the early and the chronic phases of critical illness

Hormones		Phase I (early)		Phase II (chronic)	
Growth hormone axis	GH (pulsatile)	↑	Peripheral resistance	↓	Pituitary dysfunction
	IGF-I	↓		↓↓	
	GH-BP	↓		↑	
Thyroid axis	TSH (pulsatile)	↑ =	Lack of peripheral activation	↓	Pituitary dysfunction
	T4	↑ =		↓	
	T3	↓		↓↓	
	rT3	↑		↑ =	
Sex hormone axis	LH (pulsatile)	↑ =	Leydig cells alterations	↓	Pituitary dysfunction
	Testosterone	↓		↓↓	
Axe corticotrope	ACTH	↑	Peripheral resistance	↓	? (endothelin)
	Cortisol	↑↑		↓ = ↑	
Prolactin	PRL (pulsatile)	↑	Hypothalamic stimulation	↓	?

early days. After the first week, mediators of inflammation are no longer found in the blood of critically ill patients [6], and the mechanisms of endocrine dysregulation are therefore essentially linked to a reduction in the synthesis of hypothalamic hormones. Mechanisms are widely different; however, the energy metabolism of the body remains profoundly altered. Free fatty acids are no longer used which results in fatty liver disease, and energetic substrates are recruited via the pursuit of increased muscle and bone proteolysis [7]. This persistent catabolic phase results in prolonged muscle weakness, with failure of ventilatory weaning. This period is associated with high susceptibility to infections and mortality in intensive care units of nearly 25% of patients [8]. Full recovery can take several years in survivors and sometimes never occurs [9].

The hypothalamic–pituitary axis is composed of five axes which can, separately or in concert, encounter a dysfunction and cause complications.

16.2.2 Growth Hormone (GH)

Resting state. The pulsatile release of GH from the pituitary gland is stimulated by hypothalamic GH-RH (GH-releasing hormone) and inhibited by somatostatin [3]. Ghrelin, a highly conserved hormone expressed in the hypothalamus and in the gut, is also a key driver of pulsatile GH release. Blood levels of GH alternate between peaks and indices within the day. The effects of GH on the body are essentially indirect, mediated by IGF-I (insulin-like growth factor) which stimulates muscle anabolism, mitogenesis, and lipolysis and is responsible of hyperglycemia by peripheral insulin resistance.

Response to stress: acute peripheral resistance. Despite the pulsatile release of GH, GH insufficiency is mediated by a reduction in the number of receptors of GH on myocytes and hepatocytes. This peripheral resistance to GH is mediated by the inflammatory cytokines produced during the systemic inflammatory response. The collapse of IGF-I and IGF-BP (IGF-binding protein) limits the negative retrocontrol on the pituitary axis and results in high blood levels of GH [10]. Theoretically, acute GH insufficiency is beneficial because initial catabolism provides endogenous energy substrates necessary for the response to aggression: increased lipolysis and blood glucose, which is parallel to the rise in blood levels of GH [11].

Response to stress: the late hypothalamic insufficiency. Blood levels of GH slightly decrease as compared to the early phase but remain higher than normal values. The loss of pulsatility of the GH release during this period is responsible of the GH insufficiency characterized by persistent low levels of IGF-I and IGF-BP [12]. The negative feedback of GH on the hypothalamus is retained, which may explain the decrease of GH-RH. During this phase, the supply of synthetic GH-RH makes it possible to raise the blood levels of GH, IGF-I, and IGF-BP, which confirms the correction of peripheral resistance to GH and suggests a hypothalamic disorder. This relative deficit in GH (loss of pulsatility by GH-RH collapse) leads to a low muscle anabolism and limits the weight-recovery capacities of critically ill patients [7, 13].

16.2.3 Pituitary–Adrenocortical Axis

Resting state. The hypothalamic cortico-releasing hormone (CRH) stimulates the pituitary secretion of adrenocorticotropin hormone (ACTH). The morning peak of ACTH stimulates the adrenal release of cortisol which therefore has a nycthemeral rhythm of secretion characterized by a peak in the morning at 8:00 and a valley at night. The negative feedback of cortisol on CRH and ACTH avoids hypercorticism.

Response to stress: the early phase. Inflammation mediators, such as Il-6, activate the hypothalamic–pituitary axis leading to early and massive release of CRH and ACTH. The nycthemeral rhythm of secretion of cortisol is thus abolished, and there is an early hypercorticism which is an essential mechanism of adaptation to stress [14]. After several days of resuscitation, there is a decrease in cortisol-binding globulin resulting in elevation of free cortisol, even though total cortisol is low. During critical illness, reduced cortisol breakdown, related to suppressed expression also and activity of cortisol-metabolizing enzymes, contributed to hypercortisolemia and hence corticotropin suppression [15]. Cortisol activates gluconeogenesis lipolysis and induces insulin resistance to favor the supply of substrates to organs with poor stock of energy such as the brain. Cortisol also plays an important role in hemodynamic homeostasis and the maintenance of an optimal blood pressure: (1) cortisol stimulated the renal angiotensin and the sympathetic nervous systems resulting in hydrosodic retention and high volemia; (2) cortisol increases systemic vascular resistance by sensitizing peripheral receptors to vasoactive amines [16], which is essential in the early hours of systemic inflammation; and (3) it lowers the threshold of maximal extraction of oxygen from the blood, which promotes tissue oxygenation even in case of low blood flow. All these phenomena increase the perfusion of organs and hasten tissue healing. Cortisol also controls the initial overwhelming systemic inflammation response [17]. In intensive care, the importance of the initial peak of cortisolemia was correlated with the amount of stress experienced by the patient. Paradoxically, in the most severe patients, low cortisol levels are a predictor of adverse outcome, a probable marker of endocrine dysregulation [18]. Depending on the condition, 25–65% of patients develop adrenal insufficiency related to resuscitation, which is defined as an insufficient elevation of cortisolemia in response to stress [19], a so-called state of "critical illness-related corticosteroid insufficiency" [20]. Its etiology is unknown; however, a genetic predisposition that alters the pituitary response to inflammatory cytokines is strongly suspected [21]. Blood levels of inflammatory cytokines are higher in critically ill patients with adrenal insufficiency than those with normal adrenal function [22, 23]. In conclusion, critical illness-related corticosteroid insufficiency is associated with hemodynamic instability, hospital-acquired infection, and increased mortality. These data suggest that hypercorticism is an essential component of the response to aggression, preventing systemic complication of an overwhelming inflammatory response.

Response to stress: the late phase. This period is characterized by persistent high levels of cortisolemia while the blood levels of ACTH are back to normal values. This late hypercorticism is probably mediated by high concentrations of endogenous endothelin [24]. During this late phase, hypercorticism can be responsible of delayed healing due to continued nitrogen catabolism.

16.2.4 Pituitary–Thyroid Axis

Resting state. The release of thyroid-stimulating hormone (TSH) is regulated by the hypothalamic thyroid-releasing hormone (TRH). The pulsatile secretion of TSH results in thyroid release of thyroxine (T4), an inactive hormone, that is converted into tri-iodothyronine (T3) which is the efficient hormone or in reverse T3 (rT3), an inactive hormone. T3 exerts inhibitory feedback on TSH and has important effects on cell growth and metabolism.

Response to stress: the acute phase. The blood levels of T3 are drastically decreased, while the levels of inactive hormones (rT3, T4, and TSH) are elevated. This hypothyroidism is correlated with severity of the acute stress [25]. Inflammatory cytokines (TNFα, IL 1, and 6) participate directly in this "low-T3 syndrome" by reducing the peripheral activation of the inactive T4 hormone. The theoretical advantage of hypothyroidism is a reduction of cell metabolism while the energy supply is jeopardized during the systemic inflammatory response.

Response to stress: late phase. Levels of T3 and T4 are diminished, while TSH one is normal. TRH gene expression in the hypothalamus of patients dead in intensive care units is low [26], demonstrating the hypothalamic origin of the late hypothyroidism in critically ill patients.

16.2.5 Pituitary–Sex Hormones Axis

Resting state. Gonadotrophin-releasing hormone (GnRH) is released by the hypothalamus and stimulates the secretion of luteinizing hormone and thus indirectly of sexocorticoids, including testosterone. Testosterone is a powerful anabolic hormone that stimulates protein synthesis, especially muscle. Prolactin (PRL) is rapidly released in response to stress. T-and B-lymphocytes possess PRL receptors which regulate their activity. Changes in PRL production are related to immune alterations in critically ill patients.

Response to stress: early phase. There is a transient increase in LH, but the testosterone level is diminished. This phenomenon contributes to the decrease of anabolism in the early days of ICU hospitalization [27]. PRL is one of the first hormones released in large quantities in the blood in response to stress, but its effect on the immune response in humans has been poorly investigated.

Response to stress: late phase. Hypogonadotropism, characterized by low levels of GnRH and of testosterone, accentuates long-term weight loss [28].

16.3 Diagnosis of Endocrine Dysfunction in Critically Ill Patients

With the exception of the pituitary–adrenocortical axis, the diagnosis of endocrine dysregulations is not specific to critically ill patients. Given the variety of mechanisms and the rapid evolution of these disorders, it is essential to simultaneously dose the pituitary hormones and the peripheral hormones before and after stimulation tests of the various neuroendocrine axes (see [29] for review).

16.3.1 Growth Hormone (GH)

Static assays should include both the GH and the IGF-I. There are two stimulation tests: the insulin test and the GH-RH test. The insulin test is based on stimulation of the somatotropic axis by iatrogenic hypoglycemia with a nadir of less than 2.2 mmol/L induced by the intravenous injection of 0.1 ui/ kg of rapid insulin. The main limitations of this insulin test are the risk of hypoglycemia in a sedated patient and the insulin resistance which can make it difficult to achieve severe hypoglycemia. The GH-RH test, which is thus the reference, consists in the intravenous injection of the hypothalamic hormone (1 μg/kg ivd) followed by four measurements of the plasmatic concentration of GH over 90 min. An increase in GH in response to GH-RH injection would confirm the hypothalamic origin of a GH defect.

16.3.2 Pituitary–Adrenocortical Axis

In intensive care units, the loss of the nycthemeral rhythm allows to test this axis without the usual time constraints. Free cortisol is the active form of the hormone and may therefore be a better reflection of the state of the adrenal axis [30]. However, there is currently no consensual threshold of free cortisolemia that defines adrenal insufficiency in ICU, and its dosage is not routinely available in clinical practice. Evaluation of adrenal function in resuscitated patients is typically done by a standard stimulation test with Synacthène® (250 μg IVD of ACTH and assay of cortisolemia at T0 and T30 T60 min). This dose of ACTH is supraphysiological and allows to stimulate the adrenals even in case of peripheral resistance to ACTH and thus evaluates the adrenal reserve in cortisol. The short corticotrophin test (using a 1 μg injection of ACTH) could be more sensitive, but this method may have a low positive predictive value for response to hydrocortisone therapy. Absolute adrenal insufficiency is characterized by a basal cortisol level below 3 μg/dL. An alteration of the response to ACTH means that the adrenal glands will no longer be able to handle a new stress and is so-called critical illness-related corticosteroid insufficiency. Most published studies define adrenal insufficiency associated with resuscitation with a baseline cortisol concentration of less than 15 μg/dL and/or an increase of less than 9 μg/dL in the corticotrophin test [31, 32]. The real threshold defining an adrenal insufficiency in intensive care units is likely to vary depending on the extent of stress and systemic inflammation, and the measurement of inflammatory mediators (such as C Reactive protein [33]) to the corticotrophin test could enhance the selection of patients requiring steroids.

16.3.3 Pituitary–Thyroid Axis

Static assays should include TSH-us, T3, and T4. For the dynamic test, TSH-us is measured 30 min after the injection of TRH (250 μg).

16.3.4 Pituitary–Sex Hormones Axis

There is no dynamic test to explore this axis. The static dosages of testosterone and of PRL are sufficient to explore these pathways.

16.3.5 Limits of Assessment Methods in Critically Ill Patients

Direct stimulation of the hypothalamic–pituitary axis by inflammatory cytokines attenuates the daily oscillations of hormonal levels. Thus the hormonal assays, in particular concerning the corticotropic axis, can be carried out without any time constraints. However, many drugs can disrupt test results. Etomidate inhibits the synthesis of cortisol. A single injection is responsible for a relative adrenal insufficiency for a period of 8–72 h [34, 35]. A Synacthene® test is therefore of significance in the diagnosis of critical illness-related corticosteroid insufficiency only if the test is performed no sooner than 12 h after an injection of etomidate. The use of dopamine also decreases secretion and anterior pituitary function, which aggravates catabolism, dysfunction of cellular immunity, and induces hypothyroidism [36]. The use of dopamine should therefore be taken into account when interpreting thyroid dosage assays.

16.4 Indications of Hormonal Treatments in Intensive Care Units

16.4.1 Growth Hormone (GH)

Takala et al. conducted a randomized clinical trial in 1999 evaluating the benefit of GH therapy in intensive care patients hospitalized more than 7 days [37]. In this study, a 14-day treatment by GH increased the blood levels of IGF-I and restored anabolism with better weight gain of patients. However, these beneficial effects were counteracted by the high incidence of treatment-related adverse events such as a blunt in the rate of hospital-acquired infections, a protraction of mechanical ventilation, and an excess in mortality (relative risk of death = 1.9, 95% CI [1.3, 2.9]).

This disappointing result is probably explained by the supraphysiological dose of GH which is known to induce digestive atrophy and hyperglycemia and to activate lipolysis. In another study, the combination of GH with glutamine therapy improved the protein balance of severe traumatized patients but increased insulin resistance and did not improve clinical outcomes [38]. For the future, a treatment with the hypothalamic hormone (GH-RH) may be more efficient than direct injection of GH because the GH-inhibitory retro-control on the pituitary gland would be preserved, ensuring a physiological adaptation of the levels of GH to the patient's needs. However, there is currently no data from the literature to validate this hypothesis.

16.4.2 Thyroid Hormones

Treatments with thyroid hormones (TRH and T3) have been proposed to treat the acute hypothyroidism observed in critically ill patients. A 5-day infusion of TRH in protracted critical illness reactivated blunted TSH secretion, with preserved peripheral responsiveness, and induces a shift toward anabolic metabolism [39]. In a clinical trial, treatment with T3 improved the cardiac function of children undergoing cardiac surgery and decreased their length of stay in intensive care unit [40]. However, there is not yet sufficient evidence to recommend such treatment in daily practice [41].

16.4.3 Androgens

In a large population of severe burn patients, testosterone administration significantly reduced protein catabolism, increased intracellular amino acid intake, and reduced muscle wasting [42]. In a non-randomized study, oxandrolone, a synthetic androgen, decreased weight loss, improved functional status, and accelerates healing of severe burn patients [43]. Since high initial blood levels of estradiol were correlated with the occurrence of infections and of organ failure in trauma patients [44], early opotherapy using these two hormones does not appear promising in this population. To date, there is no treatment with androgens that is not recommended in critically ill patients.

16.4.4 Hydrocortisone

In 2000, Annane et al. showed that the response to a standard synacthen test was correlated with mortality in septic shock patients [18]. In this study, the rate of mortality was higher in patients with an increase in total cortisol levels smaller than 9 μg/dL after stimulation with 250 μg IVD of ACTH and/or basal cortisol levels below 15 μg/dL (so-called non-responders) than in patients with a basal cortisolemia between 15 and 34 μg/dL and a delta bigger than 9 μg/dL after the stimulation. Two years later, the same authors demonstrated that a treatment with "physiological" dose of hydrocortisone (200 mg/day for 7 days) associated with a mineralocorticoid (fludrocortisone) reduced the mortality from 63 to 53% (RR 0.67, 95% CI [0.47–0.95]) in non-responder septic shock patients [45]. In 2008, the CORTICUS study [34] failed to reproduce these results, since this time mortality was not altered by treatment (39% vs. 36%, $p = 0.69$) [46]. Three important remarks may explain why CORTICUS did not validate the results obtained previously: (1) the inclusion of all the initially planned patients was not performed due to the result of an intermediate analysis; (2) mortality in the control group is lower than in the initial study (63% vs. 39%), which reflects the inclusion of patients less severe than in the princeps study; and (3) the time to inclusion of patients is greater in CORTICUS (8 h vs. 72 h after onset of septic shock). In these two studies, the incidence of side effects with the treatment was low, and hydrocortisone accelerated the weaning of vasoactive amines, probably because it increases the sensitivity to 1-adrenoceptor stimulation and of its effects on salt retention [47, 48]. When analyzing the effects of glucocorticoids in septic patients, it is of major importance to consider both the regimen dose and the duration of the treatment. In a review of literature with meta-analysis, prolonged (7–10 days) low dose (200 mg/day) of hydrocortisone has been associated with a reduced rate of mortality, while short course (2 days) of higher doses was ineffective to prevent death of septic patients [49]. Glucocorticoid treatment induces hyperglycemia, but the addition of intensive insulinotherapy to hydrocortisone did not improve mortality of septic patients [50]. Moreover, the addition of mineralocorticoid appears optional [50].

Other patient populations are affected by critical illness-related corticosteroid insufficiency such as trauma [17], brain injury [19], and cardiac surgery patients [20]. In cardiac surgery patients, hydrocortisone administration reduced the durations of catecholamine support and of the intensive care length of stay [51], and dexamethasone may reduce the rate of postoperative atrial fibrillation [52]. In severe burn patients, hydrocortisone reduces the duration of vasopressor treatment without delaying skin healing [53]. In severe trauma patients [54] and in severe traumatic brain injured patients [55], prolonged low dose of hydrocortisone reduced the occurrence of hospital-acquired pneumonia and the duration of mechanical ventilation. This surprising effect is explained by the immunological effects of hydrocortisone in patients suffering from systemic inflammation [56]. Indeed, hydrocortisone counteracts the development of critical illness-related immunosuppression such as the formation of suppressive natural killer cells [57] and to prevent an overwhelming inflammatory response to secondary infection [58]. Finally, glucocorticoid administration may prevent long-term psychological disorder which is frequently observed in critically ill patients (such as post-traumatic stress disorder) [59, 60]. Taking these results altogether, treatment of critically ill patients with prolonged low dose of hydrocortisone is probably beneficial in case of refractory shock, of high risk of post-traumatic pneumonia, or of high risk of death septic patients.

Conclusions

The neuroendocrine dysfunctions observed in critically ill patients initiate a phase of intense catabolism and a state of acquired-immunosuppression, both of them are responsible of hospital-acquired infections, difficult weaning of mechanical ventilation, and late mortality [3, 8]. Usual cares, such as early enteral nutrition [61], are insufficient to reverse the complications associated with neuroendocrine dysregulations observed in patients, thus supplementations with hormonal treatments are thus appealing.

It is important to understand the mechanisms of these neuroendocrine dysfunctions to timely diagnose them. In the acute phase of the response to severe stress, the pituitary hormones are actively secreted, but the effector organs are resistant to their effects. For instance, blood levels of cortisol higher than in healthy controls do not exclude critical illness-related corticosteroid insufficiency [32]. During the chronic period, which can last for several months, the pituitary production of hormones drops, and the blood levels of the effector hormones remain low. Given the rapid modifications between these two periods, the interpretations of blood test results are tricky, and the selection of patients requiring treatment remains challenging.

To date, clinical trials evaluating hormone therapy in intensive care units have most often given disappointing results, perhaps because they have only evaluated the treatment of one hormonal axis, neglecting the potential combination of hormonal defects in patients. The rapid reactivation of the somatotropic, thyrotropic, and gonadal axes is likely to increase anabolism and stop the intense catabolism of resuscitation patients, but few trials have been conducted on these axes. Treatment with hydrocortisone improves the prognosis of subgroup of patients without treating all the endocrine alterations listed in this review. Treatments with hypothalamic hormones are likely to reactivate the pituitary as a whole but also to induce the production of peripheral effector hormones such as IGF-1 or T3. Randomized clinical trials using synthetic extracts of hypothalamic hormones, and/or combining simultaneous opotherapy of several endocrine axes, are expected in the near future.

References

1. Kaukonen K-M, Bailey M, Suzuki S, Pilcher D, Bellomo R (2014) Mortality related to severe sepsis and septic shock among critically ill patients in Australia and New Zealand, 2000-2012. JAMA 311(13):1308–1309
2. Singer M, De Santis V, Vitale D, Jeffcoate W (2004) Multiorgan failure is an adaptive, endocrine-mediated, metabolic response to overwhelming systemic inflammation. Lancet 364(9433):545–548
3. Van den Berghe G (2016) On the Neuroendocrinopathy of critical illness: perspectives for feeding and novel treatments. Am J Respir Crit Care Med 194(11):1337–1348
4. Reid CL, Campbell IT, Little RA (2004) Muscle wasting and energy balance in critical illness. Clin Nutr 23(2):273–280
5. Van den Berghe G, de Zegher F, Bouillon R (1998) Clinical review 95: acute and prolonged critical illness as different neuroendocrine paradigms. J Clin Endocrinol Metab 83(6):1827–1834
6. Roquilly A, Braudeau C, Cinotti R, Dumonte E, Motreul R, Josien R et al (2013) Impaired blood dendritic cell numbers and functions after aneurysmal subarachnoid hemorrhage. PLoS One 8(8):e71639
7. Orford NR, Lane SE, Bailey M, Pasco JA, Cattigan C, Elderkin T et al (2016) Changes in bone mineral density in the year after critical illness. Am J Respir Crit Care Med 193(7):736–744

8. van Vught LA, Klein Klouwenberg PMC, Spitoni C, Scicluna BP, Wiewel MA, Horn J et al (2016) Incidence, risk factors, and attributable mortality of secondary infections in the intensive care unit after admission for sepsis. JAMA 315(14):1469–1479
9. Herridge MS, Tansey CM, Matté A, Tomlinson G, Diaz-Granados N, Cooper A et al (2011) Functional disability 5 years after acute respiratory distress syndrome. N Engl J Med 364(14):1293–1304
10. Hermansson M, Wickelgren RB, Hammarqvist F, Bjarnason R, Wennström I, Wernerman J et al (1997) Measurement of human growth hormone receptor messenger ribonucleic acid by a quantitative polymerase chain reaction-based assay: demonstration of reduced expression after elective surgery. J Clin Endocrinol Metab 82(2):421–428
11. Vanhorebeek I, Van den Berghe G (2004) Hormonal and metabolic strategies to attenuate catabolism in critically ill patients. Curr Opin Pharmacol 4(6):621–628
12. Ross R, Miell J, Freeman E, Jones J, Matthews D, Preece M et al (1991) Critically ill patients have high basal growth hormone levels with attenuated oscillatory activity associated with low levels of insulin-like growth factor-I. Clin Endocrinol 35(1):47–54
13. Moss M, Nordon-Craft A, Malone D, Van Pelt D, Frankel SK, Warner ML et al (2015) A randomized trial of an intensive physical therapy program for acute respiratory failure patients. Am J Respir Crit Care Med 193(10):1101–1110
14. Naito Y, Fukata J, Tamai S, Seo N, Nakai Y, Mori K et al (1991) Biphasic changes in hypothalamo-pituitary-adrenal function during the early recovery period after major abdominal surgery. J Clin Endocrinol Metab 73(1):111–117
15. Boonen E, Vervenne H, Meersseman P, Andrew R, Mortier L, Declercq PE et al (2013) Reduced cortisol metabolism during critical illness. N Engl J Med 368(16):1477–1488
16. Hoen S, Mazoit J-X, Asehnoune K, Brailly-Tabard S, Benhamou D, Moine P et al (2005) Hydrocortisone increases the sensitivity to alpha1-adrenoceptor stimulation in humans following hemorrhagic shock. Crit Care Med 33(12):2737–2743
17. Hoen S, Asehnoune K, Brailly-Tabard S, Mazoit J-X, Benhamou D, Moine P et al (2002) Cortisol response to corticotropin stimulation in trauma patients: influence of hemorrhagic shock. Anesthesiology 97(4):807–813
18. Annane D, Sebille V, Troché G, Raphaël JC, Gajdos P, Bellissant E (2000) A 3-level prognostic classification in septic shock based on cortisol levels and cortisol response to corticotropin. JAMA 283(8):1038–1045
19. Cohan P, Wang C, McArthur DL, Cook SW, Dusick JR, Armin B et al (2005) Acute secondary adrenal insufficiency after traumatic brain injury: a prospective study. Crit Care Med 33(10):2358–2366
20. Marik PE (2009) Critical illness-related corticosteroid insufficiency. Chest 135(1):181–193
21. Prigent H, Maxime V, Annane D (2004) Science review: mechanisms of impaired adrenal function in sepsis and molecular actions of glucocorticoids. Crit Care 8(4):243–252
22. Woiciechowsky C, Schöning B, Cobanov J, Lanksch WR, Volk H-D, Döcke W-D (2002) Early IL-6 plasma concentrations correlate with severity of brain injury and pneumonia in brain-injured patients. J Trauma 52(2):339–345
23. Woiciechowsky C, Schöning B, Lanksch WR, Volk HD, Döcke WD (1999) Mechanisms of brain-mediated systemic anti-inflammatory syndrome causing immunodepression. J Mol Med 77(11):769–780
24. Roth-Isigkeit A, Dibbelt L, Eichler W, Schumacher J, Schmucker P (2001) Blood levels of atrial natriuretic peptide, endothelin, cortisol and ACTH in patients undergoing coronary artery bypass grafting surgery with cardiopulmonary bypass. J Endocrinol Investig 24(10):777–785
25. Arem R, Wiener GJ, Kaplan SG, Kim HS, Reichlin S, Kaplan MM (1993) Reduced tissue thyroid hormone levels in fatal illness. Metab Clin Exp 42(9):1102–1108
26. Fliers E, Wiersinga WM, Swaab DF (1998) Physiological and pathophysiological aspects of thyrotropin-releasing hormone gene expression in the human hypothalamus. Thyroid 8(10):921–928
27. Guo H, Calkins JH, Sigel MM, Lin T (1990) Interleukin-2 is a potent inhibitor of Leydig cell steroidogenesis. Endocrinology 127(3):1234–1239

28. Van den Berghe G, de Zegher F, Lauwers P, Veldhuis JD (1994) Luteinizing hormone secretion and hypoandrogenaemia in critically ill men: effect of dopamine. Clin Endocrinol 41(5):563–569
29. Van den Berghe G (2003) Endocrine evaluation of patients with critical illness. Endocrinol Metab Clin N Am 32(2):385–410
30. Hamrahian AH, Oseni TS, Arafah BM (2004) Measurements of serum free cortisol in critically ill patients. N Engl J Med 350(16):1629–1638
31. Marik PE, Pastores SM, Annane D, Meduri GU, Sprung CL, Arlt W et al (2008) Recommendations for the diagnosis and management of corticosteroid insufficiency in critically ill adult patients: consensus statements from an international task force by the American College of Critical Care Medicine. Crit Care Med 36(6):1937–1949
32. Annane D, Maxime V, Ibrahim F, Alvarez JC, Abe E, Boudou P (2006) Diagnosis of adrenal insufficiency in severe sepsis and septic shock. Am J Respir Crit Care Med 174(12):1319–1326
33. Torres A, Sibila O, Ferrer M, Polverino E, Menendez R, Mensa J et al (2015) Effect of corticosteroids on treatment failure among hospitalized patients with severe community-acquired pneumonia and high inflammatory response. JAMA 313(7):677–610
34. Asehnoune K, Mahe PJ, Seguin P, Jaber S, Jung B, Guitton C et al (2012) Etomidate increases susceptibility to pneumonia in trauma patients. Intensive Care Med 38(10):1673–1682
35. Vinclair M, Broux C, Faure P, Brun J, Genty C, Jacquot C et al (2008) Duration of adrenal inhibition following a single dose of etomidate in critically ill patients. Intensive Care Med 34(4):714–719
36. Arafah BM (2006) Hypothalamic pituitary adrenal function during critical illness: limitations of current assessment methods. J Clin Endocrinol Metab 91(10):3725–3745
37. Takala J, Ruokonen E, Webster NR, Nielsen MS, Zandstra DF, Vundelinckx G et al (1999) Increased mortality associated with growth hormone treatment in critically ill adults. N Engl J Med 341(11):785–792
38. Duška F, Fric M, Waldauf P, Pažout J, Anděl M, Mokrejš P et al (2008) Frequent intravenous pulses of growth hormone together with glutamine supplementation in prolonged critical illness after multiple trauma: effects on nitrogen balance, insulin resistance, and substrate oxidation. Crit Care Med 36(6):1707–1713
39. Van den Berghe G, Wouters P, Weekers F, Mohan S, Baxter RC, Veldhuis JD et al (1999) Reactivation of pituitary hormone release and metabolic improvement by infusion of growth hormone-releasing peptide and thyrotropin-releasing hormone in patients with protracted critical illness. J Clin Endocrinol Metab 84(4):1311–1323
40. Bettendorf M, Schmidt KG, Grulich-Henn J, Ulmer HE, Heinrich UE (2000) Tri-iodothyronine treatment in children after cardiac surgery: a double-blind, randomised, placebo-controlled study. Lancet 356(9229):529–534
41. Dimmick S, Badawi N, Randell T (2004) Thyroid hormone supplementation for the prevention of morbidity and mortality in infants undergoing cardiac surgery. Cochrane Database Syst Rev 3:CD004220
42. Ferrando AA, Sheffield-Moore M, Wolf SE, Herndon DN, Wolfe RR (2001) Testosterone administration in severe burns ameliorates muscle catabolism. Crit Care Med 29(10):1936–1942
43. Demling RH (1999) Comparison of the anabolic effects and complications of human growth hormone and the testosterone analog, oxandrolone, after severe burn injury. Burns 25(3):215–221
44. Gee AC, Sawai RS, Differding J, Muller P, Underwood S, Schreiber MA (2007) The influence of sex hormones on coagulation and inflammation in the trauma patient. Shock 29(3):334–341
45. Annane D, Sébille V, Charpentier C, Bollaert PE, François B, Korach J-M et al (2002) Effect of treatment with low doses of hydrocortisone and fludrocortisone on mortality in patients with septic shock. JAMA 288(7):862–871
46. Sprung CL, Annane D, Keh D, Moreno R, Singer M, Freivogel K et al (2008) Hydrocortisone therapy for patients with septic shock. N Engl J Med 358(2):111–124
47. Laviolle B, Le Maguet P, Verdier M-C, Massart C, Donal E, Lainé F et al (2010) Biological and hemodynamic effects of low doses of fludrocortisone and hydrocortisone, alone or in combination, in healthy volunteers with hypoaldosteronism. Clin Pharmacol Ther 88(2):183–190

48. Laviolle B, Annane D, Fougerou C, Bellissant E (2012) Gluco- and mineralocorticoid biological effects of a 7-day treatment with low doses of hydrocortisone and fludrocortisone in septic shock. Intensive Care Med 38(8):1306–1314
49. Annane D, Bellissant E, Bollaert PE, Briegel J, Confalonieri M, De Gaudio R et al (2009) Corticosteroids in the treatment of severe sepsis and septic shock in adults: a systematic review. JAMA 301(22):2362–2375
50. Study Investigators COIITSS, Annane D, Cariou A, Maxime V, Azoulay E, D'honneur G et al (2010) Corticosteroid treatment and intensive insulin therapy for septic shock in adults: a randomized controlled trial. JAMA 303(4):341–348
51. Weis F, Beiras-Fernandez A, Schelling G, Briegel J, Lang P, Hauer D et al (2009) Stress doses of hydrocortisone in high-risk patients undergoing cardiac surgery: effects on interleukin-6 to interleukin-10 ratio and early outcome. Crit Care Med 37(5):1685–1690
52. Halonen J, Halonen P, Järvinen O, Taskinen P, Auvinen T, Tarkka M et al (2007) Corticosteroids for the prevention of atrial fibrillation after cardiac surgery: a randomized controlled trial. JAMA 297(14):1562–1567
53. Venet F, Plassais J, Textoris J, Cazalis M-A, Pachot A, Bertin-Maghit M et al (2015) Low-dose hydrocortisone reduces norepinephrine duration in severe burn patients: a randomized clinical trial. Crit Care 19(1):21–29
54. Roquilly A, Mahe PJ, Seguin P, Guitton C, Floch H, Tellier AC et al (2011) Hydrocortisone therapy for patients with multiple trauma: the randomized controlled HYPOLYTE study. JAMA 305(12):1201–1209
55. Asehnoune K, Seguin P, Allary J, Feuillet F, Lasocki S, Cook F et al (2014) Hydrocortisone and fludrocortisone for prevention of hospital-acquired pneumonia in patients with severe traumatic brain injury (Corti-TC): a double-blind, multicentre phase 3, randomised placebo-controlled trial. Lancet Respir Med 2(9):706–716
56. Keh D, Boehnke T, Weber-Cartens S, Schulz C, Ahlers O, Bercker S et al (2003) Immunologic and hemodynamic effects of "low-dose" hydrocortisone in septic shock: a double-blind, randomized, placebo-controlled, crossover study. Am J Respir Crit Care Med 167(4):512–520
57. Roquilly A, Broquet A, Jacqueline C, Masson D, Segain JP, Braudeau C et al (2014) Hydrocortisone prevents immunosuppression by interleukin-10+ natural killer cells after trauma-hemorrhage. Crit Care Med 42(12):e752–e761
58. Jamieson AM, Yu S, Annicelli CH, Medzhitov R (2010) Influenza virus-induced glucocorticoids compromise innate host defense against a secondary bacterial infection. Cell Host Microbe 7(2):103–114. Elsevier
59. McFarlane AC, Atchison M, Yehuda R (1997) The acute stress response following motor vehicle accidents and its relation to PTSD. Ann N Y Acad Sci 821:437–441
60. Delahanty DL, Raimonde AJ, Spoonster E (2000) Initial posttraumatic urinary cortisol levels predict subsequent PTSD symptoms in motor vehicle accident victims. Biol Psychiatry 48(9):940–947
61. Reintam Blaser A, Starkopf J, Alhazzani W, Berger MM, Casaer MP, Deane AM et al (2017) Early enteral nutrition in critically ill patients: ESICM clinical practice guidelines. Intensive Care Med 43(3):380–398

Hyperglycemia in ICU

17

Carole Ichai and Jean-Charles Preiser

17.1 Introduction

Stress hyperglycemia refers usually to a transient elevation of blood glucose level (BGL) which occurs during acute diseases in patients without previous evidence of diabetes. This metabolic disorder is frequent and can reach up to 50% of critically ill patients [1, 2]. Many data support the relationship between stress hyperglycemia and an increased morbidity and mortality. A great enthusiasm has been triggered in 2001 after the first clinical trial showing that a tight glycemic control (TGC) in intensive care unit (ICU) reduced significantly the mortality rate and improved several other outcome variables in critically ill patients [3]. However, further studies failed to confirm these results leading to question about the real benefit and external validity of a TGC in ICU [4–8]. The recent discussions and controversies revealed the complexity of the metabolic response to stress.

C. Ichai (✉)
Intensive Care Unit, Hôpital Pasteur 2, 30 Voie Romaine, 06001 Nice, Cédex 1, France

IRCAN (INSERM U1081, CNRS UMR 7284), University Hospital of Nice, Nice, France
e-mail: ichai@unice.fr

J-C. Preiser
Department of Intensive Care, Erasme University Hospital, Université libre de Bruxelles, Brussels, Belgium

C. Ichai et al. (eds.), *Metabolic Disorders and Critically Ill Patients*,
http://doi.org/10.1007/978-3-319-64010-5_17

17.2 Blood Glucose Level in Physiological and Pathological Conditions

17.2.1 Regulation of Glycemia

The regulation of BGL results from three essential mechanisms [1, 9]:

- The hormonal regulation consists in an equilibrium between the hypoglycemic insulin hormone and the counter-regulatory hyperglycemic hormones (glucagon, epinephrine, cortisol).
- The neurological regulation is triggered by glucose sensors which are located in various cells and which activate or inhibit different messages and pathways.
- The liver via an autoregulation.

These signals modulate carbohydrates metabolism by controlling glucose turnover and pathways, especially endogenous glucose production (EGP) and glucose entry in the cells. The translocation of glucose transporters (GLUT) represents the essential mechanism by which glucose crosses the membrane and enters into the cells [1, 10] (Table 17.1). Among these transporters, GLUT-1 is particularly involved in non-insulin-mediated tissues [1, 9]. GLUT-2 regulates the flux of glucose through hepatic cell membranes. GLUT-4 is mainly regulated by insulin and regulates therefore the entry of glucose in insulin-mediated tissues, i.e., adipose tissue, heart, and skeletal muscles (Fig. 17.1a).

Table 17.1 Different types, localization, and functions of GLUT transporters

Name	Tissue expression	Substrate affinity
Class I		
• GLUT-1 • GLUT-2 • GLUT-3 • GLUT-4	• Red blood cell, brain • Renal tubular cells, β-pancreatic, epithelial, and intestinal cells • Neurons, placenta • Adipose tissue, skeletal and cardiac muscles	• Stimulated by the decrease of glycemia and by cytokines (glucose uptake by non-insulin-mediated tissues) • Low affinity • High affinity • Glucose uptake on insulin-mediated tissues
Class II		
• GLUT-5 • GLUT-7 • GLUT-9 • GLUT-11	• Testis, intestine, muscle • Testis, intestine, muscle, prostate • Liver, kidneys • Placenta, kidneys, muscle, pancreas	• Fructose transportation • Glucose transportation outside the endoplasmic reticulum
Class III		
• GLUT-6 • GLUT-8 • GLUT-10 • GLUT-12	• Brain, spleen, leukocytes • Brain, adipocytes, testis • Liver, pancreas • Heart, prostate, breast cancer	Unknown

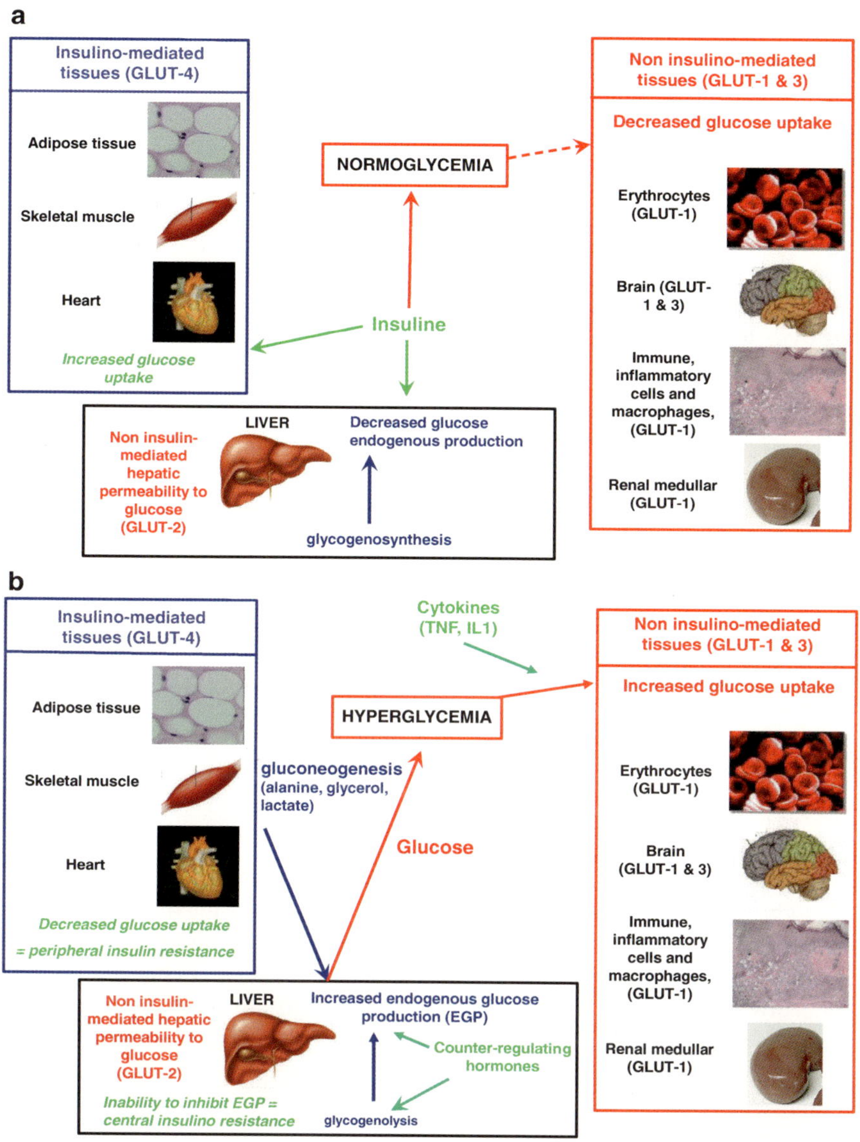

Fig. 17.1 (**a**) Insulin and glycemia in physiological condition. Insulin allows the entry of glucose in insulin-mediated tissues (heart, skeletal muscles, and adipose tissue) by activating GLUT-4 transporters leading to reduce glycemia (insulin is a hypoglycemic hormone). Consequently, the entry of glucose in non-insulin-mediated tissues via GLUT-1 (and 3) transporters decreases, as well as in the liver (GLUT-2). (**b**) Stress hyperglycemia and insulin resistance. The decreased glucose uptake by insulin-mediated tissues via GLUT-4 transporters defines peripheral insulin resistance. In the liver, the endogenous glucose production (EGP) is maintained by glycogenolysis and gluconeogenesis (alanine, glycerol, lactate) which are stimulated by the counter-regulatory hormones: this is the central insulin resistance. The resulting hyperglycemia increases in turn glucose uptake by the non-insulin-mediated tissues (GLUT-1 and GLUT-3), a phenomenon which is accentuated by proinflammatory cytokines

17.2.2 Mechanisms of Hyperglycemia in ICU

On a theoretical point of view, stress hyperglycemia and hyperglycemia caused by diabetes (essentially type 2) appears as two different situations. Diabetes-related hyperglycemia is caused by the association of an insulin resistance and the inability of the pancreatic ß cells to secrete a sufficient amount of insulin to overcome insulin resistance, leading to a chronic high BGL. Stress hyperglycemia is induced by transient complex interactions between counter-regulatory hormones, insulin, and proinflammatory mediators (cytokines) that lead to an acute elevated BGL secondary to an activation of EGP and a peripheral insulin resistance (Fig. 17.1b) [1, 11, 12]. The severity of stress hyperglycemia is variable within time, according to the type, severity of the disease, the inflammation, and the stage of illness [13]. The divergences between the two pathophysiological patterns are probably overestimated, since the preexistence of type 2 diabetes is often overlooked and as ICU-acquired diabetes is frequent [2, 14, 15].

17.2.2.1 Increase in Glucose Production

Glucose production is increased under the influence of catecholamines and maintained by the counter-regulatory hormones and inflammatory mediators [1, 9]. The hepatic glucose production results from gluconeogenesis and in a less proportion from glycogenolysis. Gluconeogenesis is essentially activated by glucagon, as compared with epinephrine and cortisol, while glycogenolysis is initiated in the early phase by catecholamines and sustained by epinephrine and cortisol. Tumor necrosis factor-α (TNFα) might favor gluconeogenesis by stimulating the release of glucagon [11].

17.2.2.2 Insulin Resistance

Two types of insulin resistance are classically described [1, 12, 16]. Peripheral insulin resistance is characterized by the inability of skeletal muscles and adipocytes to uptake glucose. This phenomenon is the consequence of an impaired post-receptor insulin signalling and a downregulation of GLUT-4 transporters. Central insulin resistance is defined by an impaired ability of insulin to suppress hepatic EGP. This latter pathway seems to be less altered than peripheral insulin resistance during stress (Fig. 17.1b). All these modifications lead to an increased entry of glucose in insulin-mediated tissues, via a cytokine-mediated upregulation of GLUT-1. Cytokines cause a complex alteration of the post-receptor insulin signalling caused by modifications of metabolic pathways and translocation of GLUT-4.

17.3 Biochemical Rational for the Control of BGL in ICU

17.3.1 Hyperglycemia and Glucotoxicity

Glucose is commonly the preferential source of energy for different organs (brain, red blood cells, immune cells) in various conditions [9, 17]. Therefore, stress hyperglycemia has been considered for a long time as a beneficial and appropriate response in critically ill patients, allowing to deliver the adequate energy demand in tissues [18]. However, such a response is triggered by severe inflammation and neuroendocrine disorders which may cause harmful and adverse effects if prolonged and severe. Because facilitative glucose transporters GLUT-1 and GLUT-3 are upregulated during critical illness, an acute excessive entry of glucose independently of insulin saturates non-insulin-mediated tissues. This abnormal upregulation is activated by numerous factors such as proinflammatory mediators, counter-regulatory hormones, and hypoxia [14]. Various mechanisms of adverse effects of high glucose concentration have been reported [1, 10]. Alterations in mitochondrial protein and an excessive oxidative stress with a high production of reactive oxygen species (ROS) develop due to a shift of glycolysis toward usual secondary metabolic pathway (pentose phosphate, hexosamines, polyols) [17]. Acute hyperglycemia causes also lipotoxicity by increasing lipolysis and exacerbates muscle catabolism. Other consequences of this abnormal signalling are the exacerbation of cellular inflammatory pathways, decrease in complement activity, modifications of the innate immune system, endothelial and hepatic mitochondrial dysfunctions, and abolition of preconditioning and of protein glycosylation [19–22]. All these tissue derangements are responsible of organ complications and failure. Glucotoxicity exacerbates the inflammatory and oxidative stress response, creating a vicious circle.

17.3.2 Potential Beneficial Effects of Insulin

Binding of insulin to its receptor triggers an autophosphorylation which activates two major signalling pathways: the metabolic pathway activates phosphoinositol 3-kinase (PI3K) via the "insulin receptor substrate (IRS)" and the mitogenic pathway induces a cascade activation of protein kinases (MAPK) via the activation of Shc/Grb2. Some beneficial effects of insulin are attributed to the higher insulin signalling associated with a muscular GLUT-4 activation. Beside these effects on glucose metabolism, insulin greatly modifies lipid metabolism: it reduces lipolysis of adipose tissues by inhibiting lipase and adiponectin activity [23]. The resulting decrease in lipid blood concentration favors the antioxidant effect and improves the insulin sensibility by reducing the proinflammatory phenomenons. Insulin exerts also protective anabolic effects which are characterized by a higher protein synthesis and a reduction in muscular proteolysis. Moreover, due to the activation of the mitogenic pathway, it exerts non-metabolic effects: regulation of cell proliferation and apoptosis resulting from a cascade of protein phosphorylations, improvement of endothelial function due to the activation of the endothelial NO synthase (e-NOS) and an inhibition of the inducible NOS (et une inhibition de la NOS inductible), anti-inflammatory effects secondary to the blockade of the NF-kappa B pathway, and reduction of lipotoxicity [19, 23].

17.4 Hyperglycemia in ICU: A Risk Factor of Poor Outcome

Numerous observational clinical trials have shown that hyperglycemia at admission in ICU is associated with an increased risk of morbi-mortality. Most of them were initially performed in diabetic patients undergoing cardiac surgery. The large observational study of Portland begun in 1987 and included 6500 patients within 12 years

[24]. During this period, the goal for glycemic control in the perioperative period progressively changed, aiming to reach at last a target of BGL < 140 mg/dL as compared with initial BGL above 200 mg/dL. Moreover, while BGL control was only performed by subcutaneous insulin perioperatively, intravenous insulin was introduced progressively, and BGL control was sustained within the 3 postoperative days. The authors showed that a glycemia <10 mmol/L was independently associated with a lower mortality and infection rate following cardiac surgery. Based on these results, they recommended to maintain BGL < 8.3 mmol/L during surgery and within the 3 following postoperative days of cardiac surgery in diabetics [25]. Other studies have confirmed the relationship between perioperative hyperglycemia and the increased risk of death and morbidity such as stroke or infections [24, 26]. In a "before-after" trial, the implementation of a protocol for controlling BGL during and after surgery has found an improved survival rate in 300 diabetic patients [27]. A retrospective study performed in diabetic patients undergoing cardiac surgery reported that a poor glycemic control was associated with a higher occurrence of postoperative complications [28]. However, the impact of a preoperative hyperglycemia in nondiabetic patients or noncardiac surgery remains controversial [29–31]. The association of a poor outcome and preoperative hyperglycemia has been reported in a retrospective trial, regardless the diabetic status of the patients [32].

The relationship between hyperglycemia and poor outcome is also well described in medical patients with myocardial infarction [33, 34], stroke, and cerebral hemorrhage [35]. Nevertheless, the increased risk of mortality associated with a high BGL on admission remains controversial in nondiabetic brain-injured patients [36, 37]. The association between hyperglycemia and a higher morbi-mortality is also reported in various types of critically ill patients, medical and surgical [37–40] as well as trauma patients [41].

17.5 Glycemic Control in ICU: From a Tight to a Moderate Control

17.5.1 The Rational

Beneficial effects of maintaining mean BGL < 8 mmol/L were suggested by retrospective analysis of a large cohort of critically ill patients [42, 43]. However, none of these trials allows to conclude about a causality between hyperglycemia and the adverse outcomes. Therefore, hyperglycemia is considered also as a marker of illness severity and might be an appropriate metabolic response.

At the beginning of the twenty-first century, Van den Berghe et al. [3] were the first to perform a large landmark interventional randomized trial aiming to assess the impact of a TGC in critically ill surgical patients. More than 1500 patients were randomized in a group targeting normoglycemia (4.4–6.1 mmol/L/80–110 mg/dL) versus a control group targeting a conventional BGL (10–12.1 mmol/L/180–210 mg/dL). Results were very impressive as in-ICU and in-hospital mortality was significantly reduced in the TGC group as compared with the noninterventional one. The beneficial effect on survival was greater in the subgroup of patients hospitalized in ICU for more than 5 days. Moreover TGC reduced also morbidity, especially infectious episodes, acute kidney injury, anemia, polyneuropathy, and length of ventilation and of stay in ICU. These data conducted in a strong enthusiasm and rapid widespread changes in our practical management of glycemic control in ICUs.

Within the following 15 years, numerous trials tried to replicate these first findings, but all failed. The Leuven team performed a second trial using the same design in medical ICU patients [44]. The comparison between groups failed to demonstrate significant difference in hospital mortality. However, morbi-mortality was lower in the interventional subgroup of patients with an ICU length of stay of >3 days. The following large trials tried to validate these results and to determine the optimal glycemic target [4–8]. All of them were designed to compare an interventional group with a strict glycemic control (normoglycemia 4.4–6.1 mmol/L) and a control group. The target BGL in the control group differed among trials: between 10 and 11 mmol/L [4–6], between 7 and 10 mmol/L [7], or below 10 mmol/L [8]. In two monocentric randomized studies, there was no difference in mortality between the two groups [4, 5]. The VISEP study [6] focused on septic critically ill patients and failed also to demonstrate a reduction in 28- and 90-day mortality in TGC group as compared with the control group. No difference in ICU mortality was found in the large multicentric Glucontrol trial which included 1078 medicosurgical ICU patients [7]. The NICE-SUGAR international randomized study published in 2009 included more than 3000 mixed critically ill patients expected to require ICU hospitalization for at least 3 days [8]. The authors reported a higher 90-day mortality in the TGC group than in the control group. Such a difference was found regardless of the subtype of patients, i.e., surgical, medical, and those with or without diabetes. However, no difference between groups was observed concerning morbidity (length of stay, number of days with mechanical ventilation, renal replacement therapy, and 28-day mortality).

Six meta-analyses have been published [45–50] and report controversial results, probably because of various inclusion criteria. The two oldest [45, 49] conclude that short-term mortality and morbidity are lower in the TGC group. In contrast, the four most recent, which include the large NICE-SUGAR study, do not report any difference in mortality between groups [46–48, 50]. Beneficial effects of TGC could be influenced by some factors. Indeed, Griesdale et al. [47] demonstrate a possible beneficial effect of TGC only in the subgroup of surgical patients. As reported in the meta-analysis of Marik et al. [48], parenteral nutrition delivering high amounts of carbohydrates and calories might be harmful, leading to a misinterpretation of beneficial glycemic control strategy. The lack of external validity of the Leuven 1 study can be related to the local practice of administration of large amounts of intravenous glucose as parenteral nutrition, thereby requiring high doses of insulin to treat the induced hyperglycemia. Early parenteral nutrition has been later assessed by the same team against late parenteral nutrition in adults [51] and children [52] and consistently associated with adverse effects. Hence, the evaluation of the effects of TGC in the absence of early PN is urgently required.

There are few randomized studies assessing the effects of TGC during surgery. TGC versus conventional glycemic control (<10 mmol/L) was evaluated in patients (with and without diabetes) undergoing cardiac surgery. Postoperative glycemic control was similar in both groups in the postoperative period. The sole intraoperative TGC did not change the outcome of patients [53].

Based on these data, the initial enthusiasm for a widespread TGC with intensive insulin therapy in ICU moved progressively to disappointment with a moderate glycemic control [54, 55].

17.5.2 Factors Influencing the Effect of Glycemic Control

Conflicting results conducted to better understand the factors involved in the potential beneficial or deleterious effects of glycemic control. Therefore, the initial simple universal sole target of mean BGL in ICU becomes now a complex individualized and personalized range of BGL with multiple measurements. Many parameters are now considered as a source of conflicting and heterogenous results and must be taken into account in the management of glycemic control in ICU [56].

17.5.2.1 The Optimal BGL Target

Only Van den Berghe et al. [3] succeeded to compare really euglycemia (4.4–6.1 mmol/L) with hyperglycemia. All following studies failed to maintain normoglycemia in the interventional group, and only morning values were reported. Moreover from 2005, due to substantial practical changes in practices, targets for BGL were lower than 10 mmol/L. As a result, an overlap in BGL and a substantial reduction in differences in glycemia between groups were present and might explain the absence of positive results. TGC is constantly associated with an increased risk of hypoglycemia, leading to question about a counter-harmful effect. Finally, results are strongly influenced by case mix (nature and severity of diseases). In clinical practice, it appears very difficult to maintain ICU patients with euglycemia without increasing the occurrence of hypoglycemia. The global consensus now is to maintain BGL lower than 10–11 mmol/L and higher than 4.4 mmol/L to avoid deleterious effects of both excessive hyperglycemia and severe hypoglycemias. The potential benefits of TGC in critically ill patients need to be assessed against standard care when technological improvements (continuous glucose monitoring, closed-loop systems) will allow a safe and effective clamp of BGL at a predefined and individualized value [57].

17.5.2.2 Impact of Hypoglycemia

The substantial increased risk of hypoglycemic episodes makes TGC very difficult. An increased risk of 5–25% is largely reported [3, 6–8, 44, 58]. The association between severe hypoglycemia (< 2.2 mmol/L) and an elevation in mortality has been found [6, 7]. In contrast, Van den Berghe et al. [3] did not found differences between patients presenting or not hypoglycemic episodes. In the NICE-SUGAR study [8], 6.8% of patients experienced at least one episode of severe hypoglycemia (15-fold increased risk), but no long-term sequelae was observed. Despite using a computerized-assisted glucose control system, hypoglycemia has been reported to be present in 69.6% of patients versus 36.1% in the control group [59]. Regardless the study group, isolated and moderate hypoglycemias were more frequent (81% of hypoglycemia) but without any serious adverse events. Multiple (>3 episodes) and severe (<2.2 mmol/L) hypoglycemic episodes were present in 19% of patients with hypoglycemia and were associated with a higher mortality.

Nevertheless, the real impact of glycemic control-related hypoglycemia on ICU patients outcome remains questioned as the causality is not established [58–61]. Many additional markers of severity are also associated with an increased risk of hypoglycemic episodes: mechanical ventilation, renal replacement therapy, sepsis, catecholamines, brain injury, etc. [5, 60, 61]. Despite a relationship between cell necrosis and acute severe hypoglycemia, other aggravating factors might be responsible for the deleterious effects. In an experimental model, Suh et al. [57] showed that neuronal injury and death occur not really during glucose deprivation but rather during the hyperglycemic rebound caused by the exogenous administration of glucose. This phenomenon is associated with a substantial increase in ROS production. At last, in patients with acute myocardial infarction, spontaneous hypoglycemia is associated with a higher occurrence of adverse events as compared with those with "iatrogenic" insulin-related hypoglycemia [58, 63, 64].

17.5.2.3 Type of Patients

Numerous data suggest that the harmful effects of hyperglycemia depend on the type of ICU population:

- *Surgical* versus *medical patients*: Beneficial effects of glycemic control seem to be higher in surgical than in medical critically ill patients [3, 45, 47]. Reasons for that remain unclear: target BGL easily reached, less severe patients, homogenous population, better monitoring, etc. A consensus seems to be accepted for controlling glycemia in cardiac surgery [24]. In this population, BGL control must be initiated during and within the 3 days following surgery or within all days in ICU.
- *Brain-injured patients*: Stress hyperglycemia is frequent in brain-injured patients [65]. The relationship between hyperglycemia and a poor outcome in patients with stroke or traumatic brain injury (TBI) is largely reported, especially with BGL exceeding 11 mmol/L [66–68]. On the other hand, hypoglycemic episodes could worsen the neurological outcome as glucose remains an important source of energy. Vespa et al. [69] showed that a reduction in extracellular glucose concentration is frequent within the 50 h following TBI and is associated with an increased poor 6 months neurological outcome. Numerous studies using cerebral microdialysis confirmed that intensive insulinotherapy targeting BGL < 6–7 mmol/L reduces extracellular brain glucose concentration and elevates in turn the risk of insufficient glucose supply [69–74]. A concomitant increase in lactate and glutamate brain interstitial concentration with a reduction of lactate-to-pyruvate ratio suggests a cerebral metabolic crisis [74]. Several randomized trials assessing the impact of BGL control in TBI failed to demonstrate an increased risk in mortality or a worsened neurological outcome [75–79]. But

all of them were associated with a higher occurrence of hypoglycemic episodes. A recent meta-analysis including 1248 brain-injured patients does not show any beneficial impact of TGC on mortality [80]. More patients present a worsened neurological outcome when BGL is >12 mmol/L. The occurrence of hypoglycemia is higher in the interventional group, but there is large heterogeneity and no more mortality in patients presenting hypoglycemia. In summary, hyperglycemia >10–11 mmol/L worsens the neurological outcome without affecting mortality rate. "Tight" glycemic control (< 8 mmol/L) does not improve the prognosis while increasing potential hypoglycemic episodes and cerebral metabolic crisis. Therefore, the range of BGL which procures safety and efficiency is between 8 and 10 mmol/L [80, 81].

– *Diabetics* versus *non diabetics*: The deleterious impact of acute hyperglycemia seems to be lower in diabetics than in nondiabetics [39, 40, 82]. In a case-control prospective trial, non-survival diabetic patients had a longer time with BGL > 11 mmol/L as compared with those surviving [40]. BGL > 10 mmol/L is not associated with a poor outcome in a cohort of critical illness diabetics compared with those without diabetes [39]. A recent retrospective cohort trial assessed the impact of hyperglycemia in 3529 critically ill patients stratified according to the presence or not of diabetes [83]. The risk of mortality in both groups was analyzed using a logistic regression and comparing two BGL targets, moderate (90–140 mg/dL) versus TGC (80–110 mg/dL). Whether moderate or TGC strategy, diabetic patients presented higher mean BGL. But, moderate glycemic control was significantly associated with a reduction in 30-day mortality risk in diabetics (OR = 0.65), while it was increased in nondiabetic patients (OR = 1.36). In both groups, the frequency of moderate and severe hypoglycemia was higher with TGC. Such results have been recently confirmed in a retrospective analysis of prospectively collected data including 44,964 patients of 23 ICUs [84]. Results shows that mean BGL ≥ 140 mg/dL is associated with an increased risk of mortality in patients without diabetes, whereas mean BGL between 110 and 180 mg/dL is associated with a decreased risk of mortality in patients with diabetes. In a before and after study, higher BGL was associated with an improved outcome of patients with type 2 diabetes [85]. All of these results underline that acute and chronic hyperglycemia cause different response [2, 86]. A recent prospective observational study supports this hypothesis [86]. Measurements of HbA1c were performed in 1000 critically ill patients allowing to distinguish patients without preexisting diabetes (< 6.5%) from those with unrecognized diabetes (> 6.5%) and those with a well-controlled or not known diabetes. Critical illness-associated hyperglycemia is the most frequent cause of high BGL, present in near 50% of patients. Normoglycemia is present in 22.7% of patients while 22% of them present known diabetes and 5.5% unrecognized preexisting diabetes. The risk of death increases by 20% for each increase in acute glycemia of 1 mmol/L in patients with stress hyperglycemia and in those with well-controlled preexisting diabetes (HbA1c < 7%). Mechanisms by which acute and chronic hyperglycemia influences the outcome of ICU patients remain unclear. Adaptative changes at the cellular level caused by chronic high BGL are evoked: a downregulation of GLUT transporters causes a reset for relative neuroglycopenia and protects the cell from an acute and massive glucose entry (glycotoxicity) [87].

17.5.2.4 Nutrition

The management of nutrition, i.e., amount of calories, route of nutrition, and glucose delivery, varies greatly among studies [46]: parenteral nutrition of 1000 kcal/day with 200 g of carbohydrates in the Leuven study [3] versus enteral nutrition of 800 kcal/day in the NICE-SUGAR one [8]. It may be hypothesized that high glucose delivery by parenteral nutrition might cause severe hyperglycemia and that intensive insulin therapy would have induced in turn beneficial effects. In the NICE-SUGAR study, the increased mortality in the BGL control might be attributed to the very early BGL normalization leading to an inappropriate inhibition of the adaptative stress hyperglycemia [16]. A recent meta-analysis reports that beneficial effects on mortality are only present when caloric delivery is performed for at least 80% parenterally [88].

17.5.2.5 Metrics or Domains of Glycemic Control

Not only high mean BGL is associated with adverse outcome in ICU. BGL variability was rapidly demonstrated to be an independent risk factor too. Egi et al. [89] firstly reported in 7049 critically ill patients that glycemic variability (identified by the standard deviation, SD) was independently associated with a higher mortality. Numerous further studies confirmed these data [89–93]. The more glycemic variability increases, the more mortality rate increases too, especially in quartiles of mean BGL between 80 and 140 mg/dL [90–92]. Such a relationship has been recently confirmed in a large retrospective trial including more than 6000 patients with and without diabetes [94]. Results show that BG variability (SD) is associated with 30-day mortality, even after adjustment for comorbidities, severity, hypoglycemia, and presence of diabetes. This association is higher in nondiabetics than in diabetics. Several mechanisms have been evoked to explain this phenomenon [89, 93]. Less BGL variability could reflect more attention in medical and nurse care or less patient severity. Another hypothesis is that great variation in glycemia would cause real biological toxicity, especially an increased oxidative stress and apoptosis [62, 94]. Nowadays it is well established that beside BGL variability, other parameters are involved in the adverse effects of hyperglycemia [95]. All of these parameters are described as glucose “metrics” or “domains” which are classified into three types: central tendency, dispersion, and metrics of hypoglycemia. Metrics of central tendency include mean and median BGL, time-averaged BGL, and hyperglycemic index. Metrics of variability are SD, mean amplitude of glycemia, coefficient of variation, glycemic lability index, maximum glucose, etc. Metrics of hypoglycemia is the minimum value of BGL. These factors have been assessed in four ICUs [95]. The authors report that all of them (except mean and median BGL) are independently associated with a higher mortality. Moreover, even independent each from the other, the association of these three metrics increases the risk of death. Finally, such an association is different among the case mix (trauma, cardiac surgery, brain injury). Differences in the impact of metrics are confirmed according to the presence or not of diabetes [83, 96]: critically ill patients presented greater glycemic variability than those without diabetes. Nevertheless, the association between these metrics and the risk of mortality is less important in patients with than those without diabetes. A recent retrospective large trial has compared the impact of time in targeted BG range on mortality between patients with and without diabetes [97]. In agreement with previous data, results support that time in BG range between 70 and 140 mg/dL is associated with a better survival in patients without diabetes. Diabetic patients have more frequently BG out of the target range, but this is not associated with a higher risk of mortality. Moreover, more of these data demonstrate the causality between metrics and the harmful effects. One should argue that the dispersion of metrics is only a marker of severity rather than the cause of mortality.

17.5.2.6 Glucose Measurements and Protocol

Techniques for BGL measurement strongly influence glycemic values. Three parameters are essentially involved: the site of sample, devices used for measurements, and continuous or intermittent techniques. BGL can be measured using point-of-care glucose meters or blood gas analyzers. All data conclude that the accuracy of glucometers is insufficient [98–102]. Rules of accuracy required by the International Health Organization were developed for all monitoring devices at home and not for critically ill patients. Such devices may interfere with various substances (ascorbic acid, acetaminophen) or conditions (hypotension, hypothermia, anemia, acid-base disorders) [98, 99, 103, 104]. Moreover, depending on the enzyme used for measurement (glucose oxidase or glucose 1-dehydrogenase), values can be over- or underestimated.

Besides the devices, sample site must be considered [98, 99] and may be a source of error. Arterial BG concentration is higher than the venous one [100, 105]. Sampling in capillary is totally inaccurate in ICU with values being between arterial and venous ones. Moreover, many parameters frequently present in critically ill patients, such as microcirculation abnormalities, vasoconstriction (catecholamines), peripheral edema, and hypotension, cause errors in BGL values. In these situations, rapid changes in BGL require a delay to reach a constant capillary concentration [106]. Measurements with point-of-care devices are on whole blood and need to be converted to plasma values which are higher. In summary, point-of-care devices and capillary and venous samples are inaccurate in unstable critically ill patients. Such management can lead to failure to recognize abnormal BGL, especially hypoglycemia which require life-threatening treatment.

Several techniques of continuous glucose monitoring are now available for critically ill patients. The technology is based on in vitro or ex vivo (vascular or interstitial site measurements). Theoretical advantages of these techniques are to detect and treat earlier changes in BGL but above all to provide trends monitoring of BGL. Delay between measures varies between 1 and 5 min, allowing a better reporting of glucose control metrics. Holzinger et al. [107], in a randomized study, failed to demonstrate any improvement in glycemic control but found a reduction in hypoglycemic episodes. But, more randomized controlled studies comparing the beneficial impact of a continuous monitoring on the intermittent measurements are needed to recommend this technique.

Glucose control requires to implement a protocol. At least, dynamic scale protocols combining glucose target and the previous value of BGL and the insulin infusion are needed. Static protocols must be prohibited [108]. Automatic model predictive control algorithm is safe and effective [109, 110]. In a randomized controlled study, including 2684 patients, the impact of a computer decision support system has been compared with a conventional method of glycemic control [111]. The authors failed to demonstrate any differences in 90-day mortality in the computerized system group despite a lower BGL than in the control group. Moreover, more hypoglycemic episodes occurred in the interventional group, and BG variability was not different between groups.

17.6 Practical Management of Glycemic Control in ICU: Recommendations

Nowadays, glycemic control in ICU raises complexing questions. Despite growing data, there is no absolute conclusive evidence, and many questions remain unanswered. Hyperglycemia and hypoglycemia are probably harmful, but unblinded studies cannot confirm totally that and will not be performed in the future. Moreover, the precise range in which glycemia fails to be protective and becomes harmful is not known. A sole universal target of mean BGL in all patients is too simple and not the right goal to improve the outcome of ICU patients. The management of glycemic control becomes more and more complex and requires to take into account various parameters: the metrics of BGL, the type of patients, and the prevention of repeated and severe hypoglycemic episodes. The general consensus is first to avoid both harmful excessive hyperglycemia by maintaining BGL < 10 mmol/L and severe hypoglycemia (<2.2 mmol/L). Most experts recommend an "intermediate or moderate glycemic control" targeting a range of mean BGL between 7.8 and 10 mmol/L in nondiabetic and well-controlled known diabetic critically ill patients [2, 55, 56, 80, 99]. In poor-controlled diabetic patients (HbA1c > 7%), a higher range of BGL seems more appropriate (up to 11 mmol/L) is acceptable. In brain-injured patients, it is strongly suggested to favor intermediate BGL in order to prevent hypoglycemic episodes and monitor BGL tightly [80]. Methods for glycemic measurements concerning the site samples and the devices as well as appropriate markers of glucose control are described by experts [55, 99]. Most important messages are that: (1) samples should be drawn from an arterial line in patients equipped with an indwelling arterial catheter, and if not possible from venous sampling, capillary samples should be avoided; (2) capillary samples are authorized in non-severe patients; (3) the reference method for BGL measurement on arterial or venous blood is the central laboratory, and blood gas analyzer can be used if delays with the laboratory are too long; (4) in not severe patients, measurements on capillary samples can be performed on glucometers; (5) each team must know the characteristics of their devices and above all the limitations for accurate measurements (interferences). Finally, each team must adapt to its glycemic control protocol taking into account its population, its target BGL, its devices for BGL measurements, and its system for performing glycemic control (computerized or noncomputerized dynamic protocol). A large French audit has reported that 80% of ICUs had implemented a protocol in 2009 and that mean BGL was maintained in the current intermediate recommended BGL [112]. The incidence of hypoglycemia was low. However, data were collected only on 1 day, and other metrics than mean BGL were not collected.

Conclusion

Harmful effects of excessive hyperglycemia are well accepted in critically ill patients. Following the first enthusiasm following the Leuven study, several studies tried to confirm these results but failed. None succeed really to compare different groups as glycemic overlap. Despite these disappointed results, the story of glycemic control continues and becomes more complex. Controversial data help us to improve our knowledge concerning the impact of glucose disorders in critically ill patients. The sole goal of controlling mean blood glucose level is insufficient, and beneficial effects of glycemic control must take into account other metrics of glucose control such as BGL variability, time in the target, occurrence of hypoglycemia, etc. The type of patients and their severity also influences the impact of such a strategy. Therefore, the precise optimal BGL is unknown and probably not universal. Nowadays, it seems reasonable to recommend a moderate glycemic control, aiming to maintain BGL between 7.8 and 10 mmol/L which represents the best deal for efficiency and safety.

Acknowledgments No conflict of interest.

References

1. Dungan KM, Braithwaite SS, Preiser JC (2009) Stress hyperglycaemia. Lancet 373:1798–1807
2. Marik PE, Egi M (2014) Treatment thresholds for hyperglycemia in critically ill patients with and without diabetes. Intensive Care Med 40:1049–1051
3. Van den Berghe G, Wouters P, Weekers F et al (2001) Intensive insulin therapy in critically ill patients. N Engl J Med 345:1359–1367
4. Arabi YM, Dabbagh OC, Tamim HM et al (2008) Intensive versus conventional insulin therapy: a randomized controlled trial in medical and surgical critically ill patients. Crit Care Med 36:3190–3197
5. De la Rosa GC, Donado JH, Restrepo AH et al (2008) Strict glycemic control in patients hospitalized in a mixed medical and surgical intensive care unit: a randomized clinical trial. Crit Care 12:R120
6. Brunkhorst FM, Engel C, Bloos F et al (2008) Intensive insulin therapy and Pentastarch resuscitation in severe sepsis. N Engl J Med 358:125–139
7. Preiser JC, Devos P, Ruiz-Santana S et al (2009) A prospective randomised multi-centre controlled trial on tight glucose control by intensive insulin therapy in adult intensive care units: the Glucontrol study. Intensive Care Med 35:1738–1748
8. The NICE-SUGAR Study Investigators, Finfer S, Chittock DR, Su SY et al (2009) Intensive versus conventional glucose control in critically ill patients. N Engl J Med 360:1283–1297

9. Von Cromphaut SJ (2009) Hyperglycemia as a part of the stress response: the underlying mechanisms. Best Pract Clin Anaesth 23:375–386
10. Scheepers A, Joost HG, Schürmann A (2004) The glucose transporter families SGLT and GLUT: molecular basis of normal and aberrant function. J Parenter Enter Nutr 28:365–374
11. Petersen KF, Shulman GI (2006) Etiology of insulin resistance. Am J Med 119(Suppl 1):S10–S16
12. Bagry HS, Raghavendran S, Carli F (2008) Metabolic syndrome and insulin resistance: perioperative considerations. Anesthesiology 108:506–523
13. Zauner A, Nimmerichter P, Anderwald C et al (2007) Severity of insulin resistance in critically ill medical patients. Metabolism 56:1–5
14. Preiser JC, de Longueville C (2017) Could type 2 diabetes be a component of the post-intensive care syndrome? Crit Care 21:26
15. Abdelhamid AY, Kar P, Finnis ME et al (2016) Stress hyperglycaemia in critically ill patients and the subsequent risk of diabetes: a systematic review and meta-analysis. Crit Care 20:301
16. Lena D, Kalfon P, Preiser JC, Ichai C (2011) Glycemic control in the intensive care unit and during the postoperative period. Anesthesiology 114:438–444
17. Leverve X (2003) Hyperglycemia and oxidative stress: complex relationships with attractive prospects. Intensive Care Med 29:511–514
18. Marik PE, Bellomo R (2013) Stress hyperglycemia: an essential survival response! Crit Care 17:305
19. Vanhorebeek I, Langouche L (2009) Molecular mechanisms behind clinical benefits of intensive insulin therapy during critical illness: glucose versus insulin. Best Pract Res Clin Anaesth 23:449–459
20. Turina M, Fry DE, Polk HC Jr (2005) Acute hyperglycemia and the innate immune system. Crit Care Med 33:1624–1633
21. Vanhorebeek I, De Vos R, Mesotten D, Wouters PJ, De Wolf-Peeters C, Van den Berghe G (2005) Protection of hepatocyte mitochondrial ultrastructure and function by strict blood glucose control with insulin in critically ill patients. Lancet 365:53–59
22. Vanhorebeek I, Ellger B, De Vos R et al (2009) Tissue-specific glucose toxicity induces mitochondrial damage in a burn injury model of critical illness. Crit Care Med 37:1355–1364
23. Avromaglu RK, Basciano H, Adeli K (2006) Lipid and lipoprotein dysregulation in insulin resistant states. Clin Chim Acta 368:1–19
24. Furnary AP, Wu Y (2006) Eliminating the diabetic disadvantage: the Portland diabetic project. Semin Thorac Cardiovasc Surg 18:302–308
25. Lazar HL, McDonnell M, Chipkin SR et al (2009) The society of thoracic surgeons practice guideline series: blood glucose management during adult cardiac surgery. Ann Thorac Surg 87:663–669
26. Doenst T, Wijeysundera D et al (2005) Hyperglycemia during cardiopulmonary bypass is an independent risk factor for mortality in patients undergoing cardiac surgery. J Thor Cardiovasc Surg 130:1144–1149
27. D'Alessandro C, Leprince P, Golmard JL et al (2007) Strict glycemic control reduces EuroSCORE expected mortality in diabetic patients undergoing myocardial revascularization. J Thorac Cardiovasc Surg 134:29–37
28. Ouattara A, Lecomte P, Le Manach Y et al (2005) Poor intraoperative blood glucose control is associated with a worsened hospital outcome after cardiac surgery in diabetic patients. Anesthesiology 103:687–694
29. Butterworth J, Wagenknecht LE, Legault C et al (2005) Attempted control of hyperglycemia during cardiopulmonary bypass fails to improve neurologic and neurobehavioral outcomes in patients without diabetes mellitus undergoing coronary artery bypass grafting. J Cardiovasc Surg 130:1319–1325
30. Malmstedt J, Wahlberg E, Jorneskog G, Swedenborg J (2006) Influence of perioperative blood glucose levels on outcome after infrainguinal bypass surgery in patients with diabetes. Br J Surg 93:1360–1367

31. Vriesendorp TM, DeVries JH, Hulscher JBF, Holleman F, van Lanschot JJ, Hoekstra JBL (2004) Early postoperative hyperglycaemia is not a risk factor for infectious complications and prolonged in-hospital stay in patients undergoing oesophagectomy: a retrospective analysis of prospective trial. Crit Care 8:R437–R442
32. Falciglia M, Freyberg RW, Almenoff PL, D'Alessio DA, Render ML (2009) Hyperglycemia-related mortality in critically ill patients varies with admission diagnosis. Crit Care Med 37:3001–3009
33. Worthley MI, Shrive FM, Anderson TJ, Traboulsi M (2007) Prognostic implication of hyperglycemia in myocardial infarction and primary angioplasty. Am J Med 120(643):e1–e7
34. Petursson P, Herlitz J, Caidahl K et al (2007) Admission glycaemia and outcome after acute coronary syndrome. Int J Cardiol 116:315–320
35. Stöllberger C, Exner I, Finsterer J, Slany J, Steger C (2005) Stroke in diabetic and non-diabetic patients: course and prognostic value of admission serum glucose. Ann Med 37:357–364
36. Capes SE, Hunt D, Malmberg K, Pathak P, Gerstein HC (2001) Stress hyperglycaemia and prognosis of stroke in nondiabetic and diabetic patients: a systematic overview. Stroke 32:2426–2432
37. Freire AX, Bridges L, Umpierrez GE, Kuhl D, Kitabchi AE (2005) Admission hyperglycemia and other risk factors as predictors of hospital mortality in a medical ICU population. Chest 128:3109–3116
38. Whitcomb BW, Pradhan EK, Pittas AG, Roghmann MC, Perencevich EN (2005) Impact of admission hyperglycemia on hospital mortality in various intensive care unit populations. Crit Care Med 33:2772–2777
39. Egi M, Bellomo R, Stachowski E et al (2008) Blood glucose concentration and outcome of critical illness: the impact of diabetes. Crit Care Med 36:2249–2255
40. Rady MY, Johnson DJ, Patel BM, Larson JS, Helmers RA (2005) Influence of individual characteristics on outcome of glycemic control in intensive care unit patients with or without diabetes mellitus. Mayo Clin Proc 80:1558–1567
41. Wahl WL, Taddonio M, Maggio PM, Arbabi S, Hemmila MR (2008) Mean glucose values predict trauma patient mortality. J Trauma 65:42–47
42. Krinsley JS (2004) Effect of an intensive glucose management protocol on the mortality of critically ill adult patients. Mayo Clin Proc 79:992–1000
43. Krinsley JS (2006) Glycemic control, diabetic status, and mortality in a heterogenous population of critically ill patients before and during the era of intensive glycemic management six and one-half years experience at a university-affiliated community hospital. Semin Thorac Cardiovasc Surg 18:317–325
44. Van den Berghe G, Wilmer A, Hermans G et al (2006) Intensive insulin therapy in the medical ICU. N Engl J Med 354:449–461
45. Pittas AG, Siegel RD, Lau J (2006) Insulin therapy and in-hospital mortality in critically ill patients: systematic review and meta-analysis of randomized controlled trials. J Parenter Enter Nutr 30:164–172
46. Wiener RS, Wiener DC, Larson RJ (2008) Benefits and risks of tight glucose control in critically ill adults. A meta-analysis JAMA 300:933–944
47. Griesdale DEG, de Souza RJ, van Dam RM et al (2009) Intensive insulin therapy and mortality among critically ill patients: a meta-analysis including NICE-SUGAR study data. CMAJ 180:821–827
48. Marik PE, Preiser JC (2010) Toward understanding tight glycaemic control in the ICU: a systematic review and metaanalysis. Chest 137:544–551
49. Ghandhi GY, Murad MH, Flynn DN et al (2008) Effect of perioperative insulin infusion on surgical morbidity and mortality: systematic review and meta-analysis of randomized trials. Mayo Clin Proc 83:418–430
50. Yamada T, Shojima N, Noma H, Yamauchi T, Kadowaki T (2017) Glycemic control, mortality, and hypoglycemia in critically ill patients: a systematic review and network meta-analysis of randomized controlled trials. Intensive Care Med 43:1–15
51. Fivez T, Kerklaan D, Mesotten D et al (2016) Early versus late parenteral nutrition in critically ill children. N Engl J Med 374:1111–1122

52. Casaer MP, Mesotten D, Hermans G et al (2011) Early versus late parenteral nutrition in critically ill adults. N Engl J Med 365:506–517
53. Ghandi GY, Nuttall GA, Abel MD et al (2007) Intensive intraoperative insulin therapy versus conventional glucose management during cardiac surgery. Ann Intern Med 146:233–243
54. Mesotten D, Preiser JC, Kosiborod M (2015) Glucose management in critically ill adults and children. Lancet Diabetes Endocrinol 3:723–733
55. Ichai C, Preiser JC, for the Sfar, Srlf and expert panel (2010) International recommendations for glucose control in adult non diabetic critically ill patients. Crit Care 14:R166
56. Preiser JC, Devos P, Chioléro R (2010) Which factors influence glycemic control in the ICU? Curr Opin Clin Nutr Metab Care 13:205–210
57. Preiser JC, Chase JG, Hovorka R et al (2016) Glucose control in the ICU: a continuing story. J Diabetes Sci Technol 10:1372–1381
58. Krinsley JS, Grover A (2007) Severe hypoglycemia in critically ill patients: risk factors and outcomes. Crit Care Med 35:2262–2267
59. Kalfon P, Le Manach Y, Ichai C et al (2015) Severe and multiple hypoglycemic episodes are associated with increased risk of death in ICU patients. Crit Care 19:153
60. Vriesendorp TM, DeVries JH, van Santen S et al (2006) Evaluation of short-term consequences of hypoglycemia in an intensive care unit. Crit Care Med 34:2714–2718
61. Arabi YM, Tamim HM, Rishu A (2009) Hypoglycemia with intensive insulin therapy in critically ill patients: predisposing factors and association with mortality. Crit Care Med 37:2536–2544
62. Suh SW, Gum ET, Hamby AM, Chan PH, Swanson RA (2007) Hypoglycemic neuronal death is triggered by glucose reperfusion and activation of neuronal NADPH oxidase. J Clin Invest 117:910–918
63. Kosiborod M, Inzucchi SE, Goyal A et al (2009) Relationship between spontaneous and iatrogenic hypoglycemia and mortality in patients hospitalized with acute myocardial infarction. JAMA 301:1556–1564
64. Di Muzio F, Presello B, Glassford NJ et al (2016) Liberal versus conventional glucose targets in critically ill diabetic patients: an exploratory safety cohort assessment. Crit Care Med 44:1683–1691
65. Sonneville R, Vanhorebeek I, den Hertog HM et al (2015) Critical illness-induced dysglycemia and the brain. Intensive Care Med 41:192–202
66. Liu-DeRyke X, Collingridge DS, Orme J, Roller D, Zurasky J, Rohney DH (2009) Clinical impact of early hyperglycemia during acute phase of traumatic brain injury. Neurocrit Care 11:151–157
67. Jeremitsky E, Omert LA, Dunham CM, Wilberger J, Rodriguez A (2005) The impact of hyperglycemia on patients with severe brain injury. J Trauma 58:47–50
68. Griesdale DE, Tremblay MH, McEwen J, Chittock DR (2009) Glucose control and mortality in patients with severe traumatic brain injury. Neurocrit Care 11:311–316
69. Vespa P, McArthur D, O'Phelan K, Glenn T et al (2003) Persistently low extracellular glucose correlates with poor outcome 6 months after human traumatic brain injury despite a lack of increased lactate: a microdialysis study. J Cereb Blood Flow Metab 23:865–877
70. Vespa P, Boonyaputthikul R, McArthur DL et al (2006) Intensive insulin therapy reduces microdialysis glucose values without altering glucose utilization or improving the lactate/pyruvate ratio after traumatic brain injury. Crit Care Med 34:850–856
71. Oddo M, Schmidt JM, Carrera E et al (2008) Impact of tight glycemic control on cerebral glucose metabolism after severe brain injury: a microdialysis study. Crit Care Med 36:3233–3238
72. Meierhans R, Bechir M, Ludwig S et al (2010) Brain metabolism is significantly impaired at blood glucose below 6 mM and brain glucose below 1 mM in patients with severe traumatic brain injury. Crit Care 14:R13
73. Oddo M, Schmidt JM, Mayer SA, Chiolero RL (2008) Glucose control after severe brain injury. Curr Opin Clin Nutr Metab Care 11:134–139
74. Vespa P, McArthur DL, Stein N et al (2012) Tight glycemic control increases metabolic distress in traumatic brain injury: a randomized controlled within-subjects trial. Crit Care Med 40:1923–1929

75. Bilotta F, Caramia R, Paoloni FP, Delfini R, Rosa G (2009) Safety and efficacy of intensive insulin therapy in critical neurosurgical patients. Anesthesiology 110:611–619
76. Bilotta F, Caramia R, Cernak I et al (2008) Intensive insulin therapy after severe traumatic brain injury: a randomized clinical trial. Neurocrit Care 9:159–166
77. Coester A, Neumann CR, Schmidt MI (2010) Intensive insulin therapy in severe traumatic brain injury: a randomized trial. J Trauma 68:904–911
78. Nice-Sugar Study Investigators for the Australian New Zealand Intensive Care Society Clinical Trials Group, the Canadian Critical Care Trials Group, Finfer S, Chittock D, Li Y et al (2015) Intensive versus conventional glucose control in critically ill patients with traumatic brain injury: long-term follow-up of a subgroup of patients from the NICE-SUGAR study. Intensive Care Med 41:1037–1047
79. Cinotti R, Ichai C, Orban JC et al (2014) Effects of tight computerized glucose control on neurological outcome in severely brain injured patients: a multicenter sub-group analysis of the randomized-controlled open-label CGAO-REA study. Crit Care 18:498
80. Kramer AH, Roberts D, Zygun DA (2012) Optimal glycemic control in neurocritical care patients: a systematic review and meta-analysis. Crit Care 16:R203
81. Billota F, Rosa G (2012) Optimal glycemic control in neurocritical care. Crit Care 16:163
82. Van den Berghe G, Wilmer W, Milants I et al (2006) Intensive insulin therapy in mixed medical/surgical intensive care units: benefit versus harm. Diabetes 55:3151–3159
83. Lanspa MJ, Hirshberg EL, Phillips GD, Holmen J, Stoddard G, Orme J (2013) Moderate glucose control is associated with increased mortality compared with tight glucose control in critically ill patients without diabetes. Chest 143:1226–1234
84. Krinsley JS, Egi M, Devendra AN et al (2013) Diabetic status and the relation of the three domains of glycemic control to mortality in critically ill patients: an international multicenter cohort study. Crit Care 17:R37
85. Plummer MP, Bellomo R, Cousins CE et al (2014) Dysglycaemia in the critically ill and the interaction of chronic and acute glycaemia with mortality. Intensive Care Med 40:973–980
86. Schlenk F, Graetz D, Nagel A, Schmidt M, Sarrafzdeh AS (2008) Insulin-related decrease in cerebral glucose despite normoglycemia in aneurysmal subarachnoid hemorrhage. Crit Care 12:R9
87. Krinsley JS, Preiser JC, Hirsch IB (2017) Safety and efficacy of personalized glycemic control in critically ill patients: a 2-year before and after interventional trial. Endocr Pract 23:318–330
88. Singer P, Berger MM, Van den Berghe G et al (2009) ESPEN guidelines on parenteral nutrition: intensive care. Clin Nutr 28:387–400
89. Egi M, Bellomo R, Stachowski E, French CJ, Hart G (2006) Variability of blood glucose concentration and short-term mortality in critically ill patients. Anesthesiology 105:244–252
90. Krinsley JS (2008) Glycemic variability: a strong independent predictor of mortality in critically ill patients. Crit Care Med 36:3008–3013
91. Ali NA, O'Brien JM, Dungan K et al (2008) Glucose variability and mortality in patients with sepsis. Crit Care Med 36:2316–2321
92. Dossett LA, Cao H, Mowery NT, Dortch MJ, Morris JM, May AK (2008) Blood glucose variability is associated with mortality in the surgical intensive care unit. Ann Surg 74:679–685
93. Egi M, Bellomo R (2009) Reducing glycemic variability in intensive care unit patients: a new therapeutic target? J Diabetes Sci Technol 3:1302–1308
94. Monnier L, Mas E, Ginet C et al (2006) Activation of oxidative stress by acute glucose fluctuations compared with sustained chronic hyperglycemia in patients with type 2 diabetes. JAMA 295:1681–1687
95. Mackenzie IMJ, Whitehouse T, Nightingale PG (2011) The metrics of glycaemic control in critical care. Intensive Care Med 37:435–443
96. Lanspa MJ, Dickerson J, Morris AH, Orme JF, Holmen J, Hirshbergb E (2014) Coefficient of glucose variation is independently associated with mortality in critically ill patients receiving intravenous insulin. Crit Care 18:R86

97. Krinsley JS, Preiser JC (2015) Time in blood glucose range 70 to 140 mg/dl > 80% is strongly associated with increased survival in non-diabetic critically ill adults. Crit Care 19:179
98. Rebel A, Rice MA, Fahy BG (2012) The accuracy of point-of-care glucose measurements. J Diabetes Sci Technol 6:396–411
99. Finfer S, Wernerman J, Preiser JC et al (2013) Clinical review: consensus recommendations on measurement of blood glucose and reporting glycemic control in critically ill adults. Crit Care 17:229
100. Kanji S, Buffie J, Hutton B et al (2005) Reliability of point-of-care testing for glucose measurement in critically ill adults. Crit Care Med 33:2778–2785
101. Hoedemaekers CW, Klein Gunnewiek JM, Prinsen MA, Willems JL, Hoeven JG (2008) Accuracy of bedside glucose measurement from three glucometers in critically ill patients. Crit Care Med 36:3062–3066
102. Vlasselaers D, Van Herpe T, Milants I et al (2008) Blood glucose measurements in arterial blood of intensive care unit patients submitted to tight glycemic control: agreement between bedside tests. J Diabetes Sci Technol 2:932–938
103. Dungan K, Chapman J, Braithwaithe SS, Buse J (2007) Glucose measurement: confounding issues in setting targets for inpatients management. Diabetes Care 30:403–409
104. D'Orazio P, Burnett RW, Fogh-Andersen N et al (2006) Approved IFCC recommendation on reporting results for blood glucose: International Federation of Clinical Chemistry and Laboratory Medicine Scientific Division, working group on selective electrodes and point-of-care testing (IFCC-SD-SEPOCT). Clin Chem Lab Med 44:1486–1490
105. Pereira AJ, Corrêa TD, Preira de Almeida F et al (2015) Inaccuracy of venous point-of-care glucose measurements in critically ill patients: a cross-sectional study. PLoS One 10:e129568
106. Desachy A, Vuagnat AC, Ghazali AD et al (2008) Accuracy of bedside glucometry in critically ill patients: influence of clinical characteristics and perfusion index. Mayo Clin Proc 83:400–405
107. Holzinger U, Warszawska J, Kitzberger R et al (2010) Real-time continuous glucose monitoring in critically ill patients. Diabetes Care 33:467–472
108. Meijering S, Corstjens AM, Tulleken JA, Meertens JHJM, Zijlstra JG, Ligtenberg JJM (2006) Towards a feasible algorithm for tight glycaemic control in critically ill patients: a systematic review of the literature. Crit Care 10:R19
109. Plank J, Blaha J, Cordingley J et al (2006) Multicentric, randomized, controlled trial to evaluate blood glucose control by the model predictive control algorithm versus routine glucose managements protocols in intensive care unit. Diabetes Care 20:271–276
110. Cordingley JJ, Vlasselaers DV, Dormand NC et al (2009) Intensive insulin therapy: enhanced model predictive control algorithm versus standard care. Intensive Care Med 35:123–128
111. Kalfon P, Giraudeau B, Ichai C et al (2014) Tight computerized versus conventional glucose control in the ICU: a randomized controlled trial. Intensive Care Med 40:171–181
112. Orban JC, Scarlatti A, Lefrant JY et al (2013) Management of glycemia: an audit in 66 ICUs. Ann Fr Anesth Réanim 32:84–88

Part VI

Energetic Metabolism, Nutrition

18 Nutritional Requirements in Intensive Care Unit

Marie-Pier Bachand, Xavier Hébuterne, and Stéphane M. Schneider

18.1 Introduction

Energy requirements are the amount of macro- and micronutrients needed to balance energy expenditure in order to maintain reserve, good metabolic, and physiologic functions. Nutritional support in the intensive care unit (ICU) is a challenge. The critically ill patients exhibit hypermetabolism, proteolysis with nitrogen loss and accelerated gluconeogenesis and glucose utilization [1]. The degree of metabolic response to aggression depends on the extent and severity of insult and is mediated through the release of cytokines and counterregulatory hormones like tumor necrosis factor, interleukins 1 and 6, catecholamines, glucagon, and cortisol. There are also many other endocrine modifications induced by stress in ICU, like insulin resistance and reduced thyroid and sex hormones secretion (see chapter x). Many factors influence metabolic needs during acute illness such as mechanical ventilation and the administration of vasoactive or sedative agents. Nutritional needs depend also on the disease, severity of illness, nutritional state before ICU, and comorbidities of the patient. Metabolism and energy needs of the critically ill

M.-P. Bachand • X. Hébuterne • S.M. Schneider (✉)
Gastroentérologie et Nutrition Clinique, Centre Hospitalier Universitaire de Nice, 151 route de Saint-Antoine, 06200 Nice, France

Faculté de Médecine, Université de Nice Sophia-Antipolis, Université Côte d'Azur, 29 avenue de Valombrose, 06100 Nice, France
e-mail: stephane.schneider@unice.fr

C. Ichai et al. (eds.), *Metabolic Disorders and Critically Ill Patients*,
http://doi.org/10.1007/978-3-319-64010-5_18

patients seem to be dynamic, changing through the continuum of the ICU stay [2]. Like Griffiths of Liverpool [3] said, *failure to give adequate oxygen to the critically ill would universally be considered unacceptable practice (...) similarly, a failure to provide food to a captive would elicit international condemnation (...) Why, then, does the provision and delivery of nutrition receive such a low profile in the ICU?* The difficulty to assess nutritional needs in critically ill patients may be the answer.

18.2 Energy Needs

For most critically ill patients, protein requirements are higher than normal. Loss of total body protein is inevitable in the first days of ICU, even with an aggressive nutritional approach, primarily due to the catabolism of muscle. On the other hand, over- and underfeeding are both noxious. Thus, it is important to clearly identify the goals of nutrition, as determined by energy requirements. The goals of nutrition support in ICU are to minimize weight loss (especially loss of lean body mass), provide nutrients to support the immune system, and obtain positive or balanced nitrogen balance. Nutrition support won't stop initial catabolism but will minimize it to allow optimal chance of maintaining muscle function. This allows patients to attain physical function and quality of life in the recovery phase. Also, the increased metabolic needs related to stress are likely to accelerate the development of malnutrition. Indeed, nutritional support in ICU has to be able to restore the nutrient deficit in malnourished patient.

18.2.1 Therapeutic Index of Energy Provision

Determining energy needs in critically ill patients is quite challenging, but underestimation and overestimation of daily energy expenditure may result in adverse outcomes [4]. The target of energy requirements has evolved in these past few years, from 40 to 25 kcal/kg/day. The last ESPEN (European Society for Clinical Nutrition and Metabolism) [5, 6] guidelines date from 2009. In 2014, guidelines by French-speaking societies: SFAR (Société Française d'Anesthésie-Réanimation), SFNEP (Société Francophone Nutrition Clinique Métabolisme), and SRLF (Société de Réanimation de Langue Française) were released [7]. Finally, in 2015, new guidelines from ASPEN (American Society for Parenteral and Enteral Nutrition) and SCCM (Society of Critical Care Medicine) were also released [8]. Current guidelines detail the optimal delivery of nutritional support and recommend specific energy and protein needs. Yet, no published data have validated these standard daily caloric intake targets. Although there is general consensus that excessive hypocaloric (< 25% recommended daily caloric intake) or hypercaloric (>125%) feeding should be avoided, controversy still exists over what feeding targets should be [9]. Some authors claim for hypocaloric feeding, although we still don't know much about the consequences of it today ([10] and [11]).

18.2.1.1 Risks of Underfeeding

A high number of acutely ill patients (30–50%) are in a malnourished state [12]. The prevalence can be as high as 45% for chronic respiratory diseases [13]. Obese people are also at risk of malnutrition in and out of the ICU; indeed, a recent study showed that sarcopenia and sarcopenic obesity were prevalent in the ICU (56% and 24% of patients, respectively, between CT imaging and SGA assessment). Misclassified individuals in ICU were predominantly male, minority, and overweight or obese patients [14]. Malnutrition can be difficult to assess in critically ill patients because traditional nutrition assessment tools (albumin, transthyretin, and anthropometry) are not validated in the ICU [8]. Also, only 50% of critically ill patients meet their caloric and protein goals on the third day of ICU stay, a percentage that decreased to 30% at day 7 [15]. Recent data reveal a 6-month mortality rate of 40% after ICU discharge for sepsis admission. Many of these deaths are believed to occur indirectly as a consequence of hypercatabolism, loss of lean body mass during ICU, lack of adequate physical activity, and, ultimately, weakness and inability to mobilize [12]. Moreover, contrary to simple lack of intake, aggression induces the most accelerated breakdown of body protein reserve causing faster malnutrition [16]. Indeed, a patient's nutritional status often becomes significantly more compromised during their ICU stay [12].

For critically ill patients, there are clear evidences that energy and protein intake are significantly associated with outcomes [17]. Impact of early enteral nutrition (EN) on patient outcome is a dose-dependent effect [8]. Indeed, the first goal of nutritional support is to obtain nitrogen equilibrium or, ideally, positive nitrogen balance to aid healing and restore lean body mass. If nutritional needs are not covered, the patient will use its own protein stores, including muscle amino acids for gluconeogenesis. Underfeeding in the ICU may therefore lead to malnutrition, muscle weakness, and impaired immunity. Despite recommendations for early EN in critically ill patients [6], in practice there is a disparity between prescribed calories supply and delivered calories [18]. This reflects many factors including cautious decision-making in the early phases of stress, absence of protocols in many ICUs, interruption of nutrition for digestive complications, investigations, large gastric aspirates, patient transfer, physical therapy, airway management, and prolonged fasting for procedures [6, 15, 19]. All pose challenges and may induce energy deficit, especially with EN. Many studies have shown that this deficit can reach 400–800 kcal per day, and there is a correlation with the rate of opportunistic infections, multi-organ failure, surgery, bedsores, longer length of stay, and mechanical ventilation days [20, 21]. This energy deficit carries short- and long-term consequences, such as a worse prognosis and more infectious complications. Moreover, a retrospective study of 295 ICU patients showed a mortality rate of 2.43 in patients receiving less than 60% of energy requirements during the first week [22]. Also, a prospective study done on 61 medical ICU patients who received EN for at least 7 days showed that the quantity of nutrition administered was 86 ± 30% of the quantity prescribed [23]. The patients in whom goals were not achieved during the first 4 days had a higher mortality rate than the other group who achieved the nutritional goals (73.3 vs. 26.1%; $p = 0.002$). In an observational study with 2772 ICU patients, the odds ratio for 60-day mortality was 0.76 (0.61–0.95) for each 1000 kcal supply and 0.84 (0.74–0.96) for each 30 g of protein supply. This benefit only concerned patients with BMI under 25 or over 40 [17]. A study on well-nourished patients showed a higher morbidity and mortality with these energy goals [24]; these results parallel the ones of the famous Veterans Administration study that showed parenteral nutrition (PN) was deleterious in non-malnourished patients (perioperative total parenteral nutrition in surgical patients [25]). Overall, before studies in favor of permissive underfeeding, ESPEN guidelines recommend that "All patients receiving less than their targeted enteral feeding after 2 days should be considered for supplementary PN" [6].

18.2.1.2 Risks of Overfeeding

Overfeeding in the ICU has been associated with increased carbon dioxide production, respiratory failure, hyperglycemia, and fat deposits in the liver. Fat accumulation also increases the production of tumor necrosis factor (TNF) and other pro-inflammatory cytokines. Excess carbohydrates induce hyperglycemia that is difficult to control with insulin therapy, and increased CO_2 production may exacerbate gaseous exchange of patients in acute respiratory distress syndrome (ARDS) if overfed (see nutritional support in specific critical illnesses). Glucose-based PN increases CO_2 production by 15% [6]. Hypertriglyceridemia exaggerates intrapulmonary shunt and hemostasis disorders in ARDS. Also, it has immunosuppressive effects; it impairs the reticuloendothelial system and increases opportunistic infections. Energy excess causes fat mass inflation with cardiac and respiratory consequences [26], longer mechanical ventilation time, and metabolic acidosis. Carbohydrate and lipid excess induce a higher thermogenesis and are the cause of liver dysfunctions on PN. An American multicentric study in 1998 has demonstrated that 32.2–92.8% of patients were overfed in ICU [27].

18.2.2 Quantitative Requirements

In a normal state, energy supply must cover total energy expenditure, which is made of resting energy expenditure (REE), diet-induced thermogenesis, and physical activity expenditure (mobilization for position changes and respiratory physiotherapy) [28]. Resting energy expenditure (REE) is defined as the amount of energy required by the body at rest during a 24-h period and represents 60–80% of calories used by the body. The metabolic response of critically ill patients is characterized by an increase in REE. However, the lack of physical activity in ICU patients explains why some of them are not hypermetabolic [29]. A precise evaluation of energy needs in these patients is essential in order to avoid underfeeding and overfeeding, as well as to avoid loss of lean body mass and worsening of any existing nutrients deficiencies. Three methods to determine energy requirements exist: indirect calorimetry, weight-based predictive equations (25 kcal/kg/day), or published predictive equations [6].

18.2.2.1 Indirect Calorimetry

The most accurate method to determine calories requirements is to measure REE with indirect calorimetry. This method is based on the principle that REE is proportional to O_2 consumption and CO_2 production and the proportion of fuels being utilized is reflected in their ratio, the respiratory quotient (RQ). The RQ provides information on substrate utilization. It is a 20-min test that requires trained personal [2]. In ICU patients, indirect calorimetry is not always accurate in situations preventing complete collection of expired gases, such as air leaks from the ventilator circuit and around endotracheal tubes and CO_2 loss across hemodialysis membranes. High settings on ventilation, including inspiratory fraction of oxygen (FiO_2) above 0.6 may result in false measurements of REE with old instruments [20]. New instruments have to be carefully chosen for mechanically ventilated patients [30]. Also, agitated and hemodynamically unstable patients will have inaccurate measurements. Therefore, this technique has to be done with small continuous quantities of nutrients, outside mobilization time, ventilation change, and fever [28]. Other than for research, indirect calorimetry is interesting in the recovery phase of the patient who has spent more than 10 days in the ICU. It is also useful at extreme ages or weights. Studies that analyzed REE in critically ill patients revealed a great disparity, from 1382 ± 130 to 2236 ± 140 kcal/day [31] (Table 18.1).

Although many nutritional experts favor indirect calorimetry for determining REE in critically ill patients, no study has yet proven that it should be adopted as a

Table 18.1 Factors affecting energy expenditure [31]

Patient related
Diagnosis
Metabolic disorder
Sepsis
Organ failure
Comorbidity (obesity, diabetes, heart, lung disease, etc.)
State of consciousness
Nutritional status
Food intake
Body temperature
Respiratory frequency
Treatment related
Medications (sedative, analgesics, etc.)
Ventilator
Surgery
Investigations and treatment (hemofiltration, etc.)
Mobilization (active or passive)
Ambient temperature
Measurement related
Time to aggression
Duration of the measurement (after equilibration)
Time of day
Fraction of inspired oxygen (FiO_2)
Air leak on the system

standard. Recently, TICACOS (tight calorie control study), a prospective, randomized controlled, pilot study in 112 mechanically ventilated patients, showed that patients receiving tight control of energy balance through the provision of energy guided by indirect calorimetry had a higher intake of calories and protein, whereas the control group (25 kcal/kg) had a negative cumulative energy balance [32].

18.2.2.2 Equations

Over 200 predictive equations have been published (Table 18.2). The best-known equation is the Harris and Benedict [33] equation that takes into account sex, age, weight, and height of the patient (Table 18.2).

Predictive equations should be used with caution, especially in obese patients in whom they provide an approximate evaluation of energy needs [8]. Also, most predictive equations are typically derived from studies of healthy non-hospitalized individuals, and few have been validated in mechanically ventilated patients. The poor accuracy of predictive equations is related to many non-static variables affecting energy expenditure in the critically ill patient. Indeed, equations may underestimate the patient's needs because of hypermetabolism and can also overestimate it because of sedation, paralyzing agents, or mechanical ventilation [48, 49]. Chills, temperature, artificial nutrition, infection, burn, catecholamines, and pharmacologic paralysis have to be taken into account when calculating the energy needs. Physical activity is negligible in ICU patients.

Much software on smartphones and computers use these formulas to estimate needs, which significantly lowers the rate of undernutrition in ICU patient [50].

18.2.2.3 Guidelines

Both ESPEN in 2009 and the French-speaking ICU and Nutrition societies in 2014 recommend 20–25 kcal/kg/day in the acute phase and 25–30 kcal/kg/day in the recovery phase [6, 7]. For patients receiving EN, ESPEN recommends reaching 25 kcal/kg/day in 3 days [5]. There are some differences between ASPEN and ESPEN guidelines (Table 18.3). In 2015, ASPEN and SCCM guidelines recommended 25–30 kcal/kg/day over the whole ICU stay, with 50–65% of the energy goals should be reached during the first week in order to achieve the clinical benefits of EN, else PN should be added [8]. Supplemental PN is indeed not recommended during the first week [52]. A study of 59 surgical or polytrauma patients has compared indirect calorimetry to Harris and Benedict equations increased by 50% to 30 kcal per kg of ideal body weight; there were no difference between these methods [53]; a lower prevalence of obesity (20%) and the use of ideal body weight for calculation may explains these results.

18.2.2.4 Which Weight?

The use of weight in equations supposes that it reflects lean body mass, which is not always the case. In practice, we take actual body weight if the patient is not overweight and without retention of salt or water (edema, ascites).

Table 18.2 Anthropometric formulas for basal energy expenditure [2]

Harris-Benedict [33]
Man: BEE = 66.5 + 13.75 × weight (kg) + 5.0 × height (cm) - 6.78 × age (years) Woman: BEE = 655.1 + 9.56 × weight (kg) + 1.85 × height (cm) - 4.68 × age (years)
Kleiber [34] [34]
Man: BEE = 71.2 × weight (kg)$^{3/4}$ × [1 + 0.004 × (30 - age (years)) + 0.01 × (height (cm)/ weight (kg)$^{1/3}$ - 43.4)] Woman: BEE = 65.8 × weight (kg)$^{3/4}$ × [1 + 0.004 × (30 - age (years)) + 0.018 × height (cm)/ weight(kg)$^{1/3}$ – 42.1)]
Harris-Benedict modified by Roza and Shizgal [35]
Man: BEE = 13.707 × weight (kg) + 4.923 × height (cm) - 6.673 × age (years) + 77.607 Woman: BEE = 9.740 × weight (kg) + 1.729 × height (cm) - 4.737 × age (years) + 667.051
Mifflin [36]
Man: BEE = 10 × weight (kg) + 6.25 × height (cm) - 5 × age(years) + 5 Woman: BEE = 10 × weight (kg) + 6.25 × height (cm) - 5 × age (years) - 161
Liu [37]
BEE = 13.88 × weight (kg) + 4.16 × height (cm) - 3.43 × age (years) – 112 × sex (man, 0. Woman, 1) + 54.34
Fusco [38]
BEE = 12.6 × height (cm) + 11 × weight (kg) - 4 × age (years) - 983
Black [39]
Man: BEE = 1.083 × weight (kg)$^{0.48}$ × height (m)$^{0.50}$ × age (years)$^{-0.13}$ × (1000/4.1855) Woman: BEE = 0.963 × weight (kg)$^{0.48}$ × height (m)$^{0.50}$ × age (years)$^{-0.13}$ × (1000/4.1855)
Fick [40]
BEE = 95.18 × cardiac output × Hb × (SaO_2 - SvO_2)
Swinamer [41]
BEE = 945 × corporal surface (m^2) - 6.4 × age (years) + 108 × T° (°C) + 24.2 × respiratory frequency (/min) + 817 × tidal volume (L) - 4349
Ireton-Jones [42]
Ventilator-dependent: Kcal/d = 1784 + 5 (weight (kg)) – 11 (age (years)) + 244 (if men) + 239 (if trauma) + 804 (if burn) Spontaneously breathing: Kcal/d = 629 – 11 (age (years)) + 25 (weight (kg)) – 609 (if BMI >27 kg/m^2)
Frankenfield [43]
BEE = 0.85 × BEE (Harris & Benedict) + 175 × T° (°C) + 33 × respiratory minute volume (L) – 6344
Raurich [44]
BEE = 105.5 × sex (man, 1; woman, 0) - 8 × age (years) + 11.7 × weight (kg) + 7.7 × height (cm) + 93.2 × T° (°C) + 123.1 × polytrauma (present, 1; absent, 0) – 145.6 × surgery (present, 1; absent, 0) – 3295
Brandi [45]
BEE = 0.96 × BEE (Harris & Benedict) + 7 × cardiac frequency (/min) + 48 × respiratory minute volume (L) – 702
Faisy [46]
BEE = 8 × weight (kg) + 14 × height (cm) + 32 × respiratory minute volume (L) + 94 × T° (°C) – 4834

(continued)

Table 18.2 (continued)

Penn-state[47]
BEE = REE(0.85) + VE (33) + Tmax(175) -6433 REE = Harris-Benedict VE = minute ventilation (L/min) Tmax = maximal body temperature (in Celsius)

BEE basal energy expenditure, *Hb* hemoglobin, SaO_2 arterial oxygen saturation, SvO_2 venous oxygen saturation, *T* body temperature

Table 18.3 Energy requirements in ICU according to the European Society for Clinical Nutrition and Metabolism (ESPEN) [5, 6, 51]

Admission disease	Energy needs (kcal/kg/j)
Initial phase	
Severe malnutrition	25–30
Normal nutritional status	20–25 (woman)
	25–30 (man)
Obesity	15
Overweight	20[a]
Exception	
– Extensive burns	40
Rehabilitation phase	
Severe malnutrition	30–35
Normal nutritional status	25–30
Obesity	15
Overweight	25[a]
Exceptions	
– Extensive burns – Severe sepsis – Polytrauma patient – Necrotizing acute pancreatitis – Cardiac, respiratory, hepatic insufficiency	40 30–35 30–35 35–40 35–40

[a]kcal/kg of ideal weight

In malnourished patients (BMI under 18.5 or 21 if over 70 years of age, loss of 5% weight in 1 month or 10% in 6 month), the use of actual body weight is a risk for refeeding syndrome.

In obese patients (BMI over 30), the use of actual body weight or ideal body weight will lead to overfeeding or underfeeding, respectively. We know that there is no correlation between weight and energy expenditure if the BMI is over 60 [54]. In obese patients, indirect calorimetry is the exam of choice to determine REE. In practice, many alternatives exist [26]: use 20 kcal/kg/day using ideal body weight, use 11–14 kcal/kg/day actual body weight for some authors [8, 55], and use a weight matching a BMI of 25, use the Hamwi equation [56]:

For men, 48 + [height (cm) – 152] × 1.06

For women, 45.4 + [height (cm) – 152] × 0.89.

Finally, we can use formulas with adjusted body weight:

Adjusted body weight = ideal body weight + 0.25 × (actual weight − ideal weight).

In the critically ill obese patients, permissive underfeeding or hypocaloric feeding containing at least 2.0 g/kg ideal body weight per day of protein (1.3–1.5 g/kg actual weight) is recommended [8, 55].

Finally, for patients who are malnourished or obese and who cannot be weighted, we can calculate ideal body weight in function of their height with tables.

18.2.2.5 Changes in Energy Requirements During Time

It is well understood that critical illness and injury is not a homogeneous disease process. The metabolic response to insult has three phases with distinct energy requirements. It is essential to anticipate the course and stay of patients at the time of ICU admission, and to assess caloric and protein intake every day.

The first phase is the acute one characterized by the classic ebb and flow phases [57] of shock and sepsis in which the patient undergoes acute resuscitation. It is marked by rapid catabolism. There is no reliable data concerning energy expenditure during the first 48 h for most serious critically ill patients, those who are hemodynamically unstable or mechanically ventilated with FiO_2 over 60%. If the patient survives, this is followed by a more chronic phase; the patient becomes more vulnerable to complications and infections. The patient is prone to return to the acute phase at this state. If not, he will enter a recovery phase, which coincides with ICU discharge and beginning of rehabilitation.

A New Zealand study demonstrated the evolution of energy expenditure in diverse diseases (polytrauma, sepsis) in ICU [58–61]. Energy expenditures are situated around 25 kcal/kg/day between the third and fifth days, then goes up to 30 kcal/kg/day on the 10th day.

Finally, in the recovery phase, energy expenditure measured by indirect calorimetry increases significantly (maybe over 40 kcal/kg/day) but is extremely variable from one patient to another, depending on muscle activity, residual muscle mass, comorbidities, and other factors [62, 63]. Individual evaluation of REE and estimation of physical activity are needed.

18.2.3 Qualitative Requirements

In critically ill patients, carbohydrates are better used than fat. Besides an important role in energy metabolism, carbohydrates are also connected to protein metabolism. In fact, amino acids released from protein breakdown in the muscle represent a source for gluconeogenesis, while fatty acids are not adequate precursors [6]. Carbohydrates represent 65–70% of energy needs (3.8–4.5 g/kg/day of glucose) [64]. The minimal amount is 2 g/kg/day [6]. Fat requirements represent 30–35% of energy needs (0.7–1.5 g/kg/day of triglyceride). Fat emulsion limits proteolysis, volume of solution and supply fat-soluble vitamins, and essential fatty acids. Fatty acids can influence inflammatory and immune process. The nature and quantity of lipid supply have an important role. The critically ill patients require 9–12 g/day of linoleic acid and 1–3 g/day of alpha-linolenic acid. In general, mixed lipid emulsions and those with olive oil are recommended. However, studies comparing olive oil based to soybean oil based in critically ill patients did not find any difference in infection rate, acute-phase proteins, or major health outcomes [6, 65]. Fish oil, on the other hand, may shorten length of stay [6]. However, most studies evaluating fish oil in ICU were conducted on heterogeneous populations [66, 67].

Moreover, additional energy provided by dextrose-containing fluids and lipid-based medications such as propofol should be accounted when calculating energy needs.

18.2.4 Disease-Related Requirements

General rules have to be adapted in function of disease. In ARDS (acute respiratory disease syndrome), energy supply will be limited to reduce production of CO_2. Parenteral fat has to be slowly infused in order to limit pulmonary hypertension and intrapulmonary shunt in these patients [68]. However, the latest ASPEN guidelines mention that high-lipid low-carbohydrate formulations designed to reduce CO_2 production are not recommended for routine use in ICU patients with ARDS [8]. Results from uncontrolled studies suggest that high-lipid low-carbohydrate formulations are only clinically significant in lowering CO_2 production in overfed ICU patients [69].

Burn injuries result in hypermetabolism and hypercatabolism. Energy demands usually peak about 5–12 days after injury. Aggressive nutritional support is necessary to aid wound healing and improve immunocompetency. Carbohydrate supply can go up to 7 g/kg/day, with parallel reduction of fat, which will represent less than 30% of energy supply [70].

In patients on renal replacement therapy, higher glucose and nitrogen supply are necessary to compensate loss in hemodialysis or continuous renal replacement therapy (CRRT) [71, 72]. There is an increased loss of amino acid (10–15 g per day) during CRRT [8]. Optimal nutritional requirements, in their quantitative and qualitative aspects, for patient with acute kidney injury remain a partially unresolved issue. Nutritional needs should be frequently assesses and individualizes [73]. Table 18.3 presents ESPEN guidelines in specific situations [5, 6].

18.3 Protein Requirements

In ICU, protein is the most important macronutrient. In the acute phase, hypercatabolism is difficult to overcome with nutrition, and there will be a negative nitrogen balance. A recent study showed that early PN did not prevent the pronounced wasting of skeletal muscle observed over the first week of critical illness [74]. Muscle catabolism is higher in burns, polytrauma, septic patients, and after surgery [75]. Amino acids are used for gluconeogenesis, protein production for immune system, healing, and maintenance of organ functions [76]. The short-term protein and lean body mass stores are probably sufficient in patients with ICU stay of 24–48 h [12]. However, patients who stay over 3 days may lose large amounts of proteins, up to 250 g of muscle protein per day (750–1000 g of muscle mass).

In ICU, determining protein requirements is difficult. While energy requirements can be assessed by indirect calorimetry, the protein requirements are difficult to assess because whole-body nitrogen balance is not a reliable index of adequate protein synthesis in the liver, gut, and immune system [6].

It is recommended in non-previously malnourished patients to provide 0.20–0.25 g/kg/day of nitrogen (1.3–1.5 g proteins/kg ideal body weight/day [6] [7] or 1.2–2.0 g/kg actual body weight/day [8]). It can be increased to 0.35 g/kg/day of nitrogen in case of previous malnutrition or important catabolism. In ICU, solutions with a higher protein-to-calorie ratio must be used, providing 100–130 kcal per gram of nitrogen. The EPaNIC trial revealed significant protein delivery deficits in ICU patients on PN [52]. This deficit was due to the utilization of a low-protein PN solution. Hypocaloric feeding in ICU participates in worsening the nitrogen balance [77].

While in acute-phase protein, supply cannot overcome muscle proteolysis, in the rehabilitation phase, on the other hand, protein supply, if it is insufficient, can constitute a limiting factor for protein synthesis. In clinic, muscle strength recuperation and weaning from the ventilator can be delayed in case of insufficient supply. On the other hand, an excess of amino acids induces an over oxidation and secretion of urea.

Pharmaconutrients, such as glutamine and arginine, are described in Chap. 19.

18.4 Micronutrient Requirements

Early in the course of stressful illness, serum levels of many micronutrients decrease significantly because they are consumed, excreted, or sequestered in the liver and the reticuloendothelial system. ICU patients are generally hypermetabolic, with increased macronutrient, traces element, and vitamin requirements. Providing micronutrients is an integral part of nutritional support. Micronutrients supply has to be adapted to each patient.

Main electrolytes (sodium, potassium) have to be monitored daily. Critically ill patients are prone to fluid and sodium overload. Therefore, no guidelines can be appropriate. Plasma levels of other electrolytes such as magnesium and phosphorus have to be monitored; their variations are frequent in ICU, especially in malnourished patients who switch to an anabolic status (refeeding syndrome).

Micronutrients, oligo-elements, and vitamins intervene in many metabolic pathways (enzymatic cofactors), and some are important for anabolism and healing, immune system, antioxidant defenses, and inflammation. Copper, zinc, selenium, manganese, and vitamins A, C, and E are the main antioxidant micronutrients. Deficiency is frequent in the ICU because of preexisting chronic illnesses, excessive losses (digestive, cutaneous, urinary), or consumption during aggression. Oxidative stress is associated with impaired prognosis [78, 79]. Thiamine deficiency is also frequent in ICU.

The real needs in micronutrients are difficult to assess and cover in ICU for many reasons:

– Nutritional supply guidelines correspond to the lower threshold for the general population to prevent deficiency [80]. This threshold is only relative in critically ill patients, who are for the majority already deficient. Also, most commercial trace element preparations available were developed for stable patients.

– Plasma/serum micronutrient measurements are long, costly, and don't reflect the real status.

– An excessive supply in iron or copper is as noxious as deficiency because of a prooxidant status in case of excess and/or in inflammatory situations [81].

Indeed, it is necessary to supply micronutrients at the beginning. EN is supplemented in micronutrients. In Europe, an enteral polymeric product supply of 1500 kcal covers general population needs. This supply is probably insufficient in ICU patients, but there is no consensus.

Commercially available PN formulas do not contain micronutrients and have to be systematically supplemented (Tables 18.4, 18.5, and 18.6).

Table 18.4 Difference in energy and protein requirements in ICU according to different nutrition societies

Nutrient	Recommendation (kg/day)	Guideline source
Energy	20–25 kcal/kg in acute phase of critical illness 25–30 kcal/kg in recovery phase	ESPEN 2009
	In the absence of indirect calorimetry, use 25–30 kcal/kg, or predictive equations	ASPEN 2015
Energy needs in obese	15 kcal/kg actual body weight/day 20 kcal /kg ideal body weight/day	ESPEN 2009
	Consider hypocaloric feeding in critically ill obese (BMI > 30kg/m^2), e.g. 65–70% of target energy requirements by indirect calorimetry, or 11–14 kcal/kg actual body weight for BMI 30–50, or 22–25 kcal/kg ideal body weight for BMI > 50	ASPEN 2015
Protein	1.3–1.5 g protein/kg	ESPEN 2009
	1.2–2.0 g protein/kg actual body weight if BMI < 30 kg/m^2 2 g/kg ideal weight if BMI 30–40 kg/m^2 2.5 g/kg ideal weight if BMI >40 kg/m^2	ASPEN 2015
Glucose	Minimum 2 g/kg	ESPEN 2009
	Maximal glucose oxidation rate is 4–7 mg/kg/min/24 h Ideally keep to ≤5 mg/kg/min/24 h	ESPEN 2009
Fat	0.7–1.5g/kg	ESPEN 2009
	Withholding or limiting SO-based IVFE during the first week following initiation of PN in the critically ill patient	ASPEN 2015

Table 18.5 Parenteral and enteral supply of trace elements compared to nutritional supply guidelines in healthy adults [82]

Elements	RDA M/W	Nutritional supply in enteral nutrition	Addamel® N® IV	Nutryelt® IV	Supplementary IV experts opinions
Chromium (μg)	65/55	25–300	10	10	
Copper (mg)	2/1.5	1.2–10	1.3	0.3	Severe burns, 3.75 mg
Fluoride (mg)	2.5/2	0–4	0.95	0.95	
Iodine (μg)	150	130–700	131	130	
Iron (mg)	9/16	10–40	1.2	1.0	
Manganese (mg)	2–3	1–10	0.3	0.055	
Molybdenum (μg)	30–50	0.48–5.8	19	20	
Selenium (μg)	1 μg/kg	50–200	30	70	Severe burns, 375 μg
					Head injury, acute pancreatitis
					500 μg
Zinc (mg)	12/10	10–30	6.5	10	Severe burns, 40 mg
					Head injury, hepatic insufficiency, transplantation, 15 mg
					Digestive fistula, diarrhea, 15–30 mg

RDA recommended dietary allowance

Important supply of antioxidants via intravenous means is discussed; a meta-analysis of 11 studies (886 patients) showed a significant reduction in mortality (relative risk RR = 0.65 [CI 0.44–0.97]) but not on infectious complications [83]. These results were not observed with antioxidant combination, and selenium seems to be the most effective. Parenteral selenium has shown a significant reduction in all-cause mortality in critically ill patients with sepsis in a 2013 meta-analysis (RR 083; CI 0.70–0.99) [84], even though a large recent international study of enteral micronutrient supplementation (300 μg of selenium, 20 mg of zinc, 10 mg of beta carotene, 500 mg of vitamin E, and 1500 mg of vitamin C) in ICU patients failed to show any clinical benefit [85]. ESPEN guidelines recommend selenium supplementation in the range of 350–1000 μg per day at initial bolus followed by continuous infusion [6]. During severe pancreatitis, the early administration of selenium (100 μg in the first 24 h and 500 μg on the following days) lowers mortality risk [86]. Vitamin C can be efficient at 1–3 g per day for 2–7 days [87]. This vitamin is rapidly deficient in ICU patients. There is less evidence about zinc supplementation [78]. Standard micronutrient admixtures will cover the needs in the majority of cases.

However, major burns have large exudative losses of copper, selenium, and zinc: randomized trials have shown clinical benefit from doses calculated supply to compensate these losses [88]. CRRT is another condition in which there is continuous effluent loss of water-soluble micronutrients.

Table 18.6 Parenteral and enteral supply of vitamins compared to nutritional supply guidelines in healthy adult [82]

Vitamins	RDA M/W	Nutritional supply in enteral nutrition	Soluvit® + Vitalipid® IV	Cernevit® IV	Supplementary IV experts opinions
A (µg)	4000/3000	700–3600	1000	1000	Healing, 2000 µg
D (µg)	200	10–50	5	5.5	
E (mg)	12	10–60	10	10.2	Severe burns, ARDS, transplantation, 100–200 mg
K (µg)	45	70–400	150	–	
B1 (mg)	1.3/1.1	1.2–10	3	3.5	
B2 (mg)	1.6/1.5	1.6–10	3.6	4.1	
B6 (mg)	1.8/1.5	1.6–10.0	4.0	4.5	
Niacin (mg)	14/11	18–60	40	46	
B12 (µg)	2.4	1.4–14	50	6	
Folates (µg)	330/300	200–1000	400	414	
Biotin (µg)	50	15–150	60	69	
C (mg)	110	45–440	100	125	Severe burns, ARDS, transplantation, 1000 mg

RDA recommended dietary allowance

Conclusion

The goals of nutritional support in the ICU are to minimize weight loss, loss of protein during the initial phase, and to provide nutrients to support the immune system and healing. Clinical evaluation of energy needs can be complex, especially for extreme BMI, and can require REE measurement by indirect calorimetry. Actual energy expenditure is important information for deciding the optimal caloric content of nutrition. If overfeeding in terms of energy is noxious, nitrogen needs are always increase. Both over- and underfeeding increase complication rates in ICU. Finally, micronutrients have to be adapted for each patient with possibility to supplement some with selenium and vitamin C.

References

1. Preiser JC, Devos P (2006) Physiopathologie du stress sévère. In: Cano N, Barnoud D, Schneider S, Vasson MP, Hasselmann M, Leverve X (eds) Traité de nutrition artificielle de l'adulte : nourrir l'homme malade, 3ème édition edn. Springer, Paris, pp 435–444

2. Raynard B (2009) Place de la calorimétrie indirecte et des formules estimant la dépense énergétique des malades de réanimation. Nutr Clin Métabol 23(4):192–197
3. Griffiths RD (1997) Feeding the critically ill—should we do better? Intensive Care Med 23(3):246–247
4. Kan MN, Chang HH, Sheu WF, Cheng CH, Lee BJ, Huang YC (2003) Estimation of energy requirements for mechanically ventilated, critically ill patients using nutritional status. Crit Care 7(5):R108–R115. doi:10.1186/cc2366
5. Kreymann KG, Berger MM, Deutz NE, Hiesmayr M, Jolliet P, Kazandjiev G, Nitenberg G, van den Berghe G, Wernerman J, Ebner C, Hartl W, Heymann C, Spies C (2006) ESPEN guidelines on enteral nutrition: intensive care. Clin Nutr 25(2):210–223. doi:10.1016/j.clnu.2006.01.021. [pii] S0261-5614(06)00041-0
6. Singer P, Berger MM, Van den Berghe G, Biolo G, Calder P, Forbes A, Griffiths R, Kreyman G, Leverve X, Pichard C, Espen (2009) ESPEN guidelines on parenteral nutrition: intensive care. Clin Nutr 28(4):387–400. doi:10.1016/j.clnu.2009.04.024. [pii] S0261-5614(09)00098-3
7. Lefrant JY, Hurel D, Cano NJ, Ichai C, Preiser JC, Tamion F (2014) Guidelines for nutrition support in critically ill patient. Ann Fr Anesth Reanim 33(3):202–218. doi:10.1016/j.annfar.2014.01.008
8. McClave SA, Taylor B, Martindale RG, Warren MM, Johnson DR, Braunschweig C, McCarthy MS, Davanos E, Rice TW, Cresci GA, Gervasio JM, Sacks GS, Roberts PR, Compher C (2015) Guidelines for the provision and assessment of nutrition support therapy in the adult critically ill patient: Society of Critical Care Medicine (SCCM) and American Society for Parenteral and Enteral Nutrition (a.S.P.E.N.) JPEN J Parenter Enteral Nutr 40(2):159–211. doi:10.1177/0148607109335234. [pii] 33/3/277
9. Stapleton RD, Jones N, Heyland DK (2007) Feeding critically ill patients: what is the optimal amount of energy ? Crit Care Med 35(suppl):S535–S540
10. Arabi YM, Aldawood AS, Haddad SH, Al-Dorzi HM, Tamim HM, Jones GJ, Mehta S, McIntyre L, Solaiman O, Sakkijha MH, Sadat M, Afesh L (2015) Permissive underfeeding or standard enteral feeding in critically ill adults. NEJM 372(25):2398–2408
11. Charles EJ, Petroze RT, Metzger R, Hranjec T, Rosenberger LH, Riccio LM, McLeod MD, Guidry CA, Stukenbor GJ, Swenon BR, Wilcutts KF, O'Donnell KB, Sawyer RG (2014) Hypocaloric compared with eucaloric nutritional support and its effect on infection rates in a surgical intensive care unit: a randomized controlled trial. Am J Clin Nutr 100:1337–1343
12. Wischmeyer PE (2013) The evolution of nutrition in critical care: how much, how soon? Crit Care 17(Suppl 1):S7. doi:10.1186/cc11505
13. McWhirter JP, Pennington CR (1994) Incidence and recognition of malnutrition in hospital. Br Med J 308(6934):945–948
14. Sheean PM, Peterson SJ, Gomez Perez S, Troy KL, Patel A, Sclamberg JS, Ajanaku FC, Braunschweig CA (2013) The prevalence of sarcopenia in patients with respiratory failure classified as normally nourished using computed tomography and subjective global assessment. J Parenter Enter Nutr 38(7):873–879. doi:10.1177/0148607113500308
15. Pasinato VF, Berbigier MC, Rubin Bde A, Castro K, Moraes RB, Perry ID (2013) Enteral nutritional therapy in septic patients in the intensive care unit: compliance with nutritional guidelines for critically ill patients. Revista Brasileira de terapia intensiva 25(1):17–24
16. Caba D, Ochoa JB (2007) How many calories are necessary during critical illness? Gastrointest Endosc Clin N Am 17(4):703–710. doi:10.1016/j.giec.2007.07.004. [pii] S1052-5157(07)00092-X
17. Alberda C, Gramlich L, Jones N, Jeejeebhoy K, Day AG, Dhaliwal R, Heyland DK (2009) The relationship between nutritional intake and clinical outcomes in critically ill patients: results of an international multicenter observational study. Intensive Care Med 35(10):1728–1737. doi:10.1007/s00134-009-1567-4
18. De Jonghe B, Appere-De-Vechi C, Fournier M, Tran B, Merrer J, Melchior JC, Outin H (2001) A prospective survey of nutritional support practices in intensive care unit patients: what is prescribed? What is delivered? Crit Care Med 29(1):8–12

19. Wandrag L, Gordon F, O'Flynn J, Siddiqui B, Hickson M (2011) Identifying the factors that influence energy deficit in the adult intensive care unit: a mixed linear model analysis. J Hum Nutr Diet 24(3):215–222. doi:10.1111/j.1365-277X.2010.01147.x
20. Dvir D, Cohen J, Singer P (2006) Computerized energy balance and complications in critically ill patients: an observational study. Clin Nutr 25(1):37–44. doi:10.1016/j.clnu.2005.10.010. [pii] S0261-5614(05)00187-1
21. Villet S, Chiolero RL, Bollmann MD, Revelly JP, RNM C, Delarue J, Berger MM (2005) Negative impact of hypocaloric feeding and energy balance on clinical outcome in ICU patients. Clin Nutr 24(4):502–509. doi:S0261-5614(05)00054-3 [pii]. doi:10.1016/j.clnu.2005.03.006
22. Tsai JR, Chang WT, Sheu CC, Wu YJ, Sheu YH, Liu PL, Ker CG, Huang MC (2010) Inadequate energy delivery during early critical illness correlates with increased risk of mortality in patients who survive at least seven days: a retrospective study. Clin Nutr 30(2):209–214. doi:10.1016/j.clnu.2010.09.003. [pii] S0261-5614(10)00176-7
23. Petros S, Engelmann L (2006) Enteral nutrition delivery and energy expenditure in medical intensive care patients. Clin Nutr 25(1):51–59. doi:10.1016/j.clnu.2005.08.013. [pii] S0261-5614(05)00146-9
24. Arabi YM, Haddad SH, Tamim HM, Rishu AH, Sakkijha MH, Kahoul SH, Britts RJ (2010) Near-target caloric intake in critically ill medical-surgical patients is associated with adverse outcomes. JPEN J Parenter Enteral Nutr 34(3):280–288. doi:10.1177/0148607109353439. [pii] 34/3/280
25. The Veterans Affairs Total Parenteral Nutrition Cooperative Study Group (1991) Perioperative total parenteral nutrition in surgical patients. N Engl J Med 325(8):525–532
26. Petit A, Tamion F (2010) Nutrition du patient obèse agressé. Réanimation 19:448–453
27. McClave SA, Lowen CC, Kleber MJ, Nicholson JF, Jimmerson SC, McConnell JW, Jung LY (1998) Are patients fed appropriately according to their caloric requirements? JPEN J Parenter Enteral Nutr 22(6):375–381
28. Malone AM (2002) Methods of assessing energy expenditure in the intensive care unit. Nutr Clin Pract 17(1):21–28. [pii] 17/1/21
29. Jeejeebhoy KN (2004) Permissive underfeeding of the critically ill patient. Nutr Clin Pract 19(5):477–480. [pii] 19/5/477
30. Sundstrom M, Tjader I, Rooyackers O, Wernerman J (2013) Indirect calorimetry in mechanically ventilated patients. A systematic comparison of three instruments. Clin Nutr 32(1):118–121. doi:10.1016/j.clnu.2012.06.004
31. Weekes CE (2007) Controversies in the determination of energy requirements. Proc Nutr Soc 66(3):367–377. doi:S0029665107005630 [pii]. doi:10.1017/S0029665107005630
32. Singer P, Anbar R, Cohen J, Shapiro H, Shalita-Chesner M, Lev S, Grozovski E, Theilla M, Frishman S, Madar Z (2011) The tight calorie control study (TICACOS): a prospective, randomized, controlled pilot study of nutritional support in critically ill patients. Intensive Care Med 37(4):601–609. doi:10.1007/s00134-011-2146-z
33. Harris JA, Benedict FG (1919) A biometric study of basal metabolism in man. Carnegie Institute of Washington, Washington
34. Kleiber M (1932) Body size and metabolism. Hilgardia 6:315–353
35. Roza AM, Shizgal HM (1984) The Harris Benedict equation reevaluated: resting energy requirements and the body cell mass. Am J Clin Nutr 40(1):168–182
36. Mifflin MD, St Jeor ST, Hill LA, Scott BJ, Daugherty SA, Koh YO (1990) A new predictive equation for resting energy expenditure in healthy individuals. Am J Clin Nutr 51(2):241–247
37. Liu HY, Lu YF, Chen WJ (1995) Predictive equations for basal metabolic rate in Chinese adults: a cross-validation study. J Am Diet Assoc 95(12):1403–1408. doi:10.1016/S0002-8223(95)00369-X. [pii] S0002-8223(95)00369-X
38. Fusco MA, Mills ME, Nelson LD (1995) Predicting caloric requirements with emphasis on avoiding overfeeding. JPEN 19(suppl):18S. (abstract)
39. Black AE, Coward WA, Cole TJ, Prentice AM (1996) Human energy expenditure in affluent societies: an analysis of 574 doubly-labelled water measurements. Eur J Clin Nutr 50(2):72–92
40. Fick A (1855) Über diffusion. Poggendorff's Annalen der Physik und Chemie 94:59–86

41. Swinamer DL, Grace MG, Hamilton SM, Jones RL, Roberts P, King EG (1990) Predictive equation for assessing energy expenditure in mechanically ventilated critically ill patients. Crit Care Med 18(6):657–661
42. Ireton-Jones CS, Turner WW Jr, Liepa GU, Baxter CR (1992) Equations for the estimation of energy expenditures in patients with burns with special reference to ventilatory status. J Burn Care Rehabil 13(3):330–333
43. Frankenfield DC, Omert LA, Badellino MM, Wiles CE 3rd, Bagley SM, Goodarzi S, Siegel JH (1994a) Correlation between measured energy expenditure and clinically obtained variables in trauma and sepsis patients. JPEN J Parenter Enteral Nutr 18(5):398–403
44. Raurich JM, Ibanez J, Marse P, Velasco J, Bergada J (1997) Energy expenditure in patients with multiple organ failure. Clin Nutr 16(6):307–312. [pii] S0261-5614(97)80016-7
45. Brandi LS, Bertolini R, Calafa M (1997) Indirect calorimetry in critically ill patients: clinical applications and practical advice. Nutrition 13(4):349–358
46. Faisy C, Guerot E, Diehl JL, Labrousse J, Fagon JY (2003) Assessment of resting energy expenditure in mechanically ventilated patients. Am J Clin Nutr 78(2):241–249
47. MacDonald A, Hildebrandt L (2003) Comparison of formulaic equations to determine energy expenditure in the critically ill patient. Nutrition 19:233–9
48. Chioléro R, Revelly JP, Tappy L (1997) Energy metabolism in sepsis and injury. Nutrition 13(9 Suppl):45S–51S
49. Frankenfield DC, Wiles CE 3rd, Bagley S, Siegel JH (1994b) Relationships between resting and total energy expenditure in injured and septic patients. Crit Care Med 22(11):1796–1804
50. Attof Y, Hachemi M, Cannesson M, Souza Neto EP, Rosamel P, Chambrier C, Bastien O, Lehot JJ (2007) De la conception à l'évaluation d'un programme d'aide à la prescription en nutrition artificielle sous Palm OS®. Ann Fr Anesth Reanim 26(12):1031–1036. doi:10.1016/j.annfar.2007.09.026. [pii] S0750-7658(07)00515-1
51. Thibault R, Pichard C (2010) Nutrition and clinical outcome in intensive care patients. Curr Opin Clin Nutr Metab Care 13(2):177–183. doi:10.1097/MCO.0b013e32833574b9
52. Casaer MP, Mesotten D, Hermans G, Wouters PJ, Schetz M, Meyfroidt G, Van Cromphaut S, Ingels C, Meersseman P, Muller J, Vlasselaers D, Debaveye Y, Desmet L, Dubois J, Van Assche A, Vanderheyden S, Wilmer A, Van den Berghe G (2011) Early versus late parenteral nutrition in critically ill adults. N Engl J Med 365(6):506–517. doi:10.1056/NEJMoa1102662
53. Davis KA, Kinn T, Esposito TJ, Reed RL 2nd, Santaniello JM, Luchette FA (2006) Nutritional gain versus financial gain: the role of metabolic carts in the surgical ICU. J Trauma 61(6):1436–1440. doi:10.1097/01.ta.0000242269.12534.79. [pii] 00005373-200612000-00021
54. Daly JM, Heymsfield SB, Head CA, Harvey LP, Nixon DW, Katzeff H, Grossman GD (1985) Human energy requirements: overestimation by widely used prediction equation. Am J Clin Nutr 42(6):1170–1174
55. Port AM, Apovian C (2010) Metabolic support of the obese intensive care unit patient: a current perspective. Curr Opin Clin Nutr Metab Care 13(2):184–191. doi:10.1097/MCO.0b013e328335f1e6
56. Hamwi GJ (1964) Therapy: changing dietary concepts. In: Danowski TS (ed) Diabetes mellitus: diagnosis and treatment, vol 1. American Diabetes Association, New York
57. Stahel PF, Flierl MA, Moore EE (2010) "metabolic staging" after major trauma - a guide for clinical decision making? Scand J Trauma Resusc Emerg Med 18:34. doi:10.1186/1757-7241-18-34
58. Ishibashi N, Plank LD, Sando K, Hill GL (1998) Optimal protein requirements during the first 2 weeks after the onset of critical illness. Crit Care Med 26(9):1529–1535
59. Plank LD, Connolly AB, Hill GL (1998) Sequential changes in the metabolic response in severely septic patients during the first 23 days after the onset of peritonitis. Ann Surg 228(2):146–158
60. Plank LD, Hill GL (2000) Sequential metabolic changes following induction of systemic inflammatory response in patients with severe sepsis or major blunt trauma. World J Surg 24(6):630–638. doi:10.1007/s002689910104
61. Plank LD, Hill GL (2003) Energy balance in critical illness. Proc Nutr Soc 62(2):545–552

62. Kreymann G, Grosser S, Buggisch P, Gottschall C, Matthaei S, Greten H (1993) Oxygen consumption and resting metabolic rate in sepsis, sepsis syndrome, and septic shock. Crit Care Med 21(7):1012–1019
63. Uehara M, Plank LD, Hill GL (1999) Components of energy expenditure in patients with severe sepsis and major trauma: a basis for clinical care. Crit Care Med 27(7):1295–1302
64. Jolliet P, Pichard C, Biolo G, Chiolero R, Grimble G, Leverve X, Nitenberg G, Novak I, Planas M, Preiser JC, Roth E, Schols AM, Wernerman J (1998) Enteral nutrition in intensive care patients: a practical approach. Working group on nutrition and metabolism, ESICM. European Society of Intensive Care Medicine. Intensive Care Med 24(8):848–859
65. Umpierrez GE, Spiegelman R, Zhao V, Smiley DD, Pinzon I, Griffith DP, Peng L, Morris T, Luo M, Garcia H, Thomas C, Newton CA, Ziegler TR (2012) A double-blind, randomized clinical trial comparing soybean oil-based versus olive oil-based lipid emulsions in adult medical-surgical intensive care unit patients requiring parenteral nutrition. Crit Care Med 40(6):1792–1798. doi:10.1097/CCM.0b013e3182474bf9
66. Friesecke S, Lotze C, Kohler J, Heinrich A, Felix SB, Abel P (2008) Fish oil supplementation in the parenteral nutrition of critically ill medical patients: a randomised controlled trial. Intensive Care Med 34(8):1411–1420. doi:10.1007/s00134-008-1072-1
67. Manzanares W, Dhaliwal R, Jurewitsch B, Stapleton RD, Jeejeebhoy KN, Heyland DK (2014) Parenteral fish oil lipid emulsions in the critically ill: a systematic review and meta-analysis. JPEN J Parenter Enteral Nutr 38(1):20–28. doi:10.1177/0148607113486006
68. Christman JW, McCain RW (1993) A sensible approach to the nutritional support of mechanically ventilated critically ill patients. Intensive Care Med 19(3):129–136
69. Radrizzani D, Iapichino G (1998) Nutrition and lung function in the critically ill patient. Clin Nutr 17(1):7–10
70. Rousseau AF, Losser MR, Ichai C, Berger MM (2013) ESPEN endorsed recommendations: nutritional therapy in major burns. Clin Nutr 32(4):497–502. doi:10.1016/j.clnu.2013.02.012
71. Bellomo R, Martin H, Parkin G, Love J, Kearley Y, Boyce N (1991) Continuous arteriovenous haemodiafiltration in the critically ill: influence on major nutrient balances. Intensive Care Med 17(7):399–402
72. Frankenfield DC, Reynolds HN, Badellino MM, Wiles CE 3rd (1995) Glucose dynamics during continuous hemodiafiltration and total parenteral nutrition. Intensive Care Med 21(12):1016–1022
73. Fiaccadori E, Regolisti G, Maggiore U (2013) Specialized nutritional support interventions in critically ill patients on renal replacement therapy. Curr Opin Clin Nutr Metab Care 16(2):217–224. doi:10.1097/MCO.0b013e32835c20b0
74. Casaer MP, Langouche L, Coudyzer W, Vanbeckevoort D, De Dobbelaer B, Guiza FG, Wouters PJ, Mesotten D, Van den Berghe G (2013) Impact of early parenteral nutrition on muscle and adipose tissue compartments during critical illness. Crit Care Med 41(10):2298–2309. doi:10.1097/CCM.0b013e31828cef02
75. Jackson NC, Carroll PV, Russell-Jones DL, Sonksen PH, Treacher DF, Umpleby AM (1999) The metabolic consequences of critical illness: acute effects on glutamine and protein metabolism. Am J Phys 276(1 Pt 1):E163–E170
76. Hasselgren PO, Pedersen P, Sax HC, Warner BW, Fischer JE (1988) Current concepts of protein turnover and amino acid transport in liver and skeletal muscle during sepsis. Arch Surg 123(8):992–999
77. Japur CC, Monteiro JP, Marchini JS, Garcia RW, Basile-Filho A (2010) Can an adequate energy intake be able to reverse the negative nitrogen balance in mechanically ventilated critically ill patients? J Crit Care 25(3):445–450. doi:10.1016/j.jcrc.2009.05.009. [pii] S0883-9441(09)00122-1
78. Heyland DK, Jones N, Cvijanovich NZ, Wong H (2008) Zinc supplementation in critically ill patients: a key pharmaconutrient? JPEN J Parenter Enteral Nutr 32(5):509–519. doi:10.1177/0148607108322402. [pii] 0148607108322402

79. Mishra V, Baines M, Wenstone R, Shenkin A (2005) Markers of oxidative damage, antioxidant status and clinical outcome in critically ill patients. Ann Clin Biochem 42(Pt 4):269–276. doi:10.1258/0004563054255461
80. Murphy SP, Barr SI, Yates AA (2006) The recommended dietary allowance (RDA) should not be abandoned: an individual is both an individual and a member of a group. Nutr Rev 64(7 Pt 1):313–315. discussion 315-318
81. Moison RM, Bloemhof FE, Geerdink JA, de Beaufort AJ, Berger HM (2000) The capacity of different infusion fluids to lower the prooxidant activity of plasma iron: an important factor in resuscitation? Transfusion 40(11):1346–1351
82. Perlot I, Preiser JC (2010) Besoins en vitamines et oligo-éléments. In: Barnoud D, Fraipont V, Hasselmann M, Preiser JC, Schneider SM (eds) Questions de nutrition clinique de l'adulte en réanimation et soins intensifs. SFNEP-SBNC-K'Noë, Paris, pp 39–49
83. Heyland DK, Dhaliwal R, Suchner U, Berger MM (2005) Antioxidant nutrients: a systematic review of trace elements and vitamins in the critically ill patient. Intensive Care Med 31(3):327–337. doi:10.1007/s00134-004-2522-z
84. Huang TS, Shyu YC, Chen HY, Lin LM, Lo CY, Yuan SS, PJ CH (2013) Effect of parenteral selenium supplementation in critically ill patients: a systematic review and meta-analysis. PLoS One 8(1):1–9
85. Heyland D, Muscedere J, Wischmeyer PE, Cook D, Jones G, Albert M, Elke G, Berger MM, Day AG, Canadian Critical Care Trials G (2013) A randomized trial of glutamine and antioxidants in critically ill patients. N Engl J Med 368(16):1489–1497. doi:10.1056/NEJMoa1212722
86. Kuklinski B, Zimmermann T, Schweder R (1995) Decreasing mortality in acute pancreatitis with sodium selenite. Clinical results of 4 years antioxidant therapy. Med Klin (Munich) 90(Suppl 1):36–41
87. Berger MM (2009) Vitamin C requirements in parenteral nutrition. Gastroenterology 137(5 Suppl):S70–S78. doi:10.1053/j.gastro.2009.08.012. [pii] S0016-5085(09)01448-6
88. Berger MM, Baines M, Raffoul W, Benathan M, Chiolero RL, Reeves C, Revelly JP, Cayeux MC, Senechaud I, Shenkin A (2007) Trace element supplementation after major burns modulates antioxidant status and clinical course by way of increased tissue trace element concentrations. Am J Clin Nutr 85(5):1293–1300

19 Pharmaconutrition in the Critically Ill Patient

Jean-Charles Preiser, Christian Malherbe, and Carlos A. Santacruz

19.1 Introduction

Critically ill patients might benefit from specialized nutrients provided in addition to macro- and micronutrients. Initially, the theoretical basis for specialized nutrition support relates to the altered immune response associated with the prolonged inflammatory status. For instance, immune-enhancing or immune-modulating nutrition formulas have been considered as logical and attractive options in critically ill patients [1]. Subsequently, changes in the composition of nutritional formulas were brought to compensate for specific deficiencies.

The clinical effects of pharmaconutrition will be reviewed and followed by a description of its individual components. Indeed, clinical results of pharmaconutrition can widely vary according to the concentration of each component and the specific type of disease they were used in.

19.2 Clinical Effects of Pharmaconutrition

Several clinical trials have been published on the use of pharmaconutrition in critical illness. Most trials have heterogeneous populations and different methodologies. Systematic reviews and meta-analyses on pharmaconutrition have been published [2, 3]. A recent publication by Marik and Zaloga [4] reported a positive effect with the use of pharmaconutrition on the rate of infection and length of stay. Older reviews [5–7] have shown similar results, with reduced infection rate and length of

J.-C. Preiser (✉) • C.A. Santacruz
Department of Intensive Care, Erasme University Hospital, 1070 Brussels, Belgium
e-mail: Jean-Charles.Preiser@erasme.ulb.ac.be

C. Malherbe
Department of dietetics, University Hospital of Liege, Liege, Belgium

C. Ichai et al. (eds.), *Metabolic Disorders and Critically Ill Patients*,
http://doi.org/10.1007/978-3-319-64010-5_19

stay in the ICU. However, the moderate quality of the individual studies decreasedv the strength of current guidelines, implying low-grade recommendations to use immunonutrients in selected categories of patients [8, 9].

Now, the issue of pharmaconutrition is not restricted to immune-modulating formulas. In fact, specific amino acids, modified lipids, and supplemental antioxidants have been marketed to meet the particular needs of critically ill patients.

19.3 Specific Amino Acids

There has been a long-standing interest for the incorporation of specific amino acids in nutrition formulas for the critically ill. Indeed, the synthetic capabilities may be altered and the stores of some amino acids may be depleted. Consequences of such deficits are related to each disease state and may vary between individuals. For example, a decreased availability of the constitutive elements of glutathione (cysteine, glutamate, and glycine) and the most active intracellular endogenous antioxidant could increase oxidative stress [9]. Likewise, taurine is another amino acid with antioxidant properties. The most studied amino acids include glutamine, arginine, and alpha-ketoglutarate ornithine, all having been assessed in prospective randomized trials.

19.3.1 Glutamine

Glutamine has some favorable clinical effects [10]. Glutamine is the most abundant nonessential amino acid in all the body. 60% of glutamine is stored in skeletal muscle in the form of free amino acid. Glutamine is also synthesized in nearly every tissue by glutamine synthetase and hydrolyzed via a glutaminase present in mitochondria. Glutamine is implicated in several physiological mechanisms: (1) transportation of proteins and protein-related waste products; (2) intermediate metabolite for the synthesis of de novo amino acids and nucleic acids, an especially important pathway in tissues with a high turnover such as immune and epithelial cells in the digestive tract; (3) antioxidant synthesis, as a precursor for glutamate and thus synthesis of glutathione; and (4) energetic substrate for ATP production (Table 19.1).

During critical illness, the stores of glutamine are rapidly depleted, as de novo synthesis is limited. Low glutamine levels are inversely related to survival in critically ill patients [11]. Moreover, parenteral nutrition solutions lack glutamine, thereby increasing the risk for a specific deficit when used exclusively.

19.3.1.1 Parenteral Glutamine Supplementation

The rationale supporting the supplementation of glutamine in patients receiving parenteral nutrition is based on the absence of this amino acid, due to its insolubility. The benefit of supplemental intravenous glutamine was demonstrated by Griffiths et al. [12] and Goeters et al. [13], who reported a 6-month survival advantage with the use of intravenous glutamine supplementation [13]. This

Table 19.1 Physiological effects of glutamine

Metabolic • Protein synthesis • Inter-organ protein and carbonic transporter • Gluconeogenesis precursor • Renal ammonic production
Immunologic • Immune cell replication • T cell helper functions • IgA synthesis
Gut function • Enterocytes life cycle • Gut-associated lymphoid tissue function (GALT)
Antioxidant • Glutathione synthesis • Taurine synthesis

benefit was attributed to a reduction in infection rate and organ failures when the ICU stay lasted more than 5 days [14], consistent with another study on 104 surgical patients [15].

19.3.1.2 Enteral Glutamine Supplementation

Enteral glutamine supplementation was suggested to preserve the immune function of the gastrointestinal tract. Even though some benefit was found in some earlier studies [16–19], the largest studies did not confirm a beneficial effect [20] or even found an increased mortality rate associated with the use of high doses of enteral and parenteral glutamine early in the course of severe critical illness [21].

19.3.1.3 Current Recommendation for the Use of Supplemental Glutamine

According to international guidelines [8, 9, 22, 23], intravenous glutamine supplementation is recommended in patients receiving exclusive parenteral nutrition, but no longer in other situations.

19.3.2 Arginine

Arginine is synthetized from citrulline by the kidneys. Important physiological roles of arginine include the production of nitric oxide (NO) by the NO synthase enzymes, the function of arginase, regulation of in gene expression, cellular proliferation, immune response, intestinal cell homeostasis, and wound healing [24, 25]. So, arginine has many pleiotropic effects and is implicated in numerous functions.

19.3.2.1 Clinical Data

Even though some trials reported an inverse correlation between arginine levels and the outcome of critically ill patients [26–28], no benefit was associated with arginine supplementation [29].

19.3.2.2 Current Recommendation

Arginine supplementation is not recommended for critically ill patients [8, 22].

19.4 Modified Lipids

Independently of their high caloric content (9 kcal/g for palmitic acid), fatty acids exert multiple roles in the inflammatory cascade, cell membrane modulation, and gene expression properties. Hence, changes of the structure of dietary lipids are supposed to influence these pathways.

19.4.1 Medium Chain Triglycerides

Theoretical benefit with the use of medium-chain triglycerides (MCT) comes from the idea of a better energetic profile than long-chain triglycerides, associated with an immediate cofactor-less metabolism. Nutrition formulas rich in MCT are a mix (usually 50/50) between long-chain triglycerides (LCT) and MCT. These kinds of lipids are not involved in cellular membrane structure and do not exert immune effect.

19.4.2 Monounsaturated Fatty Acids

Theoretical advantages of monounsaturated fatty acids rely on a lower risk of oxidation than polyunsaturated fatty acids, in relation with the susceptibility of double bonds to oxidative process. Lipid formulas built on a mixture of olive oil (80%) and soybean are considered to be low on polyunsaturated fatty acids, while lipid formulas based on soybean oil can contain up to 60% of polyunsaturated fatty acids. Current trials have failed to demonstrate a clinical impact on mortality with the use of lipid rich formulas.

19.4.3 Lipid Formulas Rich in ω-3 Fatty Acids

The theoretical benefit of ω-3 fatty acid supplementation is the modulation of inflammation and immunity. Generally, lipid-rich enteral or parenteral formulas contain eicosapentaenoic (C20: 5 ω-3) and docosahexaenoic (C22: 6 ω-3) fatty acids. Benefit is thought to derive from inflammatory and immune modulation.

The incorporation of these types ω-3 fatty acids in cell membranes is followed by a series of functional changes [30], a reduction in the synthesis of eicosanoids and inflammatory immunosuppressive, change in the composition "lipid rafts" (microdomains rich in cholesterol and sphingolipids involved in membrane signal transduction) [27], reduction of TNF-α, IL-1β, and IL-6 production by macrophages and IL-2-stimulated lymphocytes, shift of the immune response toward a Th2 phenotype, and decreased lymphocyte production of cytokines.

19.4.4 Clinical Data

A large-scale retrospective study demonstrated that intake from 0.15 to 0.20 g. $kg^{-1} \bullet I^{-1}$ fish oil in critically ill patients resulted in a reduction in mortality, infection, prescription of antibiotics, and ICU length of stay [31]. A prospective confirmation of these beneficial effects of parenteral solutions enriched in ω-3 is expected. Preoperative conditioning by supplementation with fish oils for 2–3 days (in abdominal surgery patients) significantly reduced mortality, the need for mechanical ventilation, and length of hospital stay compared with patients who did not have supplementation [32].

Enteral solutions are enriched with ω-3 fatty acids and antioxidants (in comparison with another high-fat control solution); administration has reduced cellularity of the pro-inflammatory profile in bronchoalveolar lavage from patients with severe acute respiratory distress syndrome, increased the PaO_2/FiO_2 ratio, and reduced the duration of mechanical ventilation and ICU length of stay [33–36]. However, these findings and these beneficial effects have not been confirmed in more recent studies, as expected [37].

19.4.5 Current Recommendations

Current data do not allow a recommendation on the use of parenteral nutrition with lipid concentration in critically ill patients. However, recommendations of the European Society of Nutrition (ESPEN) [37] suggest the use of mixtures of fatty acids (long and medium chains, olive oil and fish oil) instead of soybean oil-based standard solutions. The use of enteral solutions enriched with modified lipids is no longer recommended [22].

19.5 Antioxidants

Oxidative stress, defined by the balance between antioxidant molecules and antioxidant defenses, is typically increased in critically ill patients, resulting in both increased oxidant production and consumption of endogenous antioxidants stocks. The effects of this increased oxidant stress are important [9, 38, 39]. For example, the bactericidal and the proper functioning of neutrophils, the first line of defense against microorganisms requires the production of oxygen free radicals. However, the same oxygen free radicals, if not effectively neutralized outside of their site of action can trigger significant molecular damage on lipid membranes, proteins, nucleic acids and carbohydrates [9, 39].

Prolonged and uncontrolled oxidative stress has been implicated in the pathogenesis of organ failure, by interference with multiple cellular processes and depletion of cellular energy stores [40]. Lipid peroxidation and oxidative damage to other molecules are at the origin of these disorders [40].

19.5.1 Clinical Effects

Clinical trials to test the effects of antioxidants are heterogeneous differing on the type of antioxidant used, antioxidant supplementation given to patients [9, 39], and timing of supplementation (early vs. late).

19.5.2 Antioxidant Vitamins

Proof of satisfactory absorption of vitamins A, C, and E (α-tocopherol) administered by the enteral route has been tested in critically ill patients and trauma patients [40–42]. In both types of patients, a reduction in the incidence of organ failure and death was found [42]. Similarly, clinical trials mentioned above in patients with acute hypoxic respiratory failure [40–44] have shown favorable results in patients receiving enteral nutrition formula enriched with antioxidant vitamins. However, no benefit of a cocktail of antioxidant vitamins and selenium was found in the largest published study [21].

19.5.3 Antioxidant Trace Elements

The effects of supplementation with trace elements, which serve as cofactors to antioxidant enzymes (selenium, zinc, copper, and manganese), were tested in different circumstances and in different forms. Of course, this procedure is less specific as vitamins, as trace elements play multiple other roles, but is potentially more efficient, since trace elements can detoxify many more free radicals than vitamins [45]. In summary, at present, the beneficial effects of the addition of selenium (500–1000 μg IV) were confirmed in the burned and traumatized patient [45], but not in septic patients [46, 47] or in patients with at least two organ failures [21].

19.5.4 Recommendations

Based on the available clinical data [9, 22] supplementation with vitamins C and E (without specifying, however, dose or timing) and selenium cannot be recommended in patients with other conditions than burn injury. However, trace elements and vitamins must be added to parenteral solutions to meet the general recommendations for daily intake [48].

Conclusion

In spite of strong and convincing rationale, the expected benefits of most pharmaconutrients were not confirmed in prospective randomized controlled trials. However, in some subsets of patients (e.g., antioxidants in burns) or situations (intravenous glutamine during exclusive parenteral nutrition), the addition of specific nutrients is clearly recommended. Still, many questions are still unsolved, including the optimal timing, dosing, and monitoring of adverse effects. Future trials need to address these issues with the same scrutiny than pharmaceutical studies.

References

1. Dupertuis YM, Meguid MM, Pichard C (2009) Advancing from immunonutrition to a pharmaconutrition: a gigantic challenge. Curr Opin Clin Nutr Metab Care 12:398–403
2. Heys SD, Schofield AC, Wahle KW (2004) Immunonutrition in clinical practice: what is the current evidence? Nutr Hosp 19:325–332
3. Heyland DK (2002) Immunonutrition in the critically ill patient: putting the cart before the horse? Nutr Clin Pract 17:267–272
4. Marik PE, Zaloga GP (2008) Immunonutrition in critically ill patients: a systematic review and analysis of the literature. Intensive Care Med 34:1980–1990
5. Beale RJ, Bryg DJ, Bihari DJ (1999) Immunonutrition in the critically ill: a systematic review on clinical outcome. Crit Care Med 27:2799–2805
6. Montejo JC, Zarazaga A, López-Martínez J et al (2003) Immunonutrition in the intensive care unit. A systematic review and consensus statement. Clin Nutr 22:221–233
7. Heyland DK, Novak F, Drover JW et al (2001) Should immunonutrition become routine in critically ill patients? A systematic review of the evidence. JAMA 22-29:944–953
8. McClave SA, Martindale RG, Vanek VW et al (2009) Guidelines for the Provision and Assessment of Nutrition Support Therapy in the Adult Critically Ill Patient: Society of Critical Care Medicine (SCCM) and American Society for Parenteral and Enteral Nutrition (A.S.P.E.N.) J Parenter Enter Nutr 33:277–316
9. Preiser JC (2012) Oxidative stress. J Parenter Enter Nutr 36:147–154
10. Preiser JC, Wernerman J (2003) Glutamine, a life-saving nutrient, but why? Crit Care Med 31:2555–2556
11. Oudemans-van Straaten HM, Bosman RJ, Treskes M et al (2001) Plasma glutamine depletion and patient outcome in acute ICU admissions. Intensive Care Med 27:84–90
12. Griffiths RD, Jones C, Palmer TEA (1997) Six month outcome of critically ill patients given glutamine-supplemented parenteral nutrition. Nutrition 13:295–302
13. Goeters C, Wenn A, Mertes N et al (2002) Parenteral L-alanyl-L-glutamine improves 6-month outcome in critically ill patients. Crit Care Med 30:2032–2037
14. Griffiths RD, Allen KD, Andrews FJ et al (2002) Infection, multiple organ failure, and survival in the intensive care unit: influence of glutamine-supplemented parenteral nutrition on acquired infection. Nutrition 18:546–552
15. Dechelotte P, Hasselmann M, Cynober L et al (2006) L-alanyl-L-glutamine dipeptide-supplemented total parenteral nutrition reduces infectious complications and glucose intolerance in critically ill patients: the French controlled, randomized, double-blind, multicenter study. Crit Care Med 34:598–604
16. Garrel D, Patenaude J, Nedelec B et al (2003) Decreased mortality and infectious morbidity in adult burn patients given enteral glutamine supplements: a prospective, controlled, randomized clinical trial. Crit Care Med 31:2444–2449
17. Zhou YP, Jiang ZM, Sun YH et al (2003) The effect of supplemental enteral glutamine on plasma levels, gut function, and outcome in severe burns: a randomized, double-blind, controlled clinical trial. J Parenter Enter Nutr 27:241–245
18. Peng X, Yan H, You Z et al (2004) Effects of enteral supplementation with glutamine granules on intestinal mucosal barrier function in severe burned patients. Burns 30:135–139
19. Houdijk AP, Rijnsburger ER, Jansen J et al (1998) Randomised trial of glutamine-enriched enteral nutrition on infectious morbidity in patients with multiple trauma. Lancet 352:772–776
20. Hall JC, Dobb G, Hall J et al (2003) Prospective randomized trial of enteral glutamine in critical illness. Intensive Care Med 29:1710–1716
21. Heyland D, Muscedere J, Wischmeyer PE et al (2013) A randomized trial of glutamine and antioxidants in critically ill patients. N Engl J Med 368:1489–1497
22. Lefrant JY, Hurel D, Cano NJ et al (2014) Guidelines for nutrition support in critically ill patient. Ann Fr Anesth Reanim 33(3):202–218
23. Mesejo A, Vaquerizo Alonso C, Acosta Escribano J et al (2011) Guidelines for specialized nutritional and metabolic support in the critically-ill patient. Update. Consensus of the Spanish

Society of Intensive Care Medicine and Coronary Units-Spanish Society of Parenteral and Enteral Nutrition (SEMICYUC-SENPE). Nutr Hosp 26(Suppl 2):1–85
24. Bansal V, Ochoa JB (2003) Arginine availability, arginase, and the immune response. Curr Opin Clin Nutr Metab Care 6:223–228
25. Vermeulen MA, van de Poll MC, Ligthart-Melis GC et al (2007) Specific amino acids in the critically ill patient—exogenous glutamine/arginine: a common denominator? Crit Care Med 35:S568–S576
26. Chiarla C, Giovannini I, Siegel JH (2006) Plasma arginine correlations in trauma and sepsis. Amino Acids 30:81–86
27. Druml W, Heinzel G, Kleinberger G (2001) Amino acid kinetics in patients with sepsis. Am J Clin Nutr 73:908–913
28. Luiking YC, Poeze M, Ramsay G et al (2009) Reduced citrulline production in sepsis is related to diminished de novo arginine and nitric oxide production. Am J Clin Nutr 89:142–152
29. Stechmiller JK, Childress B, Porter T (2004) Arginine immunonutrition in critically ill patients: a clinical dilemma. Am J Crit Care 13:17–23
30. Waitzberg DL, Torrinhas RS (2009) Fish oil lipid emulsions and immune response: what clinicians need to know. Nutr Clin Pract 24:487–499
31. Heller AR, Rössler S, Litz RJ (2006) Omega-3 fatty acids improve the diagnosis-related clinical outcome. Crit Care Med 34:972–979
32. Tsekos E, Reuter C, Stehle P et al (2004) Perioperative administration of fish oil supplements in a routine clinical setting improves patient outcome after major abdominal surgery. Clin Nutr 23:325–330
33. Gadek JE, DeMichele SJ, Karlstad MD et al (1999) Effect of enteral feeding with eicosapentaenoic acid, gamma-linolenic acid, and antioxidants in patients with acute respiratory distress syndrome. Crit Care Med 27:1409–1420
34. Singer P, Theilla M, Fisher H et al (2006) Benefit of an enteral diet enriched with eicosapentaenoic acid and gamma-linolenic acid in ventilated patients with acute lung injury. Crit Care Med 34:1033–1038
35. Pontes-Arruda A, Aragão AM, Albuquerque JD (2006) Effects of enteral feeding with eicosapentaenoic acid, gamma-linolenic acid, and antioxidants in mechanically ventilated patients with severe sepsis and septic shock. Crit Care Med 34:2325–2333
36. Pontes-Arruda A, DeMichele S, Seth A et al (2008) The use of an inflammation modulating diet in patients with acute lung injury or acute respiratory distress syndrome: a meta-analysis evaluation of outcome data. J Parenter Enter Nutr 32:596–605
37. Preiser JC (2008) Nutrition therapy for the acute respiratory distress syndrome. J Parenter Enter Nutr 32:669–670
38. Goodyear-Bruch C, Pierce JD (2002) Oxidative stress in critically ill patients. Am J Crit Care 11:543–551
39. Lovat R, Preiser JC (2003) Antioxidant therapy in intensive care. Curr Opin Crit Care 9:266–270
40. Motoyama T, Okamoto K, Kukita I et al (2003) Possible role of increased oxidant stress in multiple organ failure after systemic inflammatory response syndrome. Crit Care Med 31:1048–1052
41. Alonso de Vega JM, Diaz J, Serrano E, Carbonell LF (2002) Oxidative stress in critically ill patients with systemic inflammatory response syndrome. Crit Care Med 30:1782–1786
42. Preiser JC, Van Gossum A, Berre J et al (2000) Enteral feeding with a solution enriched with antioxidant vitamins A, C, and E enhances the resistance to oxidative stress. Crit Care Med 28:3828–3832
43. Nathens AB, Neff MJ, Jurkovich GJ et al (2002) Randomized, prospective trial of antioxidant supplementation in critically ill surgical patients. Ann Surg 236:814–822
44. Crimi E, Liguori A, Condorelli M et al (2004) The beneficial effects of antioxidant supplementation in enteral feeding in critically ill patients: a prospective, randomized, double-blind, placebo-controlled trial. Anesth Analg 99:857–863

45. Berger MM, Shenkin A (1998) Trace elements in trauma and burns. Curr Opin Clin Nutr Metab Care 1:513–517
46. Berger MM, Chiolero RL (2007) Antioxidant supplementation in sepsis and systemic inflammatory response syndrome. Crit Care Med 35:S584–S590
47. Angstwurm MW, Engelmann L, Zimmermann T et al (2007) Selenium in intensive care (SIC): results of a prospective randomized, placebo-controlled, multiple-center study in patients with severe systemic inflammatory response syndrome, sepsis, and septic shock. Crit Care Med 35:118–126
48. Singer P, Berger MM, Van den Berghe G et al (2009) ESPEN guidelines in parenteral nutrition: Intensive Care. Clin Nutr 28:387–400
49. Kreymann KG, Berger MM, Deutz NEP et al (2006) ESPEN guidelines on enteral nutrition: intensive care. Clin Nutr 25:210–223

Oxygen and Oxidative Stress 20

Jean-Christophe Orban and Mervyn Singer

20.1 Introduction

Oxygen is a structural and functional compound essential to life. Evoking the toxicity of this molecule could seem inappropriate or even provocative. After its discovery by Priestley in 1774, Lavoisier named it "oxygen" from the Greek words *oxys* and *gennan* meaning "generating acid". At the same time, he demonstrated its essential role in respiration. This emphasized immediately the duality of this molecule to which the vast majority of living organisms have had to adapt, especially as, in particular circumstances, oxygen can be harmful because of its oxidative characteristics.

20.2 Reactive Oxygen Species, Antioxidant Defences and Oxidative Stress [1–3]

20.2.1 Reactive Oxygen Species

Oxygen is a weak reactive free radical, mostly found as dioxygen. It is utilized in the generation of reactive oxygen species (ROS), levels of which can rise markedly in certain pathological conditions such as ischaemia-reperfusion injury and sepsis. ROS molecules are numerous, with some existing as free radicals (containing an

J.-C. Orban (✉)
Intensive Care Unit, Hôpital Pasteur 2, 30 Voie Romaine, 06001 Nice, Cedex, France
e-mail: orban.jc@chu-nice.fr

M. Singer
Bloomsbury Institute of Intensive Care Medicine, University College London,
Cruciform Building, Gower Street, London WC1E 6BT, UK

C. Ichai et al. (eds.), *Metabolic Disorders and Critically Ill Patients*,
http://doi.org/10.1007/978-3-319-64010-5_20

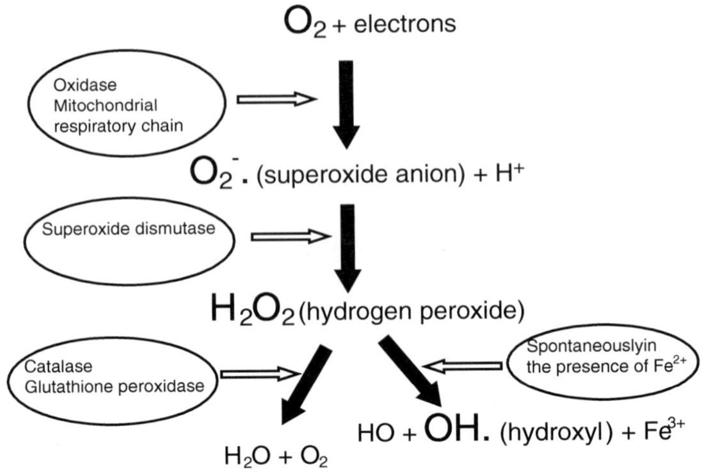

Fig. 20.1 Main reactive oxygen species and antioxidant enzymes

unpaired valence electron). The most important ROS are superoxide ion, hydrogen peroxide, hydroxyl radical, hypochlorite and peroxynitrite (Fig. 20.1). Superoxide ion can form spontaneously, from various enzymes (e.g. NADPH oxidase) or from the mitochondrial electron transport chain. It is converted by superoxide dismutase to the less reactive hydrogen peroxide which, in turn, is transformed to water and oxygen by catalase and glutathione peroxidase. In the presence of transition metals in free form (iron and copper), hydroxyl radical – the most reactive and thus most toxic ROS – may result.

Mitochondria are the main source of ROS within the body. In health, nearly 2% of oxygen used by the mitochondrial respiratory chain generates ROS. Other enzymes are also responsible for ROS generation such as oxidases (NADPH oxidase, myeloperoxidase), and these are involved in the neutrophil respiratory burst.

Some conditions lead to an excessive ROS production, in particular those related to inflammation and ischaemia-reperfusion. This latter phenomenon is characterized by the succession of an ischaemia phase (no energetic substrate and oxygen) by reperfusion, with restoration of normal (or even supranormal due to increased blood flow) oxygen conditions. Contrary to what is commonly assumed, ischaemia is often less deleterious than reperfusion. Thus, elevated production of ROS occurs during ischaemia [4] and this is sharply increased during reperfusion [5, 6]. Here, mitochondria and xanthine oxidoreductase generate large amounts of ROS. This latter enzyme normally uses NAD as electron acceptor; however, after ischaemia-reperfusion, it uses oxygen resulting in the production of superoxide.

Deleterious effects of ROS are well known as they react with lipids, proteins and DNA leading to structural and functional changes. However, ROS are also involved in essential physiological processes such as the phagocyte respiratory burst and intracellular signalling [7] and also play a protective role in ischemic preconditioning [8].

20.2.2 Antioxidants

An antioxidant is a molecule or enzyme that, in small amounts, can prevent or delay substrate oxidation [9]. Several types of antioxidant defences can be distinguished:

20.2.2.1 Enzymatic Antioxidant Defences

Three enzymes play an essential role in ROS scavenging.

Superoxide dismutase (SOD) catalyses conversion of two superoxide ions and two protons into hydrogen peroxide and oxygen [10]. SOD is found in numerous species [11]. In humans, three isoforms are described depending on their metal cofactor and location. SOD1 and SOD3 have copper/zinc cofactors. SOD1 is located in the cytosol and the nucleus, while SOD3 is extracellular and thought to play an important role in the vascular tone regulated by nitric oxide by preventing superoxide accumulation [12]. SOD2 has a manganese cofactor and is located within the mitochondria. It is essential to tamper oxidative stress coming from the respiratory chain.

Catalase transforms hydrogen peroxide into oxygen and water, decreasing its half-life and also generation of hydroxyl radicals. It is a tetrameric complex containing a heme and is located mainly in peroxisomes. Catalase is linked to NADPH that protects and enhances its activity [13].

Glutathione peroxidase oxidizes glutathione by taking an electron from hydrogen peroxide [4]. It can also react with other substrates such as lipids, thus explaining its protective effects against lipid peroxidation. The active site contains a selenium molecule. This ubiquitous enzyme is found mainly in cytosol and mitochondria and represents one of the most important antioxidant defences of the organism.

20.2.2.2 Non-enzymatic Antioxidant Defences

Glutathione is a tripeptide composed of cysteine, glutamine and glycine. Quantitatively, it is the most important antioxidant defence molecule as intracellular concentrations are high (1–10 mM). The reduced form (GSH) has direct antioxidant properties, and it is also the cofactor for glutathione peroxidase. Once oxidized to glutathione disulphide (GSSG), it is reduced by glutathione reductase in the presence of NADPH. The glutathione disulphide/glutathione couple is the main thiol involved in intracellular redox balance.

Albumin is the main plasma thiol compound and is a major antioxidant. Vitamins A, C and E also have antioxidant properties. Vitamins C and E regenerate mutually after oxidation. Other natural compounds have antioxidant properties such as flavonoids, carotenoids, thioredoxin and some metalloproteins.

20.2.2.3 Pharmacological Defences

Numerous drugs used commonly in intensive care unit or operating theatre environments offer antioxidant properties. N-Acetylcysteine is a compound containing combination of a sulfhydryl (thiol) and acetyl groups. The thiol group is responsible for the molecule's activity, whereas the acetyl group stabilizes the compound. As a source of cysteine, the antioxidant activity of acetylcysteine comes from increases in glutathione synthesis and in glutathione-S-transferase activity and by a direct action on ROS. It replenishes glutathione stocks and enhances its synthesis when utilization is increased. Propofol has a structure close to that of vitamin E explaining its antioxidant properties.

Halogenates trigger pharmacological preconditioning, exercising protective effects through reducing oxidative stress as well as via other mechanisms. Allopurinol inhibits xanthine oxidase activity that is responsible of ROS generation after, for example, ischaemia-reperfusion. Iron-binding compounds diminish the Fenton reaction and thus reduce hydroxyl radical production.

20.2.3 Oxidative Stress

While ROS are being generated continually, this phenomenon is balanced by antioxidant production. Any imbalance in favour of ROS results in an oxidative stress. This arises from an increase in ROS generation and/or decrease in antioxidant levels/activity. In critical illness this disequilibrium is often acute but, in numerous diseases, may be chronic (COPD, heart failure, renal failure, diabetes mellitus, etc.…).

Direct measurement of ROS levels is very difficult due to their extremely short half-life, (approximately 1 ns). Only complex laboratory techniques such as spin resonance or spin trapping permit direct measurement; however, these techniques are difficult to use in clinical practice. Thus, markers of oxidative injury or reductions in antioxidant levels be it enzymatic (SOD, catalase, GPX) or non-enzymatic (glutathione, thiols, vitamins, etc.) are most frequently measured as indicators of oxidative stress. The effects of ROS on different structures can be demonstrated in different ways. Terminal lipid peroxidation can be evaluated by isoprostane or TBARS (thiobarbituric acid reactive species) levels. Malondialdehyde, commonly measured in numerous clinical studies, is a TBARS. Carbonyls result from protein alterations, while nitration, chlorination and hydroxylation of amino acids indicate the action of ROS on different protein structures. Levels of 8-hydroxydeoxyguanosine evaluate DNA modifications.

20.3 Clinical Data

20.3.1 Oxidative Stress and Diseases

The importance of oxidative stress is being increasingly recognized in the pathophysiology of cardiovascular diseases, cancer, infectious diseases, diabetes and ageing [14–17].

Oxidative stress is associated with many situations in the ICU. In shock states oxidative stress results from ischaemia-reperfusion and activation of inflammatory cells. An increase in ROS generation correlated with clinical severity during both haemorrhagic [18] and septic [19] shock. Multiple organ failure is characterized by a decrease in antioxidant defences [20] and an increase in markers of lipid peroxidation [21] and is associated with a poor prognosis [21] though cause and effect remains uncertain.

Severe lung diseases such as ARDS and ALI are also associated with oxidative stress as assessed by increases in lipid peroxidation [22, 23] and protein carbonylation [24] and decreases in plasma thiols [25]. Here the cause of oxidative stress appears to be the activation of inflammatory cells and the use of high fractions of inspired oxygen.

Oxidative stress has also been demonstrated in brain injury and subarachnoid haemorrhage. In trauma patients, ischaemia increases ROS production, while in subarachnoid haemorrhage, the process differs due to iron released from haemoglobin in the subarachnoid space generating large amounts of hydroxyl radical [26]. This may potentially explain the presence of arterial vasospasm after subarachnoid haemorrhage, with the degree of oxidative stress being correlated with a poor outcome [27, 28].

The best example of whole-body ischaemia-reperfusion injury is resuscitated cardiac arrest. This should be associated with a major oxidative stress; however, to date, only one study has reported an increase in lipid peroxidation markers [29]. Indirect proof is however provided by a recent retrospective study showing a relationship between high partial pressures of oxygen on arrival in critical care and poor outcome after resuscitated cardiac arrest [30]. One possible explanation could be increased oxidative stress due to hyperoxia.

During surgery, oxidative stress is present in situations involving ischaemia-reperfusion. Release of a limb tourniquet results in a significant oxidative stress over the first few minutes after deflation but has no systemic impact [31], while the sequence of vascular occlusion and recirculation during vascular or cardiovascular surgery is also associated with increased oxidative stress [32]. Solid organ transplantation also represents a quasi-experimental ischaemia-reperfusion. Harvested organs from brain-dead donors are exposed to ischaemia but remain under protection due to hypothermia. After grafting, reperfusion leads to an increase in oxidative stress [33]. Increased malondialdehyde is reported soon after recirculation of kidney transplants [34], while, after liver transplantation, elevation of malondialdehyde begins in the first hour and can last for up to a week afterwards [35]. Antioxidant enzymes also increase post-transplant yet exhibit different kinetics.

20.3.2 Antioxidant Treatments

As reactive oxygen species are involved in the pathophysiology of many diseases, it is an obvious step to evaluate treatments that reduce or protect against oxidative stress.

N-acetylcysteine is, by far, the most tested molecule because of its good antioxidant properties increasing glutathione synthesis and its lack of severe side effects. It is best known as an antidote to acetaminophen poisoning where high doses replenish low glutathione levels. However, similar doses given in septic shock patients yielded unconvincing results. Obviously, n-acetylcysteine increases antioxidant defences, but the effect on cytokines is inconsistent [36, 37]. Only one study has reported a mortality benefit albeit in a small sample size [38]. All of these studies utilized high-dose acetaminophen, but it is now known that high antioxidant levels can lead to detrimental pro-oxidant effects. Several studies have evaluated the impact of low-dose acetaminophen on renal function after major surgery, but no benefit could be ascertained on meta-analysis [39]. This emphasizes the point that oxidative stress is not a "common" phenomenon that could be treated by a "common" antioxidant therapy.

Albumin infusion has been assessed in ARDS and septic patients [25]. It restores the balance between ROS and antioxidants by replenishing the thiol pool. However, this intervention did not improve morbidity and mortality. Recent randomized controlled studies (ALBIOS and EARSS) assessing albumin supplementation in septic shock patients have yet to be published.

The antioxidant effects of several vitamins are well known. Supplemental administration of vitamins C and E decreased mortality (45.7% vs. 67.5%) in ICU patients [40]; however, the control group received lower vitamin supplementation than usually recommended (50 mg vitamin C and 10 IU vitamin E). This study may have simply demonstrated harm from vitamin deficiency. The REDOXS study recently evaluated glutamine and an antioxidant mix of vitamins (beta-carotene, vitamins C and E) and minerals (selenium and zinc) on mortality in a general (albeit mainly medical) ICU population [41]. While antioxidants had no effect, there was a higher mortality rate in those receiving glutamine. In trauma patients, high-dose vitamins decreased ICU and hospital stay and mortality, with benefit appearing to be greater in the most severe patients [42, 43]. Taken together these results indicate that antioxidant deprivation is deleterious while supplementation is questionable.

Propofol infusion during surgery using a pneumatic tourniquet reduces oxidative stress after deflation [44], yet the clinical significance remains unknown. Another means of decreasing oxidative stress is by ischemic preconditioning. This consists of short periods of ischaemia which allows organs to cope better with longer periods of ischaemia. A decrease in oxidative stress is one of the beneficial effects of ischemic preconditioning reported after reperfusion [45]. Originally reported in dog myocardium [46], it has been replicated in varied organs such as the liver, brain or kidney. In clinical practice, ischemic preconditioning enhanced myocardial contractile function post-cardiac surgery and decreased ventricular fibrillation and tachyarrhythmia and cellular injury [47, 48]. Remote ischemic preconditioning can be induced by initiating the process on an arm, thereby inducing a protective effect on a distant organ. Three sequences of inflation/deflation of a cuff placed on an arm resulted in lower troponin levels after cardiac surgery [49] and renal injury after major aortic surgery [49]. The beneficial effects of ischemic preconditioning can be reproduced using drugs such as halogenates and may be as efficient [50].

Conclusions

Oxygen is a deadly poison yet is essential to life. Numerous physiological defences control this "fire"; however, oxidative stress may result from an imbalance occurring in numerous pathological situations. Knowledge of all underlying mechanisms remains incomplete. Reactive oxygen species also have essential physiological functions. While in some cases, the modulation of oxidative stress is beneficial, in others it has no effect or may be harmful. Many outstanding questions surround antioxidant treatments, in particular related to timing of commencement, duration of treatment, dosage and type.

References

1. Favier A (2006) Stress oxydant et pathologie humaine. Ann Pharm Fr 64:390–396
2. Kohen R, Nyska A (2002) Oxidation of biological systems: oxidative stress phenomena, antioxidants, redox reactions, and methods for their quantification. Toxicol Pathol 30:620–650
3. Droge W (2002) Free radicals in the physiological control of cell function. Physiol Rev 82:47–95
4. Levraut J, Iwase H, Shao ZH, Vanden Hoek TL, Schumacker PT (2003) Cell death during ischemia: relationship to mitochondrial depolarization and ROS generation. Am J Physiol Heart Circ Physiol 284:549–558
5. Piper HM, Garcia-Dorado D, Ovize M (1998) A fresh look at reperfusion injury. Cardiovasc Res 38:291–300
6. Vanden Hoek TL (2002) Preconditioning and postresuscitation injury. Crit Care Med 30:S172–S175
7. Dahlgren C, Karlsson A (1999) Respiratory burst in human neutrophils. J Immunol Methods 232:3–14
8. Lebuffe G, Schumacker PT, Shao ZH, Anderson T, Iwase H, Vanden Hoek TL (2003) ROS and NO trigger early preconditioning: relationship to mitochondrial KATP channel. Am J Physiol Heart Circ Physiol 284:H299–H308
9. Halliwell B, Gutteridge JM (1988) Free radicals and antioxidants protection: mechanisms and significance in toxicology and disease. Hum Toxicol 7:7–13
10. Fridovich I (1995) Superoxide radical and superoxide dismutases. Annu Rev Biochem 64:97–112
11. Richier S, Merle PL, Furla P, Pigozzi D, Sola F, Allemand D (2003) Characterization of superoxide dismutases in anoxia- and hyperoxia-tolerant symbiotic cnidarians. Biochim Biophys Acta 1621:84–91
12. Schnackenberg CG, Welch WJ, Wilcox CS (1998) Normalization of blood pressure and renal vascular resistance in SHR with a membrane-permeable superoxide dismutase mimetic: role of nitric oxide. Hypertension 32:59–64
13. Kirkman HN, Rolfo M, Ferraris AM, Gaetani GF (1999) Mechanisms of protection of catalase by NADPH. Kinetics and stoichiometry J Biol Chem 274:13908–13914
14. Giacco F, Brownlee M (2010) Oxidative stress and diabetic complications. Circ Res 107:1058–1070
15. Briones AM, Touyz RM (2010) Oxidative stress and hypertension: current concepts. Curr Hypertens Rep 12:135–142
16. Khaper N, Bryan S, Dhingra S, Singal R, Bajaj A, Pathak CM, Singal PK (2010) Targeting the vicious inflammation-oxidative stress cycle for the management of heart failure. Antioxid Redox Signal 13:1033–1049
17. Romano AD, Serviddio G, de Matthaeis A, Bellanti F, Vendemiale G (2010) Oxidative stress and aging. J Nephrol 23:S29–S36

18. Laplace C, Huet O, Vicaut E, Ract C, Martin L, Benhamou D, Duranteau J (2005) Endothelial oxidative stress induced by serum from patients with severe trauma hemorrhage. Intensive Care Med 31:1174–1180
19. Huet O, Obata R, Aubron C, Spraul-Davit A, Charpentier J, Laplace C, Nguyen-Khoa T, Conti M, Vicaut E, Mira JP, Duranteau J (2007) Plasma-induced endothelial oxidative stress is related to the severity of septic shock. Crit Care Med 35:821–826
20. Fläring UB, Rooyackers OE, Hebert C, Bratel T, Hammarqvist F, Wernerman J (2005) Temporal changes in whole-blood and plasma glutathione in ICU patients with multiple organ failure. Intensive Care Med 31:1072–1078
21. Motoyama T, Okamoto K, Kukita I, Hamaguchi M, Kinoshita Y, Ogawa H (2003) Possible role of increased oxidant stress in multiple organ failure after systemic inflammatory response syndrome. Crit Care Med 31:1048–1052
22. Carpenter CT, Price PV, Christman BW (1998) Exhaled breath condensate isoprostanes are elevated in patients with acute lung injury or ARDS. Chest 114:1653–1659
23. Quinlan GJ, Lamb NJ, Evans TW, Gutteridge JM (1996) Plasma fatty acid changes and increased lipid peroxidation in patients with adult respiratory distress syndrome. Crit Care Med 24:241–246
24. Lamb NJ, Quinlan GJ, Westerman ST, Gutteridge JM, Evans TW (1999) Nitration of proteins in bronchoalveolar lavage fluid from patients with acute respiratory distress syndrome receiving inhaled nitric oxide. Am J Respir Crit Care Med 160:1031–1034
25. Quinlan GJ, Mumby S, Martin GS, Bernard GR, Gutteridge JM, Evans TW (2004) Albumin influences total plasma antioxidant capacity favorably in patients with acute lung injury. Crit Care Med 32:755–759
26. Asano T (1999) Oxyhemoglobin as the principal cause of cerebral vasospasm: a holistic view of its actions. Crit Rev Neurosurg 9:303–318
27. Polidori MC, Mecocci P, Frei B (2001) Plasma vitamin C levels are decreased and correlated with brain damage in patients with intracranial hemorrhage or head trauma. Stroke 32:898–902
28. Gaetani P, Pasqualin A, Rodriguez y Baena R, Borasio E, Marzatico F (1998) Oxidative stress in the human brain after subarachnoid hemorrhage. J Neurosurg 89:748–754
29. Déroche D, Orban JC, Garrel C, Ferrari P, Levraut J, Ichai C (2009) Evaluation du stress oxydant après cardiaque extra-hospitalier traité par hypothermie. Ann Fr Anesth Réanim 28:S170
30. Kilgannon JH, Jones AE, Shapiro NI, Angelos MG, Milcarek B, Hunter K, Parrillo JE, Trzeciak S, Emergency Medicine Shock Research Network (EMShockNet) Investigators (2010) Association between arterial hyperoxia following resuscitation from cardiac arrest and in-hospital mortality. JAMA 303:2165–2171
31. Mathru M, Dries DJ, Barnes L, Tonino P, Sukhani R, Rooney MW (1996) Tourniquet-induced exsanguination in patients requiring lower limb surgery. An ischemia-reperfusion model of oxidant and antioxidant metabolism. Anesthesiology 84:14–22
32. Kretzschmar M, Klein U, Palutke M, Schirrmeister W (1996) Reduction of ischemia-reperfusion syndrome after abdominal aortic aneurysmectomy by N-acetylcysteine but not mannitol. Acta Anaesthesiol Scand 40:657–664
33. Basu S, Meisert I, Eggensperger E, Krieger E, Krenn CG (2007) Time course and attenuation of ischaemia-reperfusion induced oxidative injury by propofol in human renal transplantation. Redox Rep 12:195–202
34. Biernacki M, Bigda J, Jankowski K, Wozniak M, Sledziński Z (2002) Increased serum levels of markers of oxidative stress during kidney transplantation. Transplant Proc 34:544–545
35. Hassan L, Bueno P, Ferrón-Celma I, Ramia JM, Garrote D, Muffak K, García-Navarro A, Mansilla A, Villar JM, Ferrón JA (2005) Time course of antioxidant enzyme activities in liver transplant recipients. Transplant Proc 37:3932–3935
36. Emet S, Memis D, Pamukçu Z (2004) The influence of N-acetyl-L-cysteine infusion on cytokine levels and gastric intramucosal pH during severe sepsis. Crit Care 8:172–179
37. Spapen H, Zhang H, Demanet C, Vleminckx W, Vincent JL, Huyghens L (1998) Does N-acetyl-L-cysteine influence cytokine response during early human septic shock? Chest 113:1616–1624

38. Ortolani O, Conti A, De Gaudio AR, Moraldi E, Cantini Q, Novelli G (2000) The effect of glutathione and N-acetylcysteine on lipoperoxidative damage in patients with early septic shock. Am J Respir Crit Care Med 161:1907–1911
39. Ho KM, Morgan DJ (2009) Meta-analysis of N-acetylcysteine to prevent acute renal failure after major surgery. Am J Kidney Dis 53:33–40
40. Crimi E, Liguori A, Condorelli M, Cioffi M, Astuto M, Bontempo P, Pignalosa O, Vietri MT, Molinari AM, Sica V, Della Corte F, Napoli C (2004) The beneficial effects of antioxidant supplementation in enteral feeding in critically ill patients: a prospective, randomized, double-blind, placebo-controlled trial. Anesth Analg 99:857–863
41. Heyland D, Muscedere J, Wischmeyer PE, Cook D, Jones G, Albert M, et al. A randomized trial of glutamine and antioxidants in critically ill patients. N Engl J Med. 2013;368:1489–97
42. Nathens AB, Neff MJ, Jurkovich GJ, Klotz P, Farver K, Ruzinski JT, Radella F, Garcia I, Maier RV (2002) Randomized, prospective trial of antioxidant supplementation in critically ill surgical patients. Ann Surg 236:814–822
43. Collier BR, Giladi A, Dossett LA, Dyer L, Fleming SB, Cotton BA (2008) Impact of high-dose antioxidants on outcomes in acutely injured patients. JPEN J Parenter Enteral Nutr 3:384–388
44. Cheng YJ, Wang YP, Chien CT, Chen CF (2002) Small-dose propofol sedation attenuates the formation of reactive oxygen species in tourniquet-induced ischemia-reperfusion injury under spinal anesthesia. Anesth Analg 94:1617–1620
45. Vanden Hoek T, Becker LB, Shao ZH, Li CQ, Schumacker PT (2000) Preconditioning in cardiomyocytes protects by attenuating oxidant stress at reperfusion. Circ Res 86:541–548
46. Murry CE, Jennings RB, Reimer KA (1986) Preconditioning with ischemia: a delay of lethal cell injury in ischemic myocardium. Circulation 74:1124–1136
47. Wu ZK, Tarkka MR, Pehkonen E, Kaukinen L, Honkonen EL, Kaukinen S (2000) Ischaemic preconditioning has a beneficial effect on left ventricular haemodynamic function after a coronary artery biopass grafting operation. Scand Cardiovasc J 34:247–253
48. Wu ZK, Iivainen T, Pehkonen E, Laurikka J, Tarkka MR (2002) Ischemic preconditioning suppresses ventricular tachyarrhythmias after myocardial revascularization. Circulation 106:3091–3096
49. Hausenloy DJ, Mwamure PK, Venugopal V, Harris J, Barnard M, Grundy E, Ashley E, Vichare S, Di Salvo C, Kolvekar S, Hayward M, Keogh B, MacAllister RJ, Yellon DM (2007) Effect of remote ischaemic preconditioning on myocardial injury in patients undergoing coronary artery bypass graft surgery: a randomised controlled trial. Lancet 370:575–579
50. Zaugg M, Lucchinetti E, Spahn DR, Pasch T, Schaub MC (2002) Volatile anesthetics mimic cardiac preconditioning by priming the activation of mitochondrial K(ATP) channels via multiple signaling pathways. Anesthesiology 97:4–14

Energy Metabolism: From the Organ to the Cell

21

Hervé Quintard, Eric Fontaine, and Carole Ichai

Our survival state depends on serial metabolic reactions needing energy. Our environmental feed is the principal source of this energy. The purpose of this chapter is to describe all the organic and cellular mechanisms involved in this production.

21.1 Organic Energy Metabolism

Energy expenditure is delivered in three principal ways: basal metabolism (BM), thermoregulation, and muscular exercise.

21.1.1 Basal Metabolism (BM)

It represents nearly 60% of total energy expenditure. It's the basal needing of our organism at rest, to maintain homeostatic cellular condition. It depends on cellular type and so on thin mass. This one is composed essentially by muscular and bone tissue. We understand so easily that this one depends on age, sex, and genetics. Moreover cutaneous tissue is an important way of exchange with environmental explaining basal metabolism depending also on cutaneous surface. Hormonal status can also impact on basal metabolism particularly thyroid status.

In medical practice basal metabolism evaluation is based on Harris and Benedict equation, using weight (W), size (S), sex, and age (A):

H. Quintard (✉) • C. Ichai
Service de Réanimation Médicochirurgicale, CHU de Nice, Hôpital Pasteur 2,
30 voie romaine, 06000 Nice, France
e-mail: quintard.h@chu-nice.fr

E. Fontaine
INSERM, U1055, Grenoble, France

Université Joseph Fourier, Grenoble, France

C. Ichai et al. (eds.), *Metabolic Disorders and Critically Ill Patients*,
http://doi.org/10.1007/978-3-319-64010-5_21

$$
\begin{aligned}
\text{Women : BM} &= 2.741 + 0.0402\text{W} + 0.711\text{S} - 0.0197\text{A} \\
\text{Men : BM} &= 0.276 + 0.0573\text{W} + 2.073\text{S} - 0.0285\text{A}
\end{aligned}
$$

with W in kg, S in m, and A in year.

21.1.2 Thermoregulation

Inversely from other species, mammals conserve at constant temperature in whatever environmental condition. This phenomenon, named thermoregulation, has an important energy cost because freezing or sweating is needed to maintain temperature. It is completely different from other species as a crocodile, for example, needs only one chicken by week because of an economic metabolism depending on environmental condition with no thermoregulation.

21.1.3 Muscular Exercise

It is the most variable part of energy metabolism depending on habitus and way of life. This muscular expenditure can raise to 1000 kCal over 8 h in particular extreme sportive conditions (ultra, triathlon, etc.). In the same way, a 5 km running corresponds to a 375 kCal expenditure (Fig. 21.1).

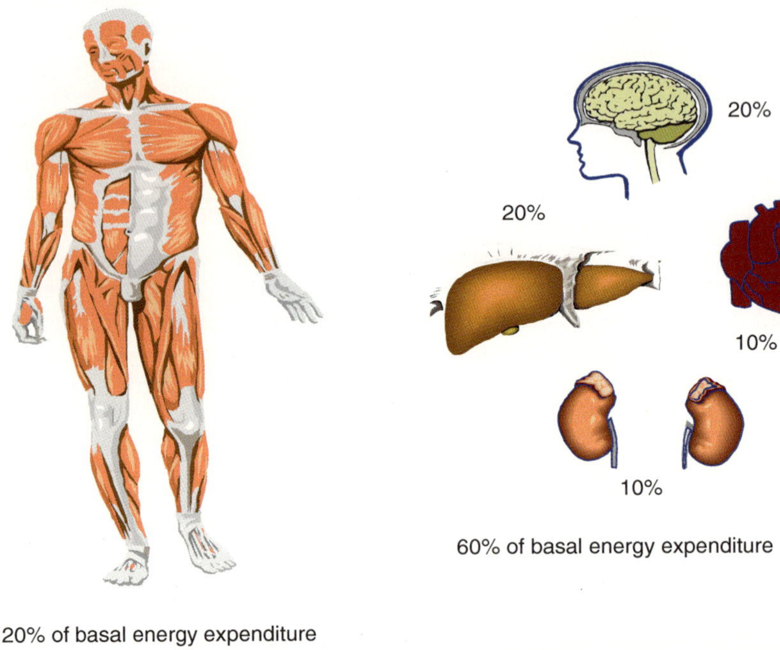

Fig. 21.1 Distribution of basal energy expenditure by different organs. While the brain, heart, liver, and kidneys account for only 5% of the total body mass, these organs alone account for nearly 60% of the basal energy expenditure. Muscle mass is much larger in terms of body mass but consumes at rest only 20% of the basal energy expenditure

Table 21.1. Energy expenditure and power developed in different physiological and pathological situations in a young 70 kg adult

Situation	Energy expenditure	Power (watts)
Resting energy expenditure	1600–1800 kcal/day	75–85 W
Daily energy expenditure	2300–2500 kcal/day	110–120 W
Cold exposure	370 kcal/3 h	Mean 150 W, max 350 W
Polytrauma	1900–2200 kcal/day	90–100 W
Serious infection	2100–2700 kcal/day	100–130 W
Great burnt	2500–3600 kcal/day	120–170 W
Weight lifting	2–5 kcal in 0.88 s	8000–25,000 W
100 m	12 kcal in 10 s	5000 W
5000 m	375 kcal in 13 min	2000 W
Marathon	3200 kcal in 2 h 10	1700 W
Triathlon	10,000 kcal in 8 h	1400 W
Tour de France	200 Mcal in 23 days	415 W

21.1.4 Variability in Energy Metabolism

As we explained before, energy expenditure depends physiologically on several parameters: BM + thermoregulation + muscular exercise. By the way, this energy expenditure can be modified by critical illness. Basal metabolism is indeed directly implicated by illness and indirectly by neurohumoral response to sepsis, for example. This energy expenditure increased by illness can be modulated by control of hyperthermia. Moreover, all the organs are not equivalent in what they need; brain, heart, liver, and kidneys represent only 5% of body weight but over 50% of energy expenditure at basal situation. Organ composition has an impact also on metabolism. Indeed, adipose tissue doesn't need a lot of energy. So energy metabolism depends on body composition and importance of metabolic tissue in thick mass (Table 21.1.).

21.2 Energy Metabolism at Cellular Level

21.2.1 Basics [1–3]

The energy contained in carbohydrates, lipids, and proteins is used by the cell. As a first approximation, this energy corresponds to the redox energy of the hydrogen atoms of these molecules. During their catabolism, the nutrients are gradually cut into smaller and smaller molecules, releasing the hydrogen atoms and providing waste (CO_2, urea, ammonia, etc.). Catabolism consists of three main steps (Fig. 21.2):

- In the first group of reactions, the large molecules are decomposed into their constituent subunits, proteins into amino acids, polysaccharides into simple carbohydrates, and lipids into fatty acids and glycerol. This first step corresponds to digestion and mainly occurs outside the cell by the action of enzymes excreted in the intestinal lumen.

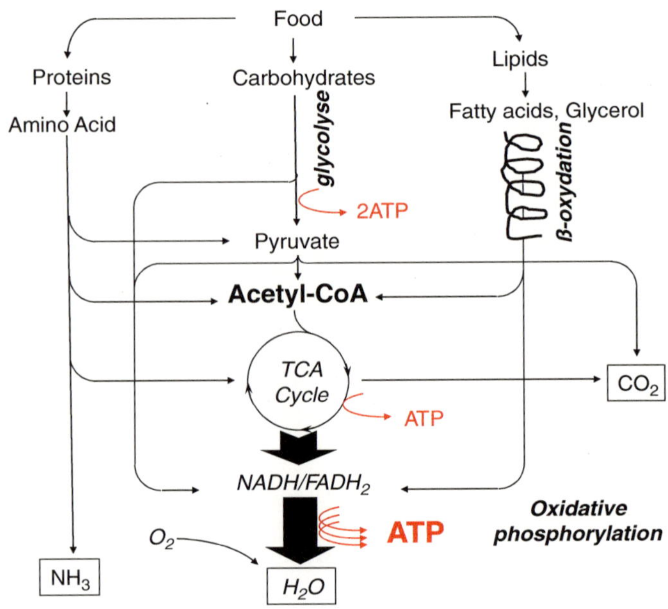

Fig. 21.2 The use of nutrients for ATP production. Fatty acids are metabolized by beta-oxidation, carbohydrates by glycolysis, and amino acids by deamination. Pyruvate is a metabolic intermediate common to carbohydrates and amino acids. Acetyl CoA is the common metabolite of all these nutrients, a metabolite that will be used in the TCA cycle. The latter allows the supply of reduced equivalents (NADH, FADH2), essential fuels for the respiratory chain, and the final production of ATP by oxidative phosphorylation. The final degradation products are water and CO_2, as well as ammonia from amino acids

- Once inside the cells, these nutrients are subsequently degraded by specific metabolic pathways: glycolysis, beta-oxidation, and deamination of amino acids. The release of energy during these reactions does not directly lead to the synthesis of ATP except during glycolysis. This second part of metabolism leads to the synthesis of acetyl CoA.
- The third group of reactions consists the TCA cycle and corresponds to a sequence in which acetyl CoA is completely degraded into CO_2 and hydrogen. CO_2, which is the thermodynamically most stable form of carbon, is eliminated from the body either as such or combined with ammonia (through ureogenesis). The hydrogen released during these various steps is not directly released in solution, but it is transferred to specific transporters: NAD+, which is reduced into NADH + H+ (simply denoted NADH) or FAD which is reduced into FADH2.

The energy in the hydrogen atoms is then released and used for ATP synthesis in a specialized intracellular organelle: the mitochondrion (Fig. 21.3). This reaction, called oxidative phosphorylation, corresponds to a set of biochemical reactions requiring two enzymatic complexes and the inner mitochondrial membrane. This membrane delimits the space inside mitochondria (the matrix). The two enzymatic complexes embedded in inner mitochondrial membrane are (Fig. 21.4):

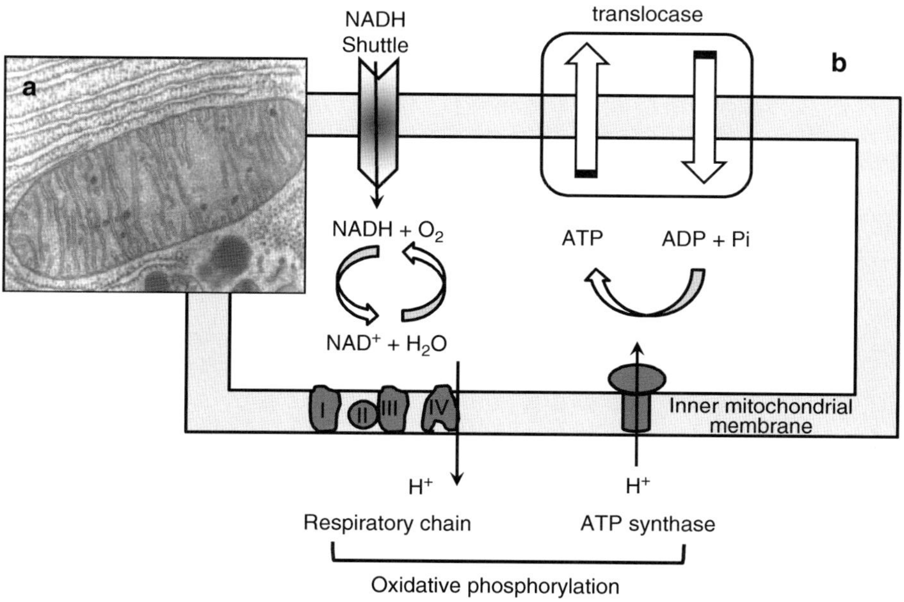

Fig. 21.3 ATP synthesis and oxygen used by mitochondria. A. Structure of a mitochondrion under electron microscopy. The mitochondria have two membranes: an outer and an inner membrane. This inner membrane is larger than the outer membrane and is therefore folded into the space delimited by the outer membrane. The inner membrane is impermeable to many solutes (including protons) and requires shuttle systems to be crossed. B. The reduced equivalents (NADH shown in the diagram) pass through the inner membrane via shuttle systems. They represent the substrates of the respiratory chain that functions in the presence of oxygen to produce a gradient of proton. The reentry of protons will release the energy necessary for ATP synthesis by the ATP synthase. ATP then comes out of the mitochondria through a transporter (ANT)

- The respiratory chain, which releases energy from hydrogen by consuming oxygen
- The ATP synthase, which uses this energy to synthesize ATP from ADP and Pi

The activity of these two enzyme complexes is coupled to a transport of protons across the membrane. The energy released during the combustion of hydrogen with oxygen is used by the respiratory chain to pump protons from the matrix, thus creating a gradient of protons from either side of the membrane. Just as the water contained in a dam is a form of energy that can be transformed into electricity, this gradient of proton is a force (a potential) pushing the protons back into the mitochondria. Since the membrane is almost impermeable to protons, they pass through the ATP synthase proton channel, thus allowing ATP synthesis. It must be to note, however, that the ATP synthase proton channel is not the only proton channel embedded in the inner membrane. Other reactions (mainly transporters) consume the gradient of proton. Consequently, the more such reactions increase, the more the yield of oxidative phosphorylation (the number of ATP synthesized per number of oxygen consumed) decreases.

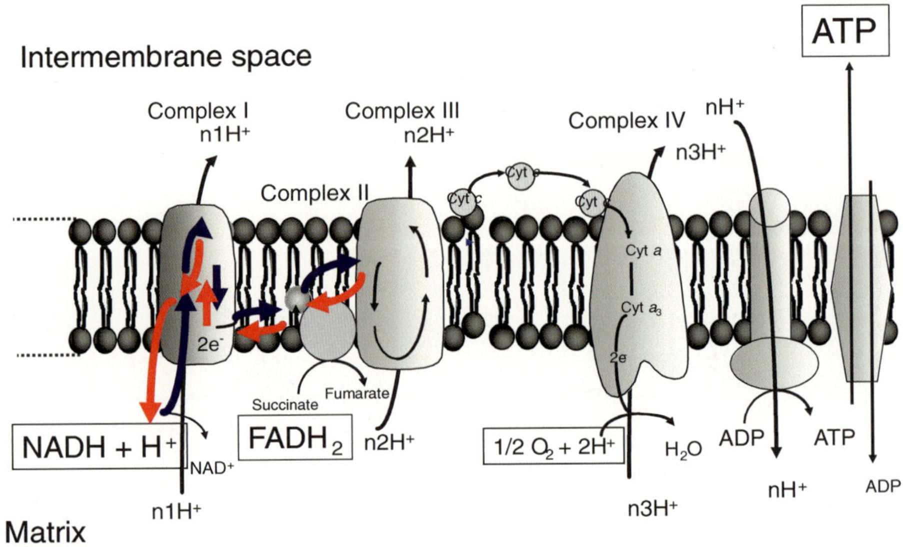

Fig. 21.4 Mitochondrial oxidative phosphorylation. The oxidative phosphorylation involves two enzymatic complexes. The first constitutes the respiratory chain, which consists of four complexes. Complexes I, III, and IV are proton pumps involved in the generation of a gradient of proton. Complex I uses NADH, whereas FADH2 enters directly at Complex II, thus bypassing Complex I. The second enzymatic complex is ATP synthase. The energy contained in the gradient of proton is then released during the reentry of protons into the matrix and used to synthesize ATP, which ultimately comes out of mitochondria through the adenine nucleotide transporter (ANT)

Besides the fact that a variable part of the gradient of proton is used for ATP synthesis, the number of protons pumped per oxygen consumed is also variable. This is due in particular to the fact that NADH and FADH2 are not thermodynamically identical and thus do not enter the respiratory chain at the same level. Without going into details, it must be remembered that NADH makes more gradient per unit of oxygen consumed than FADH2. Far from being anecdotal, this phenomenon explains the fundamental energy difference between carbohydrates and lipids. Indeed, the complete metabolism of carbohydrates (glycolysis plus TCA cycle) and lipids (beta-oxidation plus TCA cycle) releases proportionately more NADH for carbohydrates than for lipids. This explains why, by volume of oxygen consumed, carbohydrates are more energetic than lipids (Table 21.2). In other words, if oxygen consumption can be related to calorie consumption (taking into account the proportion of lipids and carbohydrates consumed), oxygen consumption can never be linked to ATP production.

Apart from the mitochondrial production, the ATP production outside mitochondria (about 5%) plays an important qualitative role. Indeed, within a cell, due to the phenomena of compartmentation and delay to diffusion, some enzymatic activities mainly depend on this ATP.

ATP synthesis outside mitochondria is classically referred to as anaerobic. This anaerobic ATP production can be "lactic" (glycolysis) or "alactic" (adenylate kinase and creatine kinase).

Table 21.2 The different energy yields obtained with different substrates

	Glucose	Lipids (palmitic acid)	Proteins
– Molecular weight (g)	180	256	2257.4
– Daily consumption (kcal)	700 (175 g)	860 (100 g)	
– O_2 used (L/g)	0.747	2.01	1.05
– CO_2 used (L/g)	0.747	1.4	0.86
– Respiratory quotient	1	0.7	0.83
– NADH produced (mole/mole)	10	30	
– FADH2 produced (mole/mole)	2	15	
– Redox quotient	0.2	0.5	
– Energy per weight (kcal/g)	3.87	9.69	4.7
– Energy per mole (kcal/mole)	456	1548	450
– Energy equivalent			
• of O_2 (kcal/L)	5.19	4.81	4.5
• of CO_2 (kcal/L)	5.19	6.92	5.44

The body consumes in quantities (grams) less fat than carbohydrates, while energy production in Kcal is quantitatively greater with lipids. Quantitatively, glucose has a lower energy yield than lipids (3.87 vs. 9.69 kcal/g). Nevertheless, due to a higher production of NADH (relative to FADH2), the energy efficiency relative to the O_2 consumption is higher with glucose than with lipids (5.19 vs. 4.81 Kcal/L). Thus, glucose is the substrate of choice in dysoxia situations

The adenylate kinase (myokinase in muscle) catalyzes the following reaction:

$$ADP + ADP \rightarrow ATP + AMP$$

This reaction is of little importance in quantitative terms because the total mass of nucleotides in human body is very small (a few hundred grams), while ATP turnover is very high (it is estimated that a man consumes his own weight of ATP per day). However, when this reaction occurs (in situation of high energy demand), the AMP formed thus triggers several signaling pathways (e.g., via AMPK activation).

Except in the liver, most tissues have another "energy-rich" compound: phosphocreatine (PCr). It is the phosphorylated form of creatine (Cr) according to the reaction:

$$Cr + ATP \rightarrow PCr + ADP$$

PCr is a reserve of energy to dampen large and abrupt variations in ATP consumption (e.g., during initiation of effort), but its full role is not yet elucidated. Indeed, the mass of PCr is low relative to the mass of ATP that can be released from the glycolysis. It is currently believed that the PCr/Cr couple actually serves to channel the diffusion of energy within the cell. The possibility that the energy-rich phosphate bond passes from PCr to ATP and then from ATP to Cr, and this is with little loss of heat, makes it possible to envisage that the PCr/Cr couple can route energy flow within the cell between production and consumption sites. In other words, energy would be preferentially transported by an enzymatic creatine kinase network, which does not carry ATP itself but carries the phosphate-rich bond. This type of metabolic pipeline would allow a faster and more spatially oriented transfer than the simple diffusion of ATP into the cytosol.

Lactic anaerobic ATP production relies on the glycolysis that takes place in the cytosol and transforms glucose (six carbon atoms) into two lactates (three carbon atoms). It releases about 7% of the energy contained in glucose by producing two molecules of ATP per glucose molecule, without using oxygen. This is the only energy source for red blood cells, which are devoid of mitochondria. From a quantitative point of view, this metabolism is not negligible at the level of the organism as a whole, considering that the red blood cells represent an anaerobic "organ" of about 2.5 kg. Certain cells in the eye, which must be transparent, are also devoid of mitochondria and also possess a strictly anaerobic metabolism. Finally, some renal medullary cells also have a predominantly anaerobic energy metabolism. In other situations and tissues, glycolysis is a complementary source of ATP. This is the case, for example, of muscle tissue in the initial phase of movement and during intense exercises. In addition, different experimental results suggest that, due to cellular compartmentation, the ATP provided by glycolysis and that provided by oxidative phosphorylation could play distinct roles. It has been suggested that ATP of mitochondrial origin is preferentially used for heart contraction, whereas glycolytic ATP is preferentially used for maintaining the membrane potential. In particular pathological situations such as chronic hypoxia, circulatory failure, metabolic changes related to tumor growth or various aggressions (infectious, traumatic, inflammatory, etc.), and the proportion between glycolytic and mitochondrial production of ATP can be altered. In the particular case of intense short-term exercise, the consumption of glucose-6-phosphate by glycolysis (which may exceed 500 mmol/min) greatly exceeds the rate at which glucose enters the cell (approximately 5 mmol/min). In such situation, the substrate of glycolysis comes almost exclusively from glycogen stores.

Parallel to ATP synthesis, the transformation of glucose (or glycogen) into pyruvate releases four hydrogen atoms. These are recovered by two molecules of NAD+ resulting in the formation of two NADH. It should be noted that if the formation of lactate is not directly related to ATP production, the reduction of pyruvate to lactate regenerates NAD+, whose pool is limited. In other words, in the absence of NAD+ regeneration, the ATP production by glycolysis would stop even in the presence of large amount of glucose (or glycogen).

In anaerobic glycolysis, pyruvate is the final hydrogen acceptor (when becoming lactate), whereas in aerobic conditions, hydrogen is transferred to the respiratory chain where oxygen is the final hydrogen acceptor (when becoming water). A deficiency in oxidative phosphorylation (hypoxia or ischemia) results not only in a decrease in ATP production but also in hydrogen accumulation (either as NADH or as lactate). It must be underlined that, in aerobic organisms such as humans, lactate is not excreted as a waste (except for small urine or sweat losses) but is used as a metabolite either in gluconeogenesis or in TCA cycle. In both cases, lactate transformation consumes oxygen (gluconeogenesis consumes six ATP provided by oxidative phosphorylation for one synthesized glucose). Therefore, if within a given cell, ATP can be synthesized anaerobically, in the whole organism no ATP is produced without oxygen being consumed (either immediately or in a deferred manner). It should also be noted that, in practice, there is no relationship between lactate concentration and its metabolism (lactate flux). In other words, apart during lactate accumulation (which is transient and reversible), the metabolism in a whole organism is strictly aerobic. When the lactate concentration is stable (at any level), there is no anaerobic production of ATP.

21.2.2 Reciprocal Control of the Synthesis and the Use of ATP [4]

It is classically considered that ATP production is dependent on its use. The great disproportion between ATP turnover and ATP content imposes a perfect match between the use and synthesis; otherwise a deficiency of synthesis, even modest, can be quickly responsible for a collapse of ATP concentration. In this classical design, the consumption of ATP results in a reduction in the phosphate potential (ATP/ADP.Pi), responsible for a stimulation of ATP synthesis consuming the gradient of proton, which in turn is maintained by an increase in oxygen consumption. Thus, it is the decrease in ATP concentration that would stimulate respiration. However, this classical design does not reflect the whole reality. For example, the drop in ATP concentration during anoxia is much less pronounced than would have been expected given the pool and turnover of ATP. This indicates that there is an adaptation of the use of ATP to the production capacities. Similarly, as some recent studies suggest, an "excess" of ATP could lead to an increase in its use by stimulating some metabolic pathways. This hypothesis has been proposed to explain, in part, the stimulation of cellular respiration after the addition of fatty acids. These two concepts are complementary and explain the perfect match between production and consumption of ATP. Production increases according to the needs and depending on substrate availability. The consumption of ATP increases with its availability, and conversely the "metabolic arbitrations" (savings) are realized when ATP availability decreases.

21.2.3 The Use of ATP: Different Items of Expenditure

At the cellular level, there are three major items of energy expenditure: active transport, synthesis, and contraction of muscle fibers. It may be considered that life, in its simplest form, begins with the constitution of a membrane limiting an internal environment different from the external environment. This difference requires active transports in order to maintain concentration gradients. In humans, at rest, all transports apparently use 30–40% of the energy consumed. This underlines the importance of these ATP consuming transports, which are responsible for:

- The net transport of different molecules (e.g., cotransport of amino acids)
- The maintenance of a membrane potential responsible for excitation phenomena (action potential)
- The regulation of the osmolarity (i.e., cell volume)
- Intracellular signals (e.g., rapid changes in intracellular calcium concentration)

The synthesis of new molecules by the cells also represents an important cost of energy. The theoretical consumption of ATP during these syntheses is known: six ATPs are required for one glucose synthesized from two lactates, four ATPs for one urea molecule formed from ammonia and aspartate, four ATPs by amino acid incorporated in a protein, one ATP by elongation of two carbons during lipogenesis, etc. However, it is much more difficult to know the real ATP cost of these syntheses in vivo. For example, the formation of urea consumes the equivalent of four ATPs but also provides one NADH (regeneration of aspartate) usable for ATP synthesis. Conversely, the actual cost of protein synthesis is higher than the four ATPs per amino acid, since the energy cost of all upstream steps, such as RNA synthesis, must be taken into account. Finally, the degradation of certain intracellular constituents is also an expensive mechanism. The best known example is that of protein degradation which is ATP-dependent. This ATP consumption occurs when labeling the proteins to be degraded (ubiquitin), when making the membranes of the vacuoles (autophagy), when maintaining the acidity of the lysosomes, and more generally when degrading the intravacuolar constituents.

The last situation of ATP consumption occurs during the contraction of the myofibrils and is observed only in muscle cells.

21.2.4 Cost in ATP

If the energy cost of an ATP varies (see above), the ATP cost for a given activity may also vary. This is particularly the case during futile cycles. During gluconeogenesis from lactate, two ATPs are consumed during the conversion of pyruvate to phosphoenolpyruvate (PEP). From PEP, gluconeogenesis can continue to glucose, but PEP can return to pyruvate. However, this reaction catalyzed by pyruvate kinase regenerates only one ATP. The pyruvate-PEP-pyruvate cycle is a futile cycle that consumes one ATP per turn. The more active this cycle is, the more glucose production consumes ATP. However, the ATP cost of this futile cycle is the price to pay for a rapid regulation of gluconeogenesis. Indeed, simply interrupt the cycle by inhibiting pyruvate kinase in order to immediately increase the production of glucose without any additional need for ATP. In fact, glucagon, which inhibits pyruvate kinase, greatly increases gluconeogenesis with a very small increase in cell respiration. This example illustrates the essential role played by futile cycles in the fine and rapid adjustment of the activity of many metabolic pathways. Futile cycles increase energy expenditure, but it is not yet clear how to assess such an increase precisely. Depending on the situations and/or the individuals, this expenditure could vary, which would have consequences on the total energy expenditure and possibly on body weight maintenance.

Similarly, the Cori cycle (lactate formation from glucose in peripheral tissues, glucose synthesis from lactate in the liver) is an ATP-consuming process but has metabolic benefits. If one glucose leads to the formation of two ATPs together with two molecules of lactate, the synthesis of one glucose from two molecules of lactate costs six ATPs. Thus, to deliver two ATPs to the periphery, it costs six ATPs in the liver. On the other hand, considering the qualitative and not only quantitative aspects, the situation is quite different: the ATP produced at the periphery is of glycolytic origin, whereas the energy used by the liver for its metabolism mainly comes from fatty acid oxidation. Thus, the Cori cycle makes it possible to provide, in fine, energy from lipids to tissues unable to metabolize them directly (e.g., red blood cells).

Conclusion

The overall energy metabolism of the body is the result of basal metabolism, thermoregulation, and muscle exercise. It varies according to age, sex, diet, and physical activity. It is also rapidly and highly altered in acutely stressed patients. Foods, by becoming nutrients, are required by the cells in order to produce ATP. Whether they are of carbohydrate, lipid, or protein origin, they will eventually lead to a common metabolite (acetyl CoA) that will integrate the TCA cycle. This TCA cycle will provide the reduced equivalents required for oxidative phosphorylation, which can only function in the presence of oxygen (aerobic metabolism). The reaction begins with the creation of a proton gradient generated by the respiratory chain. The reentry of the protons allows the final step of ATP synthesis by the ATP synthase. ATP synthesis can also be provided (in much smaller quantities) by extramitochondrial anaerobic metabolism. ATP is then used for many cellular functions in all organs.

References

1. LaNoue KF, Schoolwerth AC (1979) Metabolite transport in mitochondria. Annu Rev Biochem 48:871–922
2. Lee YP, Lardy HA (1965) Influence of thyroid hormones on L-alpha-glycerophosphate dehydrogenases and other dehydrogenases in various organs of the rat. J Biol Chem 240:1427–1436
3. Saks V, Favier R, Guzun R, Schlattner U, Wallimann T (2006) Molecular system bioenergetics: regulation of substrate supply in response to heart energy demands. J Physiol 577:769–777
4. Brown GC (1992) Control of respiration and ATP synthesis in mammalian mitochondria and cells. Biochem J 284(Pt 1):1–13

Ischemia-Reperfusion Concepts of Myocardial Preconditioning and Postconditioning

22

Pascal Chiari, Stanislas Ledochowski, and Vincent Piriou

22.1 Ischemia Reperfusion of the Myocardium

The heart is an organ that requires a significant energy input for its contractile function. Energy reserves being low, it is dependent on blood supply. Myocardial ischemia results from an imbalance between intake and myocardial oxygen requirements.

22.1.1 Determinants of Ischemia

Ischemia is a dynamic process that depends on its duration, the size of the area at risk, and the degree of reduction of the myocardial blood flow.

The duration of the ischemic assault is a major determinant. We distinguish a first phase of reversible ischemia in the onset seconds of the process. The myocardium, which shortens and thickens during systole, undergoes a passive thinning and dilation. There is a decrease in intracellular glycogen clusters and a development of a cellular edema. In case of early reperfusion, the cardiac cells regain a normal metabolism and function in a matter of hours or days. If the ischemic assault persists, irreversible damage appears. The subendocardium, which is the most vulnerable region and receives the least collateral perfusion, is the first to suffer. Necrosis gradually spreads from the endocardium to the epicardium in a "wave front" manner.

P. Chiari (✉)
CarMeN Laboratory, Inserm U 1060, Claude Bernard Lyon1 University, Lyon, France

Department of Anaesthesia and Intensive Care, Louis Pradel Hospital, Hospices Civils de Lyon, 69395 Bron, France
e-mail: pascal.chiari@chu-lyon.fr

S. Ledochowski • V. Piriou
Department of Anesthesiology and Intensive Care, Claude Bernard Lyon1 University, Centre Hospitalier Lyon Sud, Hospices Civils de Lyon, 69495 Pierre Bénite, France
e-mail: stanislas.ledochowski@chu-lyon.fr; vincent.piriou@chu-lyon.fr

C. Ichai et al. (eds.), *Metabolic Disorders and Critically Ill Patients*,
http://doi.org/10.1007/978-3-319-64010-5_22

The size of the area at risk of infarction, which corresponds to the hypoperfused territory normally vascularized by the occluded coronary artery, is another key parameter. The more proximal the occlusion occurs, the greater the hypoperfused zone will be, resulting in a more extensive damage.

Collateral flow is blood flow which persists in the hypoperfused zone after coronary occlusion. Adjacent areas, unaffected by ischemia and, therefore, normally perfused, supply the area at risk mainly from epicardial arteriolar connections. Human quantification of this parameter, which varies according to age and disease, can be made by positron-emission tomography.

22.1.2 Reperfusion

Coronary reperfusion reduces the size of the ischemic lesion, provided that it happens early enough. Given the dynamic process leading to necrosis, which follows a sigmoid curve, there is a critical time to save the cardiac myocytes. In humans, myocardial tissue is recognized as permanently lost after 6 h of ischemia.

Reperfusion is, however, a "two-edged sword" as it is responsible for its own specific secondary damage [1]. Reperfusion is accompanied by an acceleration of the necrotic process started during ischemia. In an experimental model of an isolated and perfused rat's heart, reoxygenation of the myocardium is accompanied by much greater cellular damage than if ischemia was maintained [2]. The suspected mechanisms are probably numerous but concern particularly a massive release of reactive oxygen species (ROS), an intracellular calcium (Ca^{++}) overload, alterations in myocardial metabolism, and endothelial dysfunction. There are four forms of reperfusion injury: reperfusion arrhythmias, stunned myocardium, vascular reperfusion injury or "no-reflow," and finally lethal reperfusion injury.

22.1.3 Consequences of Ischemia-Reperfusion

22.1.3.1 On Myocardial Energy Metabolism

In normoxic conditions, the main source of ATP is beta-oxidation of fatty acids that represent up to 60% of myocardial oxygen consumption. Under certain conditions, such as a high intake of carbohydrates, there is an increase in glucose metabolism, through the mobilization and use of GLUT-1 and GLUT-4 glucose transporters. There is, in fact, a competition between the different energetic substrates (fatty acids, glucose, and lactate), since the oxidation of fatty acids produces citrate, which blocks glycolysis. In normoxic conditions, however, glycolysis is inhibited by high levels of citrate and ATP. Substrates that produce energy only by mitochondrial metabolism, such as fatty acids and lactate, are therefore preferred to glucose, which can also produce oxygen by anaerobic glycolysis.

In the case of a moderate ischemia, the oxidation of pyruvate and the fatty acids beta-oxidation decreases, while the contribution of anaerobic glycolysis to produce ATP increases. This removal of the inhibition of glucose utilization arises from the stimulation of phosphofructokinase (PFK), the key enzyme of glycolysis, which is stimulated by the fall of ATP (Pasteur effect). The glucose metabolized during glycolysis comes from both myocardial glycogen degradation (glycogenolysis) and glucose uptake from the blood. Ischemia leads to a large increase in the uptake of blood glucose, which reflects an improved ability of glucose transport through the sarcolemmal membrane. As a result, reduction in the supply of glucose caused by the ischemic assault is partly offset by a better membrane conductance through the increase in the number of GLUT-1 and GLUT-4 transporters. Under these conditions, lactate production increases, resulting in an increase in the amount of intramyocardial lactate.

In the case of severe ischemia, glucose oxidation and fatty acids beta-oxidation virtually cease. Uptake of blood glucose collapses due to the fall of the coronary flow, and intracellular glycogen becomes the sole source of ATP production. The oxidation of pyruvate, which is conventionally converted into acetyl CoA by pyruvate dehydrogenase (PDH), ceases, resulting in the accumulation of 2 H^+ protons for every molecule of pyruvate formed (decoupling of anaerobic glycolysis and oxidation of pyruvate). The decreased blood flow prevents further disposal of the by-products of anaerobic glycolysis, and lactate and protons accumulate, resulting in intracellular acidosis.

During reperfusion, the heart is exposed to a significant increase in blood levels of fatty acids whose oxidation becomes the main source of ATP production, providing 80–90% of myocardial energy needs [3]. The preferential use of this substrate contributes to a decrease in myocardial efficiency as ATP production from fatty acids is more expensive in terms of oxygen consumption than glucose (it takes about 11% more oxygen to produce the same amount of ATP from fatty acids that from glucose). If the oxidation of glucose is stimulated during reperfusion, myocardial efficiency is significantly increased and cardiac function improved [4].

22.1.4 Ionic Cellular Alterations

In normal oxygenation conditions, the H^+ protons produced by the hydrolysis of ATP are immediately used in its resynthesis, maintaining the intracellular pH stable. On the other hand, when ATP is formed during anaerobic glycolysis, the H^+ ions produced are no longer consumed and, therefore, lie in excess. Furthermore, the persistence of a residual mitochondrial respiration, triglyceride hydrolysis, and degradation of adenyl nucleotides also contribute to cellular acidification. The body will then seek to restore the intracellular pH balance quickly. Among the mechanisms of pH regulation, stimulation of the sodium-proton (Na^+/H^+) exchanger at the time of reperfusion is a major contributor to the release of H^+ ions from the cell but at the cost of an inflow of Na^+ ions. This resulting accumulation of Na^+ ions causes a slowing of the operation of the Na^+/Ca^{++} exchanger, or even a reversal of this exchange, leading to an entry of Ca^{++} ions into the cell.

22.2 Preconditioning and Postconditioning of the Myocardium

The traditional approach to myocardial ischemia is to restore a balance between the needs and supply of myocardial oxygen. From a pharmacological point of view, an extensive literature has discussed the particular interest of the beta-blockers during the perioperative stage [5]. Another way to approach this is to analyze the mechanical, metabolic, and electrophysiological disorders induced by ischemia-reperfusion and try to jam these phenomena by applying cardioprotective techniques acting on the inner workings of ischemia-reperfusion [6].

22.2.1 Early Preconditioning (Figs. 22.1, 22.2, and 22.3)

It has been known since 1986 that the use of short sequences of ischemia-reperfusion (too short to induce myocyte necrosis) applied just before a prolonged ischemia (sufficient to cause myocardial infarction) reduces dramatically (50–75%) the final infarct size [7]. This phenomenon, which results from the activation of an endogenous protection pathway, is called ischemic preconditioning (PreC). This concept

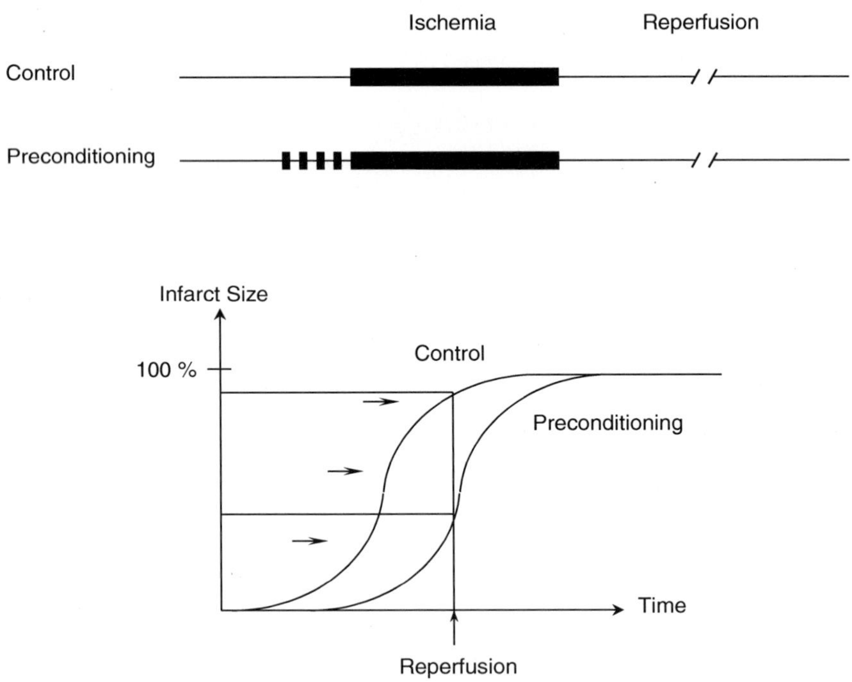

Fig. 22.1 Ischemic preconditioning. Preconditioning involves the application of brief ischemia-reperfusion sequences before a prolonged coronary occlusion followed by reperfusion. It delays the onset of infarction by shifting the curve to the right of the kinetics of the appearance of necrosis

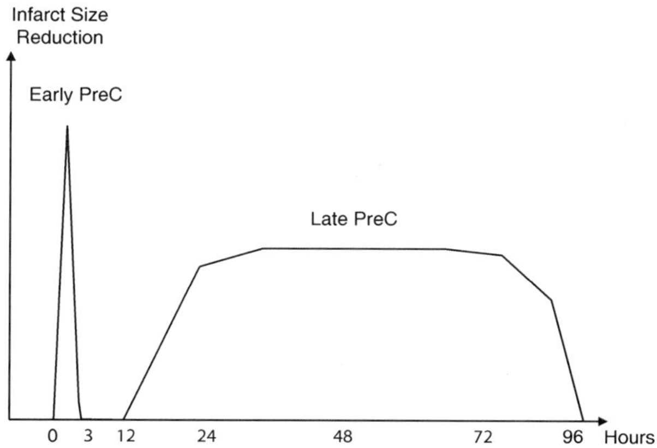

Fig. 22.2 Early and late preconditioning. Two preconditioning (PreC) windows have been described: an early window (1–2 h after the assault) and a late window which lasts between 24 and 72 h after the ischemic assault. These time spans define the time elapsed between the triggering signal and definitive ischemia

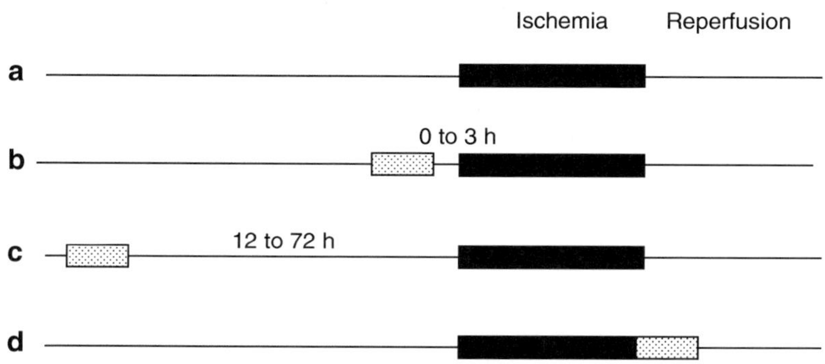

Fig. 22.3 Preconditioning and postconditioning. Compared to ischemic conditions (**a**), early preconditioning (**b**) consists in triggering a signal that increases tolerance to the deleterious myocardial ischemia just before its onset. Late preconditioning (**c**) is defined by the triggering of this signal 12–72 h before the ischemic process. Postconditioning (**d**) leads to a similar protection by applying a protective signal during the very first moments of reperfusion

has since been confirmed in many animal models and in humans. This experimental finding has also clinical implications, since a number of patients have recurrent episodes of angina or silent ischemia in the hours or days preceding a myocardial infarction. It has been shown that heart attacks occurring in such patients or those with prior angina pectoris are less extensive than when they occur primarily [8].

22.2.2 Late Preconditioning (Figs. 22.2 and 22.3)

When the time between the inducing signal (brief ischemia-reperfusion sequences) and the deleterious ischemia increases beyond 2–3 h, the protective phenomenon disappears, defining a first "preconditioning window" known as early PreC or classical PreC. It is then followed by a period of vulnerability that lasts around 12 h before the reappearance of cardioprotective capabilities. This second phenomenon perdures until the third or fourth day, defining a "second window of preconditioning" known as late PreC. These two windows are related, the latter being dependent on the former during which heat shock proteins (HSP), nitric oxide synthases (NOS), or cyclooxygenases-2 (COX-2), among others, are synthesized [9].

22.2.3 Remote Ischemic Preconditioning (RIPC)

Przyklenk et al. showed that regional myocardial ischemia induced a protective effect on an adjacent portion of the heart muscle [10]. Similarly, Dickson et al., demonstrating that ischemic PreC is transferable to another myocardium through shared blood in an isolated perfused heart model (Langendorff model), have shown the existence of a humoral phenomenon behind this protection [11]. In the same vein, ischemia of a distant organ such as the kidney, intestine, liver, lung, brain, or skeletal muscle can induce cardioprotection [12, 13]. These organs are also able to protect themselves after PreC. Hence, there is a ubiquitous phenomenon protecting against tissue ischemia [14].

22.2.4 Postconditioning (Fig. 22.3)

More recently, Vinten-Johansen's team have shown that the application of brief ischemia-reperfusion sequences, not before lethal ischemia as in the ischemic PreC but during the first moments of reperfusion, also induced cardioprotection, a phenomenon they called analogy postconditioning (PostC) [15]. But one must keep in mind that the time span during which it is possible to protect the myocardium during reperfusion is very limited. It has been reported that if the PostC is started even 1 min after reperfusion, then cardioprotection is ineffective [16]. This latter type of cardioprotection has grown considerably, particularly in the field of interventional cardiology. It has been shown that it is possible to protect the myocardium of patients with acute coronary syndrome during coronary angioplasty, through the use of four cycles of 1-min inflation and 1-min deflation of the angioplasty balloon within the first minute after stent implantation [17]. This strategy, implemented in the first minute of reperfusion, reduced up to 30 or 40% the size of myocardial necrosis. This beneficial effect persisted at 6 months and was associated with an improved left ventricular ejection fraction at 1 year [18].

22.2.5 Nature of the Protective Signal

This endogenous myocardial protection, typically triggered by a short sublethal ischemia, can also be induced by a wide variety of non-pharmacological stimuli such as hypoxia, heat stress, pacing, or through the involvement of mechanoreceptors during rapid volemic myocardial distension (stretch). Several pharmacological interventions can also trigger this protective signal such as the administration of adenosine (involvement of A1 and A3 receptors), acetylcholine (M2), bradykinin

(B2), endothelin (ET1), angiotensin (AT1) receptor, or adrenergic receptor agonists (α1). Activators of ATP-dependent potassium channels (K_{ATP}) have a similar effect. Finally cyclosporin A, regardless of its immunosuppressive properties, has a protective effect via the inhibition of cyclophilin D, a key protein of this protective signaling [19]. In the anesthetic arsenal, two agents are known to be cardioprotective opioids (δ and κ receivers) and halogenated anesthetics [14, 20, 21].

22.2.6 Mechanistic Approach

Literature that addresses the mechanisms of these cardioprotective phenomena is both abundant and complex. The aim of these works is to decipher the phenomenon, to understand it, and to ultimately be able to pharmacologically reproduce and amplify it [22]. Depending on its nature (brief ischemia, pharmacological or other manipulation), the intensity and duration of the initial stimulus or the studied species differences may appear in the chain of protective signaling. Signaling of ischemic PreC and anesthetic PreC certainly involves common elements, but differences have been suggested by genomic studies [23, 24]. It is quite likely that PreC and PostC use common signaling pathways. The heart being located in the blood stream probably also participates in the protective mechanism. The ischemia-reperfusion sequence generates deleterious leukocyte recruitment, particularly through endothelial dysfunction, ROS production, and activation of thrombotic phenomena. PreC protects from this effect through decreased neutrophil adhesion and ROS production [25]. However, the myocardial tissue itself, as shown by studies on isolated perfused heart models (Langendorff model), presents a complex cascade of intracellular events (Fig. 22.4).

Intracellular signaling:

- The cellular mechanisms are initiated through the activation of membrane receptors by autacoids substances (autacoid triggers) such as adenosine, bradykinin, opioid derivatives, natriuretic peptides (ANP, BNP), growth factor peptides (IGF-1), or TNF-α, for example [26]. K_{ATP} channels have also been identified as involved in this mechanism several years ago [27]. These channels are present at the sarcolemmal level where patch-clamp studies have shown that their activation induces potassium output to the extracellular space, thus reducing the action potential and maintaining the intracellular pool of ATP. These channels may also be present on the inner mitochondrial membrane, but their mechanism of action at this level is more hypothetical [28].
- Several pathways transmit the signal within the cell. The reperfusion injury salvage kinase (RISK) pathway, which involves protein kinase B (Akt) and ERK1/2, is well described [29]. It leads to an inhibition of glycogen synthase kinase-3β (GSK-3β), an enzyme having a direct effect on mitochondria. Other routes such as the survivor activating factor enhancement (SAFE) could also contribute to the transmission of the protective signal (Fig. 22.4).
- All these pathways lead to end effectors that are responsible for the protection itself. Research has been focusing for several years on the mitochondria and in particular on one of its functions called mitochondrial permeability transition [30].

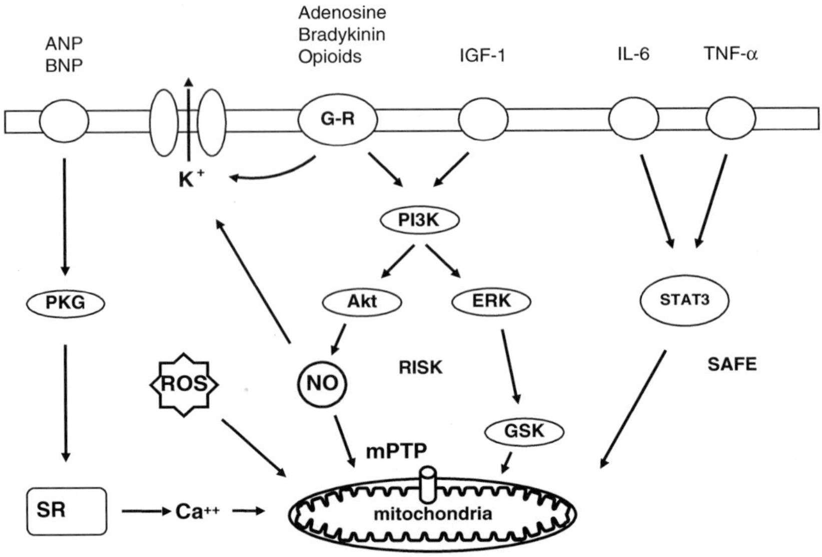

Fig. 22.4 Signaling pathways. *ANP* and *BNP*, atrial and brain natriuretic peptides; *IGF-1*, insulin-like growth factor; *IL-6*, interleukine 6; *TNF-α*, tumor necrosis factor-α; *G-R*, G-protein-coupled receptor; *PI3K*, phosphatidylinositol-3-kinase; *PKG*, protein kinase G; *Akt*, protein kinase B; *ERK* p42/p44, extracellular signal-regulated kinase; *STAT3*, signal transducer and activator of transcription 3; *ROS*, reactive oxygen species; *NO*, nitric oxide; *RISK*, reperfusion injury salvage kinase pathway; *SAFE*, survivor activating factor enhancement pathway; *GSK*, glycogen synthase kinase-3β; *SR*, sarcoplasmic reticulum; *mPTP*, mitochondrial permeability transition pore

The mitochondrial permeability transition: Mitochondria, which store energy in the form of ATP, may, following an assault such as ischemia-reperfusion, direct the cell to necrosis and/or apoptosis via the permeability transition.

These organelles are delimited by two membranes, the relatively conventional external membrane and the inner membrane, folded into numerous invaginations and characterized by its imperviousness to molecules and ions. These two membranes define two compartments: the intermembrane space, whose chemical composition is relatively close to the cytosol, and that of the mitochondrial matrix containing the genome that encodes the synthesis of the necessary metabolic enzymes (citric acid cycle, β-oxidation of fatty acids, etc.).

The permeability transition is characterized by the loss of the constitutional permeability of the inner mitochondrial membrane, thus providing a free communication between the matrix and the cytosol [31, 32]. It causes a swelling of the matrix and a collapse of the mitochondrial membrane potential (Δψm). This swelling impacts ATP synthesis and is even responsible for ATP hydrolysis as the mitochondrial enzyme runs in reverse and degrades ATP. It also leads to a rupture of the outer membrane, more fragile, causing a leak in the cytoplasm of molecules including cytochrome c, which is an activating agent of proapoptotic caspases leading to the final pathway of apoptosis.

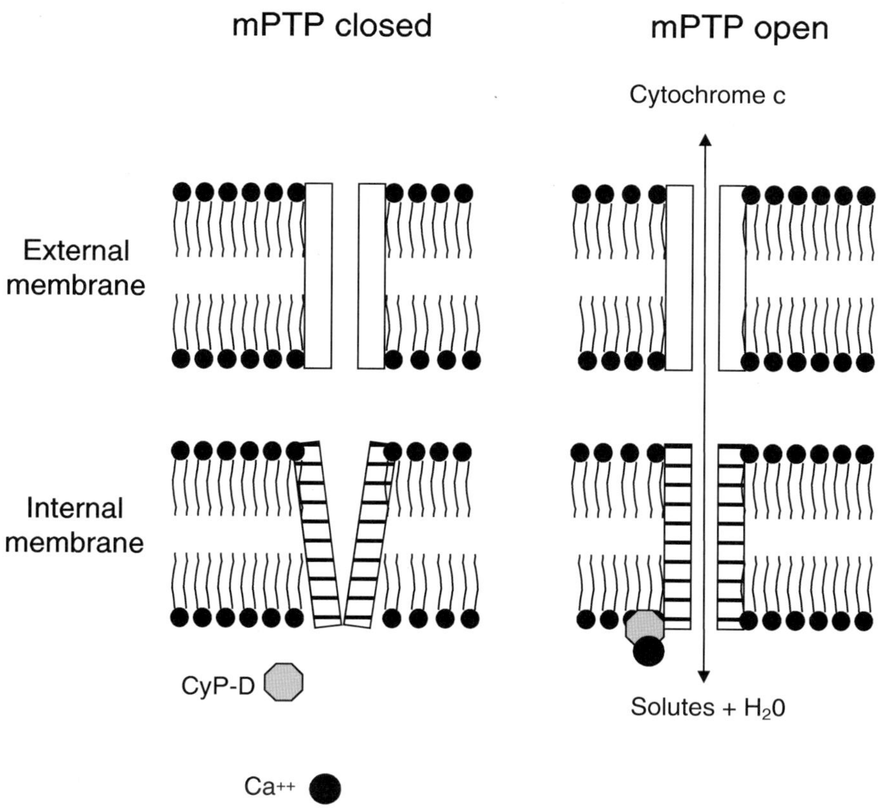

Fig. 22.5 Structure of the mitochondrial permeability transition pore (mPTP). The exact structure of the mPTP is unknown. Cyclophilin D (Cyp-D) is one of the most relevant components of this multi-protein assembly. Its opening is facilitated by a calcic overload, an ROS burst, and/or a correction of intracellular acidosis. Cyp-D, a protein situated in the mitochondrial matrix, migrates toward the internal membrane, thus altering its constitutional impermeability

This unsealing of the inner membrane is a result of the opening of a nonselective megachannel called mitochondrial permeability transition pore (mPTP) (Fig. 22.5). It is a multi-protein assembly whose precise constitution is still unknown. Cyclophilin D, located in the mitochondrial matrix, is one of the most relevant components of the mPTP. However, other proteins are probably involved in the permeability transition such as the adenine nucleotide transporter (ANT), porin (VDAC voltage-dependent anion channel), creatine kinase (CK), hexokinase, the benzodiazepine receptor, and proapoptotic proteins of the Bcl-2 family such as BAX [31]. The complex 1 of the respiratory chain also probably plays a role in the opening sensitivity of mPTP and is possibly even one of its direct components [33–35].

Modulation of the permeability transition: Many compounds are capable of influencing the opening of the mPTP, either through its activation or inhibition. Ca^{++} is the main inducer of permeability transition. Ca^{++} mitochondrial overload induces mPTP opening, while the use of a Ca^{++} chelator such as EGTA inhibits it. Intracellular Ca^{++} shifts, particularly during ischemia-reperfusion, are closely related to the sarcoplasmic reticulum. Numerous studies have examined the relationship between mitochondria and reticulum, particularly focusing on their contact zones, the mitochondria-associated membranes (MAM), which could be one of the key points of cell protection [36, 37]. The matrix pH is also an important element of this regulation since its acidification decreases the opening probability of the mPTP. ROS are also potent activators of the mitochondrial permeability transition. Cyclosporin A, by binding to cyclophilin D, prevents its attachment to the ANT and thus delays the opening of the mPTP [19, 31, 38, 39].

mPTP opening during ischemia-reperfusion: Ischemia is accompanied by a very significant acidosis which maintains mPTP closed. It was really only during reperfusion that the conditions for the opening of the mPTP are met. Na^+/H^+ and Na^+/Ca^{++} exchangers quickly correct acidosis at the cost of a high Ca^{++} overload of the mitochondrial matrix. There is an associated ROS "burst" due to the replenishment of oxygen in the respiratory chain. Reperfusion, by combining the optimal conditions for the opening of mPTP, is a decisive step in the generation of cellular damage from ischemia-reperfusion injury.

22.3 Perioperative Cardioprotection

Cardiovascular complications of perioperative myocardial ischemia are a leading cause of morbidity and mortality, both in cardiac and noncardiac surgery. Aortic clamping, necessary in cardiac surgery, induces a sequence of myocardial ischemia-reperfusion. Several studies have shown that elevated postoperative troponin I is an independent prognostic factor of morbi-mortality up to 36 months after cardiac surgery [40, 41]. Major noncardiac surgery, such as arterial vascular surgery, especially when performed on a coronary artery disease patient, may be complicated by a perioperative myocardial infarction whose prognosis remains poor (close to 40% mortality) [42]. Extensive research has been done on the perioperative setting to try to stop this process. Pharmacological protective strategies by beta-blockers and statins in particular have been developed. However, this issue of perioperative cardioprotection was clearly marked by the discovery in 1997 of the PreC effect of halogenated anesthetic agents [6].

22.3.1 Halogenated Agents and Cardioprotection

Experimental data. On an in vivo animal model, administration of isoflurane prior to a sequence of ischemia reperfusion reduced the size of myocardial infarction by 50% [43]. This effect is inhibited by glibenclamide, a sulfonylurea which blocks the opening of K_{ATP} channels, thereby confirming the role played by these channels. These early works were confirmed by a multitude of animal model studies (in vivo, ex vivo, and in vitro) as well as tissue from human atria removed during cardiac surgery [20, 21]. All halogenated agents (from the oldest, enflurane, halothane, and isoflurane, to the most recent, sevoflurane and desflurane) are cardioprotective to varying degrees depending on experimental conditions. It is considered that here is a class effect. There is a dose of anesthetic PreC as there is one for ischemic PreC. However, it is not useful to administer a dose greater than one MAC (minimum alveolar concentration) to trigger a protective signal. Furthermore, these anesthetics are also capable of inducing a late PreC, since their administration induces a myocardial resistance to ischemia for days [44]. Finally, a protective effect was found when a halogenated agent was administered during the first moments of reperfusion, defining a PostC effect [45, 46].

Clinical studies. So far, the cardioprotective effect of a halogenated agent has been mainly studied in the context of cardiac surgery. Despite promising early works in terms of reducing postoperative troponin I levels, more recent studies have since tempered the enthusiasm by revealing a positive effect only on secondary postoperative outcomes such as BNP or cardiac index [47–50]. Despite this, three meta-analyses demonstrate the protective effects of halogenated agents [51–53]. These studies, based only on small studies, are not consistent in their findings. Some found a positive effect in terms of postoperative troponin I elevation, while others in terms of mortality.

For noncardiac surgery, two recent studies found no beneficial effect of halogenated compared to intravenous general anesthesia [54, 55]. However, many confounding factors may explain this apparent lack of effectiveness [56].

The discrepancy between the experimental studies, all clearly in favor of halogenated agents, and clinical studies may be disturbing. However, this difference is probably due to the inherent complexity of clinical research. Clinical studies necessarily mix population with varying ages, conditions, and operating settings (type of surgery, different operators, multicenter study, heterogeneous coronary anatomy, etc.) with various pathologies and associated treatments.

22.3.2 Clinical Factors Modulating this Anesthetic Cardioprotection

Age modulates PreC since it has been shown that the senescent myocardium becomes less sensitive to the protective effect of a halogenated agent [57]. Estrogens have a protective effect (possibly via an effect on the K_{ATP} channels and NO production) [58]. Diabetes and hyperglycemia abolish PreC, probably through an ROS overproduction [59]. Sulfonylureas, inhibiting the opening of K_{ATP} channels, have a potentially negative effect on the tolerance to myocardial ischemia and should therefore be stopped 24–48 h before surgery [43]. The perioperative phase involves many treatments whose effects are variable (e.g., anti-protective effects of theophylline or anti-COX-2, protective effects of nicorandil, insulin, nitrates, or sildenafil). General anesthesia also combines anti-protecting agents such as midazolam and proven protective agents such as morphine [60, 61]. Ketamine, according to studies, could have a positive or a negative effect on PreC [62]. Statins, by acting very early in the synthetic pathway of cholesterol, inhibit other proteins such as protein Rho, which interacts with signaling pathways of cell death. Many studies have demonstrated that the beneficial effects of statins are well beyond their cholesterol-lowering effects (pleiotropic effects) [63]. In addition, the discontinuation of statin therapy may induce a rebound effect. Indeed, it has been shown that a discontinuation of statins in the postoperative phase of an aortic vascular surgery may increase the risk of perioperative myocardial infarction by 2.9 [64]. These examples only bear witness to the difficulties to prove a statistically significant cardioprotective effect.

Conclusion

The actual trend is to apply a multifocal strategy to protect high-risk patients from perioperative myocardial ischemia. Cardioprotective attitudes include the use of halogenated agents for anesthesia, glycemic control through insulin therapy, continuation of statins, discontinuation of sulfonylureas, and control of alkalosis and hyperglycemia. Only large multicenter studies with a sufficient number of patients could ultimately determine whether the beneficial effects of PreC and PostC, clearly detectable in experimental conditions, could represent a clinically significant protective gain.

References

1. Yellon DM, Hausenloy DJ (2007) Myocardial reperfusion injury. N Engl J Med 357:1121–1135
2. Hearse DJ (1977) Reperfusion of the ischemic myocardium. J Mol Cell Cardiol 9:605–616
3. Stanley WC, Lopaschuk GD, Hall JL, McCormack JG (1997) Regulation of myocardial carbohydrate metabolism under normal and ischaemic conditions. Potential for pharmacological interventions. Cardiovasc Res 33:243–257
4. Lopaschuk GD, Stanley WC (1997) Glucose metabolism in the ischemic heart. Circulation 95:313–315
5. Fleisher LA, Beckman JA, Brown KA, Calkins H, Chaikof EL, Fleischmann KE, Freeman WK, Froehlich JB, Kasper EK, Kersten JR, Riegel B, Robb JF (2009) 2009 ACCF/AHA focused update on perioperative beta blockade incorporated into the ACC/AHA 2007 guidelines on perioperative cardiovascular evaluation and care for noncardiac surgery: a report of the American college of cardiology foundation/American heart association task force on practice guidelines. Circulation 120:e169–e276
6. Warltier DC, Pagel PS, Kersten JR (2000) Approaches to the prevention of perioperative myocardial ischemia. Anesthesiology 92:253–259
7. Murry CE, Jennings RB, Reimer KA (1986) Preconditioning with ischemia: a delay of lethal cell injury in ischemic myocardium. Circulation 74:1124–1136
8. Ishihara M, Sato H, Tateishi H, Kawagoe T, Shimatani Y, Kurisu S, Sakai K, Ueda K (1997) Implications of prodromal angina pectoris in anterior wall acute myocardial infarction: acute angiographic findings and long-term prognosis. J Am Coll Cardiol 30:970–975
9. Bolli R (2000) The late phase of preconditioning. Circ Res 87:972–983
10. Przyklenk K, Bauer B, Ovize M, Kloner RA, Whittaker P (1993) Regional ischemic 'preconditioning' protects remote virgin myocardium from subsequent sustained coronary occlusion. Circulation 87:893–899
11. Dickson EW, Lorbar M, Porcaro WA, Fenton RA, Reinhardt CP, Gysembergh A, Przyklenk K (1999) Rabbit heart can be "preconditioned" via transfer of coronary effluent. Am J Phys 277:H2451–H2457

12. Lee HT (1999) Mechanisms of ischemic preconditioning and clinical implications for multiorgan ischemic-reperfusion injury. J Cardiothorac Vasc Anesth 13:78–91
13. Walsh SR, Tang T, Sadat U, Dutka DP, Gaunt ME (2007) Cardioprotection by remote ischaemic preconditioning. Br J Anaesth 99:611–616
14. Yellon DM, Downey JM (2003) Preconditioning the myocardium: from cellular physiology to clinical cardiology. Physiol Rev 83:1113–1151
15. Zhao ZQ, Corvera JS, Halkos ME, Kerendi F, Wang NP, Guyton RA, Vinten-Johansen J (2003) Inhibition of myocardial injury by ischemic postconditioning during reperfusion: comparison with ischemic preconditioning. Am J Physiol Heart Circ Physiol 285:579–588
16. Kin H, Zhao ZQ, Sun HY, Wang NP, Corvera JS, Halkos ME, Kerendi F, Guyton RA, Vinten-Johansen J (2004) Postconditioning attenuates myocardial ischemia-reperfusion injury by inhibiting events in the early minutes of reperfusion. Cardiovasc Res 62:74–85
17. Staat P, Rioufol G, Piot C, Cottin Y, Cung TT, L'Huillier I, Aupetit JF, Bonnefoy E, Finet G, Andre-Fouet X, Ovize M (2005) Postconditioning the human heart. Circulation 112:2143–2148
18. Thibault H, Piot C, Staat P, Bontemps L, Sportouch C, Rioufol G, Cung TT, Bonnefoy E, Angoulvant D, Aupetit JF, Finet G, Andre-Fouet X, Macia JC, Raczka F, Rossi R, Itti R, Kirkorian G, Derumeaux G, Ovize M (2008) Long-term benefit of postconditioning. Circulation 117:1037–1044
19. Hausenloy DJ, Maddock HL, Baxter GF, Yellon DM (2002) Inhibiting mitochondrial permeability transition pore opening: a new paradigm for myocardial preconditioning? Cardiovasc Res 55:534–543
20. Tanaka K, Ludwig LM, Kersten JR, Pagel PS, Warltier DC (2004) Mechanisms of cardioprotection by volatile anesthetics. Anesthesiology 100:707–721
21. Frassdorf J, De Hert S, Schlack W (2009) Anaesthesia and myocardial ischaemia/reperfusion injury. Br J Anaesth 103:89–98
22. Eltzschig HK, Eckle T (2011) Ischemia and reperfusion--from mechanism to translation. Nat Med 17:1391–1401
23. Hausenloy DJ, Yellon DM (2007) Preconditioning and postconditioning: united at reperfusion. Pharmacol Ther 116:173–191
24. Sergeev P, da Silva R, Lucchinetti E, Zaugg K, Pasch T, Schaub MC, Zaugg M (2004) Trigger-dependent gene expression profiles in cardiac preconditioning. Evidence for distinct genetic programs in ischemic and anesthetic preconditioning. Anesthesiology 100:474–488
25. Biao Z, Zhanggang X, Hao J, Changhong M, Jing C (2005) The in vitro effect of desflurane preconditioning on endothelial adhesion molecules and mRNA expression. Anesth Analg 100:1007–1013
26. Ovize M, Baxter GF, Di Lisa F, Ferdinandy P, Garcia-Dorado D, Hausenloy DJ, Heusch G, Vinten-Johansen J, Yellon DM, Schulz R (2010) Postconditioning and protection from reperfusion injury: where do we stand? Position paper from the working Group of Cellular Biology of the heart of the European society of cardiology. Cardiovasc Res 87:406–423
27. Gross GJ, Fryer RM (1999) Sarcolemmal versus mitochondrial ATP-sensitive K+ channels and myocardial preconditioning. Circ Res 84:973–979
28. Hanley PJ, Drose S, Brandt U, Lareau RA, Banerjee AL, Srivastava DK, Banaszak LJ, Barycki JJ, Van Veldhoven PP, Daut J (2005) 5-Hydroxydecanoate is metabolised in mitochondria and creates a rate-limiting bottleneck for beta-oxidation of fatty acids. J Physiol 562:307–318
29. Hausenloy DJ, Yellon DM (2004) New directions for protecting the heart against ischaemia-reperfusion injury: targeting the reperfusion injury salvage kinase (RISK)-pathway. Cardiovasc Res 61:448–460
30. Murphy E, Steenbergen C (1813) What makes the mitochondria a killer? Can we condition them to be less destructive? Biochim Biophys Acta 2011:1302–1308
31. Halestrap AP, Clarke SJ, Javadov SA (2004) Mitochondrial permeability transition pore opening during myocardial reperfusion--a target for cardioprotection. Cardiovasc Res 61:372–385
32. Di Lisa F, Carpi A, Giorgio V, Bernardi P (1813) The mitochondrial permeability transition pore and cyclophilin D in cardioprotection. Biochim Biophys Acta 2011:1316–1322

33. Juhaszova M, Wang S, Zorov DB, Nuss HB, Gleichmann M, Mattson MP, Sollott SJ (2008) The identity and regulation of the mitochondrial permeability transition pore: where the known meets the unknown. Ann N Y Acad Sci 1123:197–212
34. De Paulis D, Chiari P, Teixeira G, Couture-Lepetit E, Abrial M, Argaud L, Gharib A, Ovize M (2013) Cyclosporine a at reperfusion fails to reduce infarct size in the in vivo rat heart. Basic Res Cardiol 108:379
35. Teixeira G, Abrial M, Portier K, Chiari P, Couture-Lepetit E, Tourneur Y, Ovize M, Gharib A (2013) Synergistic protective effect of cyclosporin a and rotenone against hypoxia-reoxygenation in cardiomyocytes. J Mol Cell Cardiol 56:55–62
36. Paillard M, Tubbs E, Thiebaut PA, Gomez L, Fauconnier J, Da Silva CC, Teixeira G, Mewton N, Belaidi E, Durand A, Abrial M, Lacampagne A, Rieusset J, Ovize M (2013) Depressing mitochondria-reticulum interactions protects cardiomyocytes from lethal hypoxia-reoxygenation injury. Circulation 128:1555–1565
37. Rizzuto R, De Stefani D, Raffaello A, Mammucari C (2012) Mitochondria as sensors and regulators of calcium signalling. Nat Rev Mol Cell Biol 13:566–578
38. Argaud L, Gateau-Roesch O, Muntean D, Chalabreysse L, Loufouat J, Robert D, Ovize M (2005) Specific inhibition of the mitochondrial permeability transition prevents lethal reperfusion injury. J Mol Cell Cardiol 38:367–374
39. Piot C, Croisille P, Staat P, Thibault H, Rioufol G, Mewton N, Elbelghiti R, Cung TT, Bonnefoy E, Angoulvant D, Macia C, Raczka F, Sportouch C, Gahide G, Finet G, Andre-Fouet X, Revel D, Kirkorian G, Monassier JP, Derumeaux G, Ovize M (2008) Effect of cyclosporine on reperfusion injury in acute myocardial infarction. N Engl J Med 359:473–481
40. Croal BL, Hillis GS, Gibson PH, Fazal MT, El-Shafei H, Gibson G, Jeffrey RR, Buchan KG, West D, Cuthbertson BH (2006) Relationship between postoperative cardiac troponin I levels and outcome of cardiac surgery. Circulation 114:1468–1475
41. Fellahi JL, Hanouz JL, Manach YL, Gue X, Monier E, Guillou L, Riou B (2009) Simultaneous measurement of cardiac troponin I, B-type natriuretic peptide, and C-reactive protein for the prediction of long-term cardiac outcome after cardiac surgery. Anesthesiology 111:250–257
42. Poldermans D, Boersma E, Bax JJ, Thomson IR, van de Ven LL, Blankensteijn JD, Baars HF, Yo TI, Trocino G, Vigna C, Roelandt JR, van Urk H (1999) The effect of bisoprolol on perioperative mortality and myocardial infarction in high-risk patients undergoing vascular surgery. Dutch echocardiographic cardiac risk evaluation applying stress echocardiography study group. N Engl J Med 341:1789–1794
43. Kersten JR, Schmeling TJ, Pagel PS, Gross GJ, Warltier DC (1997) Isoflurane mimics ischemic preconditioning via activation of K(ATP) channels: reduction of myocardial infarct size with an acute memory phase. Anesthesiology 87:361–370
44. Tanaka K, Ludwig LM, Krolikowski JG, Alcindor D, Pratt PF, Kersten JR, Pagel PS, Warltier DC (2004) Isoflurane produces delayed preconditioning against myocardial ischemia and reperfusion injury. Anesthesiology 100:525–531
45. Preckel B, Schlack W, Comfere T, Obal D, Barthel H, Thamer V (1998) Effects of enflurane, isoflurane, sevoflurane and desflurane on reperfusion injury after regional myocardial ischaemia in the rabbit heart in vivo. Br J Anaesth 81:905–912
46. Chiari PC, Bienengraeber MW, Pagel PS, Krolikowski JG, Kersten JR, Warltier DC (2005) Isoflurane protects against myocardial infarction during early reperfusion by activation of phosphatidylinositol-3-kinase signal transduction: evidence for anesthetic-induced postconditioning in rabbits. Anesthesiology 102:102–109
47. De Hert SG, Van der Linden PJ, Cromheecke S, Meeus R, Nelis A, Van Reeth V, ten Broecke PW, De Blier IG, Stockman BA, Rodrigus IE (2004) Cardioprotective properties of sevoflurane in patients undergoing coronary surgery with cardiopulmonary bypass are related to the modalities of its administration. Anesthesiology 101:299–310
48. Julier K, da Silva R, Garcia C, Bestmann L, Frascarolo P, Zollinger A, Chassot PG, Schmid ER, Turina MI, von Segesser LK, Pasch T, Spahn DR, Zaugg M (2003) Preconditioning by sevoflurane decreases biochemical markers for myocardial and renal dysfunction in coronary artery

bypass graft surgery: a double-blinded, placebo-controlled, multicenter study. Anesthesiology 98:1315–1327
49. Piriou V, Mantz J, Goldfarb G, Kitakaze M, Chiari P, Paquin S, Cornu C, Lecharny JB, Aussage P, Vicaut E, Pons A, Lehot JJ (2007) Sevoflurane preconditioning at 1 MAC only provides limited protection in patients undergoing coronary artery bypass surgery: a randomized bi-centre trial. Br J Anaesth 99:624–631
50. De Hert S, Vlasselaers D, Barbe R, Ory JP, Dekegel D, Donnadonni R, Demeere JL, Mulier J, Wouters P (2009) A comparison of volatile and non volatile agents for cardioprotection during on-pump coronary surgery. Anaesthesia 64:953–960
51. Symons JA, Myles PS (2006) Myocardial protection with volatile anaesthetic agents during coronary artery bypass surgery: a meta-analysis. Br J Anaesth 97:127–136
52. Yu CH, Beattie WS (2006) The effects of volatile anesthetics on cardiac ischemic complications and mortality in CABG: a meta-analysis. Can J Anaesth 53:906–918
53. Landoni G, Biondi-Zoccai GG, Zangrillo A, Bignami E, D'Avolio S, Marchetti C, Calabro MG, Fochi O, Guarracino F, Tritapepe L, De Hert S, Torri G (2007) Desflurane and sevoflurane in cardiac surgery: a meta-analysis of randomized clinical trials. J Cardiothorac Vasc Anesth 21:502–511
54. Lurati Buse GA, Schumacher P, Seeberger E, Studer W, Schuman RM, Fassl J, Kasper J, Filipovic M, Bolliger D, Seeberger MD (2012) Randomized comparison of sevoflurane versus propofol to reduce perioperative myocardial ischemia in patients undergoing noncardiac surgery. Circulation 126:2696–2704
55. Zangrillo A, Testa V, Aldrovandi V, Tuoro A, Casiraghi G, Cavenago F, Messina M, Bignami E, Landoni G (2011) Volatile agents for cardiac protection in noncardiac surgery: a randomized controlled study. J Cardiothorac Vasc Anesth 25:902–907
56. Kersten JR (2012) A recipe for perioperative cardioprotection: what matters most? The ingredients or the chef? Circulation 126:2671–2673
57. Mio Y, Bienengraeber MW, Marinovic J, Gutterman DD, Rakic M, Bosnjak ZJ, Stadnicka A (2008) Age-related attenuation of isoflurane preconditioning in human atrial cardiomyocytes: roles for mitochondrial respiration and sarcolemmal adenosine triphosphate-sensitive potassium channel activity. Anesthesiology 108:612–620
58. Wang C, Chiari PC, Weihrauch D, Krolikowski JG, Warltier DC, Kersten JR, Pratt PF Jr, Pagel PS (2006) Gender-specificity of delayed preconditioning by isoflurane in rabbits: potential role of endothelial nitric oxide synthase. Anesth Analg 103:274–280
59. Kehl F, Krolikowski JG, Mraovic B, Pagel PS, Warltier DC, Kersten JR (2002) Hyperglycemia prevents isoflurane-induced preconditioning against myocardial infarction. Anesthesiology 96:183–188
60. Rivo J, Raphael J, Drenger B, Berenshtein E, Chevion M, Gozal Y (2006) Flumazenil mimics whereas midazolam abolishes ischemic preconditioning in a rabbit heart model of ischemia-reperfusion. Anesthesiology 105:65–71
61. Gross GJ (2003) Role of opioids in acute and delayed preconditioning. J Mol Cell Cardiol 35:709–718
62. Mullenheim J, Frassdorf J, Preckel B, Thamer V, Schlack W (2001) Ketamine, but not S(+)-ketamine, blocks ischemic preconditioning in rabbit hearts in vivo. Anesthesiology 94:630–636
63. Ray KK, Cannon CP (2005) The potential relevance of the multiple lipid-independent (pleiotropic) effects of statins in the management of acute coronary syndromes. J Am Coll Cardiol 46:1425–1433
64. Le Manach Y, Godet G, Coriat P, Martinon C, Bertrand M, Fleron MH, Riou B (2007) The impact of postoperative discontinuation or continuation of chronic statin therapy on cardiac outcome after major vascular surgery. Anesth Analg 104:1326–1333

Targeted Temperature Management in Severe Brain-Injured Patient

23

Hervé Quintard and Alain Cariou

Hyperthermia has been consistently shown to exacerbate brain injuries in animal models [1] and has been associated with poor outcome in human studies [2]. Indeed hyperthermia can improve excitotoxicity, metabolic dysfunction, inflammation, etc. Control of fever is so a basic principle in brain injury cares [3] and will not be discussed here. However, several recent data described that decrease temperature to lower level (32–36 °C), even in case of normothermia, could be helpful to protect the brain from injuries. Indeed this targeted temperature management (TTM) is an established tool used to protect the central nervous system during surgery for long years [4]. Part of this protection is mainly due to a decrease in metabolism [5] and in oxygen consumption [6], but also to a decrease in cerebral blood flow [7]. Lot of other neuroprotective effects have been described previously as on integrity of blood-brain barrier [8], excitotoxic [9], or inflammation mechanism control (Fig. 23.1). It has only recently achieved a mainstream role in clinical practice, especially in post-cardiac arrest syndrome. Indeed the decrease in core temperature improved neurologic recovery after cardiac arrest syndrome as described, 10 years ago, by randomized control trials [10]. These observations conducted to a real change in ICU management of patients after cardiac arrest and have opened an important way of search. Use of TTM in other brain injuries is less conclusive. Severe brain injury, secondary to traumatic brain injury (TBI), subarachnoid hemorrhage (SAH), stroke, meningitis, or intracerebral hemorrhage (ICH), can be complicated by several mechanisms that induce brain edema and increase in intracranial pressure (ICP) [11]. The question to induce hypothermic state in this context is quite discussed and can have conflicting aspect.

H. Quintard, M.D., Ph.D. (✉)
Intensive Care Unit, Pasteur 2 Hospital (CHU Nice), 30 voie romaine, 06000 Nice, France
e-mail: quintard.h@chu-nice.fr

A. Cariou, M.D., Ph.D.
Intensive Care Unit, Cochin Hospital (AP-HP), 75000 Paris, France

C. Ichai et al. (eds.), *Metabolic Disorders and Critically Ill Patients*,
http://doi.org/10.1007/978-3-319-64010-5_23

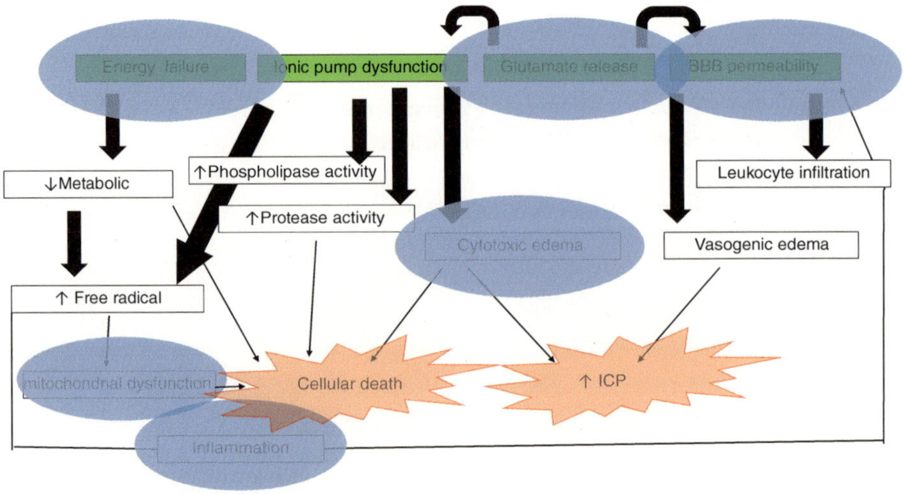

Fig. 23.1 Mechanisms involved in secondary brain injuries and neuroprotective mechanisms of hypothermia (*blue circles*)

23.1 Cardiac Arrest

Sudden cardiac death remains a major public health issue, as highlighted by epidemiological data, showing that nearly 40,000 people are supported for out-of-hospital cardiac arrest (CA) in France each year. Even more problematic, only a very low proportion of resuscitated patients will recover and will leave the hospital without major neurological impairments [12]. The evidence of further cerebral damage occurring during the reperfusion phase encouraged intense research aiming to limit the worsening of the neurological lesions occurring during the post-CA period. Post-resuscitation fever has been rapidly identified as having a major detrimental effect [13]. This culminated 10 years ago with the demonstration that post-CA cooling was an effective treatment in these patients.

Many animal models of cardiac arrest (CA) demonstrated that mild hypothermia can provide neuroprotective effects through different mechanisms of action such as a decrease in cerebral oxygen consumption, a reduction in apoptosis activation and mitochondrial dysfunction, a decrease in cerebral excitatory cascade, a decrease in local inflammatory response, a reduction in the production of free oxygen radicals production, and a decrease in vascular and membrane permeability. These convergent experimental effects translated into clinical effects as revealed in the two landmark studies published in 2002 [10, 14]. In these two pivotal trials, the implementation of induced hypothermia (between 32 and 34 °C) permitted to achieve a significantly higher survival rate without major sequel as compared with no specific temperature management. These studies were decisive and led to a rapid change in international guidelines regarding the management of comatose patients after CA. Until recently, it has been strongly recommended to routinely induce a moderate hypothermia (32–34 °C) for 12–24 h in all adults still comatose after restoration of spontaneous circulation.

Over the last decade, several clinical findings challenged this recommendation in different ways. The most important point that is debated is the level of temperature that should be targeted. The targeted temperature management (TTM) trial randomized 950 comatose patients after CA who were randomly assigned to 33 °C or 36 °C over the first 24 h [14]. This large multicenter study did not retrieve any significant difference in any outcome criteria, including survival rate and neurological outcome. As a consequence, the most recent guidelines considered that a range of temperature between 32 and 36 °C can be used in this setting. Another consequence was that the appellation "TTM" is now widely accepted as referring to all intervention aiming to obtain and maintain a targeted level of temperature in this situation.

The population that might benefit from induced hypothermia also became an important concern. If numerous observational studies further confirmed the benefit of this treatment in highly selected patients (i.e., those resuscitated from an out-of-hospital ventricular fibrillation or a pulseless ventricular tachycardia), the level of evidence remains weaker in patients presenting an initial non-shockable rhythm (i.e., those resuscitated from pulseless electrical activity or asystole) and in patients resuscitated from an in-hospital CA [15, 16]. In these patients, data are conflicting, and if present, the clinical benefit of TTM is highly suspected to be very minor. Considering that the risk-benefit ratio is sufficiently favorable, 2015 guidelines still recommend discussing the use of TTM in these patients. Ongoing randomized studies focusing on these non-shockable patients will probably provide more information.

The way to perform an adequate TTM is also a matter of debate. Even if based on low quality of evidence, it is generally recommended to use servo-controlled devices (i.e., devices driven by a feedback on patient's temperature). These systems are known to faster reach the targeted temperature and to provide a greater stability during the maintenance phase [17]. Whether an external or internal device should be preferred, it is at that time unknown as no adequately designed studies compared these two options.

23.2 Traumatic Brain Injury

Experimental trauma studies described promising results of hypothermia in control of increase ICP [11] and neuroprotective properties [8]. Several mechanisms seem to be involved. Phillips et al. described action on apoptosis with a decrease in calcium entry via the N-methyl-D-aspartate and ryanodine receptors in cultured hippocampal neurons of brain submitted to trauma [18]. Control of inflammation seems to be also involved in protection mechanisms encountered with hypothermia [19].

Clinical studies described hypothermia as a promising therapy in TBI patients [20, 21]. In a cohort of 82 patients, Marion et al. described that moderate hypothermia (33 °C) conducted for 24 h in patients with severe brain injury and Glasgow score between 5 and 7 improved the outcome [20]. Unfortunately, these promising results were contrasted by several data. Clifton et al. [22] conducted a study on 392 patients randomized in a normothermic group and a 33 °C group for 48 h but didn't find any effect of hypothermia on recovery; moreover the hypothermic group had much more hypotensive episodes. The limit of this study could be the prolonged delay reported to hypothermic temperature target, 8 ± 3 h, but the NABISH II study, which reduced this time, didn't find any benefits of hypothermia on recovery. Two studies conducted in pediatric population didn't find neither any interest in therapeutic hypothermia in a population of severe injured patients with moreover a trendy to a worth neurologic prognosis and an increase in mortality in the group hypothermia [23, 24].

The main problem of these several studies is the non-selection of TBI population for hypothermia and the heterogeneity of hypothermic methods used. Effect of hypothermia on intracranial hypertension (HTIC), which is an independent mortality risk factor, has been described in the different previous studies [25, 26]. However beneficial effect on recovery is not confirmed. In a multicenter randomized control study, Shiozaki et al. confirmed the lack of interest of hypothermia in a subpopulation of patient with low ICP [21]. In a large multicenter study of 347 patients, in patients with an intracranial pressure of more than 20 mm Hg after traumatic brain injury, therapeutic hypothermia plus standard care to reduce intracranial pressure did not result in outcomes better than those with standard care alone [27].

23.3 Subarachnoid Hemorrhage (SAH)

Delayed ischemic events can occur after SAH, secondary in part to vasospasm episodes. As the greatest neuroprotective effects of TTM are seen when treatment is initiated before the onset of ischemia, the use of hypothermia to prevent delayed cerebral ischemia after subarachnoid hemorrhage (SAH) has been proposed. The risk of coagulopathy [28] induced by hypothermia could be a limit, but several data described no bleeding risk in this context. Indeed Torok et al. described in an experimental subarachnoid model conducted in rat that mild hypothermia realized up to 3 h after the event can be neuroprotective and improve functional outcome without reported bleeding complications [29]. Moreover several surgical reports have also been conducted during aneurysm surgery (clipping surgery), with promising results, and no bleeding problem were also reported. This improvement of neurologic outcome was not however confirmed in a study conducted in 1001 patients needing a craniotomy for aneurysm clipping randomized in a normothermic and hypothermic group during procedure [30]. Few clinical studies have been conducted in clinical SAH. In a group of patient experiencing intracranial hypertension or vasospasm, Seule et al. considered mild hypothermia as the last resort treatment, even an important rate of complications was reported [31]. Indeed they reported important rate of electrolyte disorders (77%) particularly hypernatremia, pneumonia (52%), thrombocytopenia (47%), and septic shock syndrome (40%). Moreover a study realized in patient with sustained intracranial hypertension and treated with barbiturates and hypothermia >72 h or <72 h didn't find any benefit in prolonged treatment [32].

So in the context of SAH, no recommendation can be done on therapy with hypothermia, but cooling is a reasonable option for controlling fever or ICP in patients when first-line interventions failed.

23.4 Acute Ischemic Stroke

TTM has been described to have positive effect in infarct volume reduction in experimental studies. However results are different depending in model of middle cerebral artery occlusion (MCAO) studied. Indeed hypothermia used in temporary MCAO seems to have better effect in infarct volume reduction than in permanent MCAO models [33]. In clinical practice, the problem is quite different. Emergency use of thrombolytic transformed the prognosis of patients after stroke. The combination treatment would take advantage of additive effect, but interaction between recanalization and neuroprotection could occur (decrease in alteplase activity in hypothermia, etc.). Combination therapies have been tested in experimental studies with a better prognosis in animals receiving thrombolytic and cooling. Several clinical studies have been conducted to confirm these data and summarized in Table 23.1. Even encouraging data reported in a recent study [34], several studies didn't find any benefits to induce hypothermia after thrombolysis [35]. Besides these poor results in neuroprotective effect, more interesting data have been reported in population of patients with malignant middle cerebral artery syndrome, decreasing intracranial pressure and improving

Table 23.1 Literature review of studies on clinical stroke

Year of publication	Reference	Population	Therapy	Time Delay post event Duration therapy
1998	Schwab	25 malignant stroke	External cooling 33 °C	14 h 48–72 h
2000	Copenhagen stroke group	17 stroke	External cooling 35 °C	12 h 6 h
2001	Schwab	50 malignant stroke	External cooling 33 °C	22 h
2001	COOLAID	19 stroke	External cooling 32 °C	6 h 12–72 h
2004	COOLAID 2	40 stroke	Endovascular cooling 33 °C	12 h
2005	ICTuS	18 stroke	Endovascular cooling 33 °C	12 h 12–24 h
2009	Martin Stella	18 stroke	Endovascular cooling 33–35 °C	5 h 24 h
2010	ICTuS-L	59 stroke	Endovascular cooling 33 °C	6 h 24 h
2014	Hong	75 stroke	Endovascular cooling 34.5 °C	As soon as possible 48 h

prognosis in a few number of patients studied [36]. Several limitations can be opposed to the published clinical data. The optimum timing for inducing hypothermia is not well defined and the prolonged time of treatment. The ongoing ICTuS 2/3, assessing combination therapy (thrombolysis and hypothermia) vs thrombolysis alone, in a large cohort of patients (1600 patients), will randomize patients in two durations of hypothermia 12 or 24 h and will probably respond to this question NCT01778855) [37].

Hypothermia is not recommended actually at the acute phase of stroke but can be proposed in critical care patients, with cerebral edema not responding to other medical therapies.

23.5 Meningitis

After meningitis, inflammatory response and increase in ICP can potentially occurred and are associated with worth prognosis. TTM could have an anti-inflammatory action in this setting. Several experimental studies described promising results by attenuating this inflammatory response induced by infection [38, 39]. In an experimental *E. coli* meningitis, newborn piglets maintained between 34 and 35 °C, presented a decrease in ICP, in lactate concentration and TNF, and an increase in glucose concentration in CSF [40]. Few data are available in clinical studies. Lepur et al. [41] in a cohort of 10 patients presenting bacterial meningitis with increase ICP (approached by transcranial Doppler) described a favorable outcome after hypothermia induced for 72–96 h between 32 and 34 °C. In a randomized study conducted in 49 centers in France, patients with documented bacterial meningitis were randomized in a normothermic and hypothermic group (32–34 °C) for 48 h. After 98 patients included, the study was stopped because of a higher mortality rate in the group of hypothermic patients [42]. Consequently, the use of hypothermia is not recommended in bacterial meningitis.

23.6 Intracerebral Hemorrhage (ICH)

ICH accounts for 10–15% of strokes but is associated with high level of mortality and morbidity. TTM could have a place in secondary mechanisms of injury following hematoma. In experimental studies, conflicting results are reported particularly depending in time of induction. When delayed hypothermia (>12 h) is realized, MacLellan [43] described an improvement in tissue loss and in functional outcome. This improvement is lost when hypothermia is induced less than 12 h after ICH. Coagulopathy induced by hypothermia is probably responsible of this difference; even no data on volume expansion have been reported. Few data are available in clinical practice. In an historical cohort of patient, Staykov described a better prognosis in patients with ICH treated with mild hypothermia for 8–10 days [44]. An ongoing study would assess the tolerability and the adverse events occurring after cooling of 32–34 °C in patients with ICH (GSW > 7) (NCT01607151) [45].

TTM seems experimentally to be an interesting approach to improve prognosis in brain-injured animals. Nevertheless few clinical data support its use at the bedside. Beside a real place for a decrease temperature in cardiac arrest and in sustained intracranial hypertension secondary to traumatic brain injury, few studies support a systematic use at the bedside in SAH, stroke, meningitis, or ICH. Moreover a real need for search in methods proposed to induce this treatment, in level of treatment, and in process for rewarming needs to be defined more accurately before proposing TTM as a standard of care in severe brain-injured patients.

References

1. Wang CX, Stroink A, Casto JM, Kattner K (2009) Hyperthermia exacerbates ischaemic brain injury. Int J Stroke 4:274–284
2. Grau AJ, Buggle F, Hacke W (1996) Infectious diseases as a cause and risk factor for cerebrovascular ischemia. Nervenarzt 67:639–649
3. Leys D, Ringelstein EB, Kaste M, Hacke W, European Stroke Initiative Executive Committee (2007) The main components of stroke unit care: results of a European expert survey. Cerebrovasc Dis Basel Switz 23:344–352
4. Sessler DI (1995) Deliberate mild hypothermia. J Neurosurg Anesthesiol 7:38–46
5. Croughwell N et al (1992) The effect of temperature on cerebral metabolism and blood flow in adults during cardiopulmonary bypass. J Thorac Cardiovasc Surg 103:549–554
6. Metz C et al (1996) Moderate hypothermia in patients with severe head injury: cerebral and extracerebral effects. J Neurosurg 85:533–541
7. Marion DW, Obrist WD, Carlier PM, Penrod LE, Darby JM (1993) The use of moderate therapeutic hypothermia for patients with severe head injuries: a preliminary report. J Neurosurg 79:354–362
8. Smith SL, Hall ED (1996) Mild pre- and posttraumatic hypothermia attenuates blood-brain barrier damage following controlled cortical impact injury in the rat. J Neurotrauma 13:1–9
9. Busto R et al (1989) Effect of mild hypothermia on ischemia-induced release of neurotransmitters and free fatty acids in rat brain. Stroke 20:904–910
10. Bernard SA et al (2002) Treatment of comatose survivors of out-of-hospital cardiac arrest with induced hypothermia. N Engl J Med 346:557–563
11. Goss JR et al (1995) Hypothermia attenuates the normal increase in interleukin 1 beta RNA and nerve growth factor following traumatic brain injury in the rat. J Neurotrauma 12:159–167
12. Bougouin W et al (2014) Characteristics and prognosis of sudden cardiac death in greater Paris: population-based approach from the Paris sudden death expertise center (Paris-SDEC). Intensive Care Med 40:846–854
13. Zeiner A et al (2001) Hyperthermia after cardiac arrest is associated with an unfavorable neurologic outcome. Arch Intern Med 161:2007–2012
14. Nielsen N et al (2013) Targeted temperature management at 33 °C versus 36 °C after cardiac arrest. N Engl J Med 369:2197–2206
15. Dumas F et al (2011) Is hypothermia after cardiac arrest effective in both shockable and nonshockable patients?: insights from a large registry. Circulation 123:877–886
16. Chan PS et al (2016) Association between therapeutic hypothermia and survival after in-hospital cardiac arrest. JAMA 316:1375–1382
17. Deye N et al (2015) Endovascular versus external targeted temperature Management for Patients with out-of-Hospital Cardiac Arrest: a randomized, controlled study. Circulation 132:182–193

18. Phillips KF, Deshpande LS, DeLorenzo RJ (2013) Hypothermia reduces calcium entry via the N-methyl-D-aspartate and ryanodine receptors in cultured hippocampal neurons. Eur J Pharmacol 698:186–192
19. Tomura S, de Rivero Vaccari JP, Keane RW, Bramlett HM, Dietrich WD (2012) Effects of therapeutic hypothermia on inflammasome signaling after traumatic brain injury. J Cereb Blood Flow Metab 32:1939–1947
20. Marion DW et al (1997) Treatment of traumatic brain injury with moderate hypothermia. N Engl J Med 336:540–546
21. Shiozaki T et al (1993) Effect of mild hypothermia on uncontrollable intracranial hypertension after severe head injury. J Neurosurg 79:363–368
22. Clifton GL et al (2001) Lack of effect of induction of hypothermia after acute brain injury. N Engl J Med 344:556–563
23. Hutchison JS et al (2008) Hypothermia therapy after traumatic brain injury in children. N Engl J Med 358:2447–2456
24. Adelson PD et al (2005) Phase II clinical trial of moderate hypothermia after severe traumatic brain injury in children. Neurosurgery 56:740–754
25. Polderman KH, Tjong Tjin Joe R, Peerdeman SM, Vandertop WP, Girbes ARJ (2002) Effects of therapeutic hypothermia on intracranial pressure and outcome in patients with severe head injury. Intensive Care Med 28:1563–1573
26. Rossi S, Zanier ER, Mauri I, Columbo A, Stocchetti N (2001) Brain temperature, body core temperature, and intracranial pressure in acute cerebral damage. J Neurol Neurosurg Psychiatry 71:448–454
27. Andrews PJD et al (2015) Hypothermia for intracranial hypertension after traumatic brain injury. N Engl J Med 373:2403–2412
28. Davenport R (2013) Pathogenesis of acute traumatic coagulopathy. Transfusion (Paris) 53(Suppl 1):23S–27S
29. Török E et al (2009) Mild hypothermia (33 degrees C) reduces intracranial hypertension and improves functional outcome after subarachnoid hemorrhage in rats. Neurosurgery 65:352–359.; discussion 359
30. Todd MM, Hindman BJ, Clarke WR, Torner JC, Intraoperative Hypothermia for Aneurysm Surgery Trial (IHAST) Investigators (2005) Mild intraoperative hypothermia during surgery for intracranial aneurysm. N Engl J Med 352:135–145
31. Seule MA, Muroi C, Mink S, Yonekawa Y, Keller E (2009) Therapeutic hypothermia in patients with aneurysmal subarachnoid hemorrhage, refractory intracranial hypertension, or cerebral vasospasm. Neurosurgery 64:86–92
32. Gasser S, Khan N, Yonekawa Y, Imhof H-G, Keller E (2003) Long-term hypothermia in patients with severe brain edema after poor-grade subarachnoid hemorrhage: feasibility and intensive care complications. J Neurosurg Anesthesiol 15:240–248
33. van der Worp HB, Sena ES, Donnan GA, Howells DW, Macleod MR (2007) Hypothermia in animal models of acute ischaemic stroke: a systematic review and meta-analysis. Brain J Neurol 130:3063–3074
34. Hong JM et al (2014) Therapeutic hypothermia after recanalization in patients with acute ischemic stroke. Stroke 45:134–140
35. Hemmen TM et al (2010) Intravenous thrombolysis plus hypothermia for acute treatment of ischemic stroke (ICTuS-L): final results. Stroke 41:2265–2270
36. Schwab S et al (1998) Moderate hypothermia in the treatment of patients with severe middle cerebral artery infarction. Stroke 29:2461–2466
37. Lyden PD, Hemmen TM, Grotta J, Rapp K, Raman R (2014) Endovascular therapeutic hypothermia for acute ischemic stroke: ICTuS 2/3 protocol. Int J Stroke 9:117–125
38. Angstwurm K et al (2000) Induced hypothermia in experimental pneumococcal meningitis. J Cereb Blood Flow Metab 20:834–838
39. Irazuzta JE et al (2000) Hypothermia as an adjunctive treatment for severe bacterial meningitis. Brain Res 881:88–97

40. Park H-P et al (2013) Predicting the appropriate uncuffed endotracheal tube size for children: a radiograph-based formula versus two age-based formulas. J Clin Anesth 25:384–387
41. Lepur D, Kutleša M, Baršić B (2011) Induced hypothermia in adult community-acquired bacterial meningitis--more than just a possibility? J Infect 62:172–177
42. Mourvillier B et al (2013) Induced hypothermia in severe bacterial meningitis: a randomized clinical trial. JAMA 310:2174–2183
43. MacLellan CL, Davies LM, Fingas MS, Colbourne F (2006) The influence of hypothermia on outcome after intracerebral hemorrhage in rats. Stroke 37:1266–1270
44. Staykov D et al (2013) Mild prolonged hypothermia for large intracerebral hemorrhage. Neurocrit Care 18:178–183
45. Rincon F, Friedman DP, Bell R, Mayer SA, Bray PF (2014) Targeted temperature management after intracerebral hemorrhage (TTM-ICH): methodology of a prospective randomized clinical trial. Int J Stroke 9:646–651

Printed by Printforce, the Netherlands